# Side Effects of Medical Cancer Therapy

D1489625

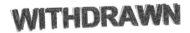

Mario A. Dicato
Editor

# Side Effects of Medical Cancer Therapy

## Prevention and Treatment

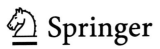 Springer

*Editor*
Mario A. Dicato, M.D.
Department
of Hematology-Oncology
Centre Hospitalier
de Luxembourg
Luxembourg

ISBN 978-0-85729-786-0     ISBN 978-0-85729-787-7    (eBook)
DOI 10.1007/978-0-85729-787-7
Springer London Heidelberg New York Dordrecht

Library of Congress Control Number: 2012954609

Printed on acid-free paper

Springer is part of Springer Science+Business Media (www.springer.com)

# Preface

The reason for publishing a book on side effects of drugs used in oncology is the fact that numerous new drugs, mostly classified as "targeted therapy," have different and very varied spectra of side effects. As standard chemotherapy drugs have not changed much over the years in their adverse effect profiles, oncologists are usually very familiar with these problems, especially because over the past 20 years only a few new chemotherapeutic drugs have been marketed.

Another aspect of oncology that has changed over the past two decades is the fact that with the increase in life expectancy, the median age at diagnosis of cancer has increased and is presently around 70 years. Therefore, comorbidities have become routine in oncological services, and many patients are being treated with multiple medications for other pathologies, which multiplies drug interactions and compliance problems.

Targeted drugs have flooded the oncological literature, and their spectrum of side effects is increasing, especially since additional drugs become available every year and are being used in several malignancies. This change of spectrum of side effects is less and less organ-limited, and a physician specialized in, for example, gastrointestinal malignancies is now confronted with cardiac (trastuzumab in gastric cancer) or dermatologic (EGFR inhibitor in colorectal cancer) toxicity. Hence, in order to make it easy to look up a problem, overlaps are unavoidable.

In putting together the layout of a book on side effects of medical cancer therapy, several problems arose. Should the side effects be grouped by organ, by drug, by type of toxicity, or by other factors? A compromise needed to be found. Therefore, the majority of the book is organ-oriented, with the exception of chapters on pharmacogenetic-pharmacokinetic, cardiac, dermatologic, and supportive care aspects.

I am grateful to the authors who spontaneously accepted the task of writing their respective chapters. Though most of them are prominent in their fields, many realized only later that more than an update of a previously studied topic was required and that they had to start anew. I thank them for complying.

Special thanks to Diane Lamsback from Springer for her untiring help in the preparation of this book.

Mario A. Dicato

# Contents

# Contributors

**Matti S. Aapro, M.D.** Department of Medical Oncology, Institut Multidisciplinaire d'Oncologie, Clinique de Genolier, Genolier, Switzerland

**Philippe G. Aftimos, M.D.** Medical Oncology Department, Institut Jules Bordet, Université Libre de Bruxelles, Bruxelles, Belgium

**Sevilay Altintas, M.D., Ph.D.** Department of Medical Oncology, Antwerp University Hospital, Edegem, Belgium

**Ahmad Awada, M.D., Ph.D.** Medical Oncology Department, Institut Jules Bordet, Brussels, Belgium

**Julie Bogaert, M.D.** Department of Digestive Oncology, University Hospitals Gasthuisberg/Leuven, Leuven, Belgium

**Irene Braña, M.D.** Medical Oncology Department, Vall d'Hebron University Hospital, Barcelona, Spain

**Sigrid Cherrier-De Wilde, M.D.** Department of Hematology, Centre Hospitalier de Luxembourg, Luxembourg, Luxembourg

**Robert E. Coleman, M.S., B.S., M.D., FRCP** Academic Unit of Clinical Oncology, Weston Park Hospital, Sheffield, South Yorkshire, UK

**Pieter-Jan Cuyle, M.D.** Department of Digestive Oncology, University Hospitals Gasthuisberg/Leuven, Leuven, Belgium

**Mario A. Dicato, M.D.** Department of Hematology-Oncology, Centre Hospitalier de Luxembourg, Luxembourg, Luxembourg

**Duhem Caroline, M.D.** Department of Hematology-Oncology, Centre Hospitalier de Luxembourg, Luxembourg, Luxembourg

**Alexander M.M. Eggermont, M.D., Ph.D.** Department of Surgical and Medical Oncology, Institut de Cancérologie Gustave Roussy, Villejuif- Paris, France

**Sonia Fatigoni, M.D.** Department of Oncology, Santa Maria Hospital, Terni, Italy

**Alessandra Curioni Fontecedro, M.D.** Department of Thoracic Surgery, University Hospital Zurich, Zurich, Switzerland

**Pere Gascon, M.D., Ph.D.** Division of Medical Oncology, Department of Hematology-Oncology, Institut Clinic de Malalties Hemato-Oncologiques, Barcelona, Spain

**Andrea Gombos, M.D.** Medical Oncology Department, Institut Jules Bordet, Université Libre de Bruxelles, Bruxelles, Belgium

**Aline Henry, M.D.** Supportive Care Department, Centre Alexis Vautrin, Vandœuvre Les Nancy, France

**Krisztian Homicsko, M.D., Ph.D.** Medical Oncology, Department of Oncology, Centre Hospitalier Universitaire Vaudois, Lausanne, Switzerland

**Didier S. Kamioner, M.D.** Department of Medical Oncology and Haematology, Hopital Prive Ouest Parisien, Trappes, France

**Ivan Krakowski, M.D.** Supportive Care Department, Centre Alexis Vautrin, Vandœuvre Les Nancy, France

**François Lokiec, Ph.D., SciD** Department of Pharmacology, Institut Curie-Hôpital René Huguenin, Saint-Cloud, France

**Christina Mateus, M.D.** Department of Dermatology, Institute Gustave Roussy, Villejuif, France

**Miriame Mino, M.D.** Internal Medicine, Centre Médico-Chirurgical de la Broye SA, Payerne, Switzerland

**Solange Peters, M.D., Ph.D.** Department of Oncology, Centre Hospitalier Universitaire Vaudois, Lausanne, Switzerland

**Martine J. Piccart, M.D., Ph.D.** Department of Medicine, Institut Jules Bordet, Université Libre de Bruxelles, Brussels, Belgium

**Laurent Plawny, M.D.** Department of Hematology, Centre Hospitalier de Luxembourg, Luxembourg, Luxembourg

**Lina Pugliano, M.D., B.Sc. (Hons), M.B.B.S., FRACP** Medical Oncology Department, Institut Jules Bordet, Université Libre de Bruxelles, Bruxelles, Belgium

**Fernand Ries, M.D.** Department of Hematology-Oncology, Centre Hospitalier de Luxembourg, Luxembourg, Luxembourg

**Caroline Robert, M.D., Ph.D.** Department of Medicine, Institute Gustave Roussy, Villejuif, France

**Fausto Roila, M.D.** Department of Oncology, Santa Maria Hospital, Terni, Italy

**Dirk L. A.L. Schrijvers, M.D., Ph.D.** Department of Medical Oncology, Ziekenhuisnetwerk Antwerpen-Middelheim, Antwerp, Belgium

**Rolf A. Stahel, M.D.** Clinic of Oncology, University Hospital Zurich,, Zurich, Switzerland

**Roger Stupp, M.D.** Departments of Neurosurgery and Clinical Neurosciences, Centre Hospitalier Universitaire Vaudois and University of Lausanne, Lausanne, Switzerland

**Josep Tabernero, M.D.** Medical Oncology Department, Vall d'Hebron University Hospital, Barcelona, Spain

**Fiona G. Taylor, B.Sc., MB ChB, MRCP** Medical Oncology, Weston Park Hospital, Sheffield, South Yorkshire, UK

**Bertrand F. Tombal, M.D., Ph.D.** Service d'Urologie, Cliniques Universitaires Saint Luc, Université Catholique de Louvain, Brussels, Belgium

**Eric Van Cutsem, M.D., Ph.D.** Department of Digestive Oncology, University Hospitals Gasthuisberg/Leuven, Leuven, Belgium

**Jan B. Vermorken, M.D., Ph.D.** Department of Medical Oncology, Antwerp University Hospital, Edegem, Belgium

**Caroline Wilson, MBChB, MRCP, M.Sc.** Academic Unit of Clinical Oncology, Weston Park Hospital, Sheffield University, Sheffield, South Yorkshire, UK

**Esther Zamora, M.D.**  Medical Oncology Department, Vall d'Hebron University Hospital, Barcelona, Spain

**Stefan Zimmermann, M.D.**  Centre Pluridisciplinaire d'Oncologie, Centre Hospitalier Universitaire Vaudois, Lausanne, Switzerland

# Chapter 1
## Drug Interactions and Pharmacogenetics

**François Lokiec**

**Abstract**  Drug interaction in cancer chemotherapy is one of the most common phenomena in cancer treatment. Cancer patients often take several medications at the same time, not only for treating their cancer, but also for side effects and other secondary illnesses. The number of comedications increases with age, and drug interactions are critical for elderly patients. Because of this, they can be at high risk for adverse drug interactions and duplicate medications. Consequences of these interactions can range from inactivation of cancer-fighting medications to severe injury or death of the patient. Pharmacogenetics studies the relationship between genetic polymorphisms and individual responses to drugs. In recent years, there has been great progress in our knowledge of the effects of drug-metabolizing enzymes and molecular target genetic polymorphisms on cancer chemotherapy. Pharmacogenetics focuses on the prediction of drug efficacy and toxicity based on a patient's genetic profile with routinely applicable genetic tests to select the most appropriate medication at optimal doses for each individual patient.

F. Lokiec, Ph.D., SciD
Department of Pharmacology, Institut Curie-Hôpital René Huguenin,
Saint-Cloud, France
e-mail: francois.lokiec@curie.net

M.A. Dicato (ed.), *Side Effects of Medical Cancer Therapy,*
DOI 10.1007/978-0-85729-787-7_1,
© Springer-Verlag London 2013

2    F. Lokiec

**Keywords**   Anticancer drugs • Drug interactions • Pharmacogenetics  •  Pharmacodynamics  •  Pharmacokinetics
Cytochromes P450

# Introduction

Drug interactions and pharmacogenetics seem to present two
different problems for the side effects of cancer chemotherapy.
In fact, we will see later in this chapter that these two
approaches are not so different.

Drug interaction in cancer chemotherapy is one of the most
common phenomena in cancer treatment. Drug interactions in
oncology are of particular importance owing to the narrow
therapeutic index and the inherent toxicity of anticancer
agents. Interactions with other medications can cause small
changes in the pharmacokinetics or pharmacodynamics of a
chemotherapy agent that could significantly alter its efficacy or
toxicity. Evaluation of drug potential interactions should not
be limited solely to the anticancer group. A drug interaction
occurs whenever the effects of one drug are modified by the
prior or concurrent administration of another pharmacologically active substance. Such interactions may result in an
antagonistic, synergistic, or unexpected response [1].

A drug interaction is defined as the pharmacologic or clinical
response to the administration or co-exposure of a drug with
another substance that modifies the patient's response to
the drug. It is reported that more than 20 % of all adverse
reactions to drugs are caused by interactions between drugs [2].
This incidence increases among the elderly and patients
who take two or more medications. Patients with cancer are
particularly at risk for drug interactions because they could
be taking many different medications as part of their cancer
treatment or for the management of other illnesses [3].

Drug interactions can occur throughout the process of drug
disposition as a result of endogenous and exogenous factors.
Drug interactions can be the result of pharmacokinetic or pharmacodynamic factors or a combination of mechanisms.
Pharmacokinetic interactions involve one drug or substance
altering the absorption, distribution, metabolism, or elimination

of another drug or substance. A common example of a pharmacokinetic interaction occurs when two drugs compete for the same metabolic pathway. When the pathway becomes saturated, neither drug can be metabolized fully, which results in higher serum concentrations of the agents and can lead to clinically unfavorable consequences. Pharmacodynamic interactions occur when two drugs or substances have similar molecular targets but do not affect the pharmacokinetic parameters of each other. When two or more drugs that have similar pharmacodynamic activity are coadministered, the additive effects might result in an excessive response or toxicity. Pharmacodynamic interactions between drugs with opposing effects can reduce the response to one or both drugs [4–6].

In this section, we have intentionally focused on the unexpected drug interactions that have been well documented in cancer patients. A special section describes interactions between anticancer drugs and resistance-modifying agents because although pharmacodynamic interactions are the aim of this kind of association, pharmacokinetic interactions can be the chief explanation for resistance reversal.

# Principles of Drug Interactions

## Physical Interactions or Chemical Incompatibilities

Cancer patients usually receive intravenous (IV) anticancer drugs plus other supportive treatment, such as antiemetics, antibiotics, and others. Special attention should be paid to the physical and chemical interactions that can occur when the drugs are given simultaneously [7].

Cancer patients usually require multiple-drug therapy. In fact, the cancer chemotherapy regimen alone often consists of three or four agents. Supportive therapy adds more drugs to the overall regimen, resulting in the (perceived) need to administer several drugs simultaneously. Also, having a steep dose–response curve, low therapeutic index, and significant toxicity, anticancer agents are particularly critical drugs. Any deviation from the dose or concentration that produces optimum activity is bound to cause problems one way or another, either through increased toxicity or loss of response. Either way the outcome may be fatal for the patient. Furthermore, one should keep in mind that chemical inactivation of anticancer drugs by the admixture of other drugs is not usually visible in terms of evident product degradation. In other words, even if an added drug does not cause clouding, precipitation, or a color change in the cytotoxic drug solution, you can never be sure that there will be no chemical inactivation. So make it a rule to always administer cytotoxic drugs alone [8].

Selected examples are presented in the following sections.

## pH Effects

Some cytotoxic drugs (e.g., fluorouracil) dissolve only at extreme pH values. Adding other drugs may cause such a shift in pH that fluorouracil will flocculate.

## Solubilizers

Other cytotoxic agents can be kept in solution only with the aid of solubilizers, which tend to be effective only within specific concentration ranges. Outside these ranges, the drugs may crystallize (e.g., etoposide, teniposide, paclitaxel).

## Plasticizers

Solubilizers may leach plasticizers from plastics, thus producing toxic effects (this is why PVC-free transfusion-giving sets must be used for paclitaxel infusions). Conversely, lipophilic cytotoxic drugs may be extracted by plasticizers from an aqueous solution.

## Sorption

Protein sorption to glass surfaces has been described in the literature. This phenomenon may cause loss of activity of biologically potent drugs, which tend to be administered in minute amounts.

## Chemical Reactions

Of the broad spectrum of possible chemical reactions, here are a few examples:
- Hydrolysis (e.g., etoposide lactone ring cleavage in basic pH range)
- Redox reactions (e.g., platinum coordination complexes and sulfite, thiols)
- Photolysis (e.g., carmustine [nitrosourea] or dacarbazine [triazene])
- Racemization (e.g., etoposide as CH-acid compound in alkaline solution)
- Formation of coordination complexes (e.g., platinum derivatives)

## Denaturation

Many proteins are stable only at specific pH values and ionic strengths (filgrastim, for instance, is unstable in normal saline). Deviations may lead to denaturation, which will not necessarily be visible as flocculation in the case of biologically potent drugs (growth factors, interferon). Loss of biologic activity will then not be macroscopically evident.

## Pharmacokinetic Interactions

Very few cytotoxic agents are administered by the oral route, but now with the tyrosine kinase inhibitor family, everything has changed; all the "small molecules" are orally administered. We should, therefore, take the pharmacokinetic interactions into consideration, including the absorption, distribution, metabolism, and elimination of anticancer drugs.

### Absorption

Many factors are able to reduce the digestive absorption of a drug. These include the degree of ionization of the drug, its contact with the digestive mucous (transit problems, defective digestive secretion), the gastric emptying, and gastrointestinal motility. Food delays gastric emptying, raises intestinal pH, increases hepatic blood flow, and slows gastrointestinal transit, so it can significantly affect the pharmacokinetic profile of some orally administered medications. Food–drug interactions can have four pharmacokinetic effects on the bioavailability of the orally administered anticancer agent: delayed, decreased, increased, or unaffected absorption.

Some orally administered anticancer agents are prodrugs, which require metabolic activation for cytotoxic activity through first-pass effects in the gastrointestinal tract and/or liver before they reach the systemic circulation. Capecitabine, altretamine, etoposide phosphate, and estramustine phosphate sodium are anticancer agents that are used in the treatment of various solid tumors (including breast, colorectal, ovarian, lung, prostate, and testicular cancer) and require such activation. Therefore, factors that alter the absorption of these medications can have profound effects on their pharmacokinetics. A decrease in the rate and extent of absorption is noted when estramustine phosphate sodium is given with food or milk, and bioavailability has been reported to decrease by 36 and 63 %, respectively [9]. Therefore, it is recommended that estramustine phosphate sodium be taken with water 1 h before or 2 h after a meal. By contrast, food has been shown to have only a minor effect on the pharmacokinetics of fluorouracil (5-FU). The rate of absorption of capecitabine (a 5-FU prodrug) is decreased in a fed state, which results in an increase in hepatic first-pass metabolism, which in turn reduces the extent of systemic absorption of the prodrug [10]. However, a greater effect is seen on the area under the concentration–time curve (AUC) of capecitabine as compared with 5′-deoxy-5′ fluorouridine (5′-DFUR), the precursor to the pharmacologically active compound 5-FU. So, the change in AUC of capecitabine is probably not clinically significant, as capecitabine itself is not the active compound.

The absorption of orally administered anticancer agents that are not prodrugs can also be altered by metabolism within the gastrointestinal tract [11]. Evidence indicates that the activity of cytochrome P450 enzymes (CYP enzymes) in the gut wall is a significant factor that alters the bioavailability of orally administered anticancer agents that are CYP3A substrates [12]. Drug–food, drug–herb, or drug–drug interactions can occur when an orally administered CYP3A substrate is given concomitantly with an inhibitor or inducer of intestinal CYP activity. One of the best described examples of a food that alters intestinal CYP3A activity is grapefruit juice. Grapefruit juice is known to be a potent inhibitor of intestinal CYP3A4 and therefore increases the bioavailability of various drugs, such as the anti-inflammatory and immunosuppressive agent cyclosporine and the calcium-channel blocker nifedipine [13–16].

## Ionization

Digestive absorption is complete when it is achieved by passive diffusion (e.g., in a non-ionized form). Most of the substances that are capable of ionizing a drug decrease its digestive absorption. Substances such as alkalinizing agents decrease the absorption of acid drugs, and acidifying drugs (citric and tartaric acid) decrease the alkaline drug absorption.

## *Complexation*

This type of interaction occurs during the digestive process, when the drug forms (with another drug or any other substance) a nonresorbable complex (e.g., aluminum colloids combined with acid drugs).

## Contact with the Digestive Mucosa

This kind of antagonism includes different physiopathologic circumstances, such as food attendance and lack of digestive secretion.

## Gastrointestinal Motility

Drugs are mainly absorbed at the intestinal level, where a wide mucous surface exists. Absorption at this level is affected all the more when gastric emptying is faster. Any substance that modifies the gastric emptying acts on the kinetics of the intestinal absorption of anticancer drugs. The anticholinergic substances slow down gastric emptying and delay the absorption of the drugs. On the other hand, metoclopramide accelerates gastric emptying and accelerates the absorption of associated drugs.

## Modifications in Drug Diffusion

These modifications become apparent in either an increase in the concentration of the free active form of the drug or a decrease in this concentration.

## *Binding to Plasma Proteins*

The competition of drugs for plasma proteins is one of the most common reasons for the occurrence of toxic side effects (methotrexate–aspirin [17, 18], methotrexate–indomethacin [19], methotrexate–trimethoprim–sulfamethoxazole [20, 21], etc.). Clinicians should be very careful with the association of drugs that are highly bound to proteins (usually albumin) because the binding sites are the same and limited in number.

## Modification of the Tissue Binding

This modification is the result of competition between two drugs for the same binding sites in a tissue. This kind of interaction is similar to the protein plasma binding but directly into the tissues.

## Metabolic Interactions

The metabolic interactions mainly occur with drugs with hepatic metabolism. The anticancer drugs involved in metabolic interactions with other drugs are those metabolized by liver enzymes, which are induced or inhibited by the associated substances. The main metabolic inducers are rifampicin, spironolactone, and phenobarbital [22, 23]; the main metabolic inhibitors are monoamine oxidase inhibitors, tricyclic antidepressants, phenothiazine neuroleptics, and allopurinol [24, 25].

## Modifications in the Elimination

Drug interactions leading to changes in the elimination of anticancer drugs mainly concern urinary drug elimination. Modifications in urinary elimination are principally due to changes of the urine pH expressing a modification in the ionization of the substances filtered by the glomerulus and secreted at the proximal tubule level. An increase in the degree of ionization of the drug corresponds to an increase in the urinary elimination of the drug. On the other hand, a decrease in drug ionization leads to a decrease in its renal elimination.

## Miscellaneous

We should always take into account the possibility that the patient is suffering from another disorder that could, by itself, interact with the pharmacokinetic behavior of the anticancer drug. For example, thyroid dysfunction may influence drug pharmacokinetics, just as the cardiovascular and respiratory systems can.

## Pharmacodynamic Interactions

Pharmacodynamic interactions involve the therapeutic power of the anticancer drug. They can enhance or decrease antineoplastic efficacy and modify the importance of the drug's toxic side effects. Pharmacodynamic interactions mainly concern the hematologic system, the liver, and the kidney.

## Terminology

The anticancer drug alone is considered as reference for the therapeutic activity. The pharmacologic consequences of drug interactions are always quantitative modifications of one or more effects of the associated drugs. Either the intensity of an effect, its duration, or both can be affected. If it is a global increase of the effect, the interaction is either synergy or enhancement. If it is a decrease of the effect, the interaction is antagonism.

## Synergy and Antagonism

Usually, we use the term "synergy" when two drugs have effects going in the same direction. The effect is additive when the observed effect is the sum of both effects. Synergy's main characteristic is that it affects only the common effects of the drugs. According to the extent of the modifications that occur, it can be described as partial, additive (the most frequent), and synergistic. Conversely, antagonisms can be observed when the effects of drug association produce a milder effect than the most active drug alone. The antagonism can be total or partial.

## Enhancement and Antagonism

Enhancement is characterized by a special phenomenon in which the increased effects all belong to the same drug. Other substances in the association do not have these effects but are capable of increasing their intensity when associated with the drug. Antagonism also exists in such situations.

It is important to note that the term "antagonism" is used to describe two phenomena, which are the contrary of synergy and the contrary of enhancement. Usually, interaction between two drugs is not defined by its mechanism but rather by its pharmacologic consequences. The interaction supervention supposes that the interaction is sufficiently intense to have a clinical translation.

It is relatively common to detect drug interactions in pharmacokinetic terms with no pharmacodynamic repercussions.

TABLE 1.1 Examples of drug–drug interactions between anticancer drugs and other active substances

| Other active substances | Examples of interactions | References |
|---|---|---|
| Antiemetics | Metoclopramide might enhance the cisplatin and the epirubicin toxicity | [26, 27] |
| Antiulcer drugs | Cimetidine increases cyclophosphamide, nitrosoureas, doxorubicin toxicities | [28–30] |
| NSAIDs | NSAIDs block the elimination of MTX through renal tubular secretion, leading to increase of MTX blood levels and toxicities | [31–34] |
| Antimicrobial agents | Penicillin delays MTX excretion | [35] |
| Anticoagulants | Warfarin has been reported to be synergistic with 5-FU | [36] |
| Psychiatric drugs | Benzodiazepines act on many anticancer drugs | [37–40] |

# Interactions Between Anticancer Drugs and Other Active Substances

Very little study has been devoted to interactions between anticancer drugs and other active substances, which is quite surprising because cancer patients usually receive a large number of pharmaceuticals and the therapeutic margin for anticancer drugs is always narrow. Mostly, the drug interactions have been reported case by case (Tables 1.1 and 1.2).

TABLE 1.2 Examples of drug–drug interactions between MTX and other anticancer drugs

| Other active substances | Examples of interactions | References |
|---|---|---|
| Penicillin | Delay of MTX excretion | [35, 41, 42] |
| Salicylates | Displacement of protein binding and increased MTX toxicity | [17, 18] |
| NSAIDs | Decrease elimination of MTX and increased toxicity | [31–34] |

## Antiemetics

Many anticancer drugs induce nausea and vomiting in cancer patients. For these reasons, antiemetics are usually used in combination with cancer treatments. The antiemetic drugs usually act at the level of the central nervous system through the dopamine or serotonin receptors. Among the antiemetics, chlorpromazine and metoclopramide seem to be the most involved in drug interactions.

### Chlorpromazine

Chlorpromazine combined with caffeine enhances cytotoxicity of alkylating agents in some rodent transplantation tumors and in the human melanoma xenograft system in mice [43]. The mechanism of its action may be related to increased retention within the tumor cells, to fixation of DNA damage, or to a nonspecific cytotoxicity. On the other hand, when chlorpromazine and caffeine have been used in patients with disseminated malignant carcinoma, no tumor cytotoxicity was enhanced [44].

### Metoclopramide

Metoclopramide might enhance antitumor activity of anticancer drugs because structurally related compounds (nicotinamide, benzamide, etc.) inhibit the chromatin-bound enzyme adenosine diphosphate ribosyl transferase [26]. This enzyme is activated by DNA-damaging agents and may play a role in DNA repair. This hypothesis was tested against a squamous cell carcinoma of the head and neck in xenografted nude mice. Metoclopramide was given at the same time as cisplatin and again 24 and 48 h later. Compared with mice not given metoclopramide, cisplatin anti-tumor activity was doubled, with no other increase in cisplatin toxicity. In another study with metoclopramide and chlorpromazine, epirubicin cytotoxic activity was enhanced when tested against Chinese hamster fibroblasts without any intrinsic cytotoxic activity [27].

## Granisetron and Ondansetron

Development of serotonin receptor antagonists gives a therapeutic class without the classic adverse reactions associated with dopamine receptor blockade, such as severe sedation or extrapyramidal side effects. Finally, of the selective 5HT3 receptor antagonists, both granisetron and ondansetron have been tested for their potential to affect drug cytotoxicity. No evidence was found that these two compounds antagonize or enhance the antitumor properties of anticancer drugs such as cisplatinum [45, 46].

## *Antiulcer Drugs*

Cimetidine and ranitidine are histamine H2 antagonists used for the treatment of diseases caused by gastric hyperacidity. Evidence has accumulated that cimetidine can alter drug metabolism through the ability to inhibit the hepatic microsomal cytochrome P450 enzyme system [47]. Ranitidine binds less avidly to microsomal enzymes and, in clinical dosage, does not appear to significantly alter microsomal metabolism [47]. Ranitidine when associated with cyclophosphamide does not change the pattern or degree of cyclophosphamide-induced leukopenia or granulocytopenia. Ranitidine administration has no significant effect on the area under the curve values for the two major oncolytic cyclophosphamide metabolites 4-hydroxycyclophosphamide and phosphoramid mustard; nevertheless, ranitidine administration is associated with significantly prolonged plasma terminal half-life and increases area under the curve for the parent drug that is not active [48].

Several anticancer drugs, including cyclophosphamide, the nitrosoureas, doxorubicin, procarbazine, and hexamethylmelamine, undergo metabolism through the hepatic oxidative microsomal enzyme system [28–30].

The result of the interaction between cimetidine and the former anticancer agents is a decrease of the antineoplastic agent clearance, leading to an increase in their activities and toxicities by typical pharmacokinetic interaction [49–51].

## Analgesics (Nonsteroidal Anti-inflammatory Drugs)

Many cases of drug interactions between nonsteroidal anti-inflammatory drugs (NSAIDs) and anticancer drugs have been reported. There have been fatal interactions between methotrexate and naproxen [52] as well as clinical and pharmacokinetic evidence of life-threatening interactions between methotrexate and ketoprofen [31]. In the latter chapter, no abnormalities in methotrexate kinetics or toxicity were noticed when ketoprofen was given at least 12 h after completion of high-dose methotrexate. The kidney was suggested to be the site of drug interaction.

A probable interaction between methotrexate and/or 5-FU and indomethacin has been reported [32]. This NSAID is known to enhance cell killing by methotrexate in vitro. Other mechanisms than renal damage are of importance in the explanation of indomethacin–methotrexate interaction such as displacement and increased transport into malignant cells [33]. Inhibition of prostaglandin synthesis seems to participate in the effect of indomethacin on methotrexate cytotoxicity.

Pharmacokinetic interaction between cisplatinum and indomethacin has been reported in vitro and in vivo [34]. The result of this interaction was an increase in free cisplatinum concentrations due to the fact that both indomethacin and cisplatinum are highly protein-bound.

Morphine, cocaine, and atropine stimulated transport of choline and nitrogen mustard into L5178Y lymphoblasts [53] and into leukemic white blood cells [54], which is interesting since the accumulation of alkylating agents is of importance for their cytotoxicity.

## Antimicrobial Agents

Antimicrobial therapy is quite common for patients treated for hematologic malignancies or solid tumors. For this reason, extensive studies have been published on the effects of anticancer agents on the antibacterial activity of antibiotics [55]. However, the effects of antibiotics on the antineoplastic activity of anticancer drugs have been considerably less discussed.

Nevertheless, there are some reports on the effects of antibiotics on the toxicity of anticancer drugs. Penicillin in combination with furosemide impaired methotrexate renal secretion and caused increased toxicity [41]. Penicillin also inhibits accumulation of methotrexate in renal slices of rabbit and monkeys and delayed the elimination of methotrexate [35]. Decreased methotrexate antitumor effect has been reported with kanamycin, neomycin, and penicillin due to a decrease of the cellular uptake of methotrexate [42]. The nephrotoxic antibiotics aminoglycoside gentamicin can enhance the toxic renal effects of methotrexate on the tubule [56].

Trimethoprim–sulfamethoxazole and netilmicin enhance the epirubicin oxygen radical formation.

Antifungal drugs such as amphotericin B potentialize the cytotoxicity of many anticancer agents (doxorubicin, vincristine, CCNU) on leukemia cells of mice [57]. Amphotericin B has also been suggested to potentialize the effect of doxorubicin, cyclophosphamide, and carmustine in human neoplasia [58].

## Miscellaneous

Anticoagulants such as dicumarol increase the enzymatic activation of mitomycin C to reactive alkylating metabolites and cause a subsequent increased cytotoxicity [59]. Warfarin, another anticoagulant, retards the growth of Lewis lung carcinoma in mice and small cell carcinoma of the lung in humans [60]. A synergistic action between 5-FU and warfarin has been also reported [36].

Psychiatric drugs are quite widely used in elderly patients being treated for cancer. The use of these psychopharmaceuticals has an influence on the activity of the antineoplastic agents. Diazepam blocks the cells in pre-S-phase and induces mitotic arrests at prometaphase by inhibiting centriolar separation [37,38]. Diazepam also causes an enhancement of doxorubicin and mitoxantrone cytotoxicity [39]. Amitriptyline, a tricyclic antidepressive, modifies the blood–brain barrier and enhances the penetration of drugs into the central nervous system [40].

Bronchodilators are often indicted in patients with airway obstruction or prominent wheezing. The main classes of bronchodilators, (beta)β-adrenoceptor agonists, and methylxanthines raise the level of 3′ 5′ cyclic AMP in mast cells and bronchial smooth muscles, thereby inhibiting mediator production and reducing muscle contractility.

As cyclic AMP is a second messenger in other cellular events, it is evident that bronchodilators might influence tumor cells and interact with cancer treatment [61]. The interaction of cyclic AMP on the cytotoxic effect of doxorubicin has been suggested [62].

# Anticancer Drug–Anticancer Drug Interactions

The interactions among anticancer drugs are of importance because the chemotherapeutic protocols include at least three different antineoplastic drugs. This is why the possibility of drug interactions should be known and taken into account.

Two aspects of drug interactions are concerned. Drug interaction may be desired for clinical modulation of an anticancer agent or undesired.

## Modulation

The modulation of an anticancer agent is accomplished by a compound that modifies some aspect of the biochemical pharmacology of the anticancer drug to improve its therapeutic index. The best example of clinical anticancer drug modulation is that of 5-FU modulation by leucovorin, which is discussed in another chapter of this book.

Another example of 5-FU modulation is the combination of methotrexate (MTX) and 5-FU [63]. The interaction of MTX and 5-FU is complex, and theoretical models for both antagonism and synergy have been postulated. By altering reduced folate pools involved in ternary complex formation, MTX may be expected to hinder 5-FU inhibition of thymidylate synthase [64, 65]. By inhibiting de novo purine synthesis, there is also less nucleic acid synthesis available for fluoropyrimidine nucleotide incorporation. However, the net balance of potential negative and positive effects appears to favor synergy. The most plausible mechanism of MTX/5-FU interaction appears to be through increased levels of phosphoribosylpyrophosphate, an intermediate needed in de novo purine synthesis, resulting from inhibition of purine synthesis [66].

## Undesired Drug Interactions

The undesired anticancer drug–anticancer drug interactions are probably fairly frequent because more than 800 polychemotherapeutic protocols have been recorded (hematologic malignancies plus solid tumors). In theory, it would seem to be an impossible task in a limited space to develop the subject of drug interactions when anticancer drugs are combined, but this is not the case in practice. In fact, very few interactions among the anticancer drug group have been reported in the literature. For this reason, it is more important to give the philosophical criteria for planning a polychemotherapeutic protocol.

In order to obtain a better antitumor response with drug association than with each drug alone, an association should discriminate between tumor sensitivity and toxic side effects. In other words, a drug association should combine the antineoplastic properties of each drug without adding their toxic side effects. One of the fundamental principles of drug combination is to combine drugs that do not have the same toxic effects.

Some impossible associations due to the same toxic effects, such as methotrexate with cisplatinum for renal toxicity, have led to second-generation drugs that do not have the same toxicities. For example, carboplatin and trimetrexate are free of the renal toxic effect of their corresponding first-generation drugs, due to the fact that the association of cisplatin with trimetrexate [67] and carboplatin with methotrexate [68] are possible and safer.

# Drug Interactions Between Anticancer Drugs and Resistance-Modifying Agents

Several systems exist by which tumor cells resist cancer chemotherapy. Numerous resistance-modifying agents are used in clinics in order to circumvent multidrug resistance (MDR), which is one of the most frequent reasons for chemotherapy failure. To reverse MDR, the combination between anticancer agents and resistance-modifying agents leads to pharmacologic interactions [69].

Pharmacodynamic interactions could be defined as desirable interactions, but the question is as follows: Are the pharmacodynamic direct interactions in target organs or are they due to pharmacokinetic modifications of the anticancer agent? In other words, the maximum tolerated dose of the antineoplastic agents when administered without the modulator is usually well established, but this is not the case for the maximum tolerated dose of the anticancer drugs when associated with the MDR-modulating drug. Clinicians should be very careful when they initiate a protocol that associates anticancer chemotherapy and MDR modulators.

## Pharmacogenetics

Pharmacogenetics relates variation in gene structure to variation in phenotypes associated with therapeutic or toxic responses to drugs and other foreign chemicals in human populations [70]. Methods of study in pharmacogenetics include the correlation of observed variation in drug pharmacokinetics or pharmacodynamics with allelic variation in individual genes encoding proteins that act as targets of drug action or mediators of drug elimination, the elucidation of biochemical and molecular mechanisms that produce variable protein function, the development of probe drug-testing procedures and predictive animal models to more precisely define the role of genetics in producing variable drug response in human populations, and the development of simple genetic tests to predict unexpected drug responses and thus to guide the clinician in the selection of appropriate drugs and drug doses [71–73].

Personalized medication management, including DNA testing, is extremely important for the proper treatment of cancer because finding the right drug and dose is so vitally important. This is not surprising to people that study genetics. Research shows that of all the clinical factors that alter a patient's response to drugs, such as age, sex, weight, general health, and liver function, genetic factors account for a significant proportion [74–76].

Early in the development of irinotecan, researchers observed that the active metabolite of the drug, SN-38, was cleared from the body through a process called glucuronidation [77]. A gene called UGT1A1 was responsible for sticking that glucuronide group onto the drug [78,79]. Once glucuronide was on a compound, it was easily excreted by the bile. So, for example, bilirubin and a number of estrogen molecules in the body are glucuronidated. Irinotecan is one of several anticancer drugs that also undergo this process. Researchers found that a subset of the population, about 10 %, has a genetic change in the UGT1A1 gene that hinders their ability to perform this glucuronidation process [80]. This change does not have an apparent phenotype; it is something that could be detected by the usual bilirubin test or by some outward manifestation of the patient. When patients with the genetic change in UGT1A1, called UGT1A1*28, receive a standard dose of irinotecan, they have a very high risk of severe or even fatal neutropenia, a condition that drastically lowers the ability of the body to fight off infection. This UGT1A1*28 genetic change is responsible for Gilbert's syndrome, which is a lack of bilirubin glucuronidation [81, 82]. In 2004, the FDA reviewed the data on UGT1A1*28 and decided that this genetic change should be included in the insert for irinotecan as a risk factor for severe toxicity. (TA)6/(TA)6 is the normal genotype; generally, there is no change in the administered dose of irinotecan provided that no other agents known to interact with irinotecan are also administered. Patients with the (TA)6/(TA)7 heterozygous genotype have intermediate UGT1A1 activity and may be at increased risk for neutropenia; however, clinical results have been variable, and such patients have been shown to tolerate normal starting doses. Patients with the (TA)7/(TA)7 homozygous genotype should have their starting dose reduced by at least one level of irinotecan [83]. However, the precise dose reduction is not known, and subsequent dose modifications should be considered based on the individual patient's tolerance to treatment.

Recent research has shown that up to 35 % of women with estrogen receptor (ER)-positive breast cancer may fail tamoxifen treatment because of drug interactions and their genetic makeup [84]. The ability of these women to convert tamoxifen to the active compound endoxifen is compromised, resulting in a greatly increased risk of relapse [85]. DNA testing and careful analysis of overall drug regimens in these patients provide evidence that can be used to improve their chances of survival. With more than 500,000 women currently taking tamoxifen, this research has wide-reaching implications.

Tamoxifen is a prodrug widely used to treat, and as prophylaxis for, ER-positive breast cancer. Out of the approximately 120,000 new ER-positive breast cancer patients per year in the IS, 41,000 of whom will die; 42,000 are predicted to fail tamoxifen treatment because of 2D6 poor metabolizer phenotype. "Hot flashes," a common side effect, is typically treated with selective serotonin reuptake inhibitors (SSRIs), many of which are potent inhibitors of CYP2D6, phenol-converting intermediate metabolizer patients into 2D6 poor metabolizers, now demonstrated as crucial to the activation of tamoxifen to endoxifen. Endoxifen has a 100 times greater receptor affinity than tamoxifen and is 30–100 times more effective. CYP2D6 genetically normal metabolizers also taking an inhibitor had 58 % lower endoxifen levels and are likely to be in the group of ~35 % of patients who do not respond to tamoxifen. CYP2D6 frank poor metabolizers, homozygous for *3, *4, *5, and *6, had endoxifen levels 26 % of WT. CYP2D6*4/*4 poor metabolizers had a 3.12 hazard ratio for breast cancer relapse. Two-year relapse-free survival is 68 % in patients with the 2D6 PM phenotype and 98 % in normal metabolizers [85, 86]. This suggests that widespread genotyping and therapeutic drug monitoring could result in successful outcomes for many of the 35 % of ER-positive breast cancer patients who currently fail tamoxifen treatment [87].

Dihydropyrimidine dehydrogenase (DPD) is the rate-limiting enzyme in the degradation of pyrimidine bases like thymidine and uracil [88]. DPD is also the main enzyme involved in the degradation of structurally related compounds like 5-fluorouracil (5-FU), a widely used anticancer drug [89, 90]. In 5-FU-based cancer chemotherapy, severe toxicities are observed at higher rates in patients who are heterozygous for a mutant DPYD allele, compared with toxicities in patients who are homozygous for the wild DPYD allele. The adverse effects of 5-FU are often lethal for patients homozygous for the mutant DPYD allele [91, 92].

On the basis of catalytic activity and on the basis of the mutation frequency, a 3 % frequency for heterozygotes ($-/+$) to DPD was predicted, projecting a 1:1,000 homozygote ($+/+$) for this mutation across racial lines.

The DPD test for 5-FU is considered appropriate for any person who is taking or considering 5-FU-based chemotherapy. It is recommended that this screening be accompanied by direct measurement of DPD activity prior to 5-FU treatment in cancer patients. Although this test looks for the most frequent genetic variation that causes DPD enzyme deficiency, this does not rule out the possibility of a decrease in DPD activity due to other factors or genetic variations [93, 94].

## Summary

Drug–drug interactions with the pharmacologic results are a really important factor. More oncologists are usually aware of antineoplastic drug associations because they know the toxic side effects of each of the associated components, but they are much less aware of the pharmacologic effects of anticancer drugs and other medical treatments.

The availability of potent and reliable genetic techniques can change the way patients will receive chemotherapy in the near future. With this perspective in mind, oncologists and clinical pharmacologists should prompt the inclusion of pharmacogenetic investigation and DNA collection into early phases of clinical drug development. Recurrent, even after dose reduction, or unexplainable toxicity can be induced by genetically reduced drug inactivation/elimination. When polymorphic genes involved in the systemic disposition of a new agent are identified, prospective phenotype/genotype correlation analysis should be performed in phase I–II clinical trials, following the example of two recent phase I and pharmacogenetic studies. Pharmacogenetics has emerged as a novel and challenging area of interest in oncology.

# References

1. Finley RS. Drug interactions in the oncology patients. Semin Oncol Nurs. 1992;8:95–101.
2. Kuhlmann J, Muck W. Clinical-pharmacologic strategies to assess drug interaction potential during drug development. Drug Saf. 2001;24:715–25.
3. Balducci L. Pharmacology of antineoplastic medications in older cancer patients. Oncology. 2009;23:78–85.
4. Evans WE, McLeod HL. Pharmacogenomics-drug disposition, drug targets, and side effects. N Engl J Med. 2003;348:538–45.
5. Weinshilboum R. Inheritance and drug response. N Engl J Med. 2003;348:529–37.
6. Scripture CD, Sparreboom A, Figg WD. Modulation of cytochrome P450 activity: implications for cancer therapy. Lancet Oncol. 2005;6:780–9.
7. William DA, Lokich J. A review on the stability and compatibility of antineoplastic drugs for multiple-drug infusions. Cancer Chemother Pharmacol. 1992;31:171–81.
8. Newton DW. Drug incompatibility chemistry. Am J Health Syst Pharm. 2009;66:348–57.
9. Gunnarsson PO, Davidson T, Andersson SB, Backman C, Johansson SA. Impairment estramustine phosphate absorption by concurrent intake of milk and food. Eur J Clin Pharmacol. 1990;38:189–93.
10. Reignier B, Verweij J, Dirix L, Cassidy J, Twelves C, Allman D, et al. Effect of food on the pharmacokinetics of capecitabine and its metabolites following oral administration in cancer patients. Clin Cancer Res. 1998;4:941–8.
11. Singh BN, Malhtrota BK. Effects of food on the clinical pharmacokinetics of anticancer agents: underlying mechanisms and implications for oral chemotherapy. Clin Pharmacokinet. 2004;43:1127–56.
12. Zhang Y, Benet LZ. The gut as a barrier to drug absorption: combined role of cytochrome P450 3A and P-glycoprotéine. Clin Pharmacokinet. 2001;40:159–68.
13. Bailey DG, Arnold JM, Spence JD. Grapefruit juice and drugs. Clin Pharmacokinet. 1994;26:91–8.
14. He K, Iyer KR, Hayes RN, Sinz MW, Woolf TF, Hollenberg PF. Inactivation of cytochrome P450 3A4 by bergamottin, a component of grapefruit juice. Chem Res Toxicol. 1998;11:252–9.
15. Edwards DJ, Bellevue III FH, Woster PM. Identification of 6',7'-dihydroxybergamottin, a cytochrome P450 inhibitor, in grapefruit juice. Drug Metab Dispos. 1996;24:1287–90.

24     F. Lokiec

16. Veronese ML, Gillen LP, Burke JP, Dorval EP, Hauck WW, Pequignot E, et al. Exposure-dependent inhibition of intestinal and hepatic CYP3A4 in vivo by grapefruit juice. J Clin Pharmacol. 2003;43:831–9.
17. Liegler DG, Henderson ES, Hahn MA. The effect of organic acids on renal clearance of methotrexate in man. Clin Pharmacol Ther. 1969;10:849–57.
18. Mandel MA. The synergistic effect of salicylates on methotrexate toxicity. Plast Reconstr Surg. 1976;57:733–9.
19. Maiche AG. Acute renal failure due to concomitant interaction between methotrexate and indomethacin. Lancet. 1986;1:1390.
20. Thomas MH, Gutterman LA. Methotrexate toxicity in a patient receiving trimethoprim-sulfamethoxazole. J Rheumatol. 1986;13: 440–1.
21. Maricic M, Davis M, Gall EP. Megaloblastic pancytopenia in a patient receiving concurrent methotrexate and trimethoprim-sulfamethoxazole treatment. Arthritis Rheum. 1986;29:133–5.
22. Burns JS, Conney AH. Enzyme stimulation and inhibition in the metabolism of drugs. Proc R Soc Med. 1965;58:955–60.
23. Remmer H. Induction of drug metabolizing enzyme system in the liver. Eur J Clin Pharmacol. 1972;5:116–36.
24. Solomon HM, Abrams WB. Interactions between digitoxin and other drugs in man. Am Heart J. 1972;83:277–80.
25. Vesell ES, Passaniti TC, Greene FE. Impairment of drug metabolism in man by allopurinol and nortriptiline. N Engl J Med. 1970;283:1484–8.
26. Kjellen E, Wennerberg J, Pero R. Metoclopramide enhances the effect of cisplatin on xenografted squamous cell carcinoma of the head and neck. Br J Cancer. 1989;59:247–50.
27. Henriksson R, Gankvist K. Epirubicin cytotoxicity but not oxygen radical formation is enhanced by four different anti-emetics. Med Oncol Tumor Pharmacother. 1989;59:175–8.
28. Dorr RT, Soble MJ, Alberts DS. Interaction of cimetidine but not ranitidine with cyclophosphamide in mice. Cancer Res. 1986;46: 1795–9.
29. Hess WA, Kornblith PL. Combination of lomustine and cimetidine in the treatment of a patient with malignant glioblastoma: a case report. Cancer Treat Rep. 1985;69:733–5.
30. Volkin RL, Shadduck RK, Winkelstein A, Ziegler ZR, Selker RG. Potentiation of carmustine-cranial irradiation induced myelosuppression by cimetidine. Arch Intern Med. 1986;142:243–5.
31. Thyss A, Milano G, Kubar J, Namer M, Schneider M. Clinical and pharmacokinetic evidence of life-threatening interaction between methotrexate and ketoprofen. Lancet. 1986;1:256–8.
32. Ellison NM, Servi RJ. Acute renal failure and death following sequential intermediate-dose methotrexate and 5-FU: a possible adverse effect due to concomitant indomethacin administration. Cancer Treat Rep. 1985;69:342–3.

33. Gaffen JD, Bennett A, Barer MR. A new method for studying cell growth in suspension, and its use to show that indomethacin enhances cell killing by methotrexate. J Pharm Pharmacol. 1985;37:261–3.
34. Ogino M, Okinaga S, Kaibara M, Ishiwata I. NSAID indomethacin enhanced cytostatic effect of cisplatinum on the proliferation of prostaglandin-producing and –nonproducing cancers in cell line. Eicosanoids and bioactive lipids in cancer and radiation injury, Detroit, 11–14 Oct 1989.
35. Nierenberg DW. Competitive inhibition of methotrexate accumulation in rabbit kidney slices by non steroidal anti-inflammatory drugs. J Pharmacol Exp Ther. 1983;226:1–6.
36. Kirsch W, Schulz D, Van Burskirk J, Young H. Effects of sodium warfarin and other cariostatic agents on malignant cells: a study of drug synergy. J Med (Basel). 1974;5:69–82.
37. Clarke GD, Ryan PJ. Tranquilizers can block mitogenesis in 3T3 cells and induce differentiation in Friend cells. Nature. 1980;287:160–1.
38. Feif C. Diazepam induces mitotic arrest at prometaphase by inhibiting centrilar separation. Nature. 1981;291:247–8.
39. Juvekar AS, Chitnis MP, Advani SH. In vitro modulation of Adriamycin and mitoxantrone cytotoxicity by hyperthermia and diazepam in human chronic myeloid leukemia cells. Neoplasma. 1987;34:199–204.
40. Raichle ME, Hartman BK, Eichling JO, Sharpe LG. Central noradrenergic regulation of cerebral blood flow and vascular permeability. Proc Natl Acad Sci. 1975;72:3726–30.
41. Nierenberg DW. Toxic reaction to methotrexate in a patient receiving penicillin and furosemide: a possible interaction. Arch Dermatol. 1983;119:449–50.
42. Zager R, Frisby S, Oliverio V. The effect of antibiotics and cancer chemotherapeutic agents in the cellular transport and antitumor activity of methotrexate in L1210 murine leukemia. Cancer Res. 1973;33:1670–6.
43. Osieka R, Glatte P, Pannenbäcker R, Schmitt CG. Enhancement of semustine-induced cytotoxicity by chlorpromazine and caffeine in a human melanoma xenograft. Cancer Treat Rep. 1986;70:1167–71.
44. Cohen MH, Schoenfeld D, Wolter J. Randomized trial of chlorpromazine, caffeine and methyl-CCNU in disseminated melanoma. Cancer Treat Rep. 1980;64:151–3.
45. Goddard PM, Jones M, Pollard LA, Valenti MR, Harrap KR. The 5-HT$_3$ antagonist BRL 43694, does not compromise the efficacy of cisplatin in tumour-bearing mice. Cancer Chemother Pharmacol. 1991;25:377–9.
46. Hall TJ, Cambridge G, James PR. Development of a co-culture system with induced HEPG2 cells and K562 cells for examining drug metabolism in vitro. Studies with cyclophosphamide, ondansetron and cisplatin. Res Commun Chem Pathol Pharmacol. 1991;72:161–8.

47. Hande K, Combs G, Swingle R, Combs GL, Anthony L. Effects of cimetidine and ranitidine on the metabolism and toxicity of hexamethylmelamine. Cancer Treat Rep. 1986;70:1443–5.
48. Alberts DS, Mason-Liddil N, Plezia PM, Roe DL, Dorr RT, Struck RF, et al. Lack of ranitidine effects on cyclophosphamide bone marrow toxicity or metabolism: a placebo-controlled clinical trial. J Natl Cancer Inst. 1991;83:1739–43.
49. Harvey VJ, Slevin ML, Dilloway MR. The influence of cimetidine on the pharmacokinetics of 5-fluorouracil. Br J Clin Pharmacol. 1984; 18:421–30.
50. Brenner DE, Collins JC, Hande KR. The effects of cimetidine upon the plasma pharmacokinetics of doxorubicin in rabbits. Cancer Chemother Pharmacol. 1986;18:219–22.
51. Dorr RT, Alberts DS. Cimetidine enhancement of cyclophosphamide antitumor activity. Br J Cancer. 1982;45:35–43.
52. Singh RR, Malaviya AN, Pandey JN, Guleria JS. Fatal interaction between methotrexate and naproxen. Lancet. 1986;1:1390.
53. Goldenberg GJ. Drug-induced stimulation of nitrogen mustard and choline transport and other system in L5178Y lymphoblasts. Cancer Res. 1974;34:2511–6.
54. Goldenberg GJ. Drug-induced stimulation of nitrogen mustard and choline by normal and leukemic human cells in vitro. Cancer Res. 1976;36:978–82.
55. Gieringer JH, Wenz AF, Just HM, Daschner FD. Effect of 5-fluorouracil, mitoxantrone, methotrexate, and vincristine on the bacterial activity of ceftriaxone, ceftazidine, cefotiam, piperacillin, and netilmicin. Chemotherapy. 1986;32:418–24.
56. Spector GN, Gleiser CA, Chan RC, Van Eys J. Effects of gentamicin and irradiation of the toxicity of high-dose methotrexate in rats. Cancer Treat Rep. 1980;64:989–91.
57. Valeriote F, Medoff G, Dieckman J. Potentiation of anticancer cytotoxicity against sensitive and resistant AKR leukemia by amphotericin B1. Cancer Res. 1979;39:2041–5.
58. Present C, Klahr C, Santala R. Amphotericin B induction sensitivity to Adriamycin, 1,3-Bis (2chloroethyl)-nitrosourea (BCNU) plus cyclophosphamide in human neoplasia. Ann Intern Med. 1977;86:47–51.
59. Keyes SR, Rockwell S, Sartorelli AC. Enhancement of mitomycin C cytotoxicity to hypoxic tumor cells by dicumarol in vivo and in vitro. Cancer Res. 1985;45:213–6.
60. Zacharski LR. Basis for selection of anticoagulant drugs for therapeutic trials in human malignancy. Haemostasis. 1986;16:300–20.
61. Grankvisk K, Berström P, Jonsson Ö, Henriksson R. Pharmacologic interactions with quinoid antitumor drugs. Free Radic Res Commun. 1990;8:383–90.
62. Di Marco A, Dasdia T, Pastori W. Interaction of calcium ions and cAMP on the cytotoxic effect of doxorubicin. Tumori. 1984;30:217–21.

63. Sotos GA, Grogan L, Allegra CJ. Preclinical and clinical aspects of biomodulation of 5-fluorouracil. Cancer Treat Rev. 1994;20:11–49.
64. Doroshow JH, Newman EM. Fluoropyrimidine biochemical modulation in colon cancer. Pharmacology relevant in both the laboratory and the clinic. J Clin Oncol. 1991;9:365–7.
65. Bertino JR, Mini E, Fernandes DJ. Sequential methotrexate and 5-fluorouracil: mechanism of synergy. Semin Oncol. 1983;10:2–5.
66. Damon LE, Cadman E, Benz C. Enhancement of 5-fluorouracil antitumor effects by the prior administration of methotrexate. Pharmacol Ther. 1989;43:155–85.
67. Hudes GR, LaCreta F, Walczak J, Tinsley P, Litwin S, Comis RL, et al. Pharmacokinetic study of trimetrexate in combination with cisplatin. Cancer Res. 1991;51:3080–7.
68. Kennedy P, Eisenberg M, Silva H, Krasnow S, Perry D, Ettinger D, et al. Toxicity of carboplatin (CBDCA) in combination with methotrexate (MTX) in patients with metastatic squamous cell carcinoma of the head and neck (SCCHN). Proc ASCO. 1987;6:136.
69. Lum BL, Fisher GA, Brophy NA, Yahanda AM, Adler KM, Kaubish S, et al. Clinical trials of modulation of multidrug resistance. Cancer. 1993;72:3503–14.
70. Boddy A, Idle J. The role of pharmacogenetics in chemotherapy: modulation of tumor response and host toxicity. Cancer Surv. 1993;17:79–104.
71. Rioux PP. Clinical trials in pharmacogenetics and pharmacogenomics: methods and applications. Am J Health Syst Pharm. 2000;57:887–98.
72. Moridani M, Maitland-van der Zee AH, Sasaki H, McKinnon R, Fleckenstein L, Shah VP. AAPS-FIP summary workshop report: pharmacogenetics in individualized medicine: methods, regulatory, and clinical applications. APPS J. 2009;11:214–6.
73. Marsh S, McLeod HL. Cancer pharmacogenetics. Br J Cancer. 2004;90:8–11.
74. Evans W, Relling M. Pharmacogenomics: translating functional genomics into rational therapeutics. Science. 1999;286:487–91.
75. Krynetski E, Evans W. Pharmacogenetics of cancer therapy: getting personal. Am J Hum Genet. 1998;63:11–6.
76. Vessel E. Advances in pharmacogenetics and pharmacogenomics. J Clin Pharmacol. 2000;40:930–8.
77. Gupta E, Leistingi TM, Mick R, Ramirez J, Vokes EE, Ratain MJ. Metabolic fate of irinotecan in humans: correlation of glucuronidation with diarrhea. Cancer Res. 1994;54:3723–5.
78. Iyer L, Whitington P, Roy SK, Ratain MJ. Genetic basis for glucuronidation of SN-38: role of UGT*1 isoform. Clin Pharmacol Ther. 1997;61:164.
79. Wasserman E, Myara A, Lokiec F, Goldwasser F, Trivin F, Mahjoubi M, et al. Severe CPT-11 toxicity in patients with Gilbert's syndrome: two cases report. Ann Oncol. 1997;8:1049–51.

80. Bosma PJ, Chowdhury JR, Bakker C, Gantla S, de Boer A, Oostra B, et al. The genetic basis of the reduced expression of bilirubin UDP-glucuronosyltransferase 1 in Gilbert's syndrome. N Engl J Med. 1995;333:1171–5.
81. Köhle C, Möhrle B, Münzel PA, Schwab M, Wernet D, Badary OA, et al. Frequent co-occurrence of the TATA box mutation associated with Gilbert's syndrome (UGT1A1*28) with other polymorphisms of the UDP-glucuronosyltransferase-1 locus (UGT1A6*2 and UGT1A7*3) in Caucasians and Egyptians. Biochem Pharmacol. 2003;65:1521–7.
82. Iyer L, Das S, Janisch L, Wen M, Ramírez J, Karrison T, et al. UGT1A1*28 polymorphism as a determinant of irinotecan disposition and toxicity. Pharmacogenomics J. 2002;2:43–7.
83. Marcuello E, Altés A, Menoyo A, Del Rio E, Gómez-Pardo M, Baiget M. UGT1A1 gene variations and irinotecan treatment in patients with metastatic colorectal cancer. Br J Cancer. 2004;9: 678–82.
84. Sachse C, Brockmoller J, Bauer S, Roots L. Cytochrome P450 2D6 variants in a Caucasian population: allele frequencies and phenotypic consequences. Am J Hum Genet. 1997;60:284–95.
85. Goetz MP, Rae JM, Suman VJ, Safgren SL, Ames MM, Visscher DW, et al. Pharmacogenetics of tamoxifen biotransformation is associated with clinical outcomes of efficacy and hot flashes. J Clin Oncol. 2005;23:9312–8.
86. Goetz MP, Knox SK, Suman VJ, Rae JM, Safgren SL, Ames MM, et al. The impact of cytochrome P450 2D6 metabolism in women receiving adjuvant tamoxifen. Breast Cancer Res Treat. 2007;101:113–21.
87. Hoskins JM, Carey LA, McLeod HL. Cyp2D6 and tamoxifen: DNA matters in breast cancer. Nat Rev Cancer. 2009;9:56–86.
88. Diasio RB, Harris BE. Clinical pharmacology of 5-fluorouracil. Clin Pharmacokinet. 1989;16:215–37.
89. Milano G, Etienne MC, Cassuto-Viguier E, Thyss A, Santini J, Fremay M, et al. Influence of sex and age on fluorouracil clearance. J Clin Oncol. 1992;10:1171–5.
90. Diasio RB, Lu Z. Dihydropyrimidine dehydrogenase activity and fluorouracil chemotherapy. J Clin Oncol. 1994;12:2239–42.
91. Fleming RA, Milano G, Gaspard MH, Bargnoux PJ, Thyss A, Plagne R, et al. Dihydropyrimidine dehydrogenase activity in cancer patients. Eur J Cancer. 1993;29A:740–4.
92. Lu ZH, Zhang R, Diasio RB. Dihydropyrimidine dehydrogenase activity in human peripheral blood mononuclear cells and liver: population characteristics, newly identified deficient patients, and clinical implication in 5-fluorouracil chemotherapy. Cancer Res. 1993;53:5433–8.
93. Albin N, Johnson MR, Diasio RB. cDNA cloning of bovine liver dihydropyrimidine dehydrogenase. DNA Seq. 1996;6:243–50.
94. Johnson MR, Wang K, Tillmanns S, Albin N, Diasio RB. Structural organization of the human dihydropyrimidine dehydrogenase gene. Cancer Res. 1997;57:1660–3.

# Chapter 2
# Breast Cancer

**Philippe G. Aftimos, Andrea Gombos, Lina Pugliano, Ahmad Awada, and Martine J. Piccart**

**Abstract** The appropriate selection of medical therapeutic interventions in breast cancer patients is a daily challenge for medical oncologists and takes into account disease characteristics such as stage at diagnosis, age and menopausal status, aggressiveness of the disease, and presence or absence of key therapeutic targets such as hormonal receptors and HER2. Knowledge of treatment-related toxicities as well as patient's comorbidities, preferences, age, and so on is a critical component of an optimal estimation of the benefit versus harm ratio of a specific therapy.

P.G. Aftimos, M.D. (✉)
Medical Oncology Department, Institut Jules Bordet,
Université Libre de Bruxelles, Bruxelles, Belgium

A. Gombos, M.D. • L. Pugliano, M.D., B.Sc. (Hons), M.B.B.S., FRACP
Medical Oncology Department, Institut Jules Bordet,
Université Libre de Bruxelles, Bruxelles, Belgium

A. Awada, M.D., Ph.D.
Medical Oncology Department, Institut Jules Bordet,
Brussels, Belgium

M.J. Piccart, M.D., Ph.D.
Department of Medicine, Institut Jules Bordet,
Université Libre de Bruxelles, Brussels, Belgium
e-mail: martine.piccart@bordet.be

M.A. Dicato (ed.), *Side Effects of Medical Cancer Therapy,*
DOI 10.1007/978-0-85729-787-7_2,
© Springer-Verlag London 2013
29

This chapter reviews the side effects of the four main medical treatment modalities for breast cancer: chemotherapy, endocrine therapy, biologic agents, and bone-modifying therapeutics in terms of frequency, monitoring, and practical management.

**Keywords**   Breast cancer • Cytotoxic chemotherapy • Endocrine treatment • Targeted agents • Bone-modifying agents • Side effects

## Introduction

Appropriate selection of medical therapies for women with breast cancer requires a careful evaluation of patient and disease characteristics. The former includes age, functional status, and comorbidities, while the latter consists of stage of the disease (early vs. metastatic breast cancer), presence of treatment targets such as hormone receptors and HER2 overexpression or amplification, previous therapies and their effectiveness, extent and location of disease sites (visceral vs. bone and soft tissues), and time course of disease.

The main objective of *adjuvant* medical treatment is to eradicate micrometastatic disease – that is, breast cancer cells that have escaped the breast and regional lymph nodes but have not yet formed a detectable metastatic deposit.

Once a patient has metastatic disease, medical treatments are essentially palliative in nature and are directed at providing symptomatic relief from disease-related symptoms and extending progression-free survival and overall survival.

Once patients have progressed through first-line therapy, their management becomes more challenging, because the probability of response to subsequent therapies decreases. This is true for sequential endocrine, anti-HER2, or chemotherapy-based approaches.

As a general rule, combination therapies have a tendency to be more highly efficacious in comparison to single-agent therapies, but this comes at a risk of significant toxicity.

At each stage of the disease, a careful assessment of benefit versus harm from a treatment modality is needed for each individual patient. Knowledge of treatment-induced side effects and serious toxicities is an essential component of this evaluation.

In this chapter the main side effects of cytotoxic chemotherapy, endocrine therapy, targeted agents, and bone-modifying agents are reviewed.

# Chemotherapy

## Classes of Chemotherapy and General Toxicities

### Antimicrotubule Agents (Taxanes, Ixabepilone, Eribulin, and Vinca Alkaloids)

Antimicrotubule agents form a large proportion of the chemotherapy agents prescribed in breast cancer patients and either promote microtubule polymerization, stabilizing microtubules and increasing the polymer mass (antimicrotubule stabilizing agents, e.g., taxanes, ixabepilone), or inhibit microtubule polymerization, destabilizing microtubules and decreasing microtubule polymer mass (antimicrotubule destabilizing agents, e.g., eribulin, the vinca alkaloid vinorelbine) [1]. These agents share the toxicities of peripheral neuropathy and myelosuppression.

### Anthracyclines (Doxorubicin, Epirubicin, Mitoxantrone, Liposomal Doxorubicin, Non-pegylated Liposomal Doxorubicin)

Anthracyclines inhibit topoisomerase II, an enzyme involved in relaxing, disentangling, and cleaving of DNA, and thereby inhibiting DNA transcription and replication. Further, anthra-cyclines can cause partial unwinding of the DNA helix through intercalation between base pairs and can lead to the formation of free radicals, which in turn have negative effects on the cell membrane [2]. These agents share the toxicities of cardiac injury, myelosuppression, and emesis.

## Antimetabolites (5-Fluorouracil, Methotrexate, Capecitabine, Gemcitabine, Pemetrexed)

Antimetabolites have structural similarity to precursors of pyrimidine or purines, which are the building blocks for DNA. Therefore, antimetabolite agents interfere with the synthesis of DNA by not allowing these molecules to be incorporated into DNA. In addition, folate and folate-derived cofactors are essential in these pathways, and antagonists to folate also provide useful cytotoxics. Three classes exist: nucleoside analogues, thymidylate synthase inhibitors, and dihydrofolate reductase inhibitors. They tend to convey greatest toxicity to cells in S-phase [3], and they have common toxicities that include mucositis, diarrhea, and myelosuppression.

## Alkylating Agents (Cyclophosphamide, Cisplatin, and Carboplatin)

Alkylating agents are cell-cycle nonspecific agents. They form covalent bonds with bases in DNA. This leads to cross-linkage of DNA strands or breaks in DNA as a result of repair efforts. Broken or cross-linked DNA is unable to complete normal replication or cell division. Furthermore, broken or cross-linked DNA is an activator of cell-cycle checkpoints, and the cell signaling that results can precipitate apoptosis [4]. As a class, they share similar toxicities: myelosuppression, gonadal dysfunction, and, rarely, pulmonary fibrosis. They also hold the ability to cause "second" neoplasms, particularly leukemia.

Table 2.1 provides a detailed review of the side effects of breast cancer chemotherapy toxicities.

The following section outlines some of the common toxicities associated with breast cancer chemotherapy and their management.

## Incidence and Management of Selected Chemotherapy Toxicities

Many of the frequent toxicities induced by cytotoxic drugs commonly prescribed to breast cancer patients, such as myelosuppression and gastrointestinal toxicity, are reviewed in other chapters of this book. Only a few toxicities are discussed in detail below.

### Febrile Neutropenia

Febrile neutropenia is a life-threatening condition of a number of chemotherapy regimens, and its proper prevention and/or management is described in another chapter in this book. As far as breast cancer chemotherapy is concerned, particular attention needs to be paid to patients receiving docetaxel, as the rate of febrile neutropenia of 15–20 % is associated with docetaxel at 100 mg/m$^2$ or anthracyclines plus taxane combinations (rates of febrile neutropenia exceeding 30 %) [31]. For the latter, prophylactic granulocyte colony-stimulating factors (G-CSF) are highly recommended.

The commonly prescribed FEC regimen (5-fluorouracil, epirubicin, cyclophosphamide) induces febrile neutropenic episodes in about 10 % of patients when the epirubicin dose is 100 mg/m$^2$. Febrile neutropenia is less common with other "popular" breast cancer chemotherapy regimens such as CMF (cyclophosphamide, methotrexate, 5-fluorouracil), weekly paclitaxel, weekly vinorelbine, or capecitabine.

TABLE 2.1 Side effects of chemotherapy

| Mechanism of action | Drug | Context of prescription (NA/A/M) and usual dose schedule | Minimum requirements for prescription | SE specific to agent | Standard special tests to modify SE |
|---|---|---|---|---|---|
| Antimicrotu-bule: stabilizer | Paclitaxel [5] | A/M (any line) | Nil | Hypersensitivity | Nil |
| | | IV dose: 80–90 mg/m$^2$ weekly or 175 mg/m$^2$ D1 q 3 weekly in metastatic setting only | | | |
| | | | | Arthralgia/myalgia | Nil |

| Risk factors and recommendation for prevention of SE | Recommendation for management of SE | In the elderly (≥65 years) | Metabolism | Excretion | Cross BBB |
|---|---|---|---|---|---|
| Premedication with corticosteroids with or without antihistamines (H1 and H2 antagonists) | Stop infusion | Reduced clearance | Hepatic cytochrome P450 enzymes, primarily CYP2C8/9 and CYP3A4 | Biliary | No |
| | Supportive therapy with oxygen and hydration if hypotension | | | | |
| | Administer IV corticosteroids and antihistamines | | | | |
| | Infusion can be recommenced at slower rate if symptoms are mild and complete recovery has occurred | | | | |
| | Treat anaphylaxis if it occurs | | | | |
| | Prophylaxis prior to next infusion with premedication: IV corticosteroids and antihistamines. Slow infusion | | | | |
| | Patients should not be rechallenged if anaphylaxis has occurred | | | | |
| Nil | Symptomatic treatment with paracetamol, NSAIDS, gabapentin, and prednisone (if severe cases) | | | | |
| | In the curative setting, dose reduction not recommended | | | | |

(continued)

TABLE 2.1 (continued)

| Mechanism of action | Drug | Context of prescription (NA/A/M) and usual dose schedule | Minimum requirements for prescription | SE specific to agent | Standard special tests to modify SE |
|---|---|---|---|---|---|
| | | | | Peripheral neuropathy (sensory) | Neurological assessments |
| | | | | Bradycardia and hypotension | Monitor vital signs |

| Risk factors and recommendation for prevention of SE | Recommendation for management of SE | In the elderly (≥65 years) | Metabolism | Excretion | Cross BBB |
|---|---|---|---|---|---|
| Previous neurotoxic chemotherapies, frequency, and severity related to cumulative doses | Mostly sensory neuropathy. Toxicity may be dose-limiting. Sensory manifestations usually resolve after several months of discontinuation | | | | |
| | Grade 2 neuropathy: reduce paclitaxel by 25 % | | | | |
| | Grade 3 and 4: omit paclitaxel | | | | |
| Nil | These are usually minor and occur during administration and do not require treatment | | | | |
| | Rare severe cardiac conduction abnormalities have been reported, and appropriate therapy should be administered with continuous cardiac monitoring | | | | |

(continued)

TABLE 2.1 (continued)

| Mechanism of action | Drug | Context of prescription (NA/A/M) and usual dose schedule | Minimum requirements for prescription | SE specific to agent | Standard special tests to modify SE |
|---|---|---|---|---|---|
| Antimicro-tubule: stabilizer | Docetaxel [6] | A/M (any line) | Nil | Hypersensitivity | Nil |
| | | IV dose: 75–100 mg/m$^2$ D1 q 3 weekly | | | |
| | | | | Fluid retention | Nil |
| | | | | Peripheral neuropathy (sensory) | Neurological assessments |
| | | | | Alopecia | Nil |

| Risk factors and recommendation for prevention of SE | Recommendation for management of SE | In the elderly (≥65 years) | Metabolism | Excretion | Cross BBB |
|---|---|---|---|---|---|
| Premedication with corticosteroids with or without antihistamines (H1 and H2 antagonists) | Stop infusion | Nil | CYP3A | Primarily biliary/fecal | Low levels found in animal studies |
| | Supportive therapy with oxygen and hydration if hypotension | | | | |
| | Administer IV corticosteroids and antihistamines | | | | |
| | Infusion can be recommenced at slower rate of infusion if symptoms are mild and complete recovery has occurred | | | | |
| | Treat anaphylaxis if it occurs | | | | |
| | Prophylaxis prior to next infusion with premedication: IV corticosteroids and antihistamines. Slow infusion | | | | |
| | Sodium cromoglycate has been used in prophylaxis in severe reactions | | | | |
| | Patients should not be rechallenged if anaphylaxis has occurred | | | | |
| Premedication with dexamethasone or methyprednisolone [7] | Slowly reversible if treatment is discontinued; however, early aggressive diuretic may be required or aspiration of fluid in pleural space for symptomatic treatment | | | | |
| Nil | Usually cumulative doses >600 mg/m² | | | | |
| | Grade 2 neuropathy: reduce docetaxel by 25 % | | | | |
| | Grade 3 and 4: omit docetaxel | | | | |
| Nil | Self-limiting. Poor hair regrowth or persistent hair loss occasionally reported | | | | |

(continued)

TABLE 2.1 (continued)

| Mechanism of action | Drug | Context of prescription (NA/A/M) and usual dose schedule | Minimum requirements for prescription | SE specific to agent | Standard special tests to modify SE |
|---|---|---|---|---|---|
| | | | | Rash/pruritus | Nil |
| | | | | Nail changes | Nil |
| | | | | Hand-foot syndrome | Nil |
| | | | | Teary/watery eyes | Nil |
| | | | | Arthralgia/myalgia | Nil |

| Risk factors and recommendation for prevention of SE | Recommendation for management of SE | In the elderly (≥65 years) | Metabolism | Excretion | Cross BBB |
|---|---|---|---|---|---|
| Avoid perfumed skin products | Self-limiting | | | | |
| | Antihistamines for pruritus | | | | |
| Some benefit from application of dark nail varnish | Cold-induced vasoconstriction by wearing frozen gloves during treatment may reduce nail toxicity | | | | |
| | Cosmetic changes disappear once treatment is withdrawn | | | | |
| | Nailbed infections are treated with topical antibiotics or antifungals, if necessary | | | | |
| Nil | May respond to administration of pyridoxine | | | | |
| Nil | Associated with cumulative dosing and occurs after a median of 400 mg/m$^2$ | | | | |
| | Treatment with artificial tears or other ocular moisturizers may ameliorate symptoms | | | | |
| | In the case of severe symptoms, lacrimal duct obstruction must be ruled out [8] | | | | |
| Nil | Symptomatic treatment with paracetamol, NSAIDS, gabapentin, and prednisone (if severe cases) | | | | |
| | In the curative setting, dose reduction is not recommended | | | | |

(continued)

TABLE 2.1 (continued)

| Mechanism of action | Drug | Context of prescription (NA/A/M) and usual dose schedule | Minimum requirements for prescription | SE specific to agent | Standard special tests to modify SE |
|---|---|---|---|---|---|
| Antimicro-tubule: stabilizer | Nanoparticle, albumin-bound paclitaxel; nab-paclitaxel; protein-bound paclitaxel [9] | M<br><br>IV dose: 300 mg/m$^2$ D1 q 3 weekly or 100–150 mg/m$^2$ weekly | After failure of combination chemotherapy for metastatic disease or relapse within 6 months of adjuvant chemotherapy | Peripheral neuropathy | Neurological assessments |
| | | | Prior therapy should have included an anthracycline unless clinically contraindicated | Ocular/visual disturbance | Nil |
| | | | | Myelosuppression (neutropenia) | Nil |

| Risk factors and recommendation for prevention of SE | Recommendation for management of SE | In the elderly (≥65 years) | Metabolism | Excretion | Cross BBB |
|---|---|---|---|---|---|
| Influenced by prior and/or concomitant therapy with neurotoxic agents | Grade-3 drug interruption until resolution followed by dose reduction for subsequent cycles | Improved compared to paclitaxel | Liver (primarily via CYP2C8, minor CYP 34A) | Extensive nonrenal | No information available |
| Dose-dependent | Severe symptoms of sensory neuropathy improve with a median of 22 days after treatment interruption [10] | | | | |
| Higher than recommended doses | Most commonly reversible keratitis and blurred vision | | | | |
| | Rare persistent optic nerve damage reported | | | | |
| Administration of granulocyte-colony-stimulating factor (G-CSF) | Usually rapidly reversible | | | | |
| Do not give therapy if neutrophil count is <1.5 × 109/L | Antimicrobials should be commenced for evidence of fever, and patients with febrile neutropenia should be treated with appropriate antibiotics | | | | |
| | Dose reductions for neutropenia lasting >1 week for subsequent cycles | | | | |

(continued)

TABLE 2.1 (continued)

| Mechanism of action | Drug | Context of prescription (NA/A/M) and usual dose schedule | Minimum requirements for prescription | SE specific to agent | Standard special tests to modify SE |
|---|---|---|---|---|---|
| Antimicro-tubule: stabilizer | Ixabepilone [11] | M | Monotherapy: after failure of taxane, anthracycline, and capecitabine chemotherapy | Peripheral neuropathy | Neurological assessments |
| | | IV dose: 40 mg/m² D1 q 3 weekly | Combination therapy with capecitabine: after failure of taxane and anthracycline chemotherapy | Myelosuppression (neutropenia) | Monitor blood count |
| | | | | Hypersensitivity | Nil |

| Risk factors and recommendation for prevention of SE | Recommendation for management of SE | In the elderly (≥65 years) | Metabolism | Excretion | Cross BBB |
|---|---|---|---|---|---|
| Patients with diabetes mellitus or preexisting peripheral neuropathy may be at increased risk of severe neuropathy Prior therapy with neurotoxic chemotherapy agents did not predict the development of neuropathy | Sensory manifestations usually resolve to baseline or grade 1,within 12 weeks upon treatment discontinuation | No effects, but limited experience in clinical trials | Liver via CYP3A4 | Feces | No information available |
| Do not give therapy if neutrophil count is <1.5 × 109/L | Delay administration of and reduce subsequent doses in patients who experience severe neutropenia or thrombocytopenia | | | | |
| Risk factor hypersensitivity reactions to polyoxyethylated castor oil or its derivatives | Stop infusion | | | | |
| Premedication with IV corticosteroids and antihistamines (H1 and H2 antagonists) | Supportive therapy with oxygen and hydration if hypotension | | | | |
| | Administer IV corticosteroids and antihistamines | | | | |
| | Infusion can be recommenced at slower rate if symptoms are mild and complete recovery has occurred | | | | |
| | Treat anaphylaxis if it occurs | | | | |
| | Prophylaxis prior to next infusion with premedication: IV corticosteroids and antihistamines. Slow infusion | | | | |
| | Patients should not be rechallenged if anaphylaxis has occurred | | | | |

(continued)

TABLE 2.1 (continued)

| Mechanism of action | Drug | Context of prescription (NA/A/M) and usual dose schedule | Minimum requirements for prescription | SE specific to agent | Standard special tests to modify SE |
|---|---|---|---|---|---|
| Antimicrotubule: destabilizer | Eribulin [12] | M (Third line and beyond)<br><br>IV dose: 1.4 mg/m$^2$ D1,8 q 3 weekly | Prior therapy should have included an anthracycline and a taxane in either the adjuvant or metastatic setting | Myelosuppression (neutropenia) | Monitor LFTs and blood counts |
| | | | | Peripheral neuropathy | Neurological assessments |
| | | | | QT prolongation | ECG monitoring in patients with congestive cardiac failure, bradyarrhythmias, drugs known to prolong the QT interval, including Class Ia and III antiarrhythmics, and electrolyte abnormalities |
| Antimicrotubule: destabilizer | Vinorelbine [13] | M (First line and beyond)<br><br>IV dose: mostly used at 20–25 mg/m$^2$ weekly | NA | Acute dyspnea and severe bronchospasm [14, 15] | Nil |
| | | | | Constipation/ileus | |
| | | | | Neuropathy | Nil |
| | | | | Chest pain | Nil |

| Risk factors and recommendation for prevention of SE | Recommendation for management of SE | In the elderly (≥65 years) | Metabolism | Excretion | Cross BBB |
|---|---|---|---|---|---|
| Elevated liver transaminases (>3x ULN) and bilirubin >1.5xULN<br><br>Do not give therapy if neutrophil is count <1.5 × 109/L | Delay administration of and reduce subsequent doses in patients who experience febrile neutropenia or grade 4 neutropenia lasting longer than 7 days | No effects, but limited experience in clinical trials | Feces | Feces | No information found |
| Nil | Withhold in patients who experience grade 3 or 4 peripheral neuropathy until resolution to grade 2 or less | | | | |
| Avoid in high-risk patients | Correct hypokalemia or hypomagnesemia prior to initiating therapy, and monitor these electrolytes periodically during therapy<br><br>Avoid in patients with congenital long QT syndrome | | | | |
| Risk factors include concurrent mitomycin | May respond to bronchodilators<br><br>Subacute pulmonary reactions characterized by cough, dyspnea, hypoxemia, and interstitial infiltration may respond to corticosteroid therapy, and oxygen may provide symptomatic relief | | Hepatic cytochrome P450 enzymes | Biliary | Brain and plasma levels are comparable in animal studies [16] |
| Prior treatment with other neurotoxic chemotherapies may result in cumulative toxicity | Mild to moderate peripheral neuropathy is usually reversible upon discontinuation<br><br>Also can cause severe constipation (G3-4), paralytic ileus, intestinal obstruction, necrosis, and/or perforation | | | | |
| Nil | Cardiovascular disease or tumor within the chest is a risk factor | | | | |

(continued)

TABLE 2.1 (continued)

| Mechanism of action | Drug | Context of prescription (NA/A/M) and usual dose schedule | Minimum requirements for prescription | SE specific to agent | Standard special tests to modify SE |
|---|---|---|---|---|---|
| | | | | Pain in tumor-containing tissue | Nil |
| Anthracyclines | Doxorubicin/epirubicin [17, 18] | A/M | N/A | Cardiotoxicity: acute, chronic, and delayed | Cardiac assessment at baseline with clinical examination, ECG, and of LVEF assessment with radionuclide angiography (MUGA scan) or serial echocardiogram |
| | | IV doses: 50–60 mg/m², 75–100 mg/m² 3 weekly for doxorubicin and epirubicin, respectively, when used in combination | | | Once cumulative dose has surpassed threshold, regular cardiac assessment should be completed as described above, and monitor for clinical symptoms of CHF prior to each cycle of anthracycline |
| | | | | Hyperuricemia (rare) | Baseline and monitor EUC |

| Risk factors and recommendation for prevention of SE | Recommendation for management of SE | In the elderly (≥65 years) | Metabolism | Excretion | Cross BBB |
|---|---|---|---|---|---|
| Nil | Acute pain syndrome within 30 min of infusion can occur at the tumor site after the first dose. It usually lasts from 1 h to several days. Management is with corticosteroids and narcotic analgesia, if necessary | | | | |
| Cumulative doses must be calculated, and monitoring is as per cumulative dose (see table) | A reduction in LVEF of 10 % to below the lower limit of normal, 20 % reduction at any level, or an absolute LVEF ≤45 % indicates deterioration in cardiac function | Doxorubicin: no information | Doxorubicin: in the liver and other tissues by an aldo-keto reductase enzyme | Doxorubicin: predominately bile | No |
| | The gold standard for diagnosis of anthracycline-induced cardiotoxicity is endomyocardial biopsy. However, it is rarely performed due to its invasive nature | Epirubicin: clearance may be decreased | Epirubicin: extensive hepatic metabolism also metabolized by other organs including RBC | Predominately hepatobiliary; rapid elimination of parent compound from plasma | |
| | Management of congestive cardiac failure This can include low-salt diet, diuretics, ACE inhibitors, or angiotensin receptor blockers, inotropes, and cardiac transplantation | | | | |
| Prophylactic treatment for high-risk patients includes aggressive hydration and discontinuation of drugs that causes hyperuricemia (e.g., thiazide diuretics) or acidic urine (e.g., salicylates); monitor electrolytes and replace as required; alkalinize the urine, allopurinol/rasburicase orally | Treatment of tumor lysis syndrome includes maintaining aggressive hydration with target urine output >100 ml/h, maintenance of urine pH at 7.0 with administration of sodium bicarbonate, allopurinol, or rasburicase monitoring, replacement, and maintenance of serum electrolytes (calcium, phosphate, renal function, LDH, and uric acid) | | | | |
| Note: allopurinol can be given IV for patients not tolerating oral medications | Hemodialysis, if necessary | | | | |

(continued)

Table 2.1 (continued)

| Mechanism of action | Drug | Context of prescription (NA/A/M) and usual dose schedule | Minimum requirements for prescription | SE specific to agent | Standard special tests to modify SE |
|---|---|---|---|---|---|
| | | | | Local extravasation | Monitor infusion site For patients with difficult venous access, consider central venous access device (CVAD) and contrast study |

| Risk factors and recommendation for prevention of SE | Recommendation for management of SE | In the elderly (≥65 years) | Metabolism | Excretion | Cross BBB |
|---|---|---|---|---|---|
| Ensure adequate peripheral access | Management of extravasation: | | | | |
| Administration time 15–20 min | Stop the injection/ infusion and disconnect the intravenous tubing | | | | |
| Monitor for erythematous streaking along vein and/or facial flushing | Withdraw as much of the drug as possible, via existing cannula or CVAD. Mark area of skin with indelible pen. Take a photograph of the area as soon as possible | | | | |
| | Elevate and apply compression to the limb | | | | |
| | If appropriate, remove the peripheral cannula (do not remove the CVAD) | | | | |
| | Utilize extravasation kit | | | | |
| | Apply cold pack | | | | |
| | Apply 98–99 % dimethyl sulfoxide (DMSO) topically to the skin within 10–25 min following local protocols | | | | |
| | Urgent assessment by plastic surgeon | | | | |

(continued)

TABLE 2.1 (continued)

| Mechanism of action | Drug | Context of prescription (NA/A/M) and usual dose schedule | Minimum requirements for prescription | SE specific to agent | Standard special tests to modify SE |
|---|---|---|---|---|---|
| Anthracyclines | Pegylated liposomal doxorubicin [19] | M | EMA but not FDA approved indication | Acute infusion reactions | Monitor first infusion |
| | | IV dose: mostly used at 40–45 mg/m$^2$ D1 q 4 weekly | | | |
| | | | | Palmar-plantar erythrodysesthesia (PPE) | Monitor patient for symptoms (numbness or tingling) |
| | | | | Stomatitis | Monitor patient for symptoms each cycle |

| Risk factors and recommendation for prevention of SE | Recommendation for management of SE | In the elderly (≥65 years) | Metabolism | Excretion | Cross BBB |
|---|---|---|---|---|---|
| Administer initial dose no faster than 1 mg/min | Slow or interrupt the rate of infusion | No pharmacokinetics effect on drug | As per doxorubicin | As per doxorubicin but significantly slower, allowing for approximately two to three orders of magnitude larger AUC than for a similar dose of conventional doxorubicin | No |
| | Antihistamines | | | | |
| | H2 blockers | | | | |
| | Steroids | | | | |
| If symptoms are present, consider increasing the dosing interval | Mild reactions resolve independently within 1–2 weeks | | | | |
| Pyridoxine (50–150 mg/day) may be used for prophylaxis without affecting the antitumor activity<br><br>Prophylactic corticosteroids may be of benefit [20] | More severe reactions may require a discontinuation of therapy, and corticosteroid use may assist in resolution | | | | |
| Avoidance of skin stressor/pressure measures to decrease PPE following infusion (e.g., avoidance of tape on skin, sun exposure, hot water, pressure, or friction on skin) | | | | | |
| Generally associated with higher doses, prior alcohol and tobacco use, poor nutritional status, and dental hygiene and concomitant use of antihistamines, anticholinergics, phenytoin, and steroids | Dose modification as per guidelines of institution | | | | |

(continued)

Table 2.1 (continued)

| Mechanism of action | Drug | Context of prescription (NA/A/M) and usual dose schedule | Minimum requirements for prescription | SE specific to agent | Standard special tests to modify SE |
|---|---|---|---|---|---|
| | | | | Cardiotoxicity: acute, chronic, and delayed | Cardiac assessment at baseline with clinical examination, ECG and of LVEF assessment with radionuclide angiography (MUGA scan) or serial echocardiogram |
| | | | | | Once cumulative dose has surpassed (see table) the threshold, regular cardiac assessment should be completed as described above, and monitor for clinical symptoms of CHF prior to each cycle of anthracycline |
| Anthracyclines | Non-pegylated liposomal doxorubicin [21] | M<br><br>IV dose 60–75 mg/m² D1 q 3 weekly | First line in combination with cyclophosphamide | Cardiotoxicity | Cardiac assessment at baseline with clinical examination, ECG, and of LVEF assessment MUGA or serial echocardiogram |

| Risk factors and recommendation for prevention of SE | Recommendation for management of SE | In the elderly (≥65 years) | Metabolism | Excretion | Cross BBB |
|---|---|---|---|---|---|
| Occurs at lower frequency than conventional doxorubicin | Treatment for congestive heart failure is as per doxorubicin/ epirubicin | | | | |
| Care should be exercised in patients who have received prior anthracycline therapy or in those patients that have a history of cardiovascular disease. LVEF assessments should be performed more frequently in this patient population | | | | | |
| Cumulative doses must be calculated and monitoring is as per cumulative dose (see table) | | | | | |
| Occurs at lower frequency than conventional doxorubicin | Treatment for congestive heart failure is as per doxorubicin/ epirubicin | Cardiac safety comparable in patients <65 years and >65 years | Hepatobiliary | Hepatobiliary | No information available |
| Care should be exercised in patients who have received prior anthracycline therapy or in those patients that have a history of cardiovascular disease. LVEF assessments should be performed more frequently in this patient population | | | | | |
| Cumulative doses must be calculated, and monitoring is as per cumulative dose (see table) | | | | | |

(continued)

TABLE 2.1 (continued)

| Mechanism of action | Drug | Context of prescription (NA/A/M) and usual dose schedule | Minimum requirements for prescription | SE specific to agent | Standard special tests to modify SE |
|---|---|---|---|---|---|
| Antimetabolite | 5-FU [22]/ capecitabine [23] | 5-FU<br><br>A | Capecitabine monotherapy after failure of taxanes or anthracycline or where anthracyclines are contraindicated | Cardiotoxicity (acute myocardial infarction, angina, dysrhythmias, cardiac arrest, cardiac failure, and ECG changes) | Consider cardiac assessment for coronary ischemia in patients who are high risk (this may include cardiac stress test and coronary angiogram) |
| | | Dose: mostly used as IV bolus 500–600 mg/m$^2$ | Capecitabine combination therapy: after failure of anthracycline-containing regimen | | |
| | | Capecitabine<br><br>M | | Capecitabine: palmar-plantar erythrodysesthesia (hand-foot skin reaction) | Nil |
| | | Oral dose: 2,000–2,500 mg/m$^2$ divided equally between morning and evening D1-14 q 3 weeks | | Hyperbilirubinemia | Monitor LFTs |
| Anti metabolite | Gemcitabine [24] | M (First line and beyond) | First line in combination with paclitaxel or single-agent palliative therapy | Elevated liver enzymes | Monitor LFTs |
| | | IV dose: 1,000 mg/m$^2$ D1, 8 q 3 weekly | | | |

| Risk factors and recommendation for prevention of SE | Recommendation for management of SE | In the elderly (≥65 years) | Metabolism | Excretion | Cross BBB |
|---|---|---|---|---|---|
| Patient screening | Risk factors include prior history of coronary artery diseases | No clinically significant difference in PK, but side effects need to be carefully monitored in this population due to impaired renal function, which should lead to a dose reduction of capecitabine | Hepatic | Renal | Limited evidence in HER2 + BC in combination with anti-HER agents |
| | Management includes discontinuation of 5-FU/capecitabine. | | | | |
| Behavioral modifications: avoid tight-fitting shoes or repetitive rubbing pressure to hands and feet; apply lanolin-containing creams to affected areas | Behavioral modifications: reactions ≥ grade 2 severity (skin changes with pain but not interfering with function), therapy should be interrupted and recommenced at a reduced dose when symptoms resolve to grade 1 | | | | |
| Nil | If hyperbilirubinemia ≥ grade 2 (serum bilirubin >1.5 times the upper limit of normal), therapy should be interrupted until hyperbilirubinemia resolves, and subsequent dose reductions may be needed for subsequent dosing | | | | |
| Nil | Usually transient and reversible elevations of liver function enzymes in about two-thirds of patients | Decreased clearance and increased half-life with increasing age | Intracellularly by nucleoside kinases | Renal | No information available |
| | Increases are rarely of clinical significance, and there is no evidence of hepatic toxicity with longer duration or cumulative doses | | | | |

(continued)

TABLE 2.1 (continued)

| Mechanism of action | Drug | Context of prescription (NA/A/M) and usual dose schedule | Minimum requirements for prescription | SE specific to agent | Standard special tests to modify SE |
|---|---|---|---|---|---|
| | | | | Hemolytic uremic syndrome (HUS) | Monitor renal function and blood count |
| | | | | Pulmonary toxicity | Nil |
| | | | | Acute dyspnea and severe pulmonary toxicities (pulmonary edema, interstitial pneumonitis, and adult respiratory distress syndrome) | |

| Risk factors and recommendation for prevention of SE | Recommendation for management of SE | In the elderly (≥65 years) | Metabolism | Excretion | Cross BBB |
|---|---|---|---|---|---|
| Nil | Onset during and shortly after gemcitabine therapy (4–8 weeks postcompletion of therapy up to several months) | | | | |
| | Monitor renal function closely, especially in patients with impaired renal function | | | | |
| | Therapies can include immunocomplex removal (plasmapheresis, immunoadsorption, or exchange transfusion) antiplatelet/ anticoagulant therapies, immunosuppressive therapies, and plasma exchange | | | | |
| | Rituximab has been successfully used in patients with chemotherapy-induced HUS | | | | |
| | Case fatality rate is high | | | | |
| Risk factors include prior irradiation to the mediastinum. Use caution when prescribing in this patient population | Acute dyspnea is usually self-limiting; symptomatic relief with oxygen | | | | |
| | Severe pulmonary toxicities usually occur after several cycles but can occur after a single cycle | | | | |
| | Discontinuation of drug and early supportive care with bronchodilators, corticosteroids, diuretics, and/or oxygen | | | | |
| | Pulmonary toxicities may be reversible, but fatal recurrences have been reported in patients rechallenged | | | | |

(continued)

TABLE 2.1 (continued)

| Mechanism of action | Drug | Context of prescription (NA/A/M) and usual dose schedule | Minimum requirements for prescription | SE specific to agent | Standard special tests to modify SE |
|---|---|---|---|---|---|
| | | | | Fever/flulike symptoms | Nil |
| | | | | Skin rash | Nil |
| | | | | Vascular toxicity (thrombotic microangiopathy, veno-occlusive disease, and digital ischemic changes and necrosis) | Nil |
| Antimetabolite | Methotrexate [25] | A/M | Nil | Hepatotoxicity | Monitor LFTs |
| | | IV dose: 40 mg/m$^2$ D1,8 q 4 weekly | | | |
| | | | | Pulmonary toxicity: acute, subacute, or chronic (inflammation, pulmonary infections, and pulmonary lymphoma [27]) | Nil |
| | | | | Neurological toxicity (intrathecal and high-dose methotrexate) | Nil |

| Risk factors and recommendation for prevention of SE | Recommendation for management of SE | In the elderly (≥65 years) | Metabolism | Excretion | Cross BBB |
|---|---|---|---|---|---|
| Nil | Symptoms are mild to transient and rarely dose-limiting | | | | |
| | Acetaminophen may provide relief | | | | |
| Nil | Not dose-limiting | | | | |
| | Responds to topical corticosteroids and antihistamines | | | | |
| Suggested to be more common after cumulative doses of 10,000 mg/m$^2$ or in the setting of combination therapy | Treat as per type of vascular toxicity | | | | |
| Avoid alcohol, medications, or herbal supplements that may increase the risk of hepatotoxicity | Liver enzymes may increase with each cycle and return to pretreatment levels after discontinuation for 1 month | | Hepatic and intracellular | Renal | Ratio of 10–30:1 for CNS concentration [26] |
| | Note: cirrhosis usually occurs with chronic low dose, and if it occurs, it should be managed as per guidelines for cirrhosis management | | | | |
| Nil | Subacute toxicity includes dyspnea, nonproductive cough, fever, crackles, cyanosis, pulmonary fibrosis, and pleural effusions. Treatment includes discontinuation of methotrexate and corticosteroid therapy. Rechallenge is not recommended | | | | |
| | Pulmonary infections with opportunistic pathogens should be treated for individual pathogen | | | | |
| | Pulmonary lymphoma regresses after discontinuation of methotrexate Rechallenge is not recommended | | | | |
| Intrathecal (IT) methotrexate | IT methotrexate | | | | |

(continued)

TABLE 2.1 (continued)

| Mechanism of action | Drug | Context of prescription (NA/A/M) and usual dose schedule | Minimum requirements for prescription | SE specific to agent | Standard special tests to modify SE |
|---|---|---|---|---|---|

| Risk factors and recommendation for prevention of SE | Recommendation for management of SE | In the elderly (≥65 years) | Metabolism | Excretion | Cross BBB |
|---|---|---|---|---|---|
| Aseptic meningitis: IT hydrocortisone or oral corticosteroids | Aseptic meningitis (onset hours): no treatment required. Patients can be rechallenged | | | | |
| Transverse myelopathy: risk factors include frequent IT methotrexate and concurrent radiotherapy | Transverse myelopathy (onset hours–days): no specific intervention and recovery variable, and patients should not be rechallenged | | | | |
| Leukoencephalopathy: risk factors include whole brain radiotherapy and IV methotrexate | Leukoencephalopathy (onset delayed): there is no uniform therapeutic approach. Available therapies include corticosteroids and leucovorin | | | | |
| | Note: other neurological sequelae include encephalopathy, seizures, neurological deficits, lumbosacral radiculopathy, neurogenic pulmonary edema, and sudden death | | | | |
| | High-dose methotrexate | | | | |
| | Acute neurotoxicity (onset within 24 h): usually spontaneous resolution | | | | |
| | Rechallenge is possible | | | | |
| | Subacute neurotoxicity – stroke-like syndrome (onset approx. 6 days after administration) resolves in minutes to days. Rechallenge is possible | | | | |
| | Leukoencephalopathy: as above | | | | |

(continued)

TABLE 2.1 (continued)

| Mechanism of action | Drug | Context of prescription (NA/A/M) and usual dose schedule | Minimum requirements for prescription | SE specific to agent | Standard special tests to modify SE |
|---|---|---|---|---|---|
| Alkylating agents | Cyclophosphamid [28] | A/M | Nil | Cardiac toxicity (ECG changes, elevation of cardiac enzymes, myocarditis, and myocardial necrosis) | Baseline ECG |
| | | IV dose: 500–600 mg/m² D1 q 3 weekly | | | |
| | | Oral dose: 100 mg/m² daily D1-14 q 4 weeks or 50 mg continuous daily dose | | | |
| | | | | Hemorrhagic cystitis | Nil |

| Risk factors and recommendation for prevention of SE | Recommendation for management of SE | In the elderly (≥65 years) | Metabolism | Excretion | Cross BBB |
|---|---|---|---|---|---|
| Risk factors include chest or mediastinal radiotherapy and anthracycline administration | Supportive treatment | No clinically significant difference in PK | Hepatic cytochrome P450 enzymes primarily CYP2B6 [29] | Enzymatic oxidation to active and inactive metabolites excreted in urine | Penetration |
| Effect is not attributable to cumulative dosing | | | | | |
| Occurs in high dose (60 mg/kg daily or 120–270 mg/kg over a few days) | | | | | |
| Risk factors include long-term use, high dose, rate of infusion, poor hydration status, decreased urine output, and concurrent exposure to other urotoxic drugs or genitourinary radiotherapy | Discontinuation of cyclophosphamide, increase fluid intake, and maintenance of platelet count at >50,000/mm³ | | | | |
| Encourage oral intake of fluids in 24–48 h prior to therapy and during therapy, frequent voiding Drug administration should be completed early in the day to avoid the drug sitting in the bladder overnight | Cystitis | | | | |
| Other measures include administration of mesna (rarely needed for doses <2 g/m²), catheter bladder drainage, bladder irrigation, intravenous diuresis, and hyperhydration (not routinely recommended) | First-line therapy: hyperhydration<br><br>Second-line therapy: bladder irrigation<br><br>Third-line therapy: prostaglandin into the bladder<br><br>Late-onset cystitis (usually due to secondary viral or bacterial infection)<br><br>Culture for bacterial pathogens, cytomegalovirus (CMV), and adenovirus<br><br>Hyperhydration +/− bladder irrigation<br><br>Treat pathogen if isolated | | | | |

(continued)

TABLE 2.1 (continued)

| Mechanism of action | Drug | Context of prescription (NA/A/M) and usual dose schedule | Minimum requirements for prescription | SE specific to agent | Standard special tests to modify SE |
|---|---|---|---|---|---|
| Alkylating agents | Cyclophosphamide | A/M | Nil | Immunogenicity: reduced skin test antigens (e.g., tuberculin-purified protein derivative) | Nil |
| | | | | Interstitial fibrosis | Nil |
| | | | | Nasal stuffiness or facial discomfort | Nil |
| | | | | Radiation recall reaction | Nil |
| | | | | SIADH | Nil |
| | | | | Secondary malignancies | Nil |
| | | | | Fluid retention and dilutional hyponatremia | Nil |

| Risk factors and recommendation for prevention of SE | Recommendation for management of SE | In the elderly (≥65 years) | Metabolism | Excretion | Cross BBB |
|---|---|---|---|---|---|
| Nil | Nil | No clinically significant difference in PK | Hepatic cytochrome P450 enzymes primarily CYP2B6 | Enzymatic oxidation to active and inactive metabolites excreted in urine | Penetration |
| Risk factors include long-term exposure, exposure to other drugs with pulmonary toxicities, and pulmonary radiotherapy | Condition may be nonreversible and fatal<br><br>Discontinuation of drug and initiation of corticosteroids<br><br>Exclude other causes of pulmonary toxicity such as opportunistic infections | | | | |
| Associated with rapid injection<br><br>Slow the infusion rate<br><br>Intermittent infusion rather than IV bolus | Analgesics, decongestants, antihistamines, intranasal steroids, or ipratropium | | | | |
| Nil | Usually resolves after several days<br><br>Treatment may include topical steroids or nonsteroidal antiinflammatories for radiation recall dermatitis | | | | |
| More common with doses of >50 mg/kg and aggravated by large volumes of hydration given to prevent hemorrhagic cystitis | Self-limiting<br><br>Diuretic therapy may be useful when the patient has stopped voiding | | | | |
| Nil | Treatment for individual malignancy | | | | |
| Associated with doses >30–40 mg/kg | Self-limiting within 24 h of therapy | | | | |

(continued)

TABLE 2.1 (continued)

| Mechanism of action | Drug | Context of prescription (NA/A/M) and usual dose schedule | Minimum requirements for prescription | SE specific to agent | Standard special tests to modify SE |
|---|---|---|---|---|---|
| Alkylating agents | Carboplatin [30] | A/M | Adjuvant HER2+ patients or metastatic | Myelosuppression (most commonly thrombocytopenia, but leukopenia, neutropenia, and anemia can also occur) | Monitor blood count |
| | | IV dose: AUC 6 | | | |
| | | | | Hypersensitivity | |
| | | | | Nephrotoxicity | Monitor renal function |

| Risk factors and recommendation for prevention of SE | Recommendation for management of SE | In the elderly (≥65 years) | Metabolism | Excretion | Cross BBB |
|---|---|---|---|---|---|
| Risk factors include prior chemotherapy, poor performance status, increasing age, impaired renal function, and concurrent myelosuppressive therapy | Anemia may be corrected with transfusions | Clearance may be reduced due to age-related renal function impairment | Intracellular | Renal | Yes |
| Dose-dependent and can be minimized by using the Calvert AUC-based dose formula | Dose as per Calvert AUC-based dose formula | | | | |
| Risk associated with repeated exposure to platinum agents especially with a second course of platinum therapy | Treatment of anaphylaxis if it occurs<br><br>Carboplatin therapy can be continued in some cases with prophylactic corticosteroid and antihistamine and/or desensitization | | | | |
| Dose as per Calvert AUC-based dose formula | Nil | | | | |

## Chemotherapy-Induced Emesis

Management of chemotherapy-induced nausea and vomiting is an essential component in the care of all patients receiving breast cancer chemotherapy and is described in another chapter in this volume. Chemotherapy regimens used in breast cancer have different potentials to induce emesis (Table 2.2) [32, 33].

## Peripheral Neuropathy

Several classes of chemotherapy agents can induce peripheral neuropathy (CIPN) (see Table 2.1 for a detailed review of agents inducing neuropathy, as well as prevention and management of this side effect). Taxanes, ixabepilone, vinorelbine, and eribulin are the most likely cause of neuropathy in breast cancer patients. Comorbidities, such as diabetes and alcohol abuse, predispose patients to toxic nerve fiber damage from chemotherapy [34]. Common symptoms include burning sensation, tingling, loss of feeling, walking difficulties, trouble using fingers, poor balance, sensitivity to temperatures, loss of reflexes, and constipation. The development of CIPN is one of the most common reasons for discontinuation of chemotherapy, and its occurrence can affect the long-term quality of life of patients. Prevention of severe CIPN is the cornerstone of management. This requires regular neurological assessment of patients prior to each scheduled chemotherapy administration. CIPN usually resolves gradually over time, but it may be irreversible.

Various small studies evaluating agents such as calcium, magnesium, vitamin E [35], glutamine [36], and glutathione [37] have been conducted mostly in oxaliplatin and cisplatin-based chemotherapy regimens. While the administration of intravenous calcium and magnesium in colon cancer patients receiving oxaliplatin appears to reduce the incidence of neuropathy while maintaining tumor response, more randomized controlled studies are required [38]. It is possible that pharmacogenetic studies will reveal particular genotypes at greater risk for CIPN [39].

See Table 2.1 for detailed management.

TABLE 2.2 Emetogenic potential of breast cancer chemotherapy agents

| Level | Agents in breast cancer |
| --- | --- |
| High emetic risk (>90 % frequency of emesis without prophylaxis) | Combination doxorubicin/epirubicin with cyclophosphamide |
| | Cyclophosphamide IV >1,500 mg/m$^2$ |
| | Doxorubicin > 60 mg/m$^2$ |
| | Epirubicin > 90 mg/m$^2$ |
| Moderate emetic risk (30–90 % frequency of emesis) | Carboplatin |
| | Cyclophosphamide IV ≤1,500 mg/m$^2$ |
| | Cyclophosphamide oral (≥100 mg/m$^2$/day) |
| | Doxorubicin ≤ 60 mg/m$^2$ |
| | Epirubicin ≤ 90 mg/m$^2$ |
| | Methotrexates IV ≥ 250 mg/m$^2$ |
| Low emetic risk (10–30 % frequency of emesis) | Docetaxel |
| | Liposomal doxorubicin |
| | 5-Flurouracil |
| | Gemcitabine |
| | Methotrexate >50 and <250 mg/m$^2$ |
| | Paclitaxel |
| | Paclitaxel-albumin |
| | Cyclophosphamide oral (<100 mg/m$^2$/day) |
| | Methotrexate oral |
| | Capecitabine |
| | Eribulin |
| | Ixabepilone |
| Minimal emetic risk (<10 % frequency of emesis) | Methotrexate < 50 mg/m$^2$ |
| | Vinorelbine |

Adapted from [32, 33]

## Cardiac Failure

Anthracyclines are highly effective drugs in breast cancer but have the significant drawback of inducing cardiac failure. In a retrospective analysis of phase III trials ($n = 613$), the estimated cumulative percentages of patients developing doxorubicin-related congestive heart failure were 5 % at a cumulative dose of 400 mg/m$^2$, 26 % at a dose of 550 mg/m$^2$, and 48 % at a dose of 700 mg/m$^2$ [40]

Due to the risk of cardiomyopathy, a lifetime maximum dose places limits on continued anthracycline administration (see Table 2.1). Acute, chronic, and delayed cardiotoxicities have been described. Acute cardiotoxicity is not dose-related, may occur immediately after a single dose of anthracycline, and usually involves ECG changes such as arrhythmias, T wave flattening, ST depression, and prolongation of QT interval. It is usually transient and does not require treatment intervention. Rarely, pericarditis, myocarditis, or cardiac failure occurs [41]. Chronic cardiac toxicity, in the form of irreversible cardiomyopathy, is dose-related and indolent in onset. It generally presents within 1 year of treatment with signs and symptoms of reduced left ventricular ejection fraction. Delayed cardiotoxicity occurring many years after exposure to anthracycline is also described and thought to be dose-related and irreversible. Table 2.1 describes the management of anthracycline-induced cardiac failure.

Cardiotoxicity may occur at lower doses in patients with prior mediastinal/pericardial irradiation, concomitant use of other cardiotoxic drugs, doxorubicin exposure at an early age, and advanced age [42]. Data also suggest that preexisting heart disease is a cofactor for increased risk of anthracycline cardiotoxicity. Coadministration with anti-HER2 agents is associated with increased risk of cardiotoxicity and is discussed further in this chapter [43].

Several approaches to reduce the cardiotoxicity of anthracyclines have been investigated. Anthracycline damage is presumed to result from the formation of anthracycline-iron complexes within myocardial cells. Dexrazoxane, a chelating agent, binds iron intracellularly. It is also thought to extract iron from the anthracycline-iron complexes [44]. Unfortunately, a phase III trial evaluating this agent in 682 patients with advanced breast cancer therapy revealed a lower objective response rate (46.8 % vs. 60.5 %, 95 % CI: –25 % to –2 %; $P=0.019$) [45]. ASCO guidelines 2008 do not recommend routine use of dexrazoxane in either the adjuvant or metastatic settings with initial doxorubicin-based chemotherapy, but it may be considered in metastatic breast cancer patients who have received more than 300 mg/m$^2$ of doxorubicin and are thought to benefit from continued doxorubicin-containing therapy [46].

The second approach involves altering the schedule of anthracyclines. A retrospective study revealed significant reduction in the probability of clinically overt cardiomyopathy occurring at a cumulative dose of 550 mg/m$^2$ when doxorubicin was given weekly as opposed to every 3 weeks [42]. A third approach consists in prolonging the anthracycline infusion time: nonrandomized data from MD Anderson Cancer Center strongly suggest a cardioprotective effect in delivering anthracyclines as a 96-h infusion versus bolus doses [47].

Two novel anthracyclines deserve specific mention owing to their reduced cardiac toxicity profile: pegylated liposomal doxorubicin (PLD) and non-pegylated liposomal doxorubicin (non-PLD). Studies in the first-line setting have shown better cardiac toxicity profile with similar antitumor effects for both agents [48, 49].

## Gastrointestinal Side Effects: Mucositis, Diarrhea, and Constipation

Diarrhea is a side effect of certain chemotherapy agents such as 5-fluorouracil (5-FU) and capecitabine. Diarrhea is associated with fluid and electrolyte loss as well as a decrease in the quality of life. Grade 3 or 4 toxicity may require dose reductions (which may affect the efficacy of the chemotherapy regimens). Other causes of diarrhea, such as infections, should always be excluded.

Assessment should include a complete blood count, blood chemistry, and stool analyses for bacterial, fungal, and parasitic, or viral pathogens. Abdominal imaging, as well as occasionally endoscopy, may be indicated to rule out confounding causes of diarrhea.

Treatment guidelines for patients with chemotherapy-induced diarrhea have been published [50]. The basis of management is fluid rehydration and electrolyte replacement, and antibiotics should be used for persistent diarrhea and/or for long-term neutropenic patients. Dietary modifications such as avoidance of lactose, caffeinated beverages, and alcohol should be encouraged [51]. Pharmacological therapies for chemotherapy-induced diarrhea involve agents such as loperamide [52]. Other agents that show benefit include opioids and octreotide [53]. Grade 3 or 4 toxicity may also require chemotherapy dose reductions (see Table 2.1 for detailed management for individual chemotherapy agents).

Chemotherapy-induced mucositis can be a dose-limiting toxicity in treatment with anthracyclines, 5-FU, capecitabine, and methotrexate. Factors that may predict for oral mucositis are previous episodes of mucositis with previous treatment cycles. It is associated with a higher risk of infection and can severely compromise nutrition and quality of life [54]. Treatment is mostly supportive, with good oral hygiene, mouthwashes, and analgesia [55]. Small trials with agents such as glutamine [56], AES-14 [57], and various growth factors [58–60] have been explored with inconclusive results. Athermic laser is effective in the prevention and management of mucositis [61].

Constipation is often associated with concomitant medication use such as 5-HT3 antagonists, antidiarrheal agents, or opioid therapy. Sinister causes for constipation such as spinal cord compression or bowel obstruction due to malignancy should be excluded with imaging. Behavioral modifications, such as increased dietary fiber, exercise, and increased fluid intake, should be encouraged. Pharmacotherapy with stool softeners may also be utilized.

## Cognitive Dysfunction

Neurotoxicity of chemotherapy agents also extends to cognitive function. Various terms have been used to describe this phenomenon: "chemo brain" or "chemo fog." Patients often describe a vagueness and difficulty in planning. A growing recognition of this occurrence has in turn resulted in extensive literature. A meta-analysis of six studies revealed that women who received adjuvant chemotherapy for breast cancer were affected by cognitive impairments [62]. Most studies tend to report a mixed diffuse cognitive pattern on neuropsychological testing, with the most compromising functions being verbal learning and memory as well as attention and concentration, which are in line with front striatal dysfunction [63–65]. This has been seen in breast cancer patients, and a study by Ahles et al. also described a dose-dependent effect with more cycles of chemotherapy linked to lower neuropsychological scores [66]. Cognitive dysfunction can persist for years after the completion of chemotherapy, and 5-FU has been implicated as a potential agent [67, 68]. To date there are no therapies for the prevention or management of this side effect. Patients and caregivers need to be educated about its occurrence, and behavioral modifications need to be encouraged

## Altered Body Image and Sexual Dysfunction

Other less recognized effects of chemotherapy include sexual dysfunction. Surgical interventions with mastectomy (with or without reconstruction) and lumpectomy have been associated with altered body image and sexuality [69, 70]. Women who undergo radiation therapy may be influenced by radiation tattoos, fatigue, or changes in breast sensation and arm mobility [71]. Chemotherapy has also been associated with sexual dysfunction [72]. In a study of 100 women, sexual dysfunction attributed to breast cancer or its treatment was assessed via a validated questionnaire, the female sexual function index (FSFI), and defined as an FSFI score <26. Sexual dysfunction was reported by 75 % of the responders. Patients attributed their sexual dysfunction to chemotherapy in 83 % of cases. Other contributors to sexual dysfunction were felt to include anxiety (by 83 % of the patients) and change in relationship with a partner (by 46 % of patients).

Assessment of sexual symptoms throughout treatment and beyond may facilitate the use of potential and specific interventions [73].

## Fertility

Adjuvant chemotherapy for breast cancer may render a premenopausal patient either temporarily or permanently amenorrheic, thus affecting her fertility. For premenopausal women this can be a significant concern, causing distress and affecting treatment-related decisions. Six hundred fifty-seven young women with breast cancer were surveyed in regards to fertility concerns; 57 % recalled substantial concern at diagnosis about becoming infertile with treatment, while 29 % of women reported that infertility concerns influenced treatment decisions [74]. Several options for potential preservation of fertility exist, such as ovarian tissue or embryo cryopreservation and luteinizing-hormone-releasing hormone agonists administered during chemotherapy. They are discussed in Chap. 14. Patients should be referred for fertility counseling to a multidisciplinary environment.

## Secondary Malignancies

Adjuvant chemotherapy with anthracyclines and/or alkylating agents has been implicated as risk factor for the development of secondary malignancies, mostly acute myeloid leukemia (AML) with or without preleukemic myelodysplastic syndrome (MDS). Often the benefit of preventing relapse from an already existing malignancy overrides the small numbers of patients that will go on to develop a second malignancy. A Danish survey [75] identified five cases of AML in 360 patients treated with epirubicin/cyclophosphamide, epirubicin/cisplatin, or alkylating agents. In a meta-analysis of 19 randomized [76] controlled trials ($N = 9,796$) of patients treated with adjuvant epirubicin in early breast cancer, the 8-year cumulative probability of AML/MDS was 0.55 % (95 % CI 0.33–0.78 %), and the risk increased in relation to the dose of epirubicin. Therefore, patients who receive standard doses of chemotherapy have a relatively low risk of AML/MDS.

# Endocrine Therapies

Endocrine therapy is the first "targeted" medical treatment in oncology with antitumor activity restricted to patients whose breast tumors express estrogen receptors (ERs) and/or progesterone receptors (PRs). It is an extremely powerful treatment modality prescribed to two-thirds of the breast cancer population, both in advanced and early disease stages.

It is also recognized as an effective prevention approach of the disease but with a low uptake by women at risk in view of its side effects.

One distinguishes three main classes of endocrine agents, based on their mechanism of action:

1. The selective estrogen receptor modulators (SERMs), which bind the ER and interfere with its transcriptional activity
2. The selective estrogen receptor downregulator fulvestrant, which binds the ER and accelerates its destruction
3. The aromatase inhibitors, which inhibit the enzyme aromatase and, as a result, profoundly reduce estrogen levels in postmenopausal women

*Tamoxifen* is the parent compound in the family of SERMs and has been in clinical use for more than 30 years. The recommended dose of tamoxifen is 20 mg daily, and its duration in the adjuvant setting is 5 years; extension beyond 5 years has no additional benefit in terms of overall survival and only modestly improves disease-free survival [77, 78]. Tamoxifen acts both as an estrogen agonist and antagonist, depending on the target organ. In breast tumor tissue, it is able to competitively block the proliferative effect of estrogen. Conversely, it displays estrogenic effects in the bone, the uterus, and the cardiovascular system.

*Fulvestrant* (Faslodex, AstraZeneca, Wilmington, DE, USA) downregulates the estrogen receptor and lacks the partial agonist effects of tamoxifen. Its clinical use is limited to the advanced setting. The currently approved dose of fulvestrant is 500 mg by intramuscular injections on days 0, 14, and 28, followed by recycling every 28 days thereafter [79].

Third-generation *aromatase inhibitors* (AIs) (exemestane, anastrozole, and letrozole) have shown superior control of advanced breast cancer when compared to tamoxifen, but no significant impact on overall survival. Adjuvant treatment with AIs in postmenopausal patients has been consistently associated with decreased risks of disease recurrence when used either upfront or after 2–3 years of tamoxifen, compared to tamoxifen alone given for 5 years [80–83]. Their impact on overall survival, however, is of small magnitude. Aromatase inhibitors are prescribed today to many postmenopausal patients newly diagnosed with hormone receptor-positive operable breast cancer, particularly when their risk of relapse is from moderate to high. Their optimal timing and duration has not yet been fully elucidated.

Data on the relative efficacy and toxicity of different AIs are beginning to emerge: the NCIC CTG MA.27 trial compared adjuvant exemestane (steroidal AI) and anastrozole (nonsteroidal AI) in postmenopausal women with hormone receptor-positive primary breast cancer and showed similar control of disease with slightly different side effect profiles [84]. Hypertriglyceridemia and hypercholesterolemia were less likely to occur in patients receiving exemestane, and patients taking exemestane were less likely to report a new diagnosis of osteoporosis. Clinical fracture rates were similar in both study arms, however. The FACE trial comparing – head-to-head – letrozole and anastrozole in about 4,000 women with ER-positive, node-positive breast cancer should also release its results soon.

Adverse effects of the three families of endocrine agents share common features, such as hot flushes related to estrogen deprivation, but also show marked differences, which is largely explained by the distinct mechanisms of action. These differences have been best studied in the very large adjuvant clinical trials that have compared, in more than 40,000 women, tamoxifen to AIs or one AI versus another (two trials of a few thousand patients). For fulvestrant, comparisons to either tamoxifen or AIs are available only in the context of smaller randomized metastatic trials involving a few hundred patients [85–87]. These toxicities are described in Table 2.3 and are discussed in more detail below.

## Gynecologic Side Effects

SERMs display estrogen agonist effects in some organs such as the uterus. Endometrial abnormalities include benign hyperplasia, benign uterine polyps, or endometrial carcinoma. The risk of endometrial cancer with long-term tamoxifen use is low and extends several years beyond treatment completion. Fewer gynecologic symptoms have been reported with fulvestrant than with tamoxifen (3.9 % vs. 6.3 %) [85]. Aromatase inhibitors are devoid of endometrial side effects, and it is therefore not surprising that gynecologic symptoms are significantly less common in patients receiving upfront AI compared to those receiving 5 years of tamoxifen in ATAC and BIG 1-98 trials [80, 81]. Fewer gynecologic symptoms are also reported in trials in which women take 2–3 years of tamoxifen in view of a switch to an AI compared to women who have pursued tamoxifen for 5 years [81, 82]. Currently, according to the recommendations of the American College of Obstetricians and Gynecologists, neither active screening by transvaginal ultrasound (TVS) nor endometrial biopsies are recommended in asymptomatic women on tamoxifen [88]. The routine follow-up of endometrial changes with TVS in 237 women taking tamoxifen found a high false-positive rate of the procedure, even with a cutoff value at 10 mm of endometrial thickness to trigger biopsy, and the price to pay was a high iatrogenic complication rate. To diagnose only one endometrial cancer in asymptomatic patients, 52 women had to undergo hysteroscopy and curettage, resulting in four uterine perforations [89]. Therefore, routine annual gynecologic

TABLE 2.3 Side effects of endocrine agent therapy

| Drug usual dose and schedule | Context of prescription | Minimal requirements for prescription | Most common side effects vs. rare ones | Special tests (if any) to monitor side effects | Recommendations for the prevention/management of side effects |
|---|---|---|---|---|---|
| Tamoxifen 20 mg PO daily | Prevention (neo) adjuvant metastatic | Presence of hormone receptors in primary tumor | Hot flushes | | Consider antidepressants such as venlafaxine or the antihypertensive centrally acting alpha-adrenergic agonist, clonidine |
| | | | Mood disturbances | | Consider psychological support |
| | | | Menstrual cycle perturbations | | Consider IUD in young and fertile women |
| | | | Fatty liver | | Monitor liver function tests from time to time |
| | | | Thromboembolic events | | Interrupt Tamoxifen a few weeks in case of surgery/immobilization |
| | | | | | Consider prophylactic anticoagulation if ≥4-h airplane travel |
| | | | Gynecologic events: vaginal discharge, uterine polyps, and endometrial abnormalities (hyperplasia, cancer) | Transvaginal ultrasonography is not recommended for active screening | Routine annual gynecologic evaluation. Any abnormal vaginal bleeding should be investigated with diagnostic hysteroscopy and endometrial biopsy |
| | | | Cataract | | Instruct patient to report visual disturbances |

| Medication | Setting | Indication | Adverse effect | Monitoring | Recommendation |
|---|---|---|---|---|---|
| Aromatase inhibitors | Adjuvant metastatic | Presence of hormone receptors in primary tumor | Arthralgias and myalgia | | Consider pain and antiinflammatory medications. If ineffective, consider shift to another AI. Anecdotal reports that glucosamine may help. Encourage patients to do regular physical exercise. For patients experiencing disabling symptoms, consider changing to Tamoxifen |
| Anastrozole 1 mg PO daily | | | Bone loss | Bone mineral density measurement by DEXA every 1–2 years | Advice on lifestyle changes. Implementation of calcium and vitamin D supplementation to prevent bone health impairment. Consider bisphosphonate therapy in osteoporotic patients but also in the case of osteopenia if risk factors for bone fracture are present, such as age older than 65 years, low BMI, family history of hip fracture, personal history of fracture under 50 years, current use of corticosteroids, or current smoking |
| Letrozole 2.5 mg PO daily | | | Cardiovascular events | | Regular screening for cardiovascular risk factors such as hypertension and hypercholesterolemia |
| Exemestane 25 mg PO daily | | | Hypercholesterolemia | | Regular lipid profile monitoring. Consider statins in the case of increased serum cholesterol level |
| | | | Hot flushes | | Consider antidepressants such as venlafaxine or the centrally acting alpha-adrenergic agonist, clonidine |
| | | | Vaginal dryness/loss of libido | | Nonhormonal local lubricants can temporarily release symptoms Estrogen-containing vaginal preparations should be avoided |
| | | | Cognitive impairment | | Instruct patients to report any memory disorder or impairments of processing speed |
| Fulvestrant 500 mg IM d0, d15, d28 then q 4 weeks | Metastatic | Presence of hormone receptors in primary tumor | Injection site reactions | | Use the proper injection technique and rotate injection site |
| | | | Joint disorders (arthralgia) | | Consider local ice or cold compresses if local complications occur; Consider pain and antiinflammatory medications; Encourage patients to do regular physical exercise |
| | | | Thromboembolic events | | Interrupt fulvestrant for a few weeks in case of surgery/immobilization; Consider prophylactic anticoagulant if ≥4-h airplane travel |
| | | | Hot flushes | | Consider antidepressants such as venlafaxine or the centrally acting alpha-adrenergic agonist, clonidine |

examination is the preferred method of monitoring women on tamoxifen. Patients should be educated to report any abnormal vaginal bleeding, discharge, or spotting. Although endometrial cancer is a rare event, it can occasionally be fatal. Therefore, every abnormal gynecologic symptom should be investigated by diagnostic hysteroscopy and endometrial biopsy. If atypical endometrial hyperplasia develops, tamoxifen treatment should be discontinued [90]. Aromatase inhibitors in this case are an alternative for postmenopausal women, but they induce vaginal dryness, contributing to the loss of libido. Nonhormonal lubricants may be used to release symptoms. Due to the risk of systemic absorption, estrogen-containing vaginal preparations should be avoided.

## Thromboembolic Disease

Several adjuvant and prevention trials have demonstrated an increased risk for venous thromboembolic events during tamoxifen treatment. With adjuvant upfront AI treatment, the frequency of thromboembolic complications is significantly lower compared to patients treated with tamoxifen [80–83]. At higher risk to develop this severe toxicity are women who need a prolonged immobilization for a surgical intervention; in this case, a treatment interruption for several weeks is highly recommended. Additionally, among patients diagnosed with tamoxifen-related venous thrombosis, the incidence of factor V Leiden mutation is nearly five times higher than in those who do develop this toxicity. Therefore, women harboring this genetic alteration are not candidates for tamoxifen [91]. A detailed personal and familial medical history in search of thromboembolic events is mandatory prior to initiating a SERM or fulvestrant. A complete blood coagulation work-up should follow in case of doubt and should consist of the following screening blood tests: resistance to activated protein C, antiphospholipid antibodies, antithrombin, and proteins C and S. Genotyping for factor V and prothrombin can be useful but should be discussed beforehand with the patient.

In the head-to-head comparison between fulvestrant and tamoxifen, the risk of developing venous thromboembolic events was comparable with both treatments [85]. Thus, in women treated with fulvestrant, the same preventive measures should be considered as in those who are treated with tamoxifen.

## Hot Flashes

Vasomotor symptoms are frequent complications consecutive to estrogen depletion in women treated for breast cancer, producing impairment of quality of life and leading to noncompliance. This adverse event seems to occur slightly more often in patients treated with tamoxifen compared to AIs in adjuvant trials and compared to fulvestrant in treatment of metastatic disease. The reported incidence across different studies is around 35–40 % [80–83]. Successful management is challenging. Nonestrogenic pharmacological interventions, such as the selective serotonin-norepinephrine reuptake inhibitor venlafaxine, at 75 mg/day, and the antihypertensive centrally acting adrenergic agonist clonidine, at 0.1 mg/day, show some efficacy in reducing hot flashes in a recent trial [92].

## Eye Problems

The rate of cataract was significantly increased by tamoxifen compared to placebo in the large NSABP P-1 preventive study. This complication occurred in 2.77 % of women treated with tamoxifen, while the incidence of cataract surgery was 1 % [93]. Women should be asked to report any visual abnormality, and ophthalmological investigations should be ordered in symptomatic patients. Four cases of retinopathy were reported in 63 patients prospectively followed for ocular toxicity. Retinal opacities were not reversible with tamoxifen withdrawal [94].

## Musculoskeletal Pain

According to toxicity data of multiple adjuvant trials, joint pain emerged as a prominent side effect of AIs, seen in about 35 % of women and representing the first cause of noncompliance. Patients should be reassured and told that symptoms can be managed, can improve over time, and are reversible upon treatment discontinuation. Patients should be encouraged to have regular physical exercise. Pharmacological interventions such as nonsteroidal antiinflammatory drugs (NSAIDs), cyclooxygenase-2 inhibitors, and the use of pain medications such as opioids can help to release symptoms [95]. A shift to another AI can be considered if pain treatment is unsuccessful, and, in the case of persisting disabling symptoms, tamoxifen might still be proposed as a suitable alternative.

## Bone Loss

Estrogen deprivation at almost undetectable levels by AIs leads to an increased bone loss and an increased risk of fractures. This is in sharp contrast to the protective effect of SERMs on bone. In the ATAC and TEAM trials, the incidence of osteoporosis ranged from 10 to 11 % among women treated with 5 years of anastrozole or exemestane [80, 83]. In the sequential arms of the IES and TEAM studies (tamoxifen followed by 2–3 years of exemestane), only 6 % of patients experienced bone loss [82, 83].

The reported fracture rate with 5 years of AI in the adjuvant setting ranges from 5 to 11 % [80, 81, 83]. Regarding fulvestrant, osteoporosis was only reported in one patient receiving the dose of 500 mg [79].

It is highly recommended that all women starting treatment with an AI undergo a bone mineral density (BMD) measurement by dual-energy x-ray absorptiometry (DEXA) and a global assessment of risk factors for developing osteoporotic fractures such as age older than 65 years, low BMI, family history of hip fracture, personal history of fracture under 50 years, current corticosteroid use, current smoking, and increased alcohol intake [96]. Those patients presenting baseline osteopenia or classified "high risk" should have their BMD monitored every 1–2 years. The implementation of lifestyle changes, and adequate supplementation of vitamin D (≥800 UI/day) and calcium (1,200–1,500 mg/day) should be considered to preserve bone health [97]. Current ASCO guidelines recommend the initiation of bisphosphonate treatment in the case of osteoporosis (T score ≤ 2.5) [96]. Lately, twice-yearly administration of 60 mg of denosumab, a fully human antibody against RANK ligand, was associated with a significant increase of BMD in women receiving adjuvant aromatase inhibitor [98].

## Cardiovascular Events

Cardiovascular events include myocardial ischemia and strokes. Monitoring of the cardiovascular safety of aromatase inhibitors has been poorly standardized in trials; in addition, data might still be immature. Individual adjuvant trials did not identify a higher risk of developing cardiac events with upfront AI compared to tamoxifen alone [80, 81]. However, a recent meta-analysis of seven adjuvant trials including 30,023 patients found that the risk of cardiovascular disease (including myocardial infarction, angina, and cardiac failure) was significantly higher with AIs upfront compared to 5 years of tamoxifen or the switching strategy (4.2 % in the AI group vs. 3.4 % in the tamoxifen group, OR = 1.26, 95 % CI = 1.10–1.43, $P < 0.001$) [99]. There is no evidence that tamoxifen increases the risk of ischemic heart disease compared to placebo in NSABP-P1 trial. Severe coronary syndromes ranged from 0.94 to 1.12 % in this study [93]. The increase in serum cholesterol level is a well-known phenomenon during AI therapy and could be one parameter for the increased risk to develop myocardial ischemia. Therefore, a regular screening for cardiovascular risk factors is highly recommended in women treated with AIs. The prescription of an AI in postmenopausal patients with a personal history of ischemic heart disease should be considered after a careful evaluation of the individual risk of breast cancer recurrence, and the sequential strategy might be preferred over upfront AI, especially for women at low or moderate risk of relapse.

## Cognitive Dysfunction

Data from large adjuvant trials regarding cognitive function are quite limited and conflicting. However, a BIG 1-98 substudy examined differences in cognitive function associated with each endocrine treatment after 5 years of treatment and 1 year after treatment cessation. Patients taking letrozole had better overall composite cognitive scores than those treated with tamoxifen [100]. An improvement was noticed after treatment withdrawal. A cross-sectional study from the TEAM trial is consistent with these findings, suggesting a better cognitive function with exemestane than tamoxifen [101]. These data are still too limited and immature to draw firm conclusions and to make recommendations on how cognitive function impairment should be monitored during long-term hormonal treatment.

# Targeted Agents

Trastuzumab (Herceptin, Genentech, South San Francisco, CA, USA) is a monoclonal IgG1 class humanized murine antibody that binds the extracellular portion of the HER2 transmembrane receptor [102]. Since its launch in 1998, trastuzumab has become the backbone of care of HER2 amplified breast cancer, both in the metastatic and early disease settings [103–108].

In 2007, a second targeted agent was approved for the treatment of HER2-positive breast cancer: lapatinib (Tykerb, GlaxoSmithKline, Philadelphia, PA, USA). This oral small molecule targets the tyrosine kinase activity of HER2 and epidermal growth factor receptor (EGFR or HER1). It is approved in combination with capecitabine or letrozole in the treatment of HER2-positive metastatic breast cancer and is currently evaluated in clinical trials in the adjuvant setting [109, 110].

A growing list of novel anti-HER2 agents is showing promising activity in women with HER2-positive disease. Pertuzumab is a monoclonal antibody that binds to the HER2 dimerization domain [111] and, as a result, inhibits the formation of HER2 dimers, including the HER2/HER3 heterodimer. Trastuzumab DM-1 is an antibody-drug conjugate linking trastuzumab with the fungal toxin maytansine (DM-1) that specifically delivers the antimicrotubule agent (DM-1) to HER2-positive cells [112]. Neratinib (HKI-272) is a potent irreversible pan-HER kinase inhibitor with efficacy shown in HER2-positive metastatic breast cancer [113]. Afatinib (Tomtovok, Boehringer Ingelheim, Ridgefield, CT, USA) is an oral, irreversible inhibitor of HER1/HER2 and is in trials in HER2-positive metastatic tumor breast cancer [114–116].

Of note, recent trials have shown promising results with "dual HER2 blockade" involving trastuzumab with either lapatinib [117] or pertuzumab [118].

Bevacizumab (Avastin, Genentech, South San Francisco, CA, USA) is the third targeted agent approved for the treatment of metastatic breast cancer. Bevacizumab is a humanized monoclonal antibody against vascular endothelial growth factor (VEGF), which is a key angiogenic factor [119]. Bevacizumab is approved by EMA for the first-line treatment of metastatic breast cancer in combination with paclitaxel or capecitabine.

Targeted therapies have toxicity profiles that differ from those of traditional cytotoxic chemotherapy. While the concept of specifically targeting malignant cells implies sparing normal cells, targeted agents have proved to have their share of side effects, often leading to dose reduction, treatment delays, and interruption. Side effects of targeted agents can be divided into "class"-specific and "agent"-specific.

Monoclonal antibodies are known to generate immediate infusion reactions, but improvement in biotechnology has lead to a significant decrease in such events.

Small molecule inhibitors often cause diarrhea and skin rash. They are mostly metabolized by cytochrome P450 3A4 and therefore are subject to multiple drug interactions, in contrast to monoclonal antibodies, which do not undergo hepatic metabolism.

All anti-HER2 agents can potentially cause left ventricular myocardial dysfunction, and caution is required when they are used in combination or sequence with cardiotoxic chemotherapy.

Toxicity of bevacizumab is typical of agents targeting the VEGF pathway and includes hypertension, bleeding, thrombosis, impaired wound healing, and, to a lesser extent, myocardial dysfunction.

Table 2.4 summarizes the indications of targeted agents used in the treatment of breast cancer [51, 120–151], major side effects, and monitoring tests. Management algorithms for some key toxicities are presented in Figs. 2.1, 2.2, and 2.3.

## Cardiovascular Toxicity

Cardiac dysfunction was the main adverse event in the first published phase III trial of trastuzumab combined with chemotherapy in the treatment of advanced HER2-positive breast cancer [103]. Its incidence was as high as 27 % in the combination with anthracyclines. This unexpected finding influenced the design of the adjuvant trials that recruited more than 12,000 patients and adopted a sequential administration of anthracyclines and trastuzumab with prospective cardiac function monitoring and stopping rules in the presence of prespecified drops in left ventricular ejection fraction. As a result, the observed incidence of cardiotoxicity was low – ranging from 0.4 to 3.6 % – and considered acceptable in view of the large reduction in breast cancer relapses and deaths [103–106]. Even though its causes are not fully elucidated,

TABLE 2.4 Side effects of targeted agents

| Drug usual dose and schedule | Context and minimal requirements for prescription | Most common side effects vs. rare ones | Incidence | Special tests (if any) to monitor side effects | Recommendations for the prevention/ management of side effects |
|---|---|---|---|---|---|
| Bevacizumab | Metastatic breast cancer in combination with paclitaxel or capecitabine | Hypertension | 0.8–17.9 %. Higher incidence with 15 mg/kg vs. 7.5 mg/kg | Blood pressure monitoring every 2–3 weeks during treatment. Target BP = 135/85 for cancer patients with comorbidities as kidney disease | Treat with appropriate antihypertensive therapy. Beware of interactions: nifedipine (use cautiously), verapamil, diltiazem, and CYP3A4 inhibitors (contraindicated). ACE inhibitors preferred mainly because of proteinuria. Discontinue bevacizumab for hypertensive crisis or hypertensive encephalopathy |
| | | | | | Hold bevacizumab for severe hypertension not controlled with medical management. Continue to monitor blood pressure at regular intervals after discontinuation of bevacizumab |
| | | Proteinuria | 0.8–3.9 % | Urine dipstick analysis for proteinuria before each administration 24-h urine collection if urine dipstick 2+ or more for proteinuria | Discontinue bevacizumab for nephrotic syndrome |
| | | | | | Hold bevacizumab for moderate to severe proteinuria (≥ 2 g/24 h) |
| | | | | | No data on bevacizumab administration in patients with moderate proteinuria |
| | | Wound-healing complications | 0.4–1.5 % | Clinical appreciation | Hold bevacizumab 28 days before elective surgery. Treat with bevacizumab 28 days after surgery if surgical wound fully healed |
| | | | | | Exclude patients with nonhealing wounds, active gastric ulcers, and bone fractures |
| | | Gastrointestinal perforation | 0.4–2.5 % | Mostly dependent on site of disease | Exclude patients with abdominal fistula, GIP, or intra-abdominal abscess in the last 6 months |
| | | | | | Discontinue bevacizumab in case of GIP |

(continued)

Table 2.4 (continued)

| Drug usual dose and schedule | Context and minimal requirements for prescription | Most common side effects vs. rare ones | Incidence | Special tests (if any) to monitor side effects | Recommendations for the prevention/ management of side effects |
|---|---|---|---|---|---|
| Bevacizumab | Metastatic breast cancer in combination with paclitaxel or capecitabine | Bleeding/ hemorrhage | 0.4–5.4 % | Clinical appreciation | Do not exclude patients with CNS metastases |
| | | | | CBC | Discontinue bevacizumab for serious bleeding events |
| | | | | | Anticoagulation should not be contraindicated |
| | | | | | Low-dose aspirin should not be contraindicated |
| | | Thromboembolic events | 0.7–6.5 % (ATE and VTE combined) | Mainly arterial thrombotic events | Prophylactic low-dose aspirin for high-risk patients (≥ 65 years old, previous arterial thrombosis or emboli) |
| | | | | | Manage by anticoagulants |
| | | | | | Discontinue bevacizumab after severe arterial thrombotic events |
| | | Cardiovascular events (CHF) | 1.6 %. No differences seen with different doses or concomitant chemotherapy agents | Echocardiography, MUGA scintigraphy every 3–4 and 6–8 months after completion of treatment. Studies on radioactive tracers, serum biomarkers, and genetic polymorphisms are ongoing | Discontinue bevacizumab Start ACE inhibitors or ARBs (aldosterone receptors blockers) + beta blockers + diuretics |
| | | Osteonecrosis of the jaw | 0.3–0.4 %. Higher in patients treated with bisphosphonates Bevacizumab does not appear to elevate the risk compared to chemotherapy | Clinical appreciation, x-ray, and CT scan | |

| Trastuzumab | HER2-positive (IHC 3+ or IHC 2+ and FISH ratio >2.2) breast cancer in the neo-adjuvant, adjuvant, and metastatic settings | Asymptomatic left ventricular systolic dysfunction | 11–17 % in the metastatic setting when combined with chemotherapy<br><br>0–18.6 % in the adjuvant setting, 4 % when combined with endocrine treatment | Echocardiography, MUGA scintigraphy every 12 weeks on treatment. Studies on radioactive tracers, serum biomarkers, and genetic polymorphisms are ongoing | Start ACE inhibitors. See algorithm of management |
|---|---|---|---|---|---|
| | | Symptomatic CHF | 2 % in the metastatic setting when combined with taxane, and 16 % when combined with anthracyclines. 0–3.8 % in the adjuvant setting, <1 % when combined with endocrine treatment. 4 % with single-agent treatment in heavily pretreated patients | | |
| | | Infusion reactions | Mild to moderate reactions <1 % 25–38 % of first infusions <1 % severe events (anaphylaxis). Includes fever, chills, and, on occasion, nausea, vomiting, pain, headache, dizziness, dyspnea, rash, and asthenia | Clinical assessment Symptoms usually occur during or within 24 h of Herceptin administration | Interrupt infusion for dyspnea or clinically significant hypotension<br><br>Monitor patients until symptoms completely resolve<br><br>Discontinue for infusion reactions manifesting as anaphylaxis, angioedema, interstitial pneumonitis, or acute respiratory distress syndrome Strongly consider permanent discontinuation in all patients with severe infusion reactions Slow infusion rate Administer acetaminophen, diphenhydramine, and/ or meperidine, corticosteroids |

(continued)

TABLE 2.4 (continued)

| Drug usual dose and schedule | Context and minimal requirements for prescription | Most common side effects vs. rare ones | Incidence | Special tests (if any) to monitor side effects | Recommendations for the prevention/management of side effects |
|---|---|---|---|---|---|
| Pertuzumab | Ongoing trials in HER2-positive (IHC 3+ or IHC 2+ and FISH ratio >2.2) breast cancer | Asymptomatic left ventricular systolic dysfunction | 6.9 % with pertuzumab alone, 3.4 % with pertuzumab in combination with non-anthracycline chemotherapy, and 6.5 % with pertuzumab in combination with trastuzumab | Echocardiography, MUGA scintigraphy every 12 weeks on treatment | See algorithm of treatment |
| | | Symptomatic CHF | 0.3 % with pertuzumab alone, 1.1 % with pertuzumab in combination with non-anthracycline chemotherapy, and 1.1 % with pertuzumab in combination with trastuzumab | | |
| | | Diarrhea | 51 % all grades and 5.4–7.3 % grade 3. 64 % when given with trastuzumab. | Patient complaint. NCI-CTC grading. | Supportive measures. Loperamide if necessary. |
| | | Nausea | 24–27 %, no grade 3 or 4. 27 % when given with trastuzumab. | Patient complaint | Antiemetics at the discretion of the treating physician |
| | | Fatigue | 22–24 %, 2.4 % grade 3. 33 % when given with trastuzumab. | Patient complaint | |
| | | Rash including allergic reaction | 20 %, no grade 3 or 4 | Clinical complaint | |
| | | Vomiting | 15 %, 2.5 % grade 3 | Patient complaint | Antiemetics at the discretion of the treating physician |

| | | | | | |
|---|---|---|---|---|---|
| T-DM-1 | Ongoing trials in HER2-positive (IHC 3+ or IHC 2+ and FISH ratio >2.2) breast cancer | Thrombocytopenia | 8 % grade 3 or 4 | CBC before administration | Dose reductions from 3.6–3 mg/kg then 2.4 mg/kg |
| | | Fatigue | 45 % grade 3 or 4. 65.2 % all grades | Patient complaint | Antiemetics at the discretion of treating physician |
| | | Nausea | 0.9 % grade 3 or 4. 50.9 % all grades | | Common analgesics |
| | | Headache | 40.2 % grade1 | | |
| | | Hypokalemia | 8.9 % grade 3 or 4. 24.1 % all grades | Chemistry before administration | K+ supplementation. Not associated with vomiting, diarrhea, or diuretic use |
| Lapatinib | Metastatic HER2-positive (IHC 3+ or IHC 2+ and FISH ratio >2.2) breast cancer in combination with capecitabine after progression on trastuzumab | Diarrhea | 19–48 % monotherapy 60 % when combined with capecitabine with 13 % grade 3/4, 60 % when combine with trastuzumab with 9 % grade 3, 63 % when combined with letrozole | Patient complaint. NCI-CTC grading | See algorithm of management |
| | | Rash | 22–44 % depending if single agent, in combination with chemotherapy or with endocrine therapy. 6 % grade 3, no grade 4 | Acne-like rash of folliculitis: inflammatory papules and pustules on the face, scalp, chest, and back | See algorithm of management. Retinoids not indicated |
| | | Other skin disorders | 1–4 % | Hair disorders, dry skin, pruritus/ urticaria, and nail disorders | Emollients, avoid sun |
| | | Hepatotoxicity | 1.5 % grade 3 ALT elevation. 0.3 % serious liver injury with hyperbilirubinemia | Monitoring of LFTs and bilirubin. Association with MHC class II allele HLA-DQA1*02:01 | Avoid drug interactions and especially CYP3A4 inducers. Screen for other causes (viral hepatitis, hemochromatosis, etc.). Withdraw treatment. |
| | | Left ventricular systolic dysfunction | | Echocardiography, MUGA scintigraphy. Cardiac biomarkers (creatinine kinase, troponin, brain natriuretic peptide)? | Reversible. See algorithm of management |

(continued)

TABLE 2-4 (continued)

| Drug usual dose and schedule | Context and minimal requirements for prescription | Most common side effects vs. rare ones | Incidence | Special tests (if any) to monitor side effects | Recommendations for the prevention/management of side effects |
|---|---|---|---|---|---|
| Neratinib | Ongoing trials in HER2-positive (IHC 3+ or IHC 2+ and FISH ratio >2.2) breast cancer | Diarrhea | 21 % grade 3 or 4, 93 % all grades | Patient complaint. NCI-CTC grading. Blood tests. Stool tests | Grade 3 lasting >2 days despite optimal medical therapy, or associated with fever or dehydration: hold neratinib until recovery to ≤grade 1 or baseline. Consider prophylactic antidiarrheal medications. If recurrence or if recovery >1 week, reduce dose to 160 mg then 120 mg |
| | | Fatigue | 2 % grade 3 or 4, 24 % all grades | Patient complaint | Grade 3 and lasting more than 3 days, hold until recovery. Dose reduction if recurrence |
| | | Nausea | 2 % grade 3 or 4, 36 % all grades | Patient complaint | Antiemetics at the discretion of treating physician. Hold treatment if grade 3 or more and dose reduction if recurrence |
| | | Vomiting | 4 % grade 3 or 4, 31 % all grades | Patient complaint | |
| | | Rash | 18 %, nongrade 3 or 4 | Clinical assessment | See rash management algorithm |
| Afatinib | Ongoing trials in HER2-positive (IHC 3+ or IHC 2+ and FISH ratio >2.2) breast cancer | Diarrhea | 87–95 %, 18–20 % grade 3 | Patient complaint. NCI-CTC grading. Blood tests. Stool tests | See algorithm of management |
| | | Skin reactions | 88–95 %, 9.8–19 % grade 3 | Clinical assessment | See algorithm of management |

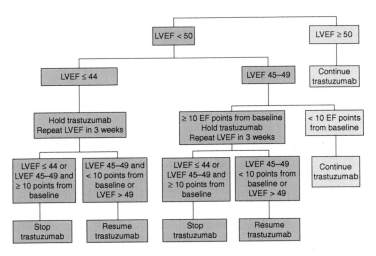

FIGURE 2.1 Management of patients showing cardiac dysfunction on trastuzumab (Reprinted from Suter et al. [152]. Reprinted with permission. © 2007 American Society of Clinical Oncology. All rights reserved)

trastuzumab-related left ventricular systolic dysfunction (LVSD) is classified as type 2 chemotherapy-related cardiotoxicity (CRCT). It is mediated by the blockade by trastuzumab of ErbB2-ErbB4 signaling in cardiac myocytes, a pathway thought to play a role in protecting cardiac myocytes from stress conditions. At the opposite of type 1 CRCT that is exemplified by anthracycline-related myocardial damage, trastuzumab LVSD is not dose-related and potentially reversible with medical therapy, and rechallenge is possible [153]. Potential risk factors influencing LVEF deterioration are older age, hypertension, and a baseline LVEF in the lower normal range [43, 103, 154]. Algorithms for initiation of therapy are proposed, as well as algorithms for monitoring and managing cardiac events (Fig. 2.1). Reporting of cardiac events in trastuzumab trials prompted close cardiac monitoring of patients on lapatinib, neratinib, and afatinib. Incidence of cardiotoxicity was found to be less with these agents, even in patients pretreated with trastuzumab and anthracycline. Furthermore, most LVEF decreases were asymptomatic and

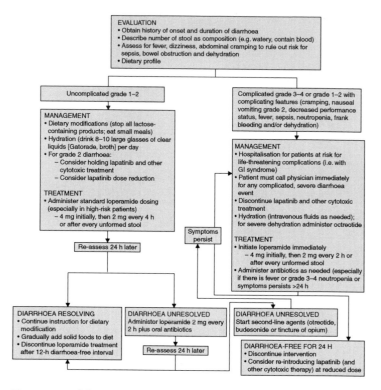

FIGURE 2.2 Management of patients experiencing diarrhea on HER1/HER2 tyrosine kinase inhibitors (Modified from [146])

almost universally reversible [150]. Even though cardiotoxicity of lapatinib seems to be type 2 CRCT, as with trastuzumab, theories are being developed to explain the lower incidence and include less potency in inhibiting the HER2/HER4 heterodimer signaling or ATP generation rather than ATP depletion [155].

Left ventricular dysfunction is also a class toxicity of agents targeting the VEGF pathway, given that VEGF plays an important role in cardiomyocyte survival after stress or injury [156]. A meta-analysis of bevacizumab trials in metastatic breast cancer demonstrated the increased incidence of congestive heart failure (CHF) in bevacizumab-treated

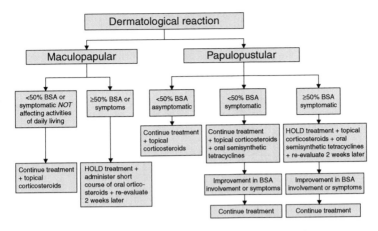

FIGURE 2.3 Management of patients experiencing skin toxicity on HER1/HER2 tyrosine kinase inhibitors (Modified from [146])

patients when compared to controls. The overall incidence, however, remains low and is not dose-dependent; nor is it associated with type of concomitant chemotherapy. Early available data show recovery of cardiac function with interruption of treatment and introduction of cardiac medications [136]. Bevacizumab is also responsible for rare arterial and venous thromboembolic events [133].

## Hypertension

Hypertension is a known class effect of antiangiogenic agents. Causal hypotheses include bevacizumab effect on kidney vasculature as well as inhibition of the generation of nitric oxide [157]. Proactive monitoring and management with commonly used antihypertensive medications are required at each cycle. Bevacizumab discontinuation is warranted for uncontrolled hypertension as well as for neurological symptoms (headache, impaired vision, etc.) that can also be caused by the very rare reversible posterior leukoencephalopathy syndrome reported with bevacizumab therapy [126].

## Infusion Reactions

Most cancer therapeutics, but most certainly monoclonal anti-bodies, carry the risk of infusion reactions. These reactions develop during the infusion or shortly thereafter. They are mostly mild to moderate with various symptoms such as fever, chills, headache, nausea, pruritus, skin rash, and so forth. Severe cases are characterized by hypotension, urticaria, bronchospasm, and, very rarely, cardiac arrest. Mechanisms by which they occur are immune-mediated – cytokine release and type 1 hypersensitivity reactions mediated by IgE. New technology is helping engineer novel, fully humanized monoclonal antibodies in order to minimize immune reactions. Trastuzumab produces one of the highest incidences of infusion reactions among the monoclonal antibodies, but these reactions are largely mild to moderate. Most patients are rechallenged successfully, with permanent discontinuation considered only in case of anaphylaxis, angioedema, or acute respiratory distress syndrome.

Incidence of such reactions is lower with bevacizumab and approaches 3.1 % in a large adjuvant trial in colorectal cancer [158]. However, there are no data here concerning the safety of rechallenge in case of a severe reaction. Physicians and nurses should be prepared when these agents are to be infused, and epinephrine, corticosteroids, intravenous antihistamines, bronchodilators, oxygen, and vasopressors should be readily available.

## Hepatotoxicity

Hepatobiliary adverse events (AEs) have been reported in patients treated with lapatinib. Hepatotoxicity is predominately hepatocellular injury [148]. A review of data from 16 clinical trials yielded an incidence of 1.5 % for grade 3 ALT/AST elevation and 0.3 % for liver injury with jaundice meeting the Hy's Law criteria [149]. One study reported four withdrawals from treatment and one toxic death by hepatic failure in 138 patients treated with lapatinib [159].

Mechanisms for severe liver toxicity are not fully understood. There might be a role for immune-mediated hypersensitivity reactions, and lapatinib has also been found to be an inactivator of CYP3A4 [160]. Furthermore, recent pharmacogenetic evaluations have identified associations between lapatinib-induced liver injury and 4 MHC class II alleles. A strong statistical association was observed with HLA-DQA1*02:01 [148]. Management depends on the severity of toxicity. Differential diagnosis must include viral hepatitis, hemochromatosis, alpha-1 antitrypsin deficiency, and liver progressive disease. Clinicians must be aware of drug interactions and avoid CYP3A4 inducers as well as other hepatotoxic drugs such as paracetamol. Liver toxicity has been reported with other tyrosine kinase inhibitors [161], and LFT elevations should alert one to possible liver toxicity of all small molecules used in breast cancer, including neratinib and afatinib.

## Gastrointestinal Perforation, Wound-Healing Complications, and Bleeding

Gastrointestinal perforation, wound-healing complications, and bleeding are typical complications of antiangiogenic therapies, but their incidence is low in metastatic breast cancer patients treated with bevacizumab, who rarely present with bulky abdominal disease. Patients with CNS metastases are not excluded anymore from antiangiogenic therapy. It is recommended to hold bevacizumab 4 weeks prior to elective surgery and until at least 28 days after in order to minimize wound-healing complications.

## Diarrhea

Diarrhea as an adverse event has been described through the entire spectrum of phase I to III trials with tyrosine kinase inhibitors. It is by far the side effect leading to most dose reductions and treatment discontinuations, and thus decreased efficacy of these small molecules [161]. Diarrhea with lapatinib appears early, during the first days of treatment (before day 6). It is rarely severe and generally does not need intervention. However, patient monitoring is crucial in order to prevent dehydration and electrolyte imbalance.

TKI-induced diarrhea responds well to conventional antidiarrheal agents. Patients should be encouraged to keep dietary measures and avoid drug interactions. Extreme cases require hospitalization for rehydration, octreotide administration, and possibly antibiotics.

Differential diagnosis includes infectious colitis and malabsorption. Secretory diarrhea is implied by a high content of sodium and chloride and with no presence of mucus, blood, leukocytes, or *Clostridium difficile* toxins. Diarrhea is also commonly described with neratinib and afatinib. The pathophysiological mechanism is secretory by inhibition of EGFR effects on chloride secretion [162]. Biopsy does not usually show mucosal damage, but analysis of tissue from a phase I trial with neratinib revealed mild duodenal mucosal gland dilatation and degeneration in the small intestine [163].

Dual HER2 blockade, using either trastuzumab and lapatinib or trastuzumab and pertuzumab, exacerbates diarrhea, which needs prompt and aggressive treatment. An algorithm (see Fig. 2.2) initially developed for management of chemotherapy-induced diarrhea is applicable once diarrhea occurs under pan-ERB TKI's therapy [50].

## Skin Rash

Skin rash has been described as a class effect toxicity of ErbB1 targeting agents. As lapatinib and afatinib target EGFR as well as HER2, breast cancer patients treated with these agents often develop a characteristic acneiform eruption that may resemble folliculitis. Rash is characterized by inflammatory papules and pustules that are found in areas with pilosebaceous glands, such as the face, scalp, chest, and back. The lack of comedones distinguishes this eruption from acne vulgaris, and histologic sections will reveal suppurative folliculitis and superficial perifolliculitis [164]. Incidence of this adverse reaction is lower during lapatinib treatment compared to other ErbB1 inhibitors. About half of patients exposed to lapatinib experience skin toxicity in the first 2 weeks of treatment. However, most are of low grade, resolve spontaneously, and almost never require interventions, dose reductions, or discontinuation.

Management depends on the type of lesions (pustular vs. papular) and extent of distribution. Therapy should be discontinued if more than 50 % of body surface is affected. An algorithm for management (see Fig. 2.3) has been developed [147, 165]. There is no clear evidence that the occurrence and severity of rash associated with agents used in breast cancer is correlated with tumor response or disease outcome, as is suggested with other anti-EGFR molecules such as cetuximab, erlotinib, and gefitinib [166, 167]. Further details on skin toxicity are considered elsewhere in this book.

## Interstitial Pneumonitis

TKI-induced interstitial pneumonitis is a very rare adverse event that can be potentially fatal. It was described with the first approved tyrosine kinase inhibitor imatinib [168]. The majority of cases were described later on with anti-EGFR tyrosine kinase inhibitors mostly used in non-small cell lung cancer, namely, erlotinib [169, 170] and gefitinib [171], as well as with mTOR inhibitors such as everolimus. Few cases were fatal [171], and the majority recovered with treatment interruption and corticosteroids [172]. Rechallenge is possible [171]. The mechanism involved in TKI-induced interstitial lung disease is unknown but is believed to be idiosyncratic, resembling hypersensitivity pneumonia, bronchiolitis obliterans, or eosinophilic pneumonia [173]. Diagnosis is one of exclusion because symptoms mimic congestive heart failure, infection, and lymphangitic carcinomatosis. Fortunately, this complication is very rarely described with TKIs used in the treatment of breast cancer. The best description comes from the expanded access program of lapatinib with 0.2 % of patients (7/4,283) developing pulmonary events: three patients experienced pneumonitis, two interstitial lung disease, and two lung infiltrations. Incidence of lapatinib-related interstitial pneumonitis is 0.3 % (36/12,795) in the overall lapatinib program [174]. All cases were reversible. Other studies with lapatinib, neratinib, and afatinib report mainly episodes of dyspnea but not interstitial lung disease specifically. One phase 1 study with afatinib [175] reported one episode of reversible pneumonitis in 53 patients. Even though TKI-induced pneumonitis is rare in breast cancer patients, it is a potentially dangerous complication that needs early recognition and management.

## Bone-Modifying Agents

Breast cancer shows a high predilection to metastasize to the skeletal system, causing multiple morbid events such as pain, hypercalcemia, and fractures, which decrease quality of life. Bisphosphonates are established therapies for preventing skeletal-related events (SREs) from bone metastases. As a result, they are very often prescribed as supportive therapy in advanced breast cancer. Their use is expected to reach the adjuvant setting soon, given the recent demonstration of the ability of zoledronic acid to reduce breast cancer relapses in a low-estrogen environment – for example, in young women on a LHRH agonist combined with either tamoxifen or anastrozole in postmenopausal women older than 55 years on adjuvant endocrine therapy [176–178].

Denosumab is a fully human monoclonal antibody that specifically binds human receptor activator of nuclear factor k-B ligand (RANKL). RANKL plays a stimulating role in osteoclast activity, thus promoting tumor cell proliferation, metastasis, and survival. By disrupting this activity, denosumab reduces bone resorption, tumor-induced bone destruction, and SREs [179, 180]. In this indication, denosumab is administered subcutaneously every 4 weeks and proved superior to zole-dronic acid in delaying or preventing SREs in patients with bone metastases from breast cancer [181]. The possible anti-metastatic role of denosumab is currently under investigation.

Bisphosphonates and RANKL monoclonal antibodies have common toxicities with different incidences, which are reviewed in detail in Chap. 16.

# References

1. Zhou J, Giannakakou P. Targeting microtubules for cancer chemo-therapy. Curr Med Chem Anticancer Agents. 2005;5:65–71.
2. Tannock IF, Hill RP, Bristow RG, Harrington L. The basic science of oncology. 4th ed. New York: McGraw-Hill Medical Publishing Division; 2005.
3. Kaye SB. New antimetabolites in cancer chemotherapy and their clinical impact. Br J Cancer. 1998;78 suppl 3:1–7.
4. Takimoto CH, Calvo E. Principles of oncologic pharmacotherapy. In: Pazdur R, Wagman LD, Camphausen KA, Hoskins WJ, editors. Cancer management: a multidisciplinary approach. 11th ed. Lawrence: CMPMedica LLC; 2008.
5. Taxol package insert. http://packageinserts.bms.com/pi/pi_taxol.pdf. Accessed on Sep 2012.
6. Taxotere package insert. http://products.sanofi.us/taxotere/taxo-tere.html. Accessed on Sep 2012.
7. Piccart MJ, Klijn J, Paridaens R, Nooij M, Mauriac L, Coleman R, et al. Corticosteroids significantly delay the onset of docetaxel-induced fluid retention: Final results of a randomized study of the European organiza-tion for research and treatment of cancer investigational drug branch for breast cancer. J Clin Oncol. 1997;15:3149–55.
8. Esmaeli B, Hidaji L, Adinin RB, Faustina M, Coats C, Arbuckle R, et al. Blockage of the lacrimal drainage apparatus as a side effect of docetaxel therapy. Cancer. 2003;98:504–7.
9. Abraxane package insert. http://www.abraxane.com/docs/Abraxane_PrescribingInformation.pdf. Accessed on Sep 2012.
10. Gradishar WJ, Tjulandin S, Davidson N, Shaw H, Desai N, Bhar P, et al. Phase III trial of nanoparticle albumin-bound paclitaxel com-pared with polyethylated castor oil-based paclitaxel in women with breast cancer. J Clin Oncol. 2005;23:7794–803.
11. Ixempra package insert. http://packageinserts.bms.com/pi/pi_ixempra.pdf. Accessed on Sep 2012.

104    P.G. Aftimos et al.

12. Eribulin package insert. http://us.eisai.com/pdf_files/HalavenPI.pdf. Accessed on Sep 2012.
13. Navelbine package insert. http://www2.pierre-fabre.com/us/file/nvb_prescribing_info_us.pdf. Accessed on Sep 2012.
14. Rouzaud P, Estivals M, Pujazon MC, Carles P, Lauque D, et al. Respiratory complications of the vinorelbine-mitomycin combination. Rev Mal Respir. 1999;16:81–4.
15. Goli AK, Osman MN, Koduri M, Byrd RP, Roy TM, et al. A case report of vinorelbine monotherapy-related acute bronchospasm and non-ST elevation acute coronary syndrome. Tenn Med. 2011;104:47–8.
16. Gregory RK, Smith IE. Vinorelbine: a clinical review. Br J Cancer. 2000;82:1907–13.
17. Adriamycin package insert. http://www.pfizer.ca/en/our_products/products/monograph/150. Accessed on Sep 2012.
18. Ellence package insert. http://labeling.pfizer.com/ShowLabeling.aspx?id=657. Accessed on Sep 2012.
19. Doxil package insert. http://www.doxil.com/assets/DOXIL_PI_Booklet.pdf. Accessed on Sep 2012.
20. Alberts DS, Muggia FM, Carmichael J, Winer EP, Jahanzeb M, Venook AP, et al. Efficacy and safety of liposomal anthracyclines in phase I/II clinical trials. Semin Oncol. 2004;31:53–90.
21. European Medicines Agency. Myocet summary of product characteristics. http://www.ema.europa.eu/docs/en_GB/document_library/EPAR_-_Product_Information/human/000297/WC500031811.pdf. Accessed on Sep 2012.
22. Fluorouracil package insert. http://hemonc.org/docs/packageinsert/fluorouracil.pdf. Accessed on Sep 2012.
23. Xeloda package insert. http://www.gene.com/gene/products/information/xeloda/pdf/pi.pdf. Accessed on Sep 2012.
24. Gemzar package insert. http://pi.lilly.com/us/gemzar.pdf. Accessed on Sep 2012.
25. Pfizer. Methotrexate product monograph. http://www.pfizer.ca/en/our_products/products/monograph/280. Accessed on Sep 2012.
26. Qin D, Ma J, Xiao J, Tang Z. Effect of brain irradiation on blood-CSF barrier permeability of chemotherapeutic agents. Am J Clin Oncol. 1997;20:263–5.
27. Ebeo CT, Girish MR, Byrd RP, Roy TM, Mehta JB. Methotrexate-induced pulmonary lymphoma. Chest. 2003;123:2150–3.
28. Cytoxan package insert. http://packageinserts.bms.com/pi/pi_cytoxan.pdf. Accessed on Sep 2012.
29. Chang TK, Weber GF, Crespi CL, Waxman DJ. Differential activation of cyclophosphamide and ifosphamide by cytochromes P-450 2B and 3A in human liver microsomes. Cancer Res. 1993;53:5629–37.

30. Paraplatin package insert. http://packageinserts.bms.com/pi/pi_paraplatin.pdf. Accessed on Sep 2012.
31. Roche H, Fumoleau P, Spielmann M, Canon JL, Delozier T, Serin D, et al. Sequential adjuvant epirubicin-based and Docetaxel chemotherapy for node positive breast cancer patients. The FNCLCC PACS 01 trial. J Clin Oncol. 2006;24(36):5664–71.
32. Hesketh PJ, Kris MG, Grunberg SM, Beck T, Hainsworth JD, Harker G, et al. Proposal for classifying the acute emetogenicity of cancer chemotherapy. J Clin Oncol. 1997;15:103–9.
33. Grunberg SM, Warr D, Gralla RJ, Rapoport BL, Hesketh PJ, Jordan K, et al. Evaluation of new antiemetic agents and definition of antineoplastic agent emetogenicity-state of the art. Support Care Cancer. 2011;19 suppl 1:S43–7.
34. Quasthoff S, Hartung HP. Chemotherapy-induced peripheral neuropathy. J Neurol. 2002;249(1):9–17.
35. Pace A, Carpano S, Galie E, Savarese A, Della Giulia M, Aschelter A, et al. Vitamin E in the neuroprotection of cisplatin induced peripheral neurotoxicity and ototoxicity. J Clin Oncol. 2007;25(18S) (June 20 Suppl). ASCO annual meeting proceedings (post-meeting edition):9114.
36. Wang WS, Lin JK, Lin TC, Chen WS, Jiang JK, Wang HS, et al. Oral glutamine is effective for preventing oxaliplatin-induced neuropathy in colorectal cancer patients. Oncologist. 2007;12(3):312–9.
37. Smyth JF, Bowman A, Perren T, Wilkinson P, Prescott RJ, Quinn KJ, et al. Glutathione reduces the toxicity and improves quality of life of women diagnosed with ovarian cancer treated with cisplatin: results of a doubleblind, randomised trial. Ann Oncol. 1997;8(6):569–73.
38. Nikcevich DA, Grothey A, Sloan JA, Kugler JW, Silberstein PT, Dentchev T, et al. A phase III randomized, placebo-controlled, double-blind study of intravenous calcium/magnesium to prevent oxaliplatin-induced sensory neurotoxicity, N04C7. J Clin Oncol. 2008 ASCO annual meeting proceedings [Abstract 4009].
39. Schneider BP, Li L, Muller K, Flockhard D, Radovich M, Hancock BA, et al. Genetic associations with taxane-induced neuropathy by a genome-wide association study (GWAS) in E5103. J Clin Oncol. 2011;29:80s (suppl; abstr 1000).
40. Swain SM, Whaley FS, Ewer MS. Congestive heart failure in patients treated with doxorubicin: a retrospective analysis of three trials. Cancer. 2003;97:2869–79.
41. Barrett-Lee PJ, Dixon JM, Farrell C, Jones A, Leonard R, Murray N, et al. Expert opinion on the use of anthracyclines in patients with advanced breast cancer at cardiac risk. Ann Oncol. 2009;20(5):816–27.
42. Von Hoff DD, Layard MW, Basa P, Davis Jr HL, Von Hoff AL, Rozencweig M, et al. Risk factors for doxorubicin induced congestive heart failure. Ann Intern Med. 1979;91:710–7.

43. Seidman A, Hudis C, Pierri MK, Shak S, Paton V, Ashby M, et al. Cardiac dysfunction in the Trastuzumab clinical trials experience. J Clin Oncol. 2002;20(5):1215–21.
44. Speyer J, Wasserheit C. Strategies for reduction of anthracycline cardiac toxicity. Semin Oncol. 1998;25:525–37.
45. Swain SM, Whaley FS, Gerber MC, Weisberg S, York M, Spicer D, et al. Cardioprotection with dexrazoxane for doxorubicin-containing therapy in advanced breast cancer. J Clin Oncol. 1997;15:1318–32.
46. Hensley ML, Hagerty KL, Kewalramani T, Green DM, Meropol NJ, Wasserman TH, et al. American Society of Clinical Oncology 2008 clinical practice guideline update: use of chemotherapy and radiation therapy protectants. J Clin Oncol. 2009;27(1):127–45.
47. Legha SS, Benjamin RS, Mackay B, Ewer M, Wallace S, Valdivieso M, et al. Reduction of doxorubicin cardiotoxicity by prolonged continuous intravenous infusion. Ann Intern Med. 1982;96:133–9.
48. O'Brien ME, Wigler N, Inbar M, Rosso R, Grischke E, Santoro A, et al. Reduced cardiotoxicity and comparable efficacy in a phase III trial of pegylated liposomal doxorubicin HCl (CAELYX/Doxil) versus conventional doxorubicin for first-line treatment of metastatic breast cancer. Ann Oncol. 2004;15(3):440–9.
49. Batist G, Ramakrishnan G, Rao CS, Chandrasekharan A, Gutheil J, Guthrie T, et al. Reduced cardiotoxicity and preserved antitumor efficacy of liposome-encapsulated doxorubicin and cyclophosphamide compared with conventional doxorubicin and cyclophosphamide in a randomized, multicenter trial of metastatic breast cancer. Clin Oncol. 2001;19(5):1444–54.
50. 3rd Benson AB, Ajani JA, Catalano RB, Engelking C, Kornblau SM, Martenson Jr JA, et al. Recommended guidelines for the treatment of cancer treatment-induced diarrhea. J Clin Oncol. 2004;22:2918.
51. Kornblau S, Benson AB, Catalano R, Champlin RE, Engelking C, Field M, et al. Management of cancer treatment-related diarrhea: issues and therapeutic strategies. J Pain Symptom Manage. 2000;19: 118–29.
52. Almer KR, Corbett CL, Holdsworth CD. Double-blind crossover study comparing loperamide, codeine and diphenoxylate in the treatment of chronic diarrhea. Gastroenterology. 1980;79:1272–5.
53. Goumas P, Naxakis S, Christopoulou A, Chrysanthopoulos C, Nikolopoulou VV, Kalofonos HP. Octreotide acetate in the treatment of fluorouracil-induced diarrhea. Oncologist. 1998;3:50–3.
54. Elting LS, Cooksley C, Chambers M, Cantor SB, Manzullo E, Rubenstein EB. The burdens of cancer therapy. Clinical and economic outcomes of chemotherapy-induced mucositis. Cancer. 2003;98:1531–8.
55. Rubenstein EB, Peterson DE, Schubert M, Keefe D, McGuire D, Epstein J, et al. Clinical practice guidelines for the prevention and treatment of cancer therapy-induced oral and gastrointestinal mucositis. Cancer. 2004;100 suppl 9:2026–46.

56. Anderson PM, Schroeder G, Skubitz KM. Oral glutamine reduces the duration and severity of stomatitis after cytotoxic cancer chemotherapy. Cancer. 1998;83:1433–9.

57. Peterson DE, Petit RG. Phase III study: AES-14 in patients at risk for mucositis secondary to anthracycline-based chemotherapy. Proc Am Soc Clin Oncol. 2004;22:731 (abstr).

58. Hejna M, Kostler W, Raderer M, Steger GG, Brodowicz T, Scheithauer W, et al. Decrease of duration and symptoms in chemotherapy-induced oral mucositis by topical GM- CSF: results of a prospective randomized trial. Eur J Cancer. 2001;37:1994–2002.

59. Gorzegno G, Cerutti S, Sperone P, et al. Effect of granulocyte macrophage colony stimulating factor (GM-CSF) mouthwash on grade III chemotherapy-induced oral mucositis. Proc Am Soc Clin Oncol. 1999;18:584a.

60. Wymenga AN, van der Graaf WT, Hofstra LS, Spijkervet FK, Timens W, Timmer-Bosscha H, et al. Phase I study of transforming growth factor-beta 3 mouthwashes for prevention of chemotherapy-induced mucositis. Clin Cancer Res. 1999;5:1363–8.

61. Bjordal JM, Bensadoun RJ, Tunèr J, Frigo L, Gjerde K, Lopes-Martins RA. A systematic review with meta-analysis of the effect of low-level laser therapy (LLLT) in cancer therapy-induced oral mucositis. Support Care Cancer. 2011;19(8):1069–77.

62. Falleti MG, Sanflippo A, Maruff P, Weih L, Phillips KA. The nature and severity of cognitive impairment associated with adjuvant chemotherapy in women with breast cancer: a meta-analysis of the current literature. Brain Cogn. 2005;59:60–70.

63. Bender CM, Pacella ML, Sereika SM, Brufsky AM, Vogel VG, Rastogi P, et al. What do perceived cognitive problems reflect? J Support Oncol. 2008;6:238–42.

64. Poppelreuter M, Weis J, Kulz AK, Tucha O, Lange KW, Bartsch HH. Cognitive dysfunction and subjective complaints of cancer patients: a cross sectional study in a cancer rehabilitation centre. Eur J Cancer. 2004;40:43–9.

65. Meyers CA. How chemotherapy damages the central nervous system. J Biol. 2008;7:11.

66. Ahles TA, Saykin AJ, Furstenberg CT, Cole B, Mott LA, Skalla K, et al. Neuropsychologic impact of standard dose systemic chemotherapy in long term survivors of breast cancer and lymphoma. J Clin Oncol. 2002;20(2):485–93.

67. Han R, Yang YM, Dietrich J, Luebke A, Mayer-Pröschel M, Noble M. Systemic 5-flurouracil treatment causes a syndrome of delayed myelin destruction in the central nervous system. J Biol. 2008;7:12.

68. Kreukels BP, Hamburger HL, de Ruiter MB, van Dam FS, Ridderinkhof KR, Boogerd W, et al. ERP amplitude and latency in breast cancer survivors treated with adjuvant chemotherapy. Clin Neurophysiol. 2008;119:533–41.

69. Schover LR, Yetman RJ, Tuason LJ. Partial mastectomy and breast reconstruction. A comparison of their effects on psychosocial adjustment, body image, and sexuality. Cancer. 1995;75:54–64.
70. Wilmoth MC, Ross JA. Women's perception: breast cancer treatment and sexuality. Cancer Pract. 1997;5:353–9.
71. Bakewell RT, Volker DL. Sexual dysfunction related to the treatment of young women with breast cancer. Clin J Oncol Nurs. 2005;9:697–702.
72. Avis NE, Crawford S, Manuel J. Psychosocial problems among younger women with breast cancer. Psychooncology. 2004;13(5): 295–308.
73. Goldfarb SB, Dickler M, Sit L, et al. Sexual dysfunction in women with breast cancer: prevalence and severity. J Clin Oncol. 2009;27(15s):Abstract 9558.
74. Partridge AH, Gelber S, Peppercorn J, Sampson E, Knudsen K, Laufer M, et al. Web-based survey of fertility issues in young women with breast cancer. J Clin Oncol. 2004;22(20):4174–83.
75. Pedersen-Bjergaard J, Sigsgaard TC, Nielson D, Gjedde SB, Philip P, Hansen M, et al. Acute monocytic or myelomonocytic leukemia with balanced chromosomal translocations to band 11q23 after therapy with 4-epidoxorubicin and cisplatin or cyclophosphamide for breast cancer. J Clin Oncol. 1992;10:1444–51.
76. Praga C, Bergh J, Bliss J, Bonneterre J, Cesana B, Coombes RC, et al. Risk of myeloid leukemia and myelodysplastic syndrome in trials of adjuvant epirubicin for early breast cancer: correlation with doses of epirubicin and cyclophosphamide. J Clin Oncol. 2005;23:4179–91.
77. Peto R, Davies C. ATLAS (Adjuvant Tamoxifen, Longer Against Shorter): international randomized trial of 10 versus 5 years of adjuvant tamoxifen among 11,500 women – preliminary results. Breast Cancer Res Treat. 2007;106(suppl 1):Abstract 48.
78. Gray RG, Rea DW, Handley K, et al. aTTom (adjuvant Tamoxifen – to offer more?): randomized trial of 10 versus 5 years of adjuvant tamoxifen among 6,934 women with estrogen receptor-positive (ER+) or ER untested breast cancer – preliminary results. J Clin Oncol. 2008;26(suppl):10s:Abstract 513.
79. Di Leo A, Jerusalem G, Petruzelka L, Torres R, Bondarenko IN, Khasanov R, et al. Results of the CONFIRM Phase III Trial Comparing fulvestrant 250 mg with fulvestrant 500 mg in post-menopausal women with estrogen receptor–positive advanced breast cancer. J Clin Oncol. 2010;28:4594–600.
80. The Arimidex, Tamoxifen, Alone or in Combination (ATAC) Trialists' Group, Buzdar A, Howell A, Cuzick J, et al. Comprehensive side-effect profile of anastrozole and tamoxifen as adjuvant treatment for early – stage breast cancer: long-term safety analysis of the ATAC trial. Lancet Oncol. 2006;7:633–43.
81. The BIG 1-98 Collaborative Group, Mouridsen H, Giobbie-Hurder A, Goldhirsch A, et al. Letrozole therapy alone or in sequence with

tamoxifen in women with breast cancer. N Engl J Med. 2009;361: 766–76.

82. Coombes RC, Kilburn LS, Snowdon CF, Paridaens R, Coleman RE, Jones SE, et al. Survival and safety of exemestane versus tamoxifen after 2-3 years' tamoxifen treatment (Intergroup Exemestane Study): a randomized controlled trial. Lancet. 2007;369:559–70.

83. van de Velde CJH, Rea D, Seynaeve C, Putter H, Hasenburg A, Vannetzel JM, et al. Adjuvant tamoxifen and exemestane in early breast cancer (TEAM): a randomized phase 3 trial. Lancet. 2011;377:321–31.

84. Goss PE, Ingle JN, Chapman J-AW, et al. Final analysis of NCIC CTG MA.27: a randomized phase iii trial of exemestane versus anastrozole in postmenopausal women with hormone receptor positive primary breast cancer (abstr. S1-1). In 33th annual San Antonio breast cancer symposium, San Antonio, 8–12 Dec 2010.

85. Howell A, Robertson JFR, Abram P, Lichinitser MR, Elledge R, Bajetta E, et al. Comparison of fulvestrant versus tamoxifen for the treatment of advanced breast cancer in postmenopausal women previously untreated with endocrine therapy: a multinational, double-blind, randomized trial. J Clin Oncol. 2004;22:1605–13.

86. Dowsett M, Cuzick J, Ingle J, Coates A, Forbes J, Bliss J, et al. Meta-analysis of breast cancer outcomes in adjuvant trials of aromatase inhibitors versus tamoxifen. J Clin Oncol. 2010;28:509–18.

87. Regan MM, Neven P, Giobbie-Hurder A, Goldhirsch A, Ejlertsen B, Mauriac L, et al. Assessment of letrozole and tamoxifen alone and in sequence for postmenopausal women with steroid receptor-positive breast cancer: the BIG 1-98 randomized clinical trial at 8.1 years median follow-up. Lancet Oncol. 2011;12;1101–8.

88. American College of Obstetricians and Gynecologists Committee on Gynecologic Practice. ACOG Committee Opinion No. 336: Tamoxifen and uterine cancer. Obstet Gynecolol. 2006;107:1475–8.

89. Gerber B, Krause A, Muller H, Reimer T, Külz T, Makovitzky J, et al. Effects of adjuvant tamoxifen on the endometrium in postmeno-pausal women with breast cancer: a prospective long-term study using transvaginal ultrasound. J Clin Oncol. 2000;18:3464–70.

90. Neri F, Maggiano T. Surveillance of endometrial pathologies espe-cially for endometrial cancer, of breast cancer patients under tamoxifen treatment. Eur J Gynaecol Oncol. 2009;30:357–60.

91. Garber JE, Halabi S, Tolaney SM. Factor V Leyden mutation and thromboembolism risk in women receiving adjuvant tamoxifen for breast cancer. J Natl Cancer Inst. 2010;102:942–9.

92. Boekhout AH, Vincent AD, Dalesio OB. Management of hot flashes in patients who have breast cancer with venlafaxine and clonidine: a randomized, double blind, placebo-controlled trial. J Clin Oncol. 2011;29:3862–8.

93. Fisher B, Constantiono JP, Wickerham L, Cecchini RS, Cronin WM, Robidoux A, et al. Tamoxifen for the prevention of breast cancer:

current status of the national surgical adjuvant breast and bowel Project P-1 Study. J Natl Cancer Inst. 2005;97:1652–62.

94. Pavlidis NA, Petris C, Briassoulis E, Klouvas G, Psilas C, Rempapis J, et al. Clear evidence that long-term, low-dose tamoxifen can induce ocular toxicity. A prospective study of 63 patients. Cancer. 1992;69:2961–4.

95. Dent SF, Gaspo R, Kissner G, Pritchard KI. Aromatase inhibitor therapy: toxicities and management strategies in the treatment of postmenopausal women with hormone-sensitive early breast cancer. Breast Cancer Res Treat. 2011;126:295–310.

96. Hillner BE, Ingle JN, Chlebowski RT, Gralow J, Yee GC, Janjan NA, et al. American Society of Clinical Oncology 2003 update on the role of bisphosphonates and bone health issues in women with breast cancer. J Clin Oncol. 2003;21:4042–57.

97. Body JJ. Prevention and treatment of side effects of systemic treatment: bone loss. Ann Oncol. 2010;21 suppl 7:vii180–5.

98. Ellis GK, Bone HG, Chlebowski R, Paul D, Spadafora S, Fan M, et al. Effect of denosumab on bone mineral density in women receiving adjuvant aromatase inhibitors for non-metastatic breast cancer: subgroup analyses of a phase 3 study. Breast Cancer Res Treat. 2009;118:81–7.

99. Amir E, Seruga B, Niraula S, Carlsson L, Ocaña A. Toxicity of adjuvant endocrine therapy in postmenopausal breast cancer patients: a systematic review and meta-analysis. J Natl Cancer Inst. 2011; 103:1299–309.

100. Phillips KA, Ribi K, Sun Z, Stephens A, Thompson A, Harvey V, et al. Cognitive function in postmenopausal women receiving adjuvant letrozole or tamoxifen for breast cancer in the BIG 1-98 randomized trial. Breast. 2010;19:388–95.

101. Schilder CM, Seynaeve C, Beex WB, Boogerd W, Linn SC, Gundy CM, et al. Effects of tamoxifen and exemestane on cognitive functioning of post-menopausal patients with breast cancer: results from the neuropsychological side study of the tamoxifen and exemestane adjuvant multinational trial. J Clin Oncol. 2010;28:1249–300.

102. Sliwkowski MX, Lofgren JA, Lewis GD, Hotaling TE, Fendly BM, Fox JA, et al. Nonclinical studies addressing the mechanism of action of trastuzumab (Herceptin). Semin Oncol. 1999;26(4 suppl 12):60–70.

103. Slamon DJ, Leyland-Jones B, Shak S, Fuchs H, Paton V, Bajamonde A, et al. Use of chemotherapy plus a monoclonal antibody against HER2 for metastatic breast cancer that overexpresses HER2. N Engl J Med. 2001;344(11):783–92.

104. Marty M, Cognetti F, Maraninchi D, Snyder R, Mauriac L, Tubiana-Hulin M, et al. Randomized phase II trial of the efficacy and safety of trastuzumab combined with docetaxel in patients with human epidermal growth factor receptor 2-positive metastatic breast cancer administered as first-line treatment: the M77001 study group. J Clin Oncol. 2005;23(19):4265–74.

105. Piccart-Gebhart MJ, Procter M, Leyland-Jones B, Goldhirsch A, Untch M, Smith I, Herceptin Adjuvant (HERA) Trial Study Team, et al. Trastuzumab after adjuvant chemotherapy in HER2-positive breast cancer. N Engl J Med. 2005;353(16):1659–72.

106. Joensuu H, Kellokumpu-Lehtinen PL, Bono P, Alanko T, Kataja V, Asola R, et al; FinHer Study Investigators. Adjuvant docetaxel or vinorelbine with or without trastuzumab for breast cancer. N Engl J Med. 2006;354(8):809–20.

107. Perez EA, Suman VJ, Davidson NE, Gralow JR, Kaufman PA, Visscher DW, et al. Sequential versus concurrent trastuzumab in adjuvant chemotherapy for breast cancer. J Clin Oncol. 2011;29(34):4491–7.

108. Slamon D, Eiermann W, Robert N, Pienkowski T, Martin M, Press M, et al; Breast Cancer International Research Group. Adjuvant trastuzumab in HER2-positive breast cancer. N Engl J Med. 2011;365(14):1273–83.

109. Geyer CE, Forster J, Lindquist D, Chan S, Romieu CG, Pienkowski T, et al. Lapatinib plus capecitabine for HER2-positive advanced breast cancer. N Engl J Med. 2006;355(26):2733–43.

110. Johnston S, Pippen Jr J, Pivot X, Lichinitser M, Sadeghi S, Dieras V, et al. Lapatinib combined with letrozole versus letrozole and placebo as first-line therapy for postmenopausal hormone receptor-positive metastatic breast cancer. J Clin Oncol. 2009;27(33): 5538–46.

111. Friedländer E, Barok M, Szöllosi J, Vereb G. ErbB-directed immunotherapy: antibodies in current practice and promising new agents. Immunol Lett. 2008;116(2):126–40.

112. Krop IE, Beeram M, Modi S, Jones SF, Holden SN, Yu W, et al. Phase I study of trastuzumab-DM1, an HER2 antibody-drug conjugate, given every 3 weeks to patients with HER2-positive metastatic breast cancer. J Clin Oncol. 2010;28(16):2698–704.

113. Burstein HJ, Sun Y, Dirix LY, Jiang Z, Paridaens R, Tan AR, et al. Neratinib, an irreversible ErbB receptor tyrosine kinase inhibitor, in patients with advanced ErbB2-positive breast cancer. J Clin Oncol. 2010;28(8):1301–7.

114. Shih J, Yang C, Su W, et al. A phase II study of BIBW 2992, a novel irreversible dual EGFR and HER2 tyrosine kinase inhibitor (TKI), in patients with adenocarcinoma of the lung and activating EGFR mutations after failure of one line of chemotherapy (LUX-Lung 2). J Clin Oncol. 2009;27(suppl; abstr 8013):15s.

115. Yang C, Shih J, Su W, et al. A phase II study of BIBW 2992 in patients with adenocarcinoma of the lung and activating EGFR mutations (LUX-Lung 2). J Clin Oncol. 2010;28(suppl; abstr 7521):15s.

116. Hickish T, Wheatley D, Lin N, Carey L, Houston S, Mendelson D, et al. Use of BIBW 2992, a novel irreversible EGFR/HER1 and

HER2 tyrosine kinase inhibitor to treat patients with HER2-positive metastatic breast cancer after failure of treatment with trastuzumab. Cancer Res. 2009;69(24 suppl):5060.

117. Blackwell KL, Burstein HJ, Storniolo AM, Rugo H, Sledge G, Koehler M, et al. Randomized study of Lapatinib alone or in combination with trastuzumab in women with ErbB2-positive, trastuzumab-refractory metastatic breast cancer. J Clin Oncol. 2010;28(7):1124–30.

118. Baselga J, Cortes J, Kim SB, Im SA, Hegg R, Im YH, et al. for the CLEOPATRA study group. Pertuzumab plus trastuzumab plus docetaxel for metastatic breast cancer. N Engl J Med. 2012;366(2):109–19. doi:10.1056NEJMoa1113216. Epub 2011 Dec 7.

119. Relf M, LeJeune S, Scott PA, Fox S, Smith K, Leek R, et al. Expression of the angiogenic factors vascular endothelial cell growth factor, acidic and basic fibroblast growth factor, tumor growth factor beta-1, platelet-derived endothelial cell growth factor, placenta growth factor, and pleiotrophin in human primary breast cancer and its relation to angiogenesis. Cancer Res. 1997;57(5): 963–9.

120. Miller K, Wang M, Gralow J, Dickler M, Cobleigh M, Perez EA, et al. Paclitaxel plus bevacizumab versus paclitaxel alone for metastatic breast cancer. N Engl J Med. 2007;357(26):2666–76.

121. Miles DW, Chan A, Dirix LY, Cortés J, Pivot X, Tomczak P, et al. Phase III study of bevacizumab plus docetaxel compared with placebo plus docetaxel for the first-line treatment of human epidermal growth factor receptor 2-negative metastatic breast cancer. J Clin Oncol. 2010;28(20):3239–47.

122. Miller KD, Chap LI, Holmes FA, Cobleigh MA, Marcom PK, Fehrenbacher L, et al. Randomized phase III trial of capecitabine compared with bevacizumab plus capecitabine in patients with previously treated metastatic breast cancer. J Clin Oncol. 2005;23(4):792–9.

123. Robert NJ, Diéras V, Glaspy J, Brufsky AM, Bondarenko I, Lipatov ON, et al. RIBBON-1: randomized, double-blind, placebo-controlled, phase III trial of chemotherapy with or without bevacizumab for first-line treatment of human epidermal growth factor receptor 2-negative, locally recurrent or metastatic breast cancer. J Clin Oncol. 2011;29(10):1252–60.

124. Brufsky A, Bondarenko IN, Smirnov V, Hurvitz S, Perez E, Ponomarova O, et al. RIBBON-2: a randomized, doubleblind, placebo-controlled, phase III trial evaluating the efficacy and safety of bevacizumab in combination with chemotherapy for second-line treatment of HER2-negative metastatic breast cancer. Cancer Res. 2009;69(suppl. 3; abstr 42):495s.

125. Hamilton EP, Blackwell KL. Safety of bevacizumab in patients with metastatic breast cancer. Oncology. 2011;80(5–6):314–25.

126. Avastin (bevacizumab) [prescribing information]. South San Francisco: Genentech; 2011.

127. Chobanian AV, Bakris GL, Black HR, Cushman WC, Green LA, Izzo JL Jr, et al; Joint National Committee on Prevention, Detection, Evaluation, and Treatment of High Blood Pressure. National Heart, Lung, and Blood Institute; National High Blood Pressure Education Program Coordinating Committee. Seventh report of the Joint National Committee on prevention, detection, evaluation, and treatment of high blood pressure. hypertension. 2003;42(6):1206–52.

128. Chen HX, Cleck JN. Adverse effects of anticancer agents that target the VEGF pathway. Nat Rev Clin Oncol. 2009;6(8):465–77.

129. Besse B, Lasserre SF, Compton P, Huang J, Augustus S, Rohr UP. Bevacizumab safety in patients with central nervous system metastases. Clin Cancer Res. 2010;16(1):269–78.

130. Nghiemphu PL, Green RM, Pope WB, Lai A, Cloughesy TF. Safety of anticoagulation use and bevacizumab in patients with glioma. Neuro Oncol. 2008;10(3):355–60.

131. Hambleton J, Skillings J, Kabbinavar F, Bergsland E, Holmgren E, Holden SN, et al. Safety of low-dose aspirin (ASA) in a pooled analysis of 3 randomized, controlled trials (RCTs) of bevacizumab (BV) with chemotherapy (CT) in patients (pts) with metastatic colorectal cancer (mCRC). J Clin Oncol. 2005;23(16s):3554. ASCO annual meeting proceedings. Part I of II (June 1 suppl).

132. Dirix LY, Romieu G, Provencher L, Grimes D, de Souzo VL, Paterson A, et al. Safety of bevacizumab (BV) plus docetaxel (D) in patients (pts) with locally recurrent (LR) or metastatic breast cancer (mBC) who developed brain metastases during the AVADO phase III study. Cancer Res. 2009;69(suppl 2; abstr 4116):292s.

133. Scappaticci FA, Skillings JR, Holden SN, Gerber HP, Miller K, Kabbinavar F, et al. Arterial thromboembolic events in patients with metastatic carcinoma treated with chemotherapy and bevacizumab. J Natl Cancer Inst. 2007;99(16):1232–9.

134. Higa GM, Abraham J. Biological mechanisms of bevacizumab-associated adverse events. Expert Rev Anticancer Ther. 2009;9(7):999–1007.

135. Choueiri TK, Mayer EL, Je Y, Rosenberg JE, Nguyen PL, Azzi GR, et al. Congestive heart failure risk in patients with breast cancer treated with bevacizumab. J Clin Oncol. 2011;29(6):632–8.

136. Monsuez JJ, Charniot JC, Vignat N, Artigou JY. Cardiac side-effects of cancer chemotherapy. Int J Cardiol. 2010;144(1):3–15.

137. Van Poznak C. Osteonecrosis of the jaw and bevacizumab therapy. Breast Cancer Res Treat. 2010;122(1):189–91.

138. Kaufman B, Mackey JR, Clemens MR, Bapsy PP, Vaid A, Wardley A, et al. Trastuzumab plus anastrozole versus anastrozole alone for the treatment of postmenopausal women with human epidermal growth factor receptor 2-positive, hormone receptor-positive

metastatic breast cancer: results from the randomized phase III TAnDEM study. J Clin Oncol. 2009;27(33):5529–37.

139. Cobleigh MA, Vogel CL, Tripathy D, Robert NJ, Scholl S, Fehrenbacher L, et al. Multinational study of the efficacy and safety of humanized anti-HER2 monoclonal antibody in women who have HER2-overexpressing metastatic breast cancer that has progressed after chemotherapy for metastatic disease. J Clin Oncol. 1999;17(9):2639–48.

140. Boxed WARNINGS and Additional Important Safety Information. http://www.herceptin.com/hcp/. Accessed on Nov 2011.

141. Chung CH. Managing premedications and the risk for reactions to infusional monoclonal antibody therapy. Oncologist. 2008;13(6): 725–32.

142. Lenihan D, Suter T, Brammer M, Neate C, Ross G, Baselga J, et al. Pooled analysis of cardiac safety in patients with cancer treated with pertuzumab. Ann Oncol. 2012;23(3):791–800. Epub 2011 Jun 10.

143. Baselga J, Gelmon KA, Verma S, Wardley A, Conte P, Miles D, et al. Phase II trial of pertuzumab and trastuzumab in patients with human epidermal growth factor receptor 2-positive metastatic breast cancer that progressed during prior trastuzumab therapy. J Clin Oncol. 2010;28(7):1138–44.

144. Gianni L, Lladó A, Bianchi G, Cortes J, Kellokumpu-Lehtinen PL, Cameron DA, et al. Open-label, phase II, multicenter, randomized study of the efficacy and safety of two dose levels of Pertuzumab, a human epidermal growth factor receptor 2 dimerization inhibitor, in patients with human epidermal growth factor receptor 2-negative metastatic breast cancer. J Clin Oncol. 2010;28(7):1131–7.

145. Burris 3rd HA, Rugo HS, Vukelja SJ, Vogel CL, Borson RA, Limentani S, et al. Phase II study of the antibody drug conjugate trastuzumab-DM1 for the treatment of human epidermal growth factor receptor 2 (HER2)-positive breast cancer after prior HER2-directed therapy. J Clin Oncol. 2011;29(4):398–405.

146. Chatsiproios D, Haidinger R, Suter T. Practical management recommendations for anti-ErbB2 therapy with lapatinib. Breast Care (Basel). 2008;3(s1):13–6.

147. Moy B, Goss PE. Lapatinib-associated toxicity and practical management recommendations. Oncologist. 2007;12(7):756–65.

148. Spraggs CF, Budde LR, Briley LP, Bing N, Cox CJ, King KS, et al. HLA-DQA1*02:01 is a major risk factor for lapatinib-induced hepatotoxicity in women with advanced breast cancer. J Clin Oncol. 2011;29(6):667–73.

149. Moy B, Rappold E, Williams L, et al. Hepatobiliary abnormalities in patients with metastatic cancer treated with lapatinib. J Clin Oncol. 2009;27(suppl; abstr 1043):15s.

150. Perez EA, Koehler M, Byrne J, Preston AJ, Rappold E, Ewer MS. Cardiac safety of lapatinib: pooled analysis of 3689 patients enrolled in clinical trials. Mayo Clin Proc. 2008;83(6):679–86.

151. Neratinib trials investigator file.
152. Suter TM, Procter M, van Veldhuisen DJ, Muscholl M, Bergh J, Carlomagno C, et al. Trastuzumab-associated cardiac adverse effects in the herceptin adjuvant trial. J Clin Oncol. 2007;25(25): 3859–65.
153. Jones AL, Barlow M, Barrett-Lee PJ, Canney PA, Gilmour IM, Robb SD, et al. Management of cardiac health in trastuzumab-treated patients with breast cancer: updated United Kingdom National Cancer Research Institute recommendations for monitoring. Br J Cancer. 2009;100(5):684–92.
154. Russell SD, Blackwell KL, Lawrence J, Pippen Jr JE, Roe MT, Wood F, et al. Independent adjudication of symptomatic heart failure with the use of doxorubicin and cyclophosphamide followed by trastuzumab adjuvant therapy: a combined review of cardiac data from the National Surgical Adjuvant breast and Bowel Project B-31 and the North Central Cancer Treatment Group N9831 clinical trials. J Clin Oncol. 2010;28(21):3416–21.
155. Azim H, Azim Jr HA, Escudier B. Trastuzumab versus lapatinib: the cardiac side of the story. Cancer Treat Rev. 2009;35(7):633–8.
156. Giordano FJ, Gerber HP, Williams SP, VanBruggen N, Bunting S, Ruiz-Lozano P, et al. A cardiac myocyte vascular endothelial growth factor paracrine pathway is required to maintain cardiac function. Proc Natl Acad Sci USA. 2001;98(10):5780–5.
157. Kamba T, McDonald DM. Mechanisms of adverse effects of anti-VEGF therapy for cancer. Br J Cancer. 2007;96(12):1788–95.
158. Allegra CJ, Yothers G, O'Connell MJ, Sharif S, Colangelo LH, Lopa SH, et al. Initial safety report of NSABP C 08: a randomized phase III study of modified FOLFOX6 with or without bevacizumab for the adjuvant treatment of patients with stage II or III colon cancer. J Clin Oncol. 2009;27(20):3385–90.
159. Gomez HL, Doval DC, Chavez MA, Ang PC, Aziz Z, Nag S, et al. Efficacy and safety of lapatinib as first-line therapy for ErbB2-amplified locally advanced or metastatic breast cancer. J Clin Oncol. 2008;26(18):2999–3005.
160. Teng WC, Oh JW, New LS, Wahlin MD, Nelson SD, Ho HK, et al. Mechanism-based inactivation of cytochrome P450 3A4 by lapatinib. Mol Pharmacol. 2010;78(4):693–703.
161. Loriot Y, Perlemuter G, Malka D, Penault-Llorca F, Boige V, Deutsch E, et al. Drug insight: gastrointestinal and hepatic adverse effects of molecular-targeted agents in cancer therapy. Nat Clin Pract Oncol. 2008;5(5):268–78.
162. Uribe JM, Keely SJ, Traynor-Kaplan AE, Barrett KE. Phosphatidylinositol 3-kinase mediates the inhibitory effect of epidermal growth factor on calcium-dependent chloride secretion. J Biol Chem. 1996;271(43):26588–95.
163. Wong KK, Fracasso PM, Bukowski RM, Lynch TJ, Munster PN, Shapiro GI, et al. A phase I study with neratinib (HKI-272), an

irreversible pan ErbB receptor tyrosine kinase inhibitor, in patients with solid tumors. Clin Cancer Res. 2009;15(7):2552–8.

164. Busam KJ, Capodieci P, Motzer R, Kiehn T, Phelan D, Halpern AC. Cutaneous side-effects in cancer patients treated with the antiepidermal growth factor receptor antibody C225. Br J Dermatol. 2001;144:1169–76.

165. Lacouture ME. Mechanisms of cutaneous toxicities to EGFR inhibitors. Nat Rev Cancer. 2006;6(10):803–12.

166. Peréz-Soler R, Saltz L. Cutaneous adverse effects with HER1/EGFR-targeted agents: is there a silver lining? J Clin Oncol. 2005;23(22):5235–46.

167. Kris MG, Natale RB, Herbst RS, Lynch Jr TJ, Prager D, Belani CP, et al. Efficacy of gefitinib, an inhibitor of the epidermal growth factor receptor tyrosine kinase, in symptomatic patients with non-small cell lung cancer: a randomized trial. JAMA. 2003;290(16):2149–58.

168. Bergeron A, Bergot E, Vilela G, Ades L, Devergie A, Espérou H, et al. Hypersensitivity pneumonitis related to imatinib mesylate. J Clin Oncol. 2002;20(20):4271–2.

169. Vahid B, Esmaili A. Erlotinib-associated acute pneumonitis: report of two cases. Can Respir J. 2007;14(3):167–70.

170. Makris D, Scherpereel A, Copin MC, Colin G, Brun L, Lafitte JJ, et al. Fatal interstitial lung disease associated with oral erlotinib therapy for lung cancer. BMC Cancer. 2007;7:150.

171. Chang SC, Chang CY, Chen CY, Yu CJ. Successful erlotinib rechallenge after gefitinib-induced acute interstitial pneumonia. J Thorac Oncol. 2010;5(7):1105–6.

172. Kuo LC, Lin PC, Wang KF, Yuan MK, Chang SC. Successful treatment of gefitinib-induced acute interstitial pneumonitis with high-dose corticosteroid: a case report and literature review. Med Oncol. 2011;28(1):79–82.

173. Yokoyama T, Miyazawa K, Kurakawa E, Nagate A, Shimamoto T, Iwaya K, et al. Interstitial pneumonia induced by imatinib mesylate: pathologic study demonstrates alveolar destruction and fibrosis with eosinophilic infiltration. Leukemia. 2004;18(3):645–6.

174. Capri G, Chang J, Chen SC, Conte P, Cwiertka K, Jerusalem G, et al. An open-label expanded access study of lapatinib and capecitabine in patients with HER2-overexpressing locally advanced or metastatic breast cancer. Ann Oncol. 2010;21(3):474–80.

175. Yap TA, Vidal L, Adam J, Stephens P, Spicer J, Shaw H, et al. Phase I trial of the irreversible EGFR and HER2 kinase inhibitor BIBW 2992 in patients with advanced solid tumors. J Clin Oncol. 2010;28(25):3965–72.

176. Gnant M, Mlineritsch B, Stoeger H, Luschin-Ebengreuth G, Heck D, Menzel C, et al. Adjuvant endocrine therapy plus zolendronic acid in premenopausal women with early-stage breast cancer:

62-month follow-up from the ABCSG-12 randomised trial. Lancet Oncol. 2011;12(7):631–41.

177. Eidtmann H, de Boer R, Bundred N, Llombart-Cussac A, Davidson N, Neven P, et al. Efficacy of zolendronic acid in postmenopausal women with early breast cancer receiving adjuvant letrozole: 36-months results of the ZO-FAST study. Ann Oncol. 2010;21:2188–94.

178. Coleman RE, Marshall H, Cameron D, Dodwell D, Burkinshaw R, Keane M, et al.; AZURE Investigators. Breast-cancer adjuvant therapy with zolendronic acid. N Engl J Med. 2011;365(15):1396–405.

179. Lacey DL, Timms E, Tan HL, Kelley MJ, Dunstan CR, Burgess T, et al. Osteoprotegerin ligand is a cytokine that regulates osteoclast differentiation and activation. Cell. 1998;93:165–76.

180. Roodman GD. Mechanisms of bone metastasis. N Engl J Med. 2004;350:1655–64.

181. Stopeck AT, Lipton A, Body JJ, Steger GG, Tonkin K, de Boer RH, et al. Denosumab compared with zolendronic acid for the treatment of bone metastases in patients with advanced breast cancer: a randomized double-blind study. J Clin Oncol. 2010;28(35):5132–9.

# Chapter 3
## Lung Cancer

**Stefan Zimmermann, Alessandra Curioni Fontecedro,
Rolf A. Stahel, and Solange Peters**

**Abstract**  Lung cancer treatment strategy relies on an accurate staging of the disease and a careful evaluation of patient characteristics, including capability of undergoing and tolerating a defined treatment plan. Therefore, a solid knowledge on all intervention-related adverse events and drug toxicities is essential for a reliable decision-making process.

Most lung cancer patients are diagnosed at an advanced stage of the disease, correlated with a dismal prognosis. Systemic therapy is the mainstay, and drug selection still strongly relies on expected toxicity profile. This chapter first

S. Zimmermann, M.D. (✉)
Centre Pluridisciplinaire d'Oncologie, Centre Hospitalier Universitaire Vaudois, Lausanne, Switzerland
e-mail: stefan.zimmermann@chuv.ch

A.C. Fontecedro, M.D.
Department of Thoracic Surgery, University Hospital Zurich, Zurich, Switzerland

R.A. Stahel, M.D.
Clinic of Oncology, University Hospital Zurich, Ramistrasse 100, Zurich, Switzerland

S. Peters, M.D., Ph.D.
Department of Oncology, Centre Hospitalier Universitaire Vaudois, Lausanne, Switzerland

M.A. Dicato (ed.), *Side Effects of Medical Cancer Therapy,*
DOI 10.1007/978-0-85729-787-7_3,
© Springer-Verlag London 2013

describes the drug standard options and their respective toxicities in this context. Side effects of more complex multimodality combined treatments of early non–small-cell lung cancer as well as small-cell lung cancer, usually involving use of the same cytotoxic agents jointly with surgery and radiotherapy, are discussed in the second part of this chapter.

**Keywords**    Non–small-cell lung cancer • Small-cell lung cancer Side effects • Tyrosine kinase inhibitor (TKI) • Platinum doublets Combined modalities

# Non–Small-Cell Lung Cancer

Lung cancer is the most common malignancy and the leading cause of human cancer deaths worldwide. Lung cancer deaths have begun to decline in men, reflecting a decrease in smoking; in contrast, it has become the main cause of cancer deaths in women in developed countries [1]. Seventy-five percent of patients are symptomatic at the time of diagnosis. The majority of patients with non–small-cell lung cancer (NSCLC) present at an advanced stage of the disease, with a poor prognosis and the absence of any curative option. For earlier-stage disease, essentially stages I and II (cT1a cN0 to cT2b cN1, according to the seventh edition of the TNM staging system), upfront surgery, followed by adjuvant chemotherapy for stage II and selected IB patients, offers the best chances for long-term survival. In stage IV, systemic palliative treatment is recommended with a series of targeted agents that constitute potential new treatment options, as they have shown promising results in a subset of selected NSCLC patients.

## Systemic Therapy in Advanced NSCLC

Decisions regarding systemic therapy for advanced NSCLC have traditionally been based on performance status of the patients, comorbidities, expected toxicity profile, and patient preferences. While this still holds true, recent developments mandate that one take additional information into account, namely, tumor histology differentiating non-squamous from squamous cell lung cancer as well as molecular tumor characteristics.

## First-Line Systemic Therapy for Advanced NSCLC

### Adenocarcinoma

In the past few years, treatment of metastatic adenocarcinoma of the lung has changed remarkably. Until a few years ago, adenocarcinoma patients were treated with standard NSCLC chemotherapy, irrespective of any histologic consideration. Nowadays patient selection has become mandatory in order to customize treatment. For adenocarcinoma, the ESMO guidelines recommend the analysis of EGFR (epithelial growth factor receptor) mutational status before making decisions about the frontline therapy [2]. In the presence of activating mutations, tyrosine kinase inhibitors (TKIs), namely, gefitinib [3, 4] or erlotinib [5–7], are recommended, because they have been associated with a higher response rate and a significantly better progression-free survival as compared to chemotherapy.

In the absence of activating mutations, a platinum-based combination with pemetrexed is preferred. Pemetrexed combined with cisplatin was associated with a better tolerability and better overall survival compared to a gemcitabine combined with cisplatin [8]. Cisplatin, if possible, should be preferred as frontline therapy owing to improved progression-free survival and overall survival when compared to carboplatin based on large meta-analyses [9]. A platinum-based doublet regimen with the addition of bevacizumab can also be considered, particularly in combination with carboplatin and paclitaxel [10, 11].

### Squamous Cell Carcinoma

The combination of a platinum-based therapy with gemcitabine can be considered as a first choice, but other doublets appear to be equally effective [12]. Molecular analysis of squamous cell lung cancer has not yet entered routine practice.

## Second-Line Systemic Therapy for Advanced NSCLC

With the exception of patients with an EGFR-mutated tumor receiving first-line erlotinib or gefitinib, second-line therapy usually consists of monotherapy with either docetaxel or erlotinib or, for patients with non-squamous NSCLC, pemetrexed, if it is not administered as first-line therapy. For patients with adenocarcinoma and an ALK gene rearrangement, the tyrosine kinase inhibitor crizotinib is emerging as a promising, and probably future standard, option [13].

## Palliative Radiotherapy

Palliative radiotherapy might be required to treat painful metastasis (bone, skin, soft tissue) and local complications due to metastasis (e.g., CNS or spinal cord compression) or related to the primary tumor (hemoptysis, vena cava compression, atelectasis due to bronchial obstruction). Usually, the relatively low dose delivered in this setting and the limited field extent strongly limits this strategy's toxicity, which consists mainly of local inflammation-related symptoms and fatigue. A rare side effect is the radiation recall syndrome (RRS), an inflammatory skin reaction that occurs in a previously irradiated body part following drug administration. This phenomenon may occur from days to years following exposure to ionizing radiation.

## Side Effects of Agents Used for the Systemic Treatment of Advanced NSCLC

### Clinical Side Effects of Tyrosine Kinase Inhibitors

The currently used EGFR TKIs, erlotinib and gefitinib, may be given for long periods in patients with sensitizing EGFR mutations and therefore might be associated with chronic side effects. The most common are cutaneous and gastrointestinal toxicities. Grade 1–2 cutaneous side effects have been reported in more than 60 % of patients, and grade 3–4 in about 15 % of patients. These include folliculitis, which can be treated, if moderate, with topical antibiotics and systemically with tetracyclines (e.g., doxycycline 100 mg/day) in case of widespread lesions. Other typical cutaneous side effects are hair changes (as trichomegaly) and paronychial inflammation. This disorder can progress from erythema to painful lateral nail fold pyogenic granuloma-like lesion. As prevention, the patient should be advised to avoid trauma to the parony-chium. In case of advanced lesions, antiseptic treatments should be applied and bacterial cultures should be sampled, if a bacterial infection is suspected. The use of steroid for cutaneous side effects remains controversial [14].

The most common gastrointestinal side effects of TKIs are diarrhea, described in about 10 % of patients and commonly treated with loperamide, and nausea [15]. Fatigue has been also reported in 5–15 % of patients [16]. Infrequent but potentially fatal complications include an acute interstitial lung disease (ILD) and acute hepatitis; treatment of these side effects includes high-dose steroids [17, 18].

Clinical Side Effects of Chemotherapy

*Cisplatin*

The most common side effects of cisplatin include nausea and fatigue, as well as neurotoxicity and ototoxicity, which have been known to sometimes last several weeks or months after treatment; neurotoxicity potentially can worsen after the end of treatment. Myelosuppression due to cisplatin occurs in about 50 % of patients and is generally mild, with only 10 % of patients experiencing grade 3–4 toxicity [19, 20]. To date there is no indication for prophylactic antibiotics or granulocyte colony-stimulating factor (G-CSF) therapy in patients receiving cisplatin-based chemotherapy. Nausea and vomiting occur very frequently; therefore, prophylactic therapy with a three-drug regimen including single doses of a 5-HT$_3$ receptor antagonist, dexamethasone, and aprepitant is recommended [21]. Ototoxicity characterized by a dose-dependent sensorineural hearing loss with tinnitus has been described to affect 15–20 %

of patients. Prevention of this complication includes a hearing assessment before treatment in order to exclude patients with hearing diseases from cisplatin-based chemotherapy. If it occurs during treatment, the recommendation is to discontinue cisplatin and to use alternative agents [22].

Nephrotoxicity may result from a direct effect of cisplatin to tubular epithelial cells as well as from vasoconstriction in the renal microvasculature and proinflammatory effects, leading to a renal function impairment and electrolyte alteration. In order to prevent this complication, intravenous isotonic saline before and after the treatment must be administered. Treatment of nephrotoxicity includes the discontinuation of cisplatin and the management of acute renal dysfunction or renal failure as for other diseases.

### Carboplatin

Carboplatin was developed to provide a less toxic, more convenient alternative to cisplatin. However, hematologic toxicity is more pronounced than with cisplatin, including severe neutropenia, anemia, and thrombocytopenia [9, 23]. The use of prophylactic G-CSF might be considered when carboplatin is combined with taxanes. Ototoxicity, neurotoxicity, and renal toxicity occur less frequently with carboplatin compared to cisplatin, but electrolyte disorders can occur in about 5 % of patients. Nausea or vomiting are largely less intense than with cisplatin; the combination of palonosetron plus dexamethasone prophylaxis is generally sufficient for prevention. Of note is the occurrence of allergic infusion reactions reported in up to 15 % of patients; interestingly, these develop more often in patients who have been extensively treated with this medication [24]. Recurrence of such reactions at readministration of carboplatin can be successfully prevented with desensitization procedures.

### Pemetrexed [8, 25, 26]

Pemetrexed is generally part of the first-line treatment for adenocarcinoma. The most common side effect of pemetrexed is myelotoxicity. The administration of vitamin B12 concurrent with folate acid has reduced its hematotoxicity to a very moderate level, with grade 3 and 4 neutropenia occurring in only about 15 % of patients. Nausea and vomiting have been reported in less than 5 % of patients. A common grade 1–2 side effect is constipation.

*Bevacizumab [11]*

The most common grade 3 or higher events reported with bevacizumab are thromboembolic events (5 %), bleeding (epistaxis, hemoptysis, CNS hemorrhage, 2–3 %), gastrointestinal perforation (1 %), hypertension (5–8 %), and proteinuria (3–6 %). Myelotoxicity is almost nonexistent as monotherapy; a slightly higher rate of neutropenia, febrile neutropenia, and thrombocytopenia has been reported when it is combined with chemotherapy as compared to chemotherapy alone [27, 28].

Renal toxicity is a rare but possible fatal side effect due to renal thrombotic microangiopathy and interstitial nephritis, leading to proteinuria and acute kidney injury. Clinically, the most important side effect is hypertension due to the production of nitric oxide as well as increase of vascular resistance through the inhibition of new blood vessel formation, as observed as a drug class effect also with other antiangiogenic molecules. Hypertension has been reported as grade 1–2 in about 15 % of patients and in 2–10 % as grade 3–4 [29, 30]. To date, there are no guidelines for treatment of hypertension in these patients; however, there are controversies regarding the use of calcium antagonists in this setting [31, 32]. Determination and management of blood pressure during therapy, with a goal of less than 140/90 mmHg for most patients, in patients with specific preexisting cardiovascular risk factors is recommended.

*Gemcitabine [33, 34]*

Toxicity of gemcitabine is generally mild and reversible after discontinuation of medication. The most common side effects are flu-like symptoms in about 50 % of patients, with fever or arthralgia. Edema (e.g., ankles) is also often observed and does not correlate with renal or cardiac dysfunction [35]. Grade 3–4 myelosuppression occurs frequently, including anemia (5 %), thrombocytopenia (1 %), leukopenia (7 %), and neutropenia (22 %), rarely resulting in neutropenia-related infection. Grade 3–4 liver toxicity can be detected in up to 10 % of patients. Nausea and vomiting often occur but are of low grade and can be prevented with a single antiemetic agent such as dexamethasone, a 5-HT$_3$ receptor antagonist, or a dopamine receptor antagonist. Of note are a few cases of severe lung toxicity, with a frequency varying in several reports from 0.1 to 5 % [36].

*Docetaxel [25, 37, 38]*

The most common side effects of docetaxel are myelotoxicity and fatigue. The rate of grade 3 or 4 neutropenia due to docetaxel varies from 40 to 60 % (according to dosage), and the risk of neutropenic fever is described in 3 % of patients. These results led to the consideration of adopting a prophylactic therapy with G-CSF, which to date is recommended in patients who had experienced a clinically significant neutropenic event with a previous cycle. Nonhematologic toxicities included alopecia, mild nausea and vomiting, and allergic manifestations such as skin rash and pruritus; therefore, pretreatment with steroids is recommended. Rare hypersensitivity reactions to docetaxel can be overcome with desensitization procedures.

# Treatment of Early NSCLC

## Surgery

Lobectomy and systematic lymph node dissection is considered standard therapy for early (stage I and II) NSCLC. Sublobar resection in the form of anatomical segmentectomy may lead to equivalent survival rates among patients with stage I NSCLC less than 1 cm in size, and is associated with fewer complications and better postoperative lung function [39]. Large wedge resections may be an option for patients who cannot tolerate a lobectomy because of severely compromised pulmonary function, advanced age, or other significant comorbidity, but they do not represent a standard of care.

Thirty-day mortality rate after lobectomy is expected to be lower than 2 % in high-volume hospitals [40]. Pretreatment pulmonary functions tests are well-known predictors of surgical risk [41–43].

Anatomical resections are currently performed according to the Bolliger and Miller algorithms that are based on forced expired volume in 1 second (FEV1) and lung carbon monoxide diffusion capacity (DLCO). Percentage of predicted FEV1 and DLCO values were shown to correlate with patient outcome (hospital and overall mortality) in patients undergoing resections. Postoperative complications and mortality were also shown to be correlated, even with a large variability, to hospital volume and surgeon skills [44]. Pneumonectomy is seldom indicated in stage I and II NSCLC, but it is associated with a higher operative mortality rate, especially for right pneumonectomy [45].

Minimally invasive video-assisted lobectomy was shown to be equivalent to open lobectomy in terms of locoregional recurrences. Data suggest a reduced systemic recurrence rate and an improved 5-year mortality rate, but since most studies were not randomized, the effect of case selection is difficult to ascertain, even if highly probable [46]. Complete mediastinal lymphadenectomy adds little morbidity to a pulmonary resection for lung cancer and possesses a prognostic impact [47, 48].

A consistent proportion of patients undergoing lung resection exhibit an important postoperative worsening in their QoL: 28 % in the physical component summary and 15 % in the mental component summary. Patients with a better preoperative physical functioning and those with worse mental health scores were those at higher risk of a relevant physical deterioration. Patients with a lower predicted postoperative forced expiratory volume in 1 second (ppoFEV1) and higher preoperative scores of social functioning and mental health were those at higher risk of a relevant emotional deterioration. Compared with the general population, nearly half of the patients displayed a depressed physical and emotional status 3 months after surgery [49]. The extent of resection, age, and adjuvant therapy was associated with a clinically relevant decline in the physical aspect of health-related quality of life 6 months after surgery [50].

## Adjuvant Chemotherapy

Despite optimum surgical management, the 5-year survival rate of resected NSCLC ranges from 25 to 75 % according to pathologic stage. A large meta-analysis by the NSCLC Collaborative Group suggests an absolute improvement in 5-year survival with platinum-based chemotherapy of 5 % (2–7) for stage IB (from 55 to 60 %), 5 % (3–8) for stage II (from 40 to 45 %), and 5 % (3–8) for stage III disease (from 30 to 35 %) [51]. Another large meta-analysis showed a detrimental effect of adjuvant chemotherapy in stage IA NSCLC [52]. The most commonly used regimens are cisplatin in combination with vinorelbine or etoposide. Cisplatin and vinorelbine adjuvant chemotherapy is associated with frequent hematologic toxic effects, including high-grade neutropenia in 85 % of patients. Common nonhematologic effects include asthenia and nausea or vomiting. There are approximately 2 % treatment-related deaths, mainly from septic shock [53]. Overall, compliance and, as a consequence, dose-intensity and total dose of adjuvant chemotherapy are disappointing. Altogether, 59 % of patients receive at least 240 mg/m$^2$ of cisplatin, this parameter being potentially more important than the choice of the second compound [52]. Regarding chemotherapy strategy, 14 % of patients received only one cycle and 10 % only two cycles, mainly because of patient refusal (35 %), toxicity (34 %), and early death or progression (9 %). The median delay between surgery and the start of chemotherapy was 39 days (>60 days in 7 % of patients) [52].

The beneficial effect of adjuvant chemotherapy on recurrences does not decrease with longer follow-up, and there is no increase in the number of secondary malignancies potentially related to a carcinogenic effect of chemotherapy. However, the maintained beneficial effect of preventing lung cancer deaths contrasts with a probable chemotherapy-induced increase in non-lung cancer mortality after 5 years that can decrease but not nullify the beneficial effect of adjuvant therapy [54]. Statistically significant causes of non-cancer deaths after cisplatin-based chemotherapy in the non-lung cancer setting were infections and circulatory and respiratory diseases [55].

## Postoperative Radiotherapy

Postoperative radiotherapy has a deleterious effect on patients with early stages I and II [56, 57]. In contrast with N2 disease, where the PORT-induced morbidity might be outweighed by the presence of residual microscopic disease, treated by radiotherapy, in patients with N0 and N1 disease, this benefit is not reproduced. With the limitation related to the availability of retrospective data only, where confounding factors in patient selection may have biased this interpretation, radiotherapy-related toxicity is probably one of the factors involved in this negative impact of PORT.

# Small-Cell Lung Cancer

Small-cell lung cancer (SCLC) accounts for approximately 15 % of primary lung carcinoma. It is invariably associated with tobacco exposure and is characterized by rapid tumor doubling time and early development of metastases. Less than 10 % of patients are asymptomatic at diagnosis. Of all histologic subtypes of lung cancer, SCLC is the most sensitive to chemotherapy and radiotherapy, but prognosis remains dismal [58]. Staging of SCLC is made according to the 7th TNM classification and according to a two-stage system developed by the Veteran's Administration Lung Cancer Study Group, dividing patients into limited (stages IA to IIIB) or extensive (stage IV) stage disease. Limited disease is thus defined as disease confined to one hemithorax (i.e., disease that can be included in a "tolerable" radiation field). Approximately one-third of patients present with clinical definition of "limited disease," but most of these patients already present with subclinical metastatic disease.

## Extensive Disease

Chemotherapy is the mainstay of treatment for patients with SCLC because of this proclivity for early dissemination. Standard chemotherapy in Caucasian patients consists of cisplatin and etoposide, having been proven equivalent and more tolerable than older regimens such as cyclophosphamide, doxorubicin, and vincristine [59].

Toxicity is mainly hematologic, especially neutropenia, 30–40 % being grade 3–4. Granulocytopenia can be effectively prevented with recombinant granulocyte colony-stimulating factor (G-CSF). Nonhematologic toxicity is essentially gastrointestinal, with little high-grade nausea or vomiting. All other clinically significant nonhematologic toxicities, excluding alopecia, were present in fewer than 4 % of patients.

## Limited Disease

The standard treatment for limited disease SCLC is combined-modality therapy consisting of thoracic radiotherapy and systemic chemotherapy. Two meta-analyses have shown an improvement of survival in patients who received chest irradiation in addition to chemotherapy compared to those receiving chemotherapy alone [60, 61], with an aim for long-term remission for a small fraction (15–25 %) of these patients. The optimal timing of radiotherapy, either concurrent or sequential, remains somehow unsettled, with compelling evidence that early radiotherapy concurrent with platinum-based chemotherapy is superior to sequential radiotherapy [62, 63].

The addition of concurrent radiotherapy to chemotherapy results in more increased myelosuppression than that observed with sequential treatment, with 88 versus 54 % high-grade leukopenia, respectively [64].

G-CSF has been controversial in this setting, with some authors advocating that primary prophylaxis with G-CSF is not indicated during chemoradiotherapy to the chest due to the increased rate of bone marrow suppression associated with an increased risk of complications and death [65]. Nonhematologic toxicities are similar, with a trend toward more infections and esophagitis. The incidence of severe pneumonitis is not significantly different between early and late chest radiotherapy, ranging between 2 and 17 % in studies with platinum-based chemotherapy. Treatment of choice consists of oral corticosteroids. The fractionation of radiotherapy might also play a role, with one trial showing a survival advantage with twice-daily versus once-daily radiotherapy, albeit with unequal biologic effective dose [66]. Hyperfractionated radiotherapy resulted in significantly more esophagitis than once-daily fractionation and may occasionally mandate tube feeding.

## Prophylactic Cranial Irradiation

Patients responding to first-line treatment, irrespective of stage, are usually offered prophylactic cranial irradiation (PCI), which has been shown to increase survival and markedly reduce the cumulative incidence of brain metastases both in patients with limited or extensive stage disease [67, 68].

PCI results in significantly more early and late (at 6 weeks and 3 months, respectively) fatigue, early and late appetite loss, nausea and vomiting, and early and late leg weakness [68].

Long-term toxicities and particularly cognitive deficits are difficult to assess, and trials yield conflicting results. A higher total dose of 36 Gy resulted in significant deterioration in neurologic function (defined as a decrease in any neuropsychological test) and increased chronic neurotoxicity (defined as deterioration in at least one neurocognitive test without documentation of brain metastases) as compared to a lower total dose of 25 Gy – without any benefit in terms of mortality and a higher incidence of subsequent brain metastases [69]. Other trials reported a negative impact on early quality of life and a limited negative impact on functioning scales of PCI, with a maximum difference in role, emotional, and cognitive functioning between 6 weeks and 3 months, then decreasing [70].

## Second-Line Therapy

Relapsing patients are offered second-line chemotherapy with the goal of survival improvement and preservation of quality of life. Oral and intravenous topotecan are classical compounds in the second-line setting. Oral topotecan extends overall survival even in patients with short (<60 days) treatment-free interval and delays deterioration of quality of life as compared to placebo [71]. Toxicity from oral topotecan is mainly hematologic, with 60 % of patients presenting with high-grade neutropenia. The most frequent nonhematologic toxicities are diarrhea and fatigue. There were fewer early deaths (<30 days) and greater likelihood of achieving symptom improvement for all symptoms, including shortness of breath, sleep interference, and fatigue.

# References

1. Jemal A, Bray F, Center MM, Ferlay J, Ward E, Forman D. Global cancer statistics. CA Cancer J Clin. 2011;61(2):69–90.
2. D'Addario G, Fruh M, Reck M, Baumann P, Klepetko W, Felip E. Metastatic non-small-cell lung cancer: ESMO Clinical Practice Guidelines for diagnosis, treatment and follow-up. Ann Oncol. 2010;21 Suppl 5:v116–9.
3. Mok TS, Wu YL, Thongprasert S, Yang CH, Chu DT, Saijo N, et al. Gefitinib or carboplatin-paclitaxel in pulmonary adenocarcinoma. N Engl J Med. 2009;361(10):947–57.
4. Sequist LV, Martins RG, Spigel D, Grunberg SM, Spira A, Janne PA, et al. First-line gefitinib in patients with advanced non-small-cell lung cancer harboring somatic EGFR mutations. J Clin Oncol. 2008; 26(15):2442–9.

5. Rosell R, Carcereny E, Gervais R, Vergnenegre A, Massuti B, Felip E, et al. Erlotinib versus standard chemotherapy as first-line treatment for European patients with advanced EGFR mutation-positive non-small-cell lung cancer (EURTAC): a multicentre, open-label, randomised phase 3 trial. Lancet Oncol. 2012;13(3):239–46.
6. Zhou C, Wu YL, Chen G, Feng J, Liu XQ, Wang C, et al. Erlotinib versus chemotherapy as first-line treatment for patients with advanced EGFR mutation-positive non-small-cell lung cancer (OPTIMAL, CTONG-0802): a multicentre, open-label, randomised, phase 3 study. Lancet Oncol. 2011;12(8):735–42.
7. Shepherd FA, Rodrigues Pereira J, Ciuleanu T, Tan EH, Hirsh V, Thongprasert S, et al. Erlotinib in previously treated non-small-cell lung cancer. N Engl J Med. 2005;353(2):123–32.
8. Scagliotti GV, Parikh P, von Pawel J, Biesma B, Vansteenkiste J, Manegold C, et al. Phase III study comparing cisplatin plus gemcitabine with cisplatin plus pemetrexed in chemotherapy-naive patients with advanced-stage non-small-cell lung cancer. J Clin Oncol. 2008;26(21): 3543–51.
9. Ardizzoni A, Boni L, Tiseo M, Fossella FV, Schiller JH, Paesmans M, et al. Cisplatin- versus carboplatin-based chemotherapy in first-line treatment of advanced non-small-cell lung cancer: an individual patient data meta-analysis. J Natl Cancer Inst. 2007;99(11):847–57.
10. Dahlberg SE, Sandler AB, Brahmer JR, Schiller JH, Johnson DH. Clinical course of advanced non-small-cell lung cancer patients experiencing hypertension during treatment with bevacizumab in combination with carboplatin and paclitaxel on ECOG 4599. J Clin Oncol. 2010;28(6):949–54.
11. Crino L, Dansin E, Garrido P, Griesinger F, Laskin J, Pavlakis N, et al. Safety and efficacy of first-line bevacizumab-based therapy in advanced non-squamous non-small-cell lung cancer (SAiL, MO19390): a phase 4 study. Lancet Oncol. 2010;11(8):733–40.
12. Schiller JH, Harrington D, Belani CP, Langer C, Sandler A, Krook J, et al. Comparison of four chemotherapy regimens for advanced non-small-cell lung cancer. N Engl J Med. 2002;346(2):92–8.
13. Kwak EL, Bang YJ, Camidge DR, Shaw AT, Solomon B, Maki RG, et al. Anaplastic lymphoma kinase inhibition in non-small-cell lung cancer. N Engl J Med. 2010;363(18):1693–703.
14. Reck M, Gutzmer R. Management of the cutaneous side effects of therapeutic epidermal growth factor receptor inhibition. Onkologie. 2010;33(8–9):470–9.
15. Wu YL, Kim JH, Park K, Zaatar A, Klingelschmitt G, Ng C. Efficacy and safety of maintenance erlotinib in Asian patients with advanced non-small-cell lung cancer: a subanalysis of the phase III, randomized SATURN study. Lung Cancer. 2012;77(2):339–45. Epub 2012 Apr 10.
16. Hesketh PJ, Chansky K, Wozniak AJ, Hirsch FR, Spreafico A, Moon J, et al. Southwest Oncology Group phase II trial (S0341) of erlotinib

(OSI-774) in patients with advanced non-small cell lung cancer and a performance status of 2. J Thorac Oncol. 2008;3(9):1026–31.

17. Inoue A, Saijo Y, Maemondo M, Gomi K, Tokue Y, Kimura Y, et al. Severe acute interstitial pneumonia and gefitinib. Lancet. 2003; 361(9352):137–9.

18. Lai YC, Lin PC, Lai JI, Hsu SY, Kuo LC, Chang SC, et al. Successful treatment of erlotinib-induced acute hepatitis and acute interstitial pneumonitis with high-dose corticosteroid: a case report and literature review. Int J Clin Pharmacol Ther. 2011;49(7):461–6.

19. Gronberg BH, Bremnes RM, Flotten O, Amundsen T, Brunsvig PF, Hjelde HH, et al. Phase III study by the Norwegian lung cancer study group: pemetrexed plus carboplatin compared with gemcitabine plus carboplatin as first-line chemotherapy in advanced non-small-cell lung cancer. J Clin Oncol. 2009;27(19):3217–24.

20. Spiro SG, Rudd RM, Souhami RL, Brown J, Fairlamb DJ, Gower NH, et al. Chemotherapy versus supportive care in advanced non-small cell lung cancer: improved survival without detriment to quality of life. Thorax. 2004;59(10):828–36.

21. Roila F, Herrstedt J, Aapro M, Gralla RJ, Einhorn LH, Ballatori E, et al. Guideline update for MASCC and ESMO in the prevention of chemotherapy- and radiotherapy-induced nausea and vomiting: results of the Perugia consensus conference. Ann Oncol. 2010;21 Suppl 5:v232–43.

22. Rademaker-Lakhai JM, Crul M, Zuur L, Baas P, Beijnen JH, Simis YJ, et al. Relationship between cisplatin administration and the development of ototoxicity. J Clin Oncol. 2006;24(6):918–24.

23. Bally C, Fadlallah J, Leverger G, Bertrand Y, Robert A, Baruchel A, et al. Outcome of acute promyelocytic leukemia (APL) in children and adolescents: an analysis in two consecutive trials of the European APL Group. J Clin Oncol. 2012;30(14):1641–6.

24. Markman M, Kennedy A, Webster K, Elson P, Peterson G, Kulp B, et al. Clinical features of hypersensitivity reactions to carboplatin. J Clin Oncol. 1999;17(4):1141.

25. Hanna N, Shepherd FA, Fossella FV, Pereira JR, De Marinis F, von Pawel J, et al. Randomized phase III trial of pemetrexed versus doc-etaxel in patients with non-small-cell lung cancer previously treated with chemotherapy. J Clin Oncol. 2004;22(9):1589–97.

26. Santoro A, O'Brien ME, Stahel RA, Nackaerts K, Baas P, Karthaus M, et al. Pemetrexed plus cisplatin or pemetrexed plus carboplatin for chemonaive patients with malignant pleural mesothelioma: results of the International Expanded Access Program. J Thorac Oncol. 2008;3(7):756–63.

27. Sandler A, Gray R, Perry MC, Brahmer J, Schiller JH, Dowlati A, et al. Paclitaxel-carboplatin alone or with bevacizumab for non-small-cell lung cancer. N Engl J Med. 2006;355(24):2542–50.

28. Reck M, von Pawel J, Zatloukal P, Ramlau R, Gorbounova V, Hirsh V, et al. Phase III trial of cisplatin plus gemcitabine with either placebo or bevacizumab as first-line therapy for nonsquamous non-small-cell lung cancer: AVAil. J Clin Oncol. 2009;27(8):1227–34.

29. Veronese ML, Mosenkis A, Flaherty KT, Gallagher M, Stevenson JP, Townsend RR, et al. Mechanisms of hypertension associated with BAY 43–9006. J Clin Oncol. 2006;24(9):1363–9.

30. Izzedine H, Ederhy S, Goldwasser F, Soria JC, Milano G, Cohen A, et al. Management of hypertension in angiogenesis inhibitor-treated patients. Ann Oncol. 2009;20(5):807–15.

31. Pande A, Lombardo J, Spangenthal E, Javle M. Hypertension secondary to anti-angiogenic therapy: experience with bevacizumab. Anticancer Res. 2007;27(5B):3465–70.

32. Mir O, Coriat R, Ropert S, Cabanes L, Blanchet B, Camps S, et al. Treatment of bevacizumab-induced hypertension by amlodipine. Invest New Drugs. 2012;30(2):702–7.

33. Anderson H, Lund B, Bach F, Thatcher N, Walling J, Hansen HH. Single-agent activity of weekly gemcitabine in advanced non-small-cell lung cancer: a phase II study. J Clin Oncol. 1994;12(9):1821–6.

34. Gridelli C, Cigolari S, Gallo C, Manzione L, Ianniello GP, Frontini L, et al. Activity and toxicity of gemcitabine and gemcitabine + vinorelbine in advanced non-small-cell lung cancer elderly patients: phase II data from the Multicenter Italian Lung Cancer in the Elderly Study (MILES) randomized trial. Lung Cancer. 2001;31(2–3): 277–84.

35. Aapro MS, Martin C, Hatty S. Gemcitabine – a safety review. Anticancer Drugs. 1998;9(3):191–201.

36. Barlesi F, Villani P, Doddoli C, Gimenez C, Kleisbauer JP. Gemcitabine-induced severe pulmonary toxicity. Fundam Clin Pharmacol. 2004;18(1):85–91.

37. Miller VA, Kris MG. Docetaxel (Taxotere) as a single agent and in combination chemotherapy for the treatment of patients with advanced non-small cell lung cancer. Semin Oncol. 2000;27(2 Suppl 3): 3–10.

38. Goodgame B, Viswanathan A, Zoole J, Gao F, Miller CR, Subramanian J, et al. Risk of recurrence of resected stage I non-small cell lung cancer in elderly patients as compared with younger patients. J Thorac Oncol. 2009;4(11):1370–4.

39. Kates M, Swanson S, Wisnivesky JP. Survival following lobectomy and limited resection for the treatment of stage I non-small cell lung cancer <=1 cm in size: a review of SEER data. Chest. 2011;139(3):491–6.

40. Cheung MC, Hamilton K, Sherman R, Byrne MM, Nguyen DM, Franceschi D, et al. Impact of teaching facility status and high-volume centers on outcomes for lung cancer resection: an examination of 13,469 surgical patients. Ann Surg Oncol. 2009;16(1):3–13.

41. Brunelli A, Refai M, Salati M, Xiume F, Sabbatini A. Predicted versus observed FEV1 and DLCO after major lung resection: a prospective evaluation at different postoperative periods. Ann Thorac Surg. 2007;83(3):1134–9.
42. Barnett SA, Rusch VW, Zheng J, Park BJ, Rizk NP, Plourde G, et al. Contemporary results of surgical resection of non-small cell lung cancer after induction therapy: a review of 549 consecutive cases. J Thorac Oncol. 2011;6(9):1530–6.
43. Ferguson MK, Vigneswaran WT. Diffusing capacity predicts morbidity after lung resection in patients without obstructive lung disease. Ann Thorac Surg. 2008;85(4):1158–64; discussion 1164–5.
44. Otake H, Yasunaga H, Horiguchi H, Matsutani N, Matsuda S, Ohe K. Impact of hospital volume on chest tube duration, length of stay, and mortality after lobectomy. Ann Thorac Surg. 2011;92(3):1069–74.
45. Wahi R, McMurtrey MJ, DeCaro LF, Mountain CF, Ali MK, Smith TL, et al. Determinants of perioperative morbidity and mortality after pneumonectomy. Ann Thorac Surg. 1989;48(1):33–7.
46. Yan TD, Black D, Bannon PG, McCaughan BC. Systematic review and meta-analysis of randomized and nonrandomized trials on safety and efficacy of video-assisted thoracic surgery lobectomy for early-stage non-small-cell lung cancer. J Clin Oncol. 2009;27(15):2553–62.
47. Allen MS, Darling GE, Pechet TT, Mitchell JD, Herndon 2nd JE, Landreneau RJ, et al. Morbidity and mortality of major pulmonary resections in patients with early-stage lung cancer: initial results of the randomized, prospective ACOSOG Z0030 trial. Ann Thorac Surg. 2006;81(3):1013–9; discussion 1019–20.
48. Saji H, Tsuboi M, Yoshida K, Kato Y, Nomura M, Matsubayashi J, et al. Prognostic impact of number of resected and involved lymph nodes at complete resection on survival in non-small cell lung cancer. J Thorac Oncol. 2011;6(11):1865–71.
49. Pompili C, Brunelli A, Xiume F, Refai M, Salati M, Sabbatini A. Predictors of postoperative decline in quality of life after major lung resections. Eur J Cardiothorac Surg. 2011;39(5):732–7.
50. Moller A, Sartipy U. Predictors of postoperative quality of life after surgery for lung cancer. J Thorac Oncol. 2012;7(2):406–11.
51. Arriagada R, Auperin A, Burdett S, Higgins JP, Johnson DH, Le Chevalier T, et al. Adjuvant chemotherapy, with or without postoperative radiotherapy, in operable non-small-cell lung cancer: two meta-analyses of individual patient data. Lancet. 2010;375(9722):1267–77.
52. Pignon JP, Tribodet H, Scagliotti GV, Douillard JY, Shepherd FA, Stephens RJ, et al. Lung adjuvant cisplatin evaluation: a pooled analysis by the LACE Collaborative Group. J Clin Oncol. 2008;26(21):3552–9.
53. Douillard JY, Rosell R, De Lena M, Carpagnano F, Ramlau R, Gonzales-Larriba JL, et al. Adjuvant vinorelbine plus cisplatin versus

observation in patients with completely resected stage IB-IIIA non-small-cell lung cancer (Adjuvant Navelbine International Trialist Association [ANITA]): a randomised controlled trial. Lancet Oncol. 2006;7(9):719–27.

54. Arriagada R, Dunant A, Pignon JP, Bergman B, Chabowski M, Grunenwald D, et al. Long-term results of the international adjuvant lung cancer trial evaluating adjuvant Cisplatin-based chemotherapy in resected lung cancer. J Clin Oncol. 2010;28(1):35–42.

55. Fossa SD, Gilbert E, Dores GM, Chen J, McGlynn KA, Schonfeld S, et al. Noncancer causes of death in survivors of testicular cancer. J Natl Cancer Inst. 2007;99(7):533–44.

56. Lally BE, Zelterman D, Colasanto JM, Haffty BG, Detterbeck FC, Wilson LD. Postoperative radiotherapy for stage II or III non-small-cell lung cancer using the surveillance, epidemiology, and end results database. J Clin Oncol. 2006;24(19):2998–3006.

57. Postoperative radiotherapy for non-small cell lung cancer. PORT Meta-analysis Trialists Group Cochrane Database Syst Rev. 2005;(2):CD002142.

58. Kelly K. New chemotherapy agents for small cell lung cancer. Chest. 2000;117(4 Suppl 1):156S–62.

59. Roth BJ, Johnson DH, Einhorn LH, Schacter LP, Cherng NC, Cohen HJ, et al. Randomized study of cyclophosphamide, doxorubicin, and vincristine versus etoposide and cisplatin versus alternation of these two regimens in extensive small-cell lung cancer: a phase III trial of the Southeastern Cancer Study Group. J Clin Oncol. 1992;10(2):282–91.

60. Pignon JP, Arriagada R, Ihde DC, Johnson DH, Perry MC, Souhami RL, et al. A meta-analysis of thoracic radiotherapy for small-cell lung cancer. N Engl J Med. 1992;327(23):1618–24.

61. Arriagada R, Pignon JP, Ihde DC, Johnson DH, Perry MC, Souhami RL, et al. Effect of thoracic radiotherapy on mortality in limited small cell lung cancer. A meta-analysis of 13 randomized trials among 2,140 patients. Anticancer Res. 1994;14(1B):333–5.

62. Pijls-Johannesma MC, De Ruysscher D, Lambin P, Rutten I, Vansteenkiste JF. Early versus late chest radiotherapy for limited stage small cell lung cancer. Cochrane Database Syst Rev. 2005;(1):CD004700.

63. Spiro SG, James LE, Rudd RM, Trask CW, Tobias JS, Snee M, et al. Early compared with late radiotherapy in combined modality treatment for limited disease small-cell lung cancer: a London Lung Cancer Group multicenter randomized clinical trial and meta-analysis. J Clin Oncol. 2006;24(24):3823–30.

64. Takada M, Fukuoka M, Kawahara M, Sugiura T, Yokoyama A, Yokota S, et al. Phase III study of concurrent versus sequential thoracic radiotherapy in combination with cisplatin and etoposide for limited-stage small-cell lung cancer: results of the Japan Clinical Oncology Group Study 9104. J Clin Oncol. 2002;20(14):3054–60.

65. Crawford J, Caserta C, Roila F. Hematopoietic growth factors: ESMO Clinical Practice Guidelines for the applications. Ann Oncol. 2010;21 Suppl 5:v248–51.
66. Turrisi 3rd AT, Kim K, Blum R, Sause WT, Livingston RB, Komaki R, et al. Twice-daily compared with once-daily thoracic radiotherapy in limited small-cell lung cancer treated concurrently with cisplatin and etoposide. N Engl J Med. 1999;340(4):265–71.
67. Auperin A, Arriagada R, Pignon JP, LePechoux C, Gregor A, Stephens RJ, et al. Prophylactic cranial irradiation for patients with small-cell lung cancer in complete remission. Prophylactic Cranial Irradiation Overview Collaborative Group. N Engl J Med. 1999;341(7): 476–84.
68. Slotman B, Faivre-Finn C, Kramer G, Rankin E, Snee M, Hatton M, et al. Prophylactic cranial irradiation in extensive small-cell lung cancer. N Engl J Med. 2007;357(7):664–72.
69. Wolfson AH, Bae K, Komaki R, Meyers C, Movsas B, Le Pechoux C, et al. Primary analysis of a phase II randomized trial Radiation Therapy Oncology Group (RTOG) 0212: impact of different total doses and schedules of prophylactic cranial irradiation on chronic neurotoxicity and quality of life for patients with limited-disease small-cell lung cancer. Int J Radiat Oncol Biol Phys. 2011;81(1): 77–84.
70. Slotman BJ, Mauer ME, Bottomley A, Faivre-Finn C, Kramer GW, Rankin EM, et al. Prophylactic cranial irradiation in extensive disease small-cell lung cancer: short-term health-related quality of life and patient reported symptoms: results of an international Phase III randomized controlled trial by the EORTC Radiation Oncology and Lung Cancer Groups. J Clin Oncol. 2009;27(1):78–84.
71. O'Brien ME, Ciuleanu TE, Tsekov H, Shparyk Y, Cucevia B, Juhasz G, et al. Phase III trial comparing supportive care alone with supportive care with oral topotecan in patients with relapsed small-cell lung cancer. J Clin Oncol. 2006;24(34):5441–7.

# Chapter 4
## Gastrointestinal Cancer: Selection of Clinically Relevant Drug-Induced Toxicities Encountered in Gastrointestinal Cancer Treatment

**Julie Bogaert, Pieter-Jan Cuyle, and Eric Van Cutsem**

**Abstract** The chemotherapeutic options have increased dramatically in patients with gastrointestinal cancer and have led to an improved outcome. With this, an in-depth understanding of the side effects of chemotherapy is becoming increasingly important in order to minimize the negative impact of the use of these agents. Chemotherapeutic agents have a long list of potential side effects. In this chapter, we focus specifically on some of the more common and/or more relevant and challenging side effects related to frequently used agents in gastrointestinal cancer. The fluoropyrimidines may cause cardiac toxicity, most frequently angina-like chest pain. The knowledge of the catabolism of fluorouracil has led to the possibility of testing for dihydropyrimidine dehydrogenase (DPD) in order to avoid serious fluorouracil-related toxicity in patients with DPD deficiency. Oxaliplatin-induced

J. Bogaert, M.D. • P.-J. Cuyle, M.D. • E. Van Cutsem, M.D., Ph.D. (✉)
Department of Digestive Oncology, University Hospitals
Gasthuisberg/Leuven, Leuven, Belgium

M.A. Dicato (ed.), *Side Effects of Medical Cancer Therapy*,
DOI 10.1007/978-0-85729-787-7_4,
© Springer-Verlag London 2013

139

neurotoxicity is probably the most important clinical problem associated with the administration of oxaliplatin. With the increasing use of oxaliplatin, hypersensitivity reactions are more frequently reported and become challenging in clinical practice. The introduction of the targeted agents in colorectal cancer led also to specific problems: the anti-VEGF-related side effects, of which gastrointestinal perforation, although relatively rare, is very relevant for the patient, and the anti-EGFR-related side effects, including skin rash, hypomagnesemia, and allergic reactions, are common. Understanding the underlying causes, mechanisms, risk factors, and developing treatment guidelines has made these side effects often more acceptable for many patients. However, the side-effect profile always has to be balanced against the activity and benefit of the anticancer agents.

**Keywords**  Fluorouracil • DPD • Oxaliplatin • Irinotecan VEGF • EGFR • Bevacizumab • Cetuximab • Panitumumab

# Fluoropyrimidines: Fluorouracil and Capecitabine

Since the late 1950s, fluorouracil (5-FU) has been used as a cytotoxic chemotherapeutic agent to treat various types of solid malignancies originating from breast, esophagus, larynx, and gastrointestinal and genitourinary tracts. Because of its variable gastrointestinal absorption and rapid degradation, 5-FU must be administered intravenously [1]. We have learned to use the most optimal regimens of 5-FU: it has been shown that infusional regimens lead to less adverse events compared to bolus regimens of 5-FU. Capecitabine (Xeloda, Roche Pharmaceuticals, Nutley, NJ, USA), an oral prodrug of 5-FU, shows a favorable toxicity profile and comparable efficacy end points in gastric and colorectal cancer [2]. Capecitabine undergoes a three-step enzymatic conversion to 5-FU that occurs primarily in the liver and tumor cells, thereby achieving high intratumoral drug concentrations.

TABLE 4.1  Common side effects of frequently used cytotoxic agents in GI cancer

| Fluorouracil (5-FU) | Capecitabine |
|---|---|
| Hematologic | Hematologic |
| Mucositis/diarrhea | Mucositis/diarrhea |
| Stomatitis | Hand-foot syndrome |
| Hand-foot syndrome | |
| Cardiac adverse events | |

| Oxaliplatin | Irinotecan |
|---|---|
| Hematologic | Hematologic |
| Nausea/vomiting | Nausea/vomiting |
| Neurotoxicity | Mucositis/diarrhea |
| Infusion reactions | Fatigue |
| | Alopecia |

Adverse events of fluorouracil and its prodrug capecitabine are summarized in Table 4.1. Fluorouracil-related severe adverse events can cause substantial morbidity and also very occasionally death, suggesting an important role for pharmacogenomics in identifying patients at risk for increased toxicity. Fluoropyrimidine-induced cardiotoxicity is relatively infrequent and generally reversible on treatment discontinuation. However, this complication can be life-threatening, and fatal outcome has been described.

## Fluorouracil-Induced Cardiac Toxicity

The incidence of 5-FU-related cardiac toxicity varies broadly throughout the literature, ranging between 1.2 and 18 % [3]. In fact, the real incidence may be even higher, as asymptomatic ischemic electrocardiography (ECG) changes do occur also [4]. This side effect may occasionally be fatal [3]. Angina-like chest pain is the most frequent presenting symptom of cardiac toxicity, and it is reported in up to 89 % of patients with cardiac toxicity [3]. Less common symptoms include palpitations, malaise, numbness of arm or neck, and loss of consciousness. Clinical pictures of congestive heart failure, cardiogenic shock, cardiac arrest, and sudden death have been reported. ECG findings may include myocardial ischemia, myocardial infarction, and cardiac arrhythmias [5]. Serum cardiac enzyme levels are usually normal, and echocardiography can reveal transient local or, more frequently, global, myocardial hypokinesia compatible with myocardial stunning [3]. Usually no significant coronary atherosclerosis is found when coronary angiography is performed. Most events occur during or within several hours after fluorouracil treatment, since the serum half-life of 5-FU is very short [3]. Symptoms are usually fully reversible shortly after treatment discontinuation.

Pathophysiologic mechanisms involved in fluorouracil-associated cardiotoxicity remain incompletely understood and are probably multifactorial. Based on the characteristic clinical and ECG presentation in the absence of relevant coronary stenosis, this phenomenon is historically attributed to fluorouracil-induced coronary vasospasm [6]. However, other mechanisms have been proposed. Data from animal models and echocardiographic studies suggest a direct toxic effect of 5-FU metabolites on the myocardial cells, resulting in toxic myocarditis and cardiomyopathy [4, 5]. Risk factors for development of fluorouracil-induced cardiotoxicity have not been specified. The impact of preexisting heart disease remains controversial [3]. Previous or current radiation involving the heart may promote cardiac toxicity. The toxic effect of 5-FU/capecitabine on the myocardium is schedule-dependent. Cardiac symptoms occur more frequently with the use of continuous 5-FU infusion, when compared to a short (bolus) administration of 5-FU [5]. Pharmacokinetics of capecitabine are comparable to that of continuous 5-FU infusion, and incidence of cardiotoxicity is reported to be similar to that of 5-FU [7].

Baseline ECG testing before starting a treatment with 5-FU-based chemotherapy could be helpful in future assessment of cardiotoxicity. Baseline echocardiography is recommended for patients with a history of heart disease [3, 4]. Patients in whom cardiotoxicity is suspected should receive cardiac monitoring because of the possible risk of life-threatening heart failure and malignant arrhythmias. Fluorouracil administration should be stopped immediately. Symptomatic treatment with nitrates and/or calcium antagonists is recommended [3]. However, the reported therapeutic efficacy of these drugs is inconsistent, and no prospective trials are available. The risk of relapse when patients are reexposed to 5-FU following previous cardiac incidents is very high, up to 82–100 % [3]. Whether the use of prophylactic antianginal medication can reduce the recurrence risk has not been established, but it is often done in patients with mild symptoms when the continuation of the fluoropyrimidine is advisable. Administration of raltitrexed (Tomudex, TDX, ZD 1694, AstraZeneca, Wilmington, DE, USA) as an alternative for 5-FU, in case of major intolerance, is suggested, although the evidence is limited [8].

## Dihydropyrimidine Dehydrogenase Deficiency

Dihydropyrimidine dehydrogenase (DPD) is the primary rate-controlling enzyme in fluoropyrimidine catabolism. Over the last two decades, the association between DPD-enzyme deficiency and the occurrence of severe fluorouracil-related toxicity has been extensively studied. Patients receiving 5-FU-based chemotherapy may develop severe to life-threatening adverse events, including neutropenia, neutropenic infections, stomatitis, diarrhea, and alopecia, and it is estimated that DPD deficiency accounts for 50–75 % of the cases of severe side effects [9].

The human dihydropyrimidine dehydrogenase (DPYD) gene, encoding DPD, is located on chromosome 1p22 and contains 23 exons. Loss-of-function mutations in this DPYD gene lead to a partial or complete lack of capacity to metabolize 5-FU or its prodrugs, explaining the risk of increased toxicity. DPD-enzyme activity is highly variable within the normal population and differs substantially between ethnic subpopulations. The prevalence of partial DPD deficiency (low DPD activity) is estimated to be 3–5 % in the overall population [10, 11]. Complete DPD deficiency was first described as an autosomal recessive disorder in pediatric patients with various neurological symptoms [10, 12].

Over 50 genetic variants have been identified in the DPYD gene coding region – however, the majority without functional consequences on enzymatic activity [9, 10]. The most prominent and most studied DPYD variant is a point mutation in the splice site of intron 14 (c.1905 + 1G>A, synonyms IVS14 + 1G>A or DPYD*2A), responsible for up to 29 % of reported grade III–V toxicities following fluorouracil administration [13]. Conflicting results were seen in a more recent prospective trial, which concluded that severe toxicities could only be marginally attributed to DPYD gene polymorphism [14]. Furthermore, it is suggested that additional enzymes and polymorphisms in various downstream acting genes may also play a role in 5-FU degradation and toxicity [9]. The pronounced variability in the DPYD coding sequence, together with contradictory results from genetic studies, causes marked difficulties in genotype-phenotype correlations and presents a major limitation to the application of a genotype-based strategy to predict severe fluorouracil toxicity in daily practice [9].

Alternatively, a number of screening tests assessing DPD functionality (phenotype-based strategy) have been developed to predict impaired fluorouracil metabolism [9, 10, 15]. Enzymatic activity can be measured ex vivo in peripheral mononuclear blood cells or can be estimated through analysis of the plasma or urine dihydrouracil/uracil (UH2/U) ratio. A noninvasive uracil breath test measuring exhaled $^{13}CO_2$ after ingestion of $2$-$^{13}C$-uracil or administration of an infratherapeutic 5-FU test dose followed by pharmacokinetic analysis are other possibilities for preliminary functional testing. Clinical data implementing systematic pretreatment functional DPD testing and subsequent DPD-based 5-FU dose tailoring are limited. However, these data suggest that this approach is feasible, reducing treatment-related severe toxicities without a loss in treatment efficacy [9, 16].

Anticipating and preventing 5-FU-related severe toxicities has been suggested to be cost-effective, to enhance patient quality of life, and to reduce chemo- or radiotherapy post-ponement, thus improving patient outcome [9]. The exact relevance of systematic DPD testing and whether genetic or functional testing is more practical and predictive in daily practice are questions that remain to be answered. Therefore, routine screening for DPD deficiency is not performed in most institutions. However, if there is a clinical picture of very severe toxicity, especially early on in the treatment of a fluoropyrimidine, DPD testing is indicated and can avoid later life-threatening toxicity.

# Oxaliplatin

Oxaliplatin (Eloxatin, Sanofi-Aventis, Bridgewater, NJ, USA), a third-generation platinum derivative, has been investigated in different types of malignancies and was shown to be particularly efficacious in the treatment of gastrointestinal neoplasms, including esophagogastric, pancreatic, and colorectal cancers [17]. Combinations of oxaliplatin with infusional fluorouracil/leucovorin (FOLFOX) or capecitabine (XELOX) have emerged as important therapeutic options in the adjuvant as well as palliative treatment of colorectal cancer [18]. Oxaliplatin has proved to be an equivalent alternative for cisplatin, with a slightly favorable toxicity profile, especially in terms of renal toxicity in gastric and pancreatic cancer. Common side effects are summarized in Table 4.1. Oxaliplatin-induced neurotoxicity and hypersensitivity infusion reactions are well-recognized dose-limiting toxicities, often encountered in clinical practice, potentially resulting in permanent discontinuation.

## Oxaliplatin-Induced Neurotoxicity

Oxaliplatin-induced neurotoxicity (OXIN) is the most frequent clinically relevant adverse event associated with the use of oxaliplatin [18]. It is a cumulative and dose-limiting complication in which symptoms are typically triggered or worsened by exposure to cold. Common terminology criteria for adverse events (CTCAE) are often used for grading and monitoring OXIN. Development of grade ≥2 neuropathy (CTCAE version 4.0) occurs in approximately half of treated patients, and 10–20 % of patients develop grade 3 neuropathy [19, 20]. In up to 90 % of patients, peripheral neuropathy reverses after oxaliplatin is discontinued – however, sometimes with a long delay. Symptom worsening is reported for up to 6 weeks after the last dose of oxaliplatin, also after surgery, and in some cases neuropathy may persist for several months or even years.

Two distinct forms of OXIN are recognized: an acute type and a chronic type [17, 18]. Acute sensory and/or motor neurotoxicity occurs during or within 1–2 days after oxaliplatin infusion. It shows a rapid onset and is characterized by paresthesia and dysesthesia affecting the acral segments of both upper and lower limbs; it is clearly exacerbated by cold exposure. The perioral and laryngopharyngeal areas may be involved as well, possibly leading to an acute sensation of respiratory discomfort. Acute motor neuropathy is associated with symptoms of muscular hyperactivity, such as jaw tightness, cramps, and fasciculations, that affect legs, thighs, hands, and jaws, hampering movements. Acute symptoms usually resolve spontaneously within a week but usually relapse with each subsequent administration of oxaliplatin, often with slightly increasing intensity after each course.

Chronic oxaliplatin-associated neuropathy is a dose-limiting chronic sensory neuropathy that involves the extremities, possibly causing functional impairment and even gait ataxia with longer treatment exposure. It becomes worse with increasing cumulative doses of oxaliplatin.

The pathophysiological mechanisms responsible for the development of OXIN remain unclear. In the acute form, oxalate, a metabolic by-product of oxaliplatin, may cause a dysfunction of the neuronal voltage-gated calcium-dependent sodium channels, disrupting intracellular homeostasis and provoking neuronal hyperexcitability [21, 22]. In the chronic form, accumulation of platinum compounds in neurons may lead to neuronal atrophy. Several studies have tried to identify pharmacogenomic markers (single nucleotide polymorphisms, or SNPs) predisposing patients to severe neurotoxicity development; however, no such marker has been validated for clinical use to this date [23, 24].

To avoid the occurrence of severe, long-lasting, and invalidating OXIN, gradual dose reductions and delay or discontinuation of oxaliplatin administration are often necessary, without a clear impact on the overall outcome. Indeed, stop-and-go strategies have been developed in metastatic colorectal cancer, mainly as a consequence of this cumulative neuropathy [25, 26]. Several trials have investigated the neuroprotective potency of calcium and magnesium infusions. As oxalate chelators, they are thought to reduce the effect of oxalate on the voltage-gated sodium channel, thereby reducing OXIN severity [27]. Although calcium and magnesium are frequently administered before and after oxaliplatin, the lack of standardization in the use and timing of objective neurotoxicity assessment and the lack of long-term neuropathy data in these studies prevent definitive conclusions; further investigation is necessary [28]. The neuroprotective efficacy of several pharmacologic agents, such as antidepressants and anticonvulsants, has been studied in a number of trials, which are nicely summarized in a recent review by Weickhart et al. [17]. Venlafaxine has been shown to reduce the incidence of acute and chronic peripheral neuropathy in patients treated with oxaliplatin in a small phase III trial [29]. At the present time, however, no strong evidence is available supporting the systematic use of these agents in the prevention or treatment of oxaliplatin-associated neuropathy. Acute oxaliplatin-induced neuropathy of the laryngopharyngeal area is often confused with allergic laryngeal angioedema but is usually manageable by prolonging oxaliplatin infusion time to 6 h, without specific antiallergic premedication.

## Oxaliplatin-Associated Hypersensitivity Infusion Reactions

Hypersensitivity to chemotherapy is historically defined as an unexpected reaction, with signs and symptoms that are inconsistent with the drug's usual toxicity profile occurring during or immediately following the administration of that drug [30, 31].

Due to the extensive use of oxaliplatin in cancer treatment over the last decade, the drug is increasingly recognized to cause hypersensitivity reactions similar to those seen with earlier generations of platinum-based compounds, at an overall incidence of 10–20 % [30–32]. However, severe grade 3–4 reactions are less common, occurring in 1.6 % of the patients, and severe anaphylaxis is reported rarely [30, 31]. Symptoms often develop acutely during oxaliplatin infusion or shortly afterward and usually occur within the first 24 h after infusion. Mild hypersensitivity reactions are characterized by skin rash, urticaria, flushing, palmar itching, burning, edema of face and hands, abdominal cramping and diarrhea, back pain, and pruritus [30]. More severe infusion reactions can present with the development of bronchospasm, tachycardia, hypo- or hypertension, angioedema, seizures, and chest pain. Hypersensitivity events are generally encountered after four to six oxaliplatin administrations [31].

Most infusion reactions seem to be IgE-mediated (type I), but type II hypersensitivity with symptoms of hemolysis and thrombocytopenia or type III allergic reactions with development of chronic urticaria, joint pain, and proteinuria have also been reported [30]. Furthermore, idiosyncratic reactions to oxaliplatin infusion, characterized by chills, fever, abdominal cramps, and chest tightness, have also been described. A recent retrospective study has identified the presence of a younger age, female sex, and the use of oxaliplatin as salvage therapy, as potential risk factors for development of oxaliplatin-associated infusion reactions [31]. However, the presence of prior allergies, disease type, and stage or treatment regimen did not seem to be associated with increased hypersensitivity.

When a hypersensitivity infusion reaction is diagnosed, the chemotherapy infusion should be interrupted promptly, followed by infusion of normal saline and administration of oxygen, systemic antihistamines, and corticosteroids. Other supportive measures should be taken as indicated until complete resolution of symptoms. The main dilemma is whether oxaliplatin can be readministered in the future. The decision should be based on the severity of the hypersensitivity reaction, on the patient's general condition, and the anticipated oncological benefit of oxaliplatin administration. In case of mild and moderate hypersensitivity reactions, reintroduction can be successful by prolonging the infusion time to 4–6 h and the use of premedication with histamine receptor antagonists and corticosteroids [32]. Nevertheless, the risk of recurrence is estimated around 30–40 %. When the reaction is relatively severe (grade ≥3), all platinum compounds should be excluded from future treatment options. Various desensitization protocols have been successfully implemented for cisplatin and carboplatin; however, oxaliplatin desensitization protocols have only been reported in a very small number of patients [30].

# Vascular Endothelial Growth Factor Inhibition: Bevacizumab

Neo-angiogenesis is crucial for tumor growth and malignant progression. In the majority of cancers, tumor vessels appear to be abnormal in structure and function, leading to a hostile microenvironment characterized by hypoxia, low pH, and high interstitial fluid pressure [33]. The spread of tumor cells, escaping through these leaky vessels, is facilitated, while, on the other hand, transport and distribution of cytotoxics and oxygen to the tumor seems to be impaired. One of the main angiogenic factors is vascular endothelial growth factor (VEGF). Blockade of VEGF signaling by pharmacologic agents can transiently repair these vascular abnormalities, thus improving oxygenation and lowering interstitial fluid pressure. This process is referred to as vascular normalization [33]. The decrease in interstitial fluid pressure improves cytotoxic drug delivery to the targeted cancer cells. Bevacizumab (Avastin, Genentech, South San Francisco, CA, USA) is a recombinant, humanized monoclonal antibody to VEGF, which inhibits binding of VEGF to its receptors, hereby suppressing downstream signaling of the VEGF pathway. The combination of bevacizumab with standard chemotherapy (irinotecan/5-FU, oxaliplatin/5-FU, or a fluoropyrimidine alone)

TABLE 4.2  Common side effects of frequently used biological agents in GI cancer

*EGFR inhibition: cetuximab and panitumumab*

Skin toxicity

Hypomagnesemia

Infusion reactions

*VEGF inhibition: bevacizumab*

Hypertension

Proteinuria

Delayed wound healing

Gastrointestinal perforation

Bleeding

Arterial thromboembolic events

has been shown to improve the clinical outcome in patients with metastatic colorectal cancer but not in the adjuvant setting [34, 35]. The clinical toxicities associated with bevacizumab use have been well described and are summarized in Table 4.2. The side effects are class-related and are also seen with other anti-VEGF targeting agents: the most important include arterial hypertension, proteinuria, mucosal bleeding, arterial thrombosis (especially in older patients with a history of arterial thrombosis), wound healing complications, and gastrointestinal perforation. Serious adverse events are relatively uncommon, and side effects are generally manageable using standard treatment. Bevacizumab does not increase the typical chemotherapy-induced side effects, such as diarrhea, stomatitis, neutropenia, and neutropenic infections, although other agents interfering with VEGF (aflibercept, VEGF tyrosine kinase inhibitors) have been reported to be associated with a higher incidence of the aforementioned chemotherapy-related side effects.

# Bevacizumab-Associated Gastrointestinal Perforation

The occurrence of gastrointestinal (GI) perforation, a potentially life-threatening complication of bevacizumab treatment, has been reported in patients with various types of solid tumors, although it is typically more frequent, for reasons that are unclear, in the management of colorectal and ovarian cancer [36]. In pivotal clinical trials and two community-based observational studies that investigated bevacizumab combination with 5-FU-based chemotherapy in advanced colorectal cancer, the estimated incidence of GI perforation was reported to be around 0–3.3 % [37]. Perforations seem to occur early in treatment, usually within 6 months after the start of bevacizumab, and can be localized anywhere along the GI tract [37]. Surgical intervention may be required, but is not always necessary. Concerns about surgical wound and anastomotic healing under bevacizumab treatment can justify a conservative approach in stable patients. Perforation rate was higher when the primary tumor was still intact, when lower GI tract endoscopy had been performed within 1 month, or if a patient had received prior abdominal radiotherapy [37]. Other risk factors included the presence of peritoneal carcinomatosis, GI obstruction, gastric ulcer disease, acute diverticulitis, and chemotherapy-associated colitis [36, 37]. However, none of these risk factors have been validated in multivariate analysis. The contribution of VEGF inhibition to the development of GI perforation is incompletely understood. Several hypotheses have been proposed, but pathophysiological mechanisms are most likely multifactorial. Among others, VEGF inhibition can induce regression of normal blood vessels in the GI tract and can cause a decreased splanchnic blood flow due to a loss of nitric oxide release [38]. Delayed healing of chemotherapy-induced mucosal damage and development of cholesterol emboli syndrome may also be involved in pathogenesis [38].

# Epidermal Growth Factor Receptor Inhibition: Cetuximab and Panitumumab

The epidermal growth factor receptor (EGFR, HER1, or ErbB1) is a glycoprotein receptor, comprising an extracellular ligand-binding domain, a transmembrane region, and an intra-cytoplasmatic domain with tyrosine kinase activity. Ligand binding of the extracellular domain results in homodimerization or heterodimerization with other members of the EGFR family (HER2, HER3, HER4) and subsequent initiation of downstream signaling pathways by autophosphorylation. These downstream signaling cascades include the mitogen-activated protein kinase (MAPK) pathway and the phosphatidylinositol-3-kinase (PI3K) pathway. EGFR regulates cellular growth, differentiation, and survival, and abnormal EGFR activation can result in uncontrolled cell proliferation, which makes this receptor an attractive target for cancer treatment. Anti-EGFR-targeted agents include antibodies and tyrosine kinase inhibitors. They play an important role in the treatment of various cancers, either as monotherapy or in combination with chemotherapy. In colorectal cancer, the tyrosine kinase inhibitors are not used, because of low or no activity. However, the anti-EGFR monoclonal antibodies cetuximab (Erbitux, ImClone Systems, New York, NY, USA) and panitumumab (Vectibix, Amgen, Thousand Oaks, CA, USA) are frequently used [39]. The clinically significant activity of cetuximab and panitumumab in metastatic colorectal cancer has been demonstrated by a number of phase III clinical trials [40]. In pancreatic cancer, the anti-EGFR tyrosine kinase inhibitor erlotinib has been approved in combination with gemcitabine, but is not widely used in Europe. Class-related adverse events are summarized in Table 4.2 and further explained in the following sections.

## EGFR Inhibitor–Associated Skin Toxicity

Dermatologic side effects are the most common class-specific adverse event reported during anti-EGFR therapy. The rash has a typical appearance (acneiform eruption on face, scalp, neck, shoulders, and upper trunk), is encountered most frequently in about 50–100 % of treated patients, and occurs rapidly after starting the antibodies [41]. Other manifestations that usually occur later in the treatment include xerosis, leading to eczema and fissures, teleangiectasia, hyperpigmentation, hair changes, and paronychia with pyogenic granuloma [41, 42].

The pathophysiology remains largely elusive. Most likely, the underlying mechanism is based on inhibition of the EGF-receptor in the skin. EGFR is expressed in the basal epidermal cells, sebaceous glands, and hair follicle outer root sheath and hair shaft [43]. There are a lot of data in different tumors with the different agents, suggesting a correlation between the severity of skin toxicity and the antitumor efficacy of EGFR-targeted treatment [41, 44]. In the EVEREST trial in chemorefractory colorectal cancer, it has been suggested that a stepwise increase in the dose of cetuximab (from weekly 250 mg/m$^2$ till 500 mg/m$^2$) may lead to increased response rate, in patients with no or only a slight rash. However, additional prospective studies are needed before one can advise this as a standard recommendation in patients who do not develop rash. The EVEREST-2 trial is ongoing to elucidate this concept further [45].

EGFR inhibitor–related skin toxicity often causes cosmetic discomfort, pruritus, or pain, thereby compromising a patient's quality of life and potentially provoking noncompliance. Therefore, adequate treatment of skin symptoms is mandatory. Although we lack evidence-based data on the treatment, many experience-based guidelines have been published, which include topical treatment as well as systemic treatment with antihistamines and antibiotics [41, 42]. A multidisciplinary cooperation of the oncologist and dermatologist is necessary to provide an optimal treatment for each individual patient. Dermatologic symptoms induced by EGFR inhibitors are generally reversible after discontinuation of treatment.

## EGFR Inhibitor–Induced Magnesium Wasting

In healthy subjects, serum magnesium ($Mg^{2+}$) levels are tightly regulated and kept within the 0.70–1.10 mmol/L range by variations in urinary $Mg^{2+}$ excretion in response to altered intestinal $Mg^{2+}$ uptake. After ultrafiltration in the kidney, magnesium is reabsorbed passively in the proximal tubule and the ascending limb of the loop of Henle. However, in the distal convoluted tubule, additional $Mg^{2+}$ reabsorption is mediated by an active transport process through the activity of the transient receptor potential cation channel TRPM6. Magnesium deficiency (serum $Mg^{2+}$ <0.70 mmol/L) may manifest with symptoms of muscle dysfunction (tetany, weakness, ataxia, spasticity, tremor, and cramps), cardiovascular disorders (prolonged QT interval and cardiac arrhythmia), or neurocognitive dysfunction (convulsion, confusion, psychosis, agitation, delirium, and depression) [46].

Clinical trials with EGFR-inhibiting monoclonal antibodies have demonstrated the occurrence of drug-induced electrolyte disorders, such as hypomagnesemia, and in patients with severe hypomagnesemia, also hypocalcemia [46]. It has been suggested that EGFR inhibition induces a TRPM6 dysfunction, comparable to the one seen in patients with hereditary loss of functional mutations in the TRPM6 gene, characterized by urinary magnesium wasting [47, 48].

Most patients with grade 1–2 hypomagnesemia seem to be asymptomatic, although the interpretation is difficult in these heavily pretreated patients with advanced cancer. Patients with severe hypomagnesemia can also develop secondary hypocalcemia through induction of parathyroid hormone (PTH) resistance or suppression [47]. A prospective analysis in patients with colorectal cancer treated with anti-EGFR antibodies showed a decrease in serum $Mg^{2+}$ concentrations in 97 % of patients during treatment [47]. The incidence of grade 3–4 hypomagnesemia varies between 4.5 and 27 % [46]. The median time to onset of hypomagnesemia is 99 days, and recovery of serum magnesium levels is usually achieved 4–6 weeks after discontinuation of EGFR inhibitors [46, 47]. Longer treatment duration with EGFR-blocking agents is associated with a higher risk of developing more severe hypomagnesemia [47, 49]. Increasing age and higher baseline serum $Mg^{2+}$ levels seem also to be related to enhanced renal magnesium wasting [47]. The available data show no difference in incidence and severity of hypomagnesemia between the cetuximab and panitumumab. The duration of treatment is an important factor that should be considered when evaluating the incidence in the different trials. The incidence of hypomagnesemia after a treatment with EGFR tyrosine kinase inhibitors seems to be very low, and this does not seem to be a clinical problem for the tyrosine kinase inhibitors.

Since symptoms of hypomagnesemia can easily remain unrecognized, serum $Mg^{2+}$ levels should be measured regularly (every 4 weeks?) in patients receiving anti-EGFR antibodies. The management is based upon the grade of severity [50]. However, oral magnesium supplementation is not well tolerated, owing to diarrhea, and is often ineffective [47, 50]. Therefore, grade 1 hypomagnesemia requires no treatment, and it is suggested that only patients with grade 2 hypomagnesemia and risk factors such as age and a history of cardiac disease should be treated [50]. Patients should be treated with high doses of oral magnesium supplementation or weekly intravenous replacement (4 g magnesium sulfate). In patients with grade 3–4 hypomagnesemia, appropriate replacement therapy should be given due to the risk of cardiac arrhythmias [50]. This can be very challenging, since serum magnesium levels tend to fall back to the low values within 3–4 days after intravenous replacement and more frequent intravenous administration of magnesium sulfate is time-consuming and socially restricting [47,50]. The best replacement strategy has yet to be determined. Dose reduction of anti-EGFR antibodies for hypomagnesemia has not been studied. A stop-and-go approach with anti-EGFR antibodies can be an alternative for patients with severe hypomagnesemia, without a large tumor burden [50].

## EGFR Inhibitor–Associated Hypersensitivity Infusion Reactions

Allergic and anaphylactic reactions during anti-EFGR antibody administration can cause severe morbidity and a risk for fatal outcome. They are encountered more frequently with the chimeric antibody, cetuximab, than with the fully humanized antibody, panitumumab. In some colorectal cancer trials, up to 5 % of the patients treated with cetuximab developed relatively severe hypersensitivity reactions, despite pretreatment with antihistamines [39]. In 0.1 % outcome was fatal [51]. The incidence of allergic reactions seen with panitumumab is much lower, with an overall incidence around 3 % and severe reactions in <1 % [39, 51]. Up to 90 % of severe reactions occur during the first dose of cetuximab [51]. More recently, it has been shown that premedication with antihistamines and corticosteroids, especially before the first administration of cetuximab, can reduce the incidence of severe infusion reactions. Therefore, prophylactic administration of antiallergic drugs is warranted prior to every cetuximab infusion, and patients should be monitored for at least 1 h after each cetuximab administration. Premedication before administration of panitumumab is not routinely recommended. The optimal prophylactic premedication to prevent hypersensitivity reactions remains unclear but probably includes a corticosteroid and an antihistamine [52].

The pathophysiology of EGFR-associated hypersensitivity is incompletely understood. The presence of IgE-antibodies against the galactose-$\alpha$ (alpha)-1,3-galactose oligosaccharide may play a role in rapid infusion reactions to cetuximab, but it does not explain the mechanisms in more delayed reactions [53]. There are no data on possible risk factors of hypersensitivity to anti-EGFR antibodies.

In case of severe grade 3–4 hypersensitivity reactions, immediate interruption of the EGFR antibody is required, followed by supportive care with administration of oxygen, corticosteroids, and antihistamines [51]. In the presence of hypotension or bronchospasm, the use of vasopressors, epinephrine, and bronchodilators may be necessary. In cases of mild to moderate grade 1–2 infusion reactions, infusion of anti-EGFR antibodies may be safely resumed at a slower infusion rate, after resolution of the allergic symptoms [54]. Because panitumumab has proven to be less allergenic compared to cetuximab, a switch to panitumumab could be a treatment option for patients who developed severe hypersensitivity reactions to cetuximab. Theoretically, there should be no crossover effect because the severe allergic reactions to cetuximab are believed to be directed against its murine component [51]. However, only scarce case reports are available that suggest this approach to be feasible and safe [51, 52].

# References

1. Walko CM, Lindley C. Capecitabine: a review. Clin Ther. 2005;27(1): 23–44.
2. Cassidy J, Saltz L, Twelves C, Van Cutsem E, Hoff P, Kang Y, et al. Efficacy of capecitabine versus 5-fluorouracil in colorectal and gastric cancers: a meta-analysis of individual data from 6171 patients. Ann Oncol. 2011;22(12):2604–9. Epub 2011 Mar 17.
3. Becker K, Erckenbrecht JF, Häussinger D, Frieling T. Cardiotoxicity of the antiproliferative compound fluorouracil. Drugs. 1999;57(4): 475–84.
4. Ang C, Kornbluth M, Thirlwell MP, Rajan RD. Capecitabine-induced cardiotoxicity: case report and review of the literature. Curr Oncol. 2010;17(1):59–63.
5. Kosmas C, Kallistratos MS, Kopterides P, Syrios J, Skopelitis H, Mylonakis N, et al. Cardiotoxicity of fluoropyrimidines in different schedules of administration: a prospective study. J Cancer Res Clin Oncol. 2008;134(1):75–82. Epub 2007 Jul 17.
6. Burger AJ, Mannino S. 5-Fluorouracil-induced coronary vasospasm. Am Heart J. 1987;114(2):433–6.
7. Van Cutsem E, Hoff PM, Blum JL, Abt M, Osterwalder B. Incidence of cardiotoxicity with the oral fluoropyrimidine capecitabine is typical of that reported with 5-fluorouracil. Ann Oncol. 2002;13(3):484–5.
8. Van Cutsem E. Raltitrexed (Tomudex). Expert Opin Investig Drugs. 1998;7(5):823–34.
9. Ciccolini J, Gross E, Dahan L, Lacarelle B, Mercier C. Routine dihydropyrimidine dehydrogenase testing for anticipating 5-fluorouracil-related severe toxicities: hype or hope? Clin Colorectal Cancer. 2010;9(4):224–8.
10. Yen JL, McLeod HL. Should DPD analysis be required prior to prescribing fluoropyrimidines? Eur J Cancer. 2007;43(6):1011–6. Epub 2007 Mar 12.
11. Etienne MC, Lagrange JL, Dassonville O, Fleming R, Thyss A, Renée N, et al. Population study of dihydropyrimidine dehydrogenase in cancer patients. J Clin Oncol. 1994;12(11):2248–53.

12. Amstutz U, Froehlich TK, Largiadèr CR. Dihydropyrimidine dehydrogenase gene as a major predictor of severe 5-fluorouracil toxicity. Pharmacogenomics. 2011;12(9):1321–36.
13. Van Kuilenburg AB, Meinsma R, Zoetekouw L, Van Gennip AH. High prevalence of the IVS14+1G>A mutation in the dihydropyrimidine dehydrogenase gene of patients with severe 5-fluorouracil-associated toxicity. Pharmacogenetics. 2002;12(7):555–8.
14. Schwab M, Zanger UM, Marx C, Schaeffeler E, Klein K, Dippon J, et al. Role of genetic and nongenetic factors for fluorouracil treatment-related severe toxicity: a prospective clinical trial by the German 5-FU Toxicity Study Group. J Clin Oncol. 2008;26(13):2131–8. Epub 2008 Feb 25.
15. Giorgio E, Caroti C, Mattioli F, Uliana V, Parodi MI, D'Amico M, et al. Severe fluoropyrimidine-related toxicity: clinical implications of DPYD analysis and UH2/U ratio evaluation. Cancer Chemother Pharmacol. 2011;68(5):1355–61. Epub 2011 Aug 11.
16. Yang CG, Ciccolini J, Blesius A, Dahan L, Bagarry-Liegey D, Brunet C, et al. DPD-based adaptive dosing of 5-FU in patients with head and neck cancer: impact on treatment efficacy and toxicity. Cancer Chemother Pharmacol. 2011;67(1):49–56. Epub 2010 Mar 5.
17. Weickhardt A, Wells K, Messersmith W. Oxaliplatin-induced neuropathy in colorectal cancer. J Oncol. 2011;2011:201593. Epub 2011 Dec 12.
18. Hoff PM, Saad ED, Costa F, Coutinho AK, Caponero R, Prolla G, et al. Literature review and practical aspects on the management of oxaliplatin-associated toxicity. Clin Colorectal Cancer. 2012;11(2):93–100. Epub 2011 Dec 6.
19. André T, Boni C, Mounedji-Boudiaf L, Navarro M, Tabernero J, Hickish T, et al. Oxaliplatin, fluorouracil, and leucovorin as adjuvant treatment for colon cancer. N Engl J Med. 2004;350(23):2343–51.
20. de Gramont A, Figer A, Seymour M, Homerin M, Hmissi A, Cassidy J, et al. Leucovorin and fluorouracil with or without oxaliplatin as first-line treatment in advanced colorectal cancer. J Clin Oncol. 2000;18(16):2938–47.
21. Gamelin L, Capitain O, Morel A, Dumont A, Traore S, le Anne B, et al. Predictive factors of oxaliplatin neurotoxicity: the involvement of the oxalate outcome pathway. Clin Cancer Res. 2007;13(21):6359–68.
22. Grolleau F, Gamelin L, Boisdron-Celle M, Lapied B, Pelhate M, Gamelin E, et al. A possible explanation for a neurotoxic effect of the anticancer agent oxaliplatin on neuronal voltage-gated sodium channels. J Neurophysiol. 2001;85(5):2293–7.
23. Won HH, Lee J, Park JO, Park YS, Lim HY, Kang WK, et al. Polymorphic markers associated with severe oxaliplatin-induced, chronic peripheral neuropathy in colon cancer patients. Cancer. 2012;118(11):2828–36. doi:10.1002/cncr.26614. Epub 2011 Oct 21.

24. Cavaletti G, Alberti P, Marmiroli P. Chemotherapy-induced peripheral neurotoxicity in the era of pharmacogenomics. Lancet Oncol. 2011; 12(12):1151–61. Epub 2011 Jun 28.

25. Tournigand C, Cervantes A, Figer A, Lledo G, Flesch M, Buyse M, et al. OPTIMOX1: a randomized study of FOLFOX4 or FOLFOX7 with oxaliplatin in a stop-and-go fashion in advanced colorectal cancer – a GERCOR study. J Clin Oncol. 2006;24(3):394–400.

26. Díaz-Rubio E, Gómez-España A, Massutí B, Sastre J, Abad A, Valladares M, et al. First-line XELOX plus bevacizumab followed by XELOX plus bevacizumab or single-agent bevacizumab as maintenance therapy in patients with metastatic colorectal cancer: The Phase III MACRO TTD Study. Oncologist. 2012;17(1):15–25. Epub 2012 Jan 10.

27. Grothey A, Nikcevich DA, Sloan JA, Kugler JW, Silberstein PT, Dentchev T, et al. Intravenous calcium and magnesium for oxaliplatin-induced sensory neurotoxicity in adjuvant colon cancer: NCCTG N04C7. J Clin Oncol. 2011;29(4):421–7. Epub 2010 Dec 28.

28. Park SB, Goldstein D, Lin CS, Krishnan AV, Friedlander ML, Kiernan MC, et al. Neuroprotection for oxaliplatin-induced neurotoxicity: what happened to objective assessment? J Clin Oncol. 2011;29(18):e553–4; author reply e555-6. Epub 2011 May 23.

29. Durand JP, Deplanque G, Montheil V, Gornet JM, Scotte F, Mir O, et al. Efficacy of venlafaxine for the prevention and relief of oxaliplatin induced acute neurotoxicity: results of EFFOX, a randomized, double-blind, placebo-controlled phase III trial. Ann Oncol. 2012;23(1):200–5. Epub 2011 Mar 22.

30. Makrilia N, Syrigou E, Kaklamanos I, Manolopoulos L, Saif MW. Hypersensitivity reactions associated with platinum antineoplastic agents: a systematic review. Met Based Drugs. 2010;2010. pii: 207084. Epub 2010 Sep 20.

31. Kim BH, Bradley T, Tai J, Budman DR. Hypersensitivity to oxaliplatin: an investigation of incidence and risk factors, and literature review. Oncology. 2009;76(4):231–8. Epub 2009 Feb 25.

32. Siu SW, Chan WL, Liu KY, Choy TS, Leung TW, Au KH. Re-challenging patients with oxaliplatin allergy: the successful use of a standardised pre-medication protocol in a single institute. Clin Oncol (R Coll Radiol). 2011;23(8):558–9. doi:10.1016/j.clon.2011.04.005. Epub 2011 Apr 23.

33. Carmeliet P, Jain RK. Principles and mechanisms of vessel normalization for cancer and other angiogenic diseases. Nat Rev Drug Discov. 2011; 10(6):417–27.

34. Jenab-Wolcott J, Giantonio BJ. Antiangiogenic therapy in colorectal cancer: where are we 5 years later? Clin Colorectal Cancer. 2010;9 Suppl 1:S7–15.

35. de Gramont A, de Gramont A, Chibaudel B, Larsen AK, Tournigand C, André T, GERCOR French Oncology Research Group. The evolution of adjuvant therapy in the treatment of early-stage colon cancer. Clin Colorectal Cancer. 2011;10(4):218–26.

160    J. Bogaert et al.

36. Hapani S, Chu D, Wu S. Risk of gastrointestinal perforation in patients with cancer treated with bevacizumab: a meta-analysis. Lancet Oncol. 2009;10(6):559–68.
37. Saif MW, Elfiky A, Salem RR. Gastrointestinal perforation due to bevacizumab in colorectal cancer. Ann Surg Oncol. 2007;14(6):1860–9. Epub 2007 Mar 14.
38. Walraven M, Witteveen PO, Lolkema MP, van Hillegersberg R, Voest EE, Verheul HM. Antiangiogenic tyrosine kinase inhibition related gastrointestinal perforations: a case report and literature review. Angiogenesis. 2011;14(2):135–41. Epub 2010 Dec 29.
39. You B, Chen EX. Anti-EGFR Monoclonal antibodies for treatment of colorectal cancers: development of cetuximab and panitumumab. J Clin Pharmacol. 2012; 52:128–55. [Epub 2011 Mar 22].
40. Prenen H, Tejpar S, Van Cutsem E. New strategies for treatment of KRAS mutant metastatic colorectal cancer. Clin Cancer Res. 2010;16(11):2921–6. Epub 2010 May 11.
41. Segaert S, Van Cutsem E. Clinical signs, pathophysiology and management of skin toxicity during therapy with epidermal growth factor receptor inhibitors. Ann Oncol. 2005;16(9):1425–33. Epub 2005 Jul 12.
42. Segaert S, Chiritescu G, Lemmens L, Dumon K, Van Cutsem E, Tejpar S. Skin toxicities of targeted therapies. Eur J Cancer. 2009;45 Suppl 1:295–308.
43. Green MR, Couchman JR. Differences in human skin between the epidermal growth factor receptor distribution detected by EGF binding and monoclonal antibody recognition. J Invest Dermatol. 1985;85(3):239–45.
44. Giovannini M, Gregorc V, Belli C, Roca E, Lazzari C, Viganò MG, et al. Clinical significance of skin toxicity due to EGFR-targeted therapies. J Oncol. 2009;2009:849051. Epub 2009 Jun 22.
45. US National Library of Medicine. ClinicalTrials.gov [online]. http://clinicaltrials.gov/ct2/show/study/NCT01251536. Accessed on sep 14, 2012.
46. Costa A, Tejpar S, Prenen H, Van Cutsem E. Hypomagnesaemia and targeted anti-epidermal growth factor receptor (EGFR) agents. Target Oncol. 2011;6(4):227–33. doi:10.1007/s11523-011-0200-y. Epub 2011 Nov 24.
47. Tejpar S, Piessevaux H, Claes K, Piront P, Hoenderop JG, Verslype C, et al. Magnesium wasting associated with epidermal-growth-factor receptor-targeting antibodies in colorectal cancer: a prospective study. Lancet Oncol. 2007;8(5):387–94.
48. Groenestege WM, Thébault S, van der Wijst J, van den Berg D, Janssen R, Tejpar S, et al. Impaired basolateral sorting of pro-EGF causes isolated recessive renal hypomagnesemia. J Clin Invest. 2007;117(8):2260–7.
49. Fakih MG, Wilding G, Lombardo J. Cetuximab-induced hypomagnesemia in patients with colorectal cancer. Clin Colorectal Cancer. 2006;6(2):152–6.

50. Fakih M. Management of anti-EGFR-targeting monoclonal antibody-induced hypomagnesemia. Oncology (Williston Park). 2008;22(1): 74–6.
51. Saif MW, Peccerillo J, Potter V. Successful re-challenge with panitumumab in patients who developed hypersensitivity reactions to cetuximab: report of three cases and review of literature. Cancer Chemother Pharmacol. 2009;63(6):1017–22. Epub 2008 Sep 10.
52. George Jr TJ, Laplant KD, Walden EO, Davis AB, Riggs CE, Close JL, et al. Managing cetuximab hypersensitivity-infusion reactions: incidence, risk factors, prevention, and retreatment. J Support Oncol. 2010;8(2):72–7.
53. Chung CH, Mirakhur B, Chan E, Le QT, Berlin J, Morse M, et al. Cetuximab-induced anaphylaxis and IgE specific for galactose-alpha-1,3-galactose. N Engl J Med. 2008;358(11):1109–17.
54. Lenz HJ. Management and preparedness for infusion and hypersensitivity reactions. Oncologist. 2007;12(5):601–9.

# Chapter 5
# Gynecologic Cancer

Sevilay Altintas, Dirk L.A.L. Schrijvers,
and Jan B. Vermorken

**Abstract** Ovarian cancer is the second most common
gynecologic malignancy, with 204,000 new cases of ovarian
cancer per year worldwide, including about 43,000 cases in
Europe and 22,000 in the United States. In the industrialized
world, a large number of these women will survive their cancer.
There have been improvements in outcomes after surgery,
chemotherapy, and radiation therapy; however, patients do
experience significant treatment-related side effects.

Besides the classical cytotoxic agents and hormonal agents,
now used for many years, the development of the newer
molecular targeted agents is currently an exciting area of
interest in the care of patients with gynecologic malignancies.

Angiogenesis seems to play an important role in gynecologic cancer pathogenesis, and elevated levels of angiogenesis
markers seem to be correlated with a worse outcome. Agents

S. Altintas, M.D., Ph.D. • J.B. Vermorken, M.D., Ph.D. (✉)
Department of Medical Oncology, Antwerp University Hospital,
Edegem, Belgium
e-mail: jan.b.vermorken@uza.be

D.L.A.L. Schrijvers, M.D., Ph.D.
Department of Medical Oncology,
Ziekenhuisnetwerk Antwerpen-Middelheim,
Antwerp, Belgium

M.A. Dicato (ed.), *Side Effects of Medical Cancer Therapy,*
DOI 10.1007/978-0-85729-787-7_5,
© Springer-Verlag London 2013

that target single or multiple pathways alone or in combination with chemotherapy are currently under study. Bevacizumab, a monoclonal antibody targeting the vascular endothelial growth factor, and the oral tyrosine kinase inhibitors such as sorafenib, sunitinib, and pazopanib are under investigation, both in the primary disease setting and in the recurrent/metastatic setting.

Challenges are careful patient and drug selection for optimizing the combination of drugs in order to obtain optimal efficacy. The latter depends on several factors: (1) the drugs used must be active as single agents against the particular tumor; (2) the drugs should have different mechanisms of action to minimize emergence of drug resistance; (3) the drugs should have a biochemical basis of at least additive and preferably synergistic effects; (4) the drugs chosen should have a different spectrum of toxicity so they can be used for maximum cell kill at full doses; and (5) the drugs chosen should be administered intermittently so that cell kill is enhanced and prolonged immunosuppression is minimized. This chapter gives an overview of the currently used treatment modalities in gynecologic cancer, their side effects, and their management.

**Keywords**   Gynecologic cancer • Chemotherapy • Targeted therapy • Hormonal therapy • Side effects

# Introduction

Systemic therapies are playing an important role in the management of many patients with gynecologic malignancies. In this present chapter, we will highlight the development in systemic therapy in various tumor types, mainly focusing on what is standard, but touch on some new developments in each of them. In some of these malignancies, a new distinction has been made between different subtypes based on distinctive morphologic and molecular genetic features, which might lead to a more personalized treatment in the future. This means that novel treatment strategies will be developed based on these characteristics (e.g., molecular targeted treatments), which will be accompanied by other and sometimes new forms of toxicity. To manage these new side effects, additional education and experience is essential.

# Epithelial Ovarian Cancer

Epithelial ovarian cancer (EOC) is the most lethal gynecologic malignancy, with a mortality in the European Union of 12/100,000 [1]. Traditionally, EOC is classified into six major histotypes (serous, mucinous, endometrioid, clear cell, transitional cell, and squamous, according to WHO); further, each of them is subdivided into benign, intermediate, and malignant. More recently, however, a subdivision into type I and type II tumors has been proposed by Kurman et al., in which type I tumors include low-grade serous, low-grade endometrioid, clear cell, and mucinous carcinomas, and type II tumors include high-grade serous, high-grade endometrioid, and undifferentiated carcinomas, differing in molecular genetic features and morphology and sensitivity to platinum compounds [2, 3]. FIGO staging is surgical (and most appropriately done by a well-trained gynecologic oncologist), separating early disease (stages I–IIA) from advanced disease (stages IIB–IV). Milestones in the treatment of EOC include (1) the application of surgical staging according to FIGO guidelines (i.e., at least lymph node sampling and peritoneal staging in early disease and upfront maximal debulking in advanced disease) and (2) the evolution in chemotherapy, with the introduction of the platinum compounds in the 1970s and the taxanes in 1990s [4].

## Cytotoxic Chemotherapy

EOC is a chemosensitive disease, and many cytotoxic agents from different classes of drugs are active in this disease, such as alkylating agents (cyclophosphamide, ifosfamide, hexame-thylmelamine), platinum compounds (cisplatin, carboplatin, oxaliplatin), taxanes (paclitaxel, docetaxel), anthracyclines (doxorubicin, epirubicin, pegylated liposomal doxorubicin [PLD]), antimetabolites (5-fluorouracil, gemcitabine), vinca alkaloids (vinorelbine), topo-I inhibitors (topotecan, irinotecan), topo-II inhibitors (etoposide), and, more recently, the minor groove binder trabectedin. Early-disease patients who are at increased risk for recurrence should receive carboplatin (six cycles) alone or the paclitaxel/carboplatin (TC) combination (three to six cycles) after surgery [5, 6]. The standard chemo-therapy approach for advanced disease is six cycles of TC. No other cytotoxic regimen has outperformed this regimen [7], but based on pretreatment conditions, both docetaxel/carbo-platin and carboplatin plus PLD could be considered an alternative to standard therapy [8, 9]. Recent data suggest that a dose-dense therapy using 3-weekly carboplatin and weekly paclitaxel might be superior than the standard TC regimen [10]. Three large randomized trials and several meta-analyses have indicated that intraperitoneal chemotherapy is the preferred approach for patients with optimal debulked disease leading to a survival advantage of about 1 year com-pared to the intravenous administration of the same drugs [11]. Many of the randomized trials performed nowadays include not only EOC but also primary peritoneal or fallopian tube cancers because these tumors behave in a similar way to systemic therapy as used so far.

## Targeted Therapy

Based on current preclinical and clinical information, out of various targets of interest (growth factors and their receptors, angiogenic pathways and extracellular matrix, signal transduction pathways, cell survival pathways, and the proteasome), the angiogenic pathways and drugs targeting these pathways appear to offer the greatest chance of success. Activity of bevacizumab has been observed as a single agent in recurrent EOC; moreover, three studies have shown progression-free survival (PFS) benefit when given in combination with cytotoxic chemotherapy, both in patients with platinum-sensitive disease and in those with platinum-resistant disease [12, 13]. Two key first-line studies, Gynecologic Oncology Group (GOG) 218 and International Collaborative Ovarian Neoplasm (ICON) 7, showed significant improvement in PFS when bevacizumab was given concurrently with the TC regimen and for 16 cycles after TC. In an updated analysis of the ICON7 study at 42 months, high-risk patients (stage III and residual disease >1 cm after surgery and stage IV) also had a better median survival (36.6 months vs. 28.8 months) [14, 15]. Several other anti-VEGF agents are under study, both in phase II and III [16]. An important question is whether these agents are preferably used in first- or second-line treatment. Further studies on this question seem warranted, considering the costs of these agents.

Another group of agents of major interest are the anti-PARP agents. These drugs have an effect in tumors deficient in BRCA1 or BRCA2 or in tumors with a phenotype like that of familial BRCA cancers. The overall frequency of this so-called BRCAness phenotype and homologous recombination dysfunction in ovarian cancer is unknown but is estimated to be up to 50 % of high-grade serous ovarian cancers. Significant improvement in PFS was observed in platinum-sensitive recurrences that were treated with olaparib as maintenance versus placebo [17]. Other PARP inhibitors are under study, both alone and in combination with cytotoxics and molecular targeted agents.

# Non-epithelial Ovarian Cancer

These rare tumors are often difficult to diagnose and therefore will be approached if they were EOC, unless tumor marker patterns ((beta) ß-hCG, AFP, LDH), clinical signs (pregnancy signs, virilization, blood loss), and clinical findings (e.g., ovarian mass and endometrial thickening) do suggest a germ cell tumor (~5 % of ovarian tumors, but >75 % in young patients) or a sex cord-stromal tumor (~5 % of ovarian tumors).

Considering the chemosensitivity of the germ cell tumors, fertility-sparing surgery is recommended. About two-thirds of cases are stage I, and in low-risk cases only careful follow-up is required. In high-risk cases and in more advanced cases, the BEP (bleomycin, etoposide, cisplatin) regimen is recommended. Also, sex cord-stromal tumors, which comprise a variety of different tumors, including granulosa cell tumors (adult and juvenile types) and the Sertoli-Leydig cell tumors, present in an early stage for which no adjuvant chemotherapy is recommended. In higher risk situations of granulosa cell tumors, such as a ruptured ovary or higher stage, adjuvant chemotherapy with EP or BEP might be considered [18]. In recurrent disease, the TC combination has shown activity, and early reports (mostly case reports) on the potential usefulness of bevacizumab and tyrosine kinase inhibitors (e.g., imatinib mesylate) are appearing. Hormonal therapies including tamoxifen, progestogens, LHRH analogues, and aromatase inhibitors have all been used with variable outcomes [18]. Carcinosarcomas previously called malignant mixed Müllerian tumors (MMMTs), which may occur in the ovary but also in the uterus, should be considered as malignant epithelial tumors, not as sarcomas, and treated as such. Adjuvant therapies are indicated in all cases, even in stage I. Based on the two components that are observed, there has been a debate about how to treat them with chemotherapy optimally – whether to use the TC regimen (as in EOC), which is reasonably well tolerated, or to use (also) anthracyclines and/or ifosfamide. The combination of cisplatin, ifosfamide, and doxorubicin (PIA) proved to be very active but too toxic for some of these patients [19].

# Cancer of the Uterine Body

Uterine fundal cancers comprise the great majority of epithelial tumors (90 %), including the typical endometrial adenocarcinomas (90 %), such as papillary endometrioid, papillary serous, clear cell, and mucinous tumors. The remaining 10 % consist of mesenchymal tumors (endometrial stromal sarcoma

[ESS], leiomyosarcoma [LMS], other nonspecific sarcomas), mixed tumors (carcinosarcomas [previously MMMT] and adenosarcomas), and secondary tumors (metastases or direct local extension [cervix, ovary, colon]).

Cancer of the endometrium is the most common gynecologic malignancy in the industrialized world, occurring in 80–90 % of postmenopausal women (median age 63 years), with 5 % occurring in women younger than 40 years old. The main etiologic factor is unopposed/excessive estrogen exposure, and predisposing factors include nulliparity, early menarche/late menopause, obesity, diabetes mellitus, hypertension, and treatment with tamoxifen. Genetic susceptibility includes the Lynch type II syndrome. The two main types of endometrial carcinoma have been recognized on the basis of clinical, pathologic, and molecular features. Type I includes the endometrioid adenocarcinomas (80 %), and type II the papillary serous tumors and clear cell tumors, differing from each other in precursor lesions, hormone sensitivity, grading, initial stage at presentation, behavior, and type of recurrence and outcome (5-year survival of type I is 85 %; of type II, 43 %). Moreover, these two types differ in molecular alterations; type I frequently shows microsatellite instability and mutations of PTEN, K-RAS, PI3K, and (beta) ß-catenin genes, while type II tumors frequently have p53 mutations and overexpression or amplification of HER2 (serous types) and chromosomal instability. Type I tumors are typically estrogen related, comprise low-grade tumors, and most express either estrogen receptors (ER) and/or progesterone receptors (PR) [20].

Contrary to the previously discussed EOCs, most of the patients with endometrial cancer are diagnosed in early stages because of abnormal uterine bleeding as the presenting symptom (90 % of cases). Similar to EOCs, endometrial cancer is surgically staged (which is not always possible due to medical reasons), but the therapeutic approach is determined by prognostic factors such as the spread of the disease, the size of the primary tumor, the degree of differentiation, and the patient's performance status. Both hormonal treatment and cytotoxic chemotherapy are playing an important role, in particular when treating patients with more advanced disease or recurrent/metastatic disease.

## Hormonal Therapy

In the setting of advanced or recurrent/metastatic disease, progestins have been the mainstay of hormonal treatment for many years. They may induce responses in a substantial number of patients, particularly in patients with PR-positive disease (37 % vs. 8 %) in PR-negative cancers [21], and overall the toxicity profile of hormonal therapies is more favorable than that of cytotoxic chemotherapy. Contrary to cytotoxic chemotherapy, hormone therapy can be given for a longer period of time, generally without cumulative and increasing toxicity. It should therefore be considered first-choice treatment in recurrent/metastatic disease. Nevertheless, these agents sometimes can be associated with significant adverse effects (see later), which may have a negative impact on the quality of life of these patients. The type of progestin and the route of administration do not seem to be of major importance; in one GOG trial in which two dosages of orally administered medroxyprogesterone acetate were compared (200 mg vs. 1,000 mg/day), the lower dose proved to be sufficient for an adequate antitumor effect [22]. Tamoxifen and aromatase inhibitors are good alternatives either as primary treatment or in those relapsing on progestins. There is sufficient literature data to discourage the use of hormonal treatment in the adjuvant setting [23, 24].

Cytotoxic chemotherapy is applied in patients failing hormonal treatment or in those with rapidly progressive disease or those known to have PR-negative tumors and poor grading. Among the different classes of cytotoxic agents, platinum compounds, anthracyclines, and taxanes are most commonly used nowadays [20]. However, 5-fluorouracil and ifosfamide (the latter significantly better than cyclophosphamide) also are active agents that can be used in appropriate cases. The TAP regimen (paclitaxel, doxorubicin, cisplatin) induces more responses and may lead to a better PFS but is too toxic for many patients. For that reason, the TC regimen (as used in the treatment of EOC) has gained popularity. It is presently the preferred regimen, both in the advanced and recurrent/metastatic disease settings, and as adjuvant in high-risk patients with early disease (type II tumors) and is presently tested in the PORTEC 3 study, which includes not only all stages of serous and clear cell carcinomas but also endometrioid carcinoma stage I grade 3 and stages II–III, comparing radiotherapy alone versus radiotherapy plus concomitant cisplatin followed by four cycles of TC.

## Targeted Therapy

As earlier mentioned, loss-of-function mutations of PTEN are common and appear to be important in the pathogenesis of type I endometrial carcinomas. Loss of PTEN causes deregulated phosphatidylinositol 3-kinase/serine-threonine kinase/mammalian target of rapamycin (PI3K/Akt/mTOR) signaling, which may provide neoplastic cells with a selective survival advantage by enhancing angiogenesis, protein translation, and cell cycle progression. Temsirolimus, an ester derivative of rapamycin that inhibits mTOR, was evaluated in this setting by Oza et al. [25] and showed encouraging single-agent activity, particularly in chemo-naive patients. However, PTEN loss and molecular markers of the PI3K/Akt/mTOR pathway did not correlate with the clinical outcome in this study. Surely, further studies in this field seem warranted.

Uterine sarcomas, although far less common than endometrial carcinomas, exhibit two features that increase the need for systemic therapy – that is, a recurrence rate of at least 50 %, even in stage I disease and a high propensity for distant failure [26]. The role of systemic therapy in patients with carcinosarcomas has been described in the section on nonepithelial ovarian cancer (see above). Numerous single agents have been tested in LMS. Chemotherapy regimens with efficacy in treating advanced uterine LMS include gemcitabine-docetaxel and doxorubicin and ifosfamide [27]. There are no studies available in patients with LMS that suggest that systemic treatment should be used in the adjuvant setting.

A large proportion of ESS is ER-positive and PR-positive, and durable responses to progestins have been reported [24]. The high percentage of aromatase positivity in low-grade ESSs may have implications for the management of patients with such tumors (i.e., patients with metastatic ESS should be considered for treatment with an aromatase inhibitor).

# Cancer of the Uterine Cervix

Cervical cancer is the second most common malignancy for women worldwide and represents the third most common cause of female mortality, responsible for about 274,000 deaths each year. High-risk persistent infection with sexually transmittable human papillomavirus is responsible for nearly all cases of cervical cancer. Therefore, risk factors for cervical cancer are the same as those for sexually transmitted disease, including early age at onset of sexual activity, multiple pregnancies, and multiple sexual partners. Also tobacco smoking is an important (co)factor for cervical cancer. In those countries where adequate screenings programs are in place, the incidence and mortality have markedly decreased. For this reason, the mortality is 10 times higher in developing countries, where approximately 80 % of new cases occur [28, 29]. In those countries where adequate screening programs are available, squamous carcinoma of the cervix in particular has decreased in the past decades, while the number of adenocarcinomas has increased and now comprises 20–25 % of all cervical cancers. Other epithelial tumors of the cervix are adenosquamous carcinoma, glassy cell carcinoma, adenoid cystic carcinoma, adenoid basal epithelioma (carcinoma), neuroendocrine tumors, carcinoid tumors, and mixed epithelial and mesenchymal tumors and sarcomas (LMS and ESS), while primary cervical melanoma occurs rarely. FIGO staging system is based on clinical evaluation; roentgenographic examination of the chest, kidneys, and skeleton; and endocervical curettage and biopsy. In the last 20 years, numerous advances have been made in the medical management of cervical cancer, including preventive vaccination, and the integration of chemotherapy in the treatment of various stages of cervical cancer.

Patients with early disease (stages I–IIA) are treated by surgery (which can be conservative and fertility sparing in some and radical in others) or radiotherapy (depending on the expertise of the institute where the patient is treated), and patients might receive postoperative concurrent chemoradiation (using cisplatin as a radioenhancer) in case of positive lymph nodes found at surgery. Patients with bulky stage I (IB2), locally advanced disease (stages II–IVA), and basically any stage (except stage IVB) with positive lymph nodes are treated with concurrent chemoradiation. For patients with recurrent and/or metastatic cervical cancer, several options are available (surgery, radiation, chemotherapy, or best supportive care only), depending on the specific situation. However, treatment of metastatic disease so far has remained palliative at best [30].

Treatment of high-risk patients changed dramatically when six randomized trials performed in the United States showed significant improvement in outcome when platinum-based chemotherapy was added to the radiation program, leading in 1999 to a NCI clinical announcement that "based on these results the incorporation of concurrent cisplatin-based chemotherapy with radiation therapy in women who require radiation therapy for cervical cancer should be strongly considered." In 2001, a systemic review and meta-analysis confirmed these data [31]. A further analysis showed that the absolute benefit at 5 years was 6 % (60 % → 66 %) but that the magnitude of benefit was significantly higher in stages I to IIB than in the higher stages [32]. The improvement in stage III/IVA was only 3 %, while for stage I–IIA this was 10 %. The majority of recurrences after concurrent chemoradiation are at distant sites; only a small percentage fail only within the pelvis. Therefore, there was a clear indication to stimulate approaches to decrease distant metastases by using systemic therapy. New approaches include the following:

1. The use of other drugs alone or in combination to enhance the effect of radiation, such as taxanes (paclitaxel), topo-I inhibitors (topotecan), and gemcitabine or targeted therapies such as cetuximab or bevacizumab.

2. The use of neoadjuvant chemotherapy, which indeed in a meta-analysis showed benefit but was highly influenced by the input of some trials from Argentina and Italy with negative other trials; therefore, it is still considered to be an experimental approach.

3. The use of adjuvant chemotherapy. Support for that was found in the meta-analysis, showing that a larger survival benefit was observed in the two trials in which chemotherapy was administered after chemoradiation [32]. Support for that can also be found in the more recent study performed by Dueñas-Gonzáles, presented at ASCO 2009 [33], treating patients during radiation with cisplatin and gemcitabine and giving two cycles of gemcitabine/cisplatin, leading to an improvement in 3-year survival of 9.1 % (69.2 % → 78.2 %). This certainly needs further study.

4. The use of hyperthermia and radiation. Experimental work has shown that hyperthermia (artificial elevation of temperature to 40–45 °C) is an effective cell-killing agent, especially cells in a hypoxic, nutrient-deprived, and low-pH environment, conditions specifically found in malignant tumors. The combination of radiotherapy with hyperthermia provides supra-additive cytotoxic effects [34, 35]. A randomized study, performed in the Netherlands, in 114 patients with locally advanced cervical cancer (stages IIB–IVA) treated with radiation alone or radiation with hyperthermia, showed that the addition of hyperthermia (given weekly) led to more complete responses (83 % vs. 57 %, $p = 0.003$), better local control rate (at 3 years 61 % vs. 41 %), and a better overall survival (at 3 years 51 % vs. 27 %, $p = 0.009$). Radiation toxicity was not enhanced by the hyperthermia, and the application of hyperthermia proved to be cost-effective, with maximum discounted cost per life-year gained of about 4,000 euro [36]. An interesting observation compared with chemoradiation is the fact that this gain in survival is obtained in a study population of more advanced disease, while the benefit with chemoradiation seems to be mainly seen in the earlier stages (see above).

5. The use of methods to overcome hypoxia during radiotherapy. An important aspect in the trials in cervical cancer

is the observation that keeping the hemoglobin level during radiation above 12 g% seems to give better results than reduced levels, irrespective of the pretreatment level [37].

## Locoregional and Metastatic Recurrence

Pelvic surgery should be considered in selected cases of central pelvic recurrence, and salvage radiotherapy should be considered in patients with a pelvic recurrence without prior irradiation. Systemic therapy (or only best supportive care) should be considered in the other cases. Lessons learned in the 1980s and 1990s when chemotherapy was given to patients with recurrent/ metastatic cervical cancer indicated that platinum-based therapies are most effective, that cisplatin seems more active than carboplatin or iproplatin, and that when higher dosages of platinum are used or combinations are used, this leads to more response, but also more toxicity, without an impact on survival; therefore, a dose 50 mg/m$^2$, administered every 3 weeks, became standard. Other newer agents showing activity in this disease are the taxanes (paclitaxel and docetaxel), the topo-I inhibitors (mainly topotecan), the vinca alkaloids (vinorelbine), and the antimetabolites (fluorouracil, gemcitabine). In a direct comparison of cisplatin versus cisplatin plus paclitaxel (GOG study 169), there was gain in PFS for the combination (not in overall survival), but when four different combinations were compared in GOG protocol 204 (cisplatin plus paclitaxel or topotecan, or vinorelbine or gemcitabine), paclitaxel/cisplatin showed a trend for having a better response and PFS, but no significant differences were observed [38, 39]. This led to further interest in targeted therapies. Single-agent bevacizumab used in patients failing one or two cytotoxic regimens showed a PFS that was better than what was available on data with cytotoxic drugs in the GOG database and therefore of interest. Also, a randomized trial of pazopanib (that targets VEGFR, PDGFR, and c-Kit) versus lapatinib (an oral EGFR-TKI with HER2 activity) showed superiority of pazopanib with comparable toxicity. So, antiangiogenesis compounds seem to be of benefit in this disease and need to be further explored [40].

# Carcinoma of the Vulva

Malignant tumors of the vulva are rare (less than 5 % of all cancers of the female genital tract). The majority of malignant vulvar cancers are squamous cell carcinomas, but melanoma, basal cell carcinoma, adenocarcinomas, and sarcomas also may occur. Finally, the vulva may be secondarily involved with malignant disease originating in the bladder, anorectum, or other genital organs [41]. Treatment consists of radical surgery (or a more individualized therapy with less morbidity, but retaining the curative potential of the radical vulvectomy operation) and postoperative irradiation in selected patients at high risk for locoregional failure. The addition of chemotherapy concurrent to radiation therapy was heavily influenced by advances in the treatment of cervical cancer (see above) and squamous cell carcinoma of the anal canal. For those patients who have unresectable primary disease or if nodes are palpably suspicious, fixed, and/or ulcerated preoperatively, chemoradiation is the preferred option. Drugs that have been used for that are 5-fluorouracil or cisplatin alone or combined. Such an approach is also attractive when it can be followed by tailored surgery, to avoid ultra-radical surgical procedures [42]. The role of chemotherapy in the metastatic disease setting is disappointing because of the fact that patients with vulvar cancer tend to be older, making them poor candidates for cytotoxic therapy, because of concomitant diseases that increase the likelihood for significant adverse effects. Nevertheless, two EORTC Gynecological Cancer Cooperative Group studies in the past showed therapeutic activity of the BMC regimen (bleomycin, methotrexate, and CCNU), inducing a response rate of the order of 60 % in the neoadjuvant setting [43, 44].

# Gestational Trophoblastic Disease

A recent review article on the current chemotherapeutic management of patients with gestational trophoblastic neoplasia (GTN) beautifully describes the chemosensitivity of this disease [45]. When in the 1950s the first patient with metastatic choriocarcinoma was successfully treated with chemotherapy at the National Cancer Institute, the late Arthur T. Hertig, professor of pathology at Harvard Medical School, called this God's first cancer and man's first cure [46]. GTN comprises a heterogeneous group of interrelated lesions that arise from abnormal proliferation of placental trophoblast. GTN lesions are histologically distinct malignant lesions that include invasive hydatiform mole, choriocarcinoma, placental site trophoblastic tumor, and epithelioid trophoblastic tumor. GTN often arises after molar pregnancies but can also occur after any gestation, including miscarriages and term pregnancies. In the United States, hydatiform moles are observed in approximately 1/600 therapeutic abortions and 1/1,000 to 2,000 pregnancies [45]. The treatment of these patients should be individualized. Once the pretreatment evaluation is completed and the extent of disease determined, the patient should be assigned a stage (FIGO stages I to IV) and a prognostic score, based on age, antecedent pregnancy, interval from index pregnancy, pretreatment serum hCG, largest tumor size, site of metastases, number of metastases, and whether or not the patient had failed on previous chemotherapy [47]. A FIGO score of 6 or less indicates low-risk GTN, whereas a score of 7 or more identifies high-risk disease. In general, low-risk patients with both metastatic and non-metastatic disease usually respond to single-agent chemotherapy, whereby the most commonly used agents are sequential methotrexate (MTX) and actinomycin D (ACT-D). In case of resistance, several combination regimens can be used, such as the MAC regimen (MTX, ACT-D, and cyclophosphamide) or the EMACO regimen (etoposide, MTX, ACT-D, cyclophosphamide, and vincristine). The high-risk patients are to be treated from the start with combination chemotherapy; for stages II or III and a FIGO prognostic score ≥7 and stage IV, preferably initially with EMACO; and in case of resistance, with drug combinations including both a platinum agent and etoposide, with or without bleomycin or ifosfamide [48].

178 S. Altintas et al.

# Cytotoxic Agents in Gynecologic Cancers

Cytotoxic agents used in gynecologic cancer are summarized in Table 5.5 [49–51].

## Alkylating Agents

Alkylating agents (Table 5.1) are so named because of their ability to alkylate many nucleophilic functional groups under conditions present in cells. They impair cell function by forming covalent bonds with the amino, carboxyl, sulfhydryl, and phosphate groups in biologically important molecules. The most important sites of alkylation are DNA, RNA, and proteins. The electron-rich nitrogen at the 7 position of guanine in DNA is particularly susceptible to alkylation. The alkylating agents depend on cell proliferation for activity but are not cell cycle phase specific. A fixed percentage of cells are killed at a given dose.

## Antitumor Antibiotics

There are many differing antitumor antibiotics (Table 5.2), but generally they prevent cell division in two ways: (1) binding to DNA, making it unable to separate, and (2) inhibiting ribonucleic acid (RNA), preventing enzyme synthesis.

## Antimetabolites

Antimetabolites (Table 5.3) masquerade as purines (azathioprine, mercaptopurine) or pyrimidines, which become the building blocks of DNA. They prevent these substances from becoming incorporated into DNA during the "S" phase of the cell cycle, stopping normal development and division. They also affect RNA synthesis. Owing to their efficacy, these drugs are the most widely used cytostatics. Antimetabolites have a nonlinear dose–response curve, such that after a certain

TABLE 5.1 Alkylating agents used for gynecologic cancer

| Cytotoxic drug | Route of administration | Treatment schedule | Treated diseases |
|---|---|---|---|
| Cisplatin | IV or IP | $10-20$ mg/m$^2$ ×5 every 3 weeks<br><br>$50-75$ mg/m$^2$ every $1-3$ weeks | Ovarian cancer, non-epithelial ovarian cancer, carcinosarcomas endometrial cancer, cervical cancer |
| Carboplatin | IV | AUC 5–AUC 7.5 | Ovarian cancer, cervical cancer, endometrial cancer |
| DTIC | IV | $2-4.5$ mg/kg/day ×10 every 4 weeks | Sarcomas |
| Cyclophosphamide | IV or oral | $1.5-3.0$ mg/kg/day oral<br><br>$10-50$ mg/kg IV every $1-4$ weeks | Ovarian cancer, sarcomas |
| Ifosfamide | IV | 5 g/m$^2$ | Cervical cancer, sarcomas, carcinosarcomas |
| Hexamethylmelamine | Oral | 260 mg/m$^2$ 14 days/4 weeks | Ovarian cancer |

TABLE 5.2 Antitumor antibiotics used for gynecologic cancer

| Cytotoxic drug | Route of administration | Treatment schedule | Treated diseases |
|---|---|---|---|
| Actinomycin D | IV | 0.3–0.5 mg/m$^2$ IV × 5 days every 3–4 weeks | Ovarian germ cell tumors, gestational trophoblastic disease, sarcomas |
| Bleomycin | IV, SC, IM | 30 mg | Cervical cancer, germ cell tumors |
| Mitomycin C | IV | 10–20 mg/m$^2$ every 6–8 weeks | Cervical cancer |
| Doxorubicin | IV | 60–90 mg/m$^2$ every 3 weeks or 20–35 mg/m$^2$ every day ×3 every 3 weeks | Ovarian cancer, endometrial cancer, sarcomas |
| Doxil/Caelyx (Liposomal doxorubicin) | IV | 30–50 mg/m$^2$ | Ovarian cancer |

TABLE 5.3  Antimetabolites used for gynecologic cancer

| Cytotoxic drug | Route of administration | Treatment schedule | Treated diseases |
|---|---|---|---|
| 5-Fluorouracil | IV | 10–15 mg/kg/week | Ovarian cancer, cervical cancer |
| Methotrexate | IV, oral, intrathecal | 240 mg/m$^2$ IV with leucovorin rescue | Gestational trophoblastic disease, ovarian cancer |
| | | 15–40 mg/day oral × 5 days | |
| | | 12–15 mg/m$^2$/week intrathecal | |
| Hydroxyurea | IV, oral | 1–2 mg/m$^2$ daily for 2–6 weeks | Cervical cancer (only in combination with RT) |
| Gemcitabine | IV | 1,000 mg/m$^2$ | Ovarian cancer, cervical cancer |

dose, no more cells are killed despite increasing doses (fluorouracil is an exception).

## Plant Alkaloids

These alkaloids (Table 5.4) are derived from plants and block cell division by preventing microtubule function. Microtubules are vital for cell division, and, without them, cell division cannot occur. The main examples are vinca alkaloids, taxanes, and podophyllotoxins.

Vinca alkaloids bind to specific sites on tubulin, inhibiting the assembly of tubulin into microtubules (M phase of the cell cycle). They are derived from the Madagascar periwinkle, *Catharanthus roseus* (formerly known as *Vinca rosea*).

Podophyllotoxin is a plant-derived compound that is said to help with digestion. It is also used to produce two other cytostatic drugs, etoposide and teniposide. They prevent the cell from entering the G1 phase (the start of DNA replication) and the replication of DNA (the S phase).

The prototype taxane is the natural product paclitaxel, originally known as Taxol and first derived from the bark of the Pacific Yew tree. Docetaxel is a semisynthetic analogue of paclitaxel. Taxanes enhance stability of microtubules, preventing the separation of chromosomes during anaphase.

## Topoisomerase Inhibitors

Topoisomerases (Table 5.5) are essential enzymes that maintain the topology of DNA. Inhibition of type I or type II topoisomerases interferes with both transcription and replication of DNA by upsetting proper DNA supercoiling. Type II topoisomerase inhibitor etoposide is extracted from the alkaloids found in the roots of mayapple plants. They work in the late S and G2 phases of the cell cycle. Etoposide's chemical makeup derives from podophyllotoxin, a toxin found in the American mayapple.

TABLE 5.4  Plant alkaloids in gynecologic cancer

| Cytotoxic drug | Route of administration | Treatment schedule | Treated diseases |
|---|---|---|---|
| *Vinca alkaloids* | | | |
| Vincristine | IV | 0.5–1.4 mg/m$^2$ (max 2 mg/m$^2$) every 1–4 weeks | Vincristine: ovarian germ cell tumors, sarcomas, cervical cancer |
| Vinblastine | IV | 5–6 mg/m$^2$ every 1–2 weeks | Vinblastine: ovarian germ cell tumors, gestational trophoblastic disease |
| *Taxanes* | | | |
| Paclitaxel | IV | 175 mg/m$^2$ 3 weekly or 70–90 mg/m$^2$ weekly | Paclitaxel: ovarian cancer, cervical cancer, endometrial cancer, sarcomas |
| Docetaxel | IV | 75 mg/m$^2$ 3 weekly | Docetaxel: ovarian cancer, cervical cancer, endometrial cancer, sarcomas |
| *Podophyllotoxins* | | | |
| Etoposide (VP-16) | IV | 300–600 mg/m$^2$ divided over 3–4 days every 3–4 weeks | Ovarian germ cell tumors, gestational trophoblastic disease |

TABLE 5.5 Topoisomerase inhibitors in gynecologic cancer

| Cytotoxic drug | Route of administration | Treatment schedule | Treated diseases |
|---|---|---|---|
| *Type I topoisomerase inhibitors* | | | |
| Topotecan | IV | 1.5 mg/m$^2$/day for 5 days, 4 weekly | Topotecan: cervical cancer |
| *Type II topoisomerase inhibitors* | | | |
| Etoposide | IV | 300–600 mg/m$^2$ divided over 3–4 days every 3–4 weeks | Ovarian germ cell tumors, gestational trophoblastic disease |

## Other Agents

### Trabectedin

Trabectedin, a marine-derived antineoplastic agent initially isolated from the tunicate *Ecteinascidia turbinata*, is currently produced synthetically. It binds covalently to the minor groove of DNA, bending DNA toward the major groove, and disrupts transcription, leading to $G_2$-M cell cycle arrest and ultimately apoptosis. Unlike platinum compounds, trabectedin is more cytotoxic in cells with an efficient transcription-coupled nucleotide excision repair system.

Trabectedin is indicated in platinum-sensitive ovarian cancer (recurrence > 6 months platinum-free interval) and sarcomas [52, 53].

### NKTR-102

NKTR-102 is a next-generation topoisomerase I inhibitor that has been engineered to provide a continuous concentration of active drug with reduced peak concentrations. NKTR-102 was designed using Nektar's Advanced Polymer Conjugate Technology platform. NKTR-102 is under investigation for platinum-resistant ovarian cancer [54].

## Side Effects of Systemic Therapy: Prevention and Treatment

Antineoplastic drugs are among the most toxic agents used in modern medicine. In the first-line setting, chemotherapy is often used with curative intent. Once the disease recurs locoregionally or at distant site, many times the main goal of cytotoxic treatment is the relief of disease-related symptoms and prolongation of PFS and overall survival while maintaining quality of life as much as possible.

Many of the side effects, particularly those to organ systems with a rapidly proliferating cell population, are dose related and predictable. In almost all instances, chemothera-peutic agents are used in doses that produce some degree of toxicity to normal tissues.

Severe systemic debility, advanced age, poor nutritional status, or direct organ involvement by primary or metastatic tumor can result in unexpected severe side effects of chemotherapy.

At each stage of the disease, careful monitoring and assessment of benefit versus harm in each individual patient is a major responsibility of the physician dealing with cyto-toxic agents [55, 56].

The commonly used agents in gynecologic cancer, their main side effects, and their prevention and management are described in the sections that follow.

## Chemotherapy

### Platinum Agents

Platinum agents include cisplatin (Platinol, Bristol-Myers-Squibb, Princeton, NJ, USA) and carboplatin (Paraplatin, Bristol-Myers-Squibb, Princeton, NJ, USA).

Platinum-based therapy plays an integral role in the first-line treatment as well as in the recurrent disease setting in several gynecologic cancers (see introduction).

Cisplatin is associated with several cumulative toxicities, including dose-dependent renal tubule toxicity and neurotoxic-ity. Extensive renal damage can occur before any detectable changes in serum creatinine levels. Renal impairment can lead to a reduction in the clearance of some co-administered cytotoxic agents and may potentially increase severe toxicities. Vigorous hydration with adequate diuresis is necessary during cisplatin administration to minimize the risk and severity of acute nephrotoxicity. Amifostine, a naturally occurring thiol that can protect cells from damage by scavenging oxygen-derived free radicals, may be considered for the prevention of nephrotoxicity in patients receiving cisplatin-based chemotherapy [57].

Peripheral neuropathy, ototoxicity, and rarely retrobulbar neuritis and blindness are known side effects of cisplatin. High doses of cisplatin are particularly likely to produce a progressive and delayed peripheral neuropathy. This defect is characterized by sensory impairment and loss of proprioception, where motor strength generally is preserved. Progression of this neuropathy 1–2 months after cessation of high-dose cisplatin has been reported. Diagnosis of neuropathy is typically based on patient history, physical examination, and if necessary an electromyography. Permanent high-tone hearing loss can occur in up to 45 % of patients receiving cisplatin therapy [58–61].

There has been lack of good evidence for the routine use of neuroprotective agents such as vitamin E, amifostine, amitriptyline, gabapentin, and other agents. Few treatment options for neuropathic pain are described, but those are not validated by large, randomized controlled trials. In small numbers of patients, gabapentin, 400 mg three times daily, and amitriptyline, 10–50 mg, have been shown to provide relief in severe neuropathic pain [57, 62].

Hypersensitivity reaction resulting in rash, bronchospasm, urticaria, and hypotension increases with continued use of cisplatin. Prophylactic treatment with steroids and antihistamines and a slow infusion rate may minimize this risk [63].

Gastrointestinal adverse events are also common with cisplatin therapy and may be acute or delayed in onset. Nausea and vomiting are the major complaints among cisplatin-treated patients. Use of 5-hydroxytryptamine-3 inhibitors (granisetron, ondansetron, and tropisetron) in combination with corticosteroids and (fos)aprepitant (NK-1 receptor antagonist) can reduce the incidence and severity of these effects [64].

Myelosuppression with leukopenia and anemia occurs in nearly half of cisplatin-treated patients with advanced ovarian cancer. Despite relatively high rates of low neutrophil counts when cisplatin is used, the rate of febrile neutropenia is low, especially when used in monotherapy. Treatment with hematopoietic growth factors such as granulocyte colony-stimulating factor (G-CSF) can be useful in some cases. The use of G-CSF for primary prophylaxis is only indicated in regimens with a risk of febrile neutropenia of 20 % (e.g., cisplatin/paclitaxel). The use of G-CSF for the treatment of febrile neutropenia is not recommended, except in settings with increased morbidity and mortality, including sepsis, tissue infection, and prolonged neutropenia [65].

Anemia can lead to many symptoms, including fatigue, subsequently impacting on patients' activities of daily living. The role of the erythropoietin-stimulating agents (ESAs) continues to be investigated. United States FDA labeling for ESAs contains a black box warning of adverse effects on survival, progression, and recurrence. Concerns regarding ESA use in a curative setting have been raised, but its use may be appropriate for patients in whom therapy is palliative [66].

The cumulative and irreversible toxicities associated with cisplatin may reduce the potential options for future treatment on relapse. Many new platinum-based formulations have been derived to minimize the severe toxicity profiles associated with cisplatin treatment. These compounds include carboplatin, which is approved for use in ovarian cancer, oxaliplatin, nedaplatin, satraplatin, and other investigational drugs [67].

As mentioned in the introduction, the current standard of care for patients with advanced (stage IIB–IV) ovarian cancer is maximal cytoreductive surgery followed by administration of systemic chemotherapy. First-line therapy consists of platinum (cisplatin or carboplatin) in combination with paclitaxel. Carboplatin is preferred over cisplatin, based on the results of the phase III trial conducted by the Gynecologic Oncology Group (GOG 158). This trial showed that carboplatin/paclitaxel treatment offered efficacy comparable with that of cisplatin/paclitaxel but did not exhibit the cumulative nephrotoxicity associated with cisplatin-based therapy. Furthermore, the International Collaborative Ovarian Neoplasm (ICON) Group studies suggested that the use of carboplatin as a single agent was an acceptable alternative first-line treatment for patients with advanced ovarian cancer [68–70]. This may be true outside trials in certain patient cohorts, but during the latest Ovarian Consensus Conference in June 2010, representatives of 23 cooperative research groups studying gynecologic cancers unanimously agreed that the basic minimum comparator in a phase III trial of advanced ovarian cancer must contain a taxane and a platinum agent given for six cycles [71].

Carboplatin is an alternative for platinum therapy that exhibits considerably lower nephrotoxicity than cisplatin. However, renal function must be monitored when determining dosage regimens to avoid acute toxicity because the renal clearance is the primary means by which carboplatin is cleared from the body. Carboplatin can cause dose-limiting and cumulative myelosuppression. Thrombocytopenia is frequent and severe, and thrombocyte transfusions can be necessary. Other side effects of carboplatin administration are neurotoxicity and hypersensitivity reactions. Hypersensitivity to carboplatin was seen in 12 % of carboplatin-treated patients in a study conducted by [72]. Because of the possibility of fatal cross-hypersensitivity, the use of cisplatin in patients who have developed hypersensitivity to carboplatin is not recommended [72–74].

Platinum agents (i.e., cisplatin and carboplatin) are the drugs of preference for the treatment of concomitant chemoradiotherapy in cervical cancer. The treatment of choice is cisplatin, 40 mg/m$^2$, administered weekly. Despite the fact that weekly cisplatin during radiation is well tolerated, its nephrotoxicity is of particular concern in a patient population that frequently has renal dysfunction as a consequence of ureteral obstruction by the disease spreading to the pelvic wall or to the bladder. Carboplatin has fewer side effects than cisplatin with significantly less gastrointestinal, neural, and renal toxicity. The activity of carboplatin given concurrently with radiotherapy for cervical cancer has been reported and is attractive, especially in terms of toxicity [75].

A particular advantage of concurrent chemotherapy with radiation is the enhancement effect on radiation, leading to better locoregional control, but an early effect on micrometastases might be an additional effect. It has been shown that this cisplatin-based chemoradiation reduces the treatment failures compared to radiotherapy alone and improves cervical cancer survival by approximately 40 % [76–78]. Patients are, however, likely to experience additive toxicities as a result of this combined treatment, and acute toxicities (hematologic toxicity, nausea, vomiting) are more common with chemoradiation than with radiation alone. Acute gastrointestinal symptoms typically involve varying degrees of diarrhea, abdominal discomfort, cramping, nausea, and vomiting. High-risk factors associated with radiotherapy complications are obesity, smoking, pelvic inflammatory disease, diverticulosis, treatment field, and dose [79].

Late toxicities include small bowel obstruction secondary to radiotherapy fibrosis, radiotherapy-induced hemorrhagic cystitis, urinary retention secondary to urethral stricture, complex fistulae, and radiotherapy enteritis and pancreatitis. Some of these late toxicities necessitate surgical intervention [79].

Chronic gastrointestinal toxicity usually occurs in the first 2 years after treatment in about 10 % of patients, with an average interval ranging from 6 to 18 months [80]. Acute gastrointestinal side effects such as diarrhea and fecal incontinence may become chronic. Acute toxicity is usually reversible, and most acute adverse events are self-limiting or resolve with medical management (hydration, loperamide, analgesics), while late effects are often permanent and affect the quality of life [81].

## Taxanes

Taxanes include paclitaxel and docetaxel.

Paclitaxel is a non-platinum-based cytotoxic agent approved for the first-line treatment of advanced ovarian cancer with high antitumor activity when used in combination with carboplatin (TC regimen). Also, in recurrent platinum-sensitive disease, this TC regimen seems to improve PFS and overall survival [68].

Carboplatin could be safely combined with paclitaxel using a dose formula based on projected renal clearance. The recommended outpatient regimen is carboplatin AUC 7.5 and paclitaxel 175 mg/m$^2$ over 3 h without initial G-CSF. However, the use of paclitaxel may be limited by cumulative peripheral neurotoxicity, and a rapid-onset sensory neuropathy can occur. The peripheral neuropathy is due to axonopathy, and also the motor and autonomic nerves appear to be affected by paclitaxel. In this case, docetaxel can be an alternative for paclitaxel, since neurotoxicity is uncommon in the combination of carboplatin/docetaxel [82, 83].

Docetaxel has been examined in several clinical trials for management of platinum-resistant and sensitive ovarian cancer, with an objective response rate of approximately 20–35 % being documented in this clinical setting. This level of activity is comparable to that of paclitaxel observed in a similar patient population.

The dose of single-agent docetaxel in these studies has been 100 mg/m$^2$, delivered on an every-3-weeks schedule. It is not known if a lower dose regimen (e.g., 60 or 80 mg/m$^2$) might result in similar response rates with reduced toxicity. The drug is generally well tolerated in this setting, with the major toxicity being neutropenia and a capillary leak syndrome with fluid accumulation that is related to the cumulative dose and number of cycles.

The toxicities caused by docetaxel use are more pronounced in patients with elevated liver function tests (i.e., transaminase levels greater than 1.5 times the upper limit of normal and alkaline phosphatase levels greater than 2.5 times the upper limit of normal) [84].

The comparison of docetaxel/carboplatin with the standard TC regimen has been studied in the SCOTROC trial, the Scottish Randomized Trial in Ovarian Cancer (paclitaxel 175 mg/m$^2$ administered for 3 h or docetaxel 75 mg/m$^2$ administered for 1 h in combination with carboplatin AUC 5), given for six cycles every 21 days. The main differences in toxicity between the two regimens related to neurotoxicity and myelosuppression, with more neurotoxicity seen with the TC regimen and more myelosuppression seen in the docetaxel plus carboplatin combination [85, 86].

Arthralgias and myalgias are well-described toxicities associated with taxanes and can be very painful and at times disabling. The natural history is to improve with each course of treatment [87]. Arthralgias/myalgias are often difficult to treat, and many patients do not respond to simple analgesics. In a phase II study reported by Markman et al., 46 patients with unacceptable myalgias and arthralgias, despite the use of nonsteroidal anti-inflammatory drugs, were treated with 10-mg twice-daily oral prednisone for 6 days. They reported that 85 % of patients experienced relief of myalgias and arthralgias [88]. Savarese et al. described a pilot study of five patients treated with oral glutamine 10 g three times a day in patients who had developed severe myalgias or arthralgias with their first cycle of paclitaxel. They reported that on glutamine there were no myalgias or arthralgias reported [89].

The acute dose-limiting toxicity of taxanes is the granulocytopenia. Other common side effects include alopecia, nausea, vomiting, diarrhea, mucositis, and hypersensitivity. To decrease the incidence and severity of hypersensitivity reactions, patients should receive pretreatment with steroids. In case of treatment with paclitaxel, the use of a H1 (promethazine or diphenhydramine) and H2 (cimetidine or zantac) receptor antagonist besides corticosteroids is recommended one-half hour before the administration of paclitaxel [90]. Moreover, concomitant steroid therapy allows paclitaxel to be administered over a 3-h infusion period, which is less myelopsuppressive than the 24-h infusion [91, 92].

Rarely, acute pneumonitis, as well as an isolated case of fatal pulmonary fibrosis, has been seen with paclitaxel use. Close monitoring of patients with underlying pulmonary disease is mandatory, and if pneumonitis develops, treatment with steroids is appropriate [93].

## Topotecan

Topotecan has efficacy in advanced ovarian cancer that is comparable with that of both paclitaxel and liposomal doxorubicin. Compared with paclitaxel and liposomal doxorubicin, the majority of topotecan's serious side effects are short-lived, reversible, and noncumulative [94]. The traditional dose schedule is 1.5 mg/m$^2$/day ×5 every 3 weeks, but more convenient weekly regimens are used also [95, 96]. In a randomized phase III trial, comparing topotecan with paclitaxel in recurrent EOC, Ten Bokkel et al. indicated that the most important adverse effect seen in all patients was myelosuppression. Grade 4 neutropenia was observed in 79 % of topotecan patients receiving second-line therapy and in 81 % of the patients who received third-line therapy. The highest incidence of grade 4 neutropenia was observed during the first course (57 % of all patients during second-line treatment and 59.3 % during third-line treatment), and this decreased in subsequent courses. Grade 4 thrombocytopenia was also higher in patients who received topotecan in both second-line and third-line treatment regimens. In the topotecan-treated group, myelosuppression was noncumulative, manageable, and resolved quickly (nadir 5–7 days). For the topotecan group, nonhematologic toxicity consisting primarily of gastrointestinal disturbances (nausea, vomiting, stomatitis, diarrhea, constipation) was generally mild or moderate (grade 1/2). Alopecia is the only cumulative toxicity reported during long-term topotecan therapy.

No end-organ toxicities, such as cardiac, neurologic, skin, or ototoxicity, were observed, and all nonhematologic toxicities were noncumulative [97].

Topotecan is not associated with significant nephrotoxicity. However, prior treatments might have compromised renal function, and because this may influence the renal clearance of topotecan (which correlates with the creatinine clearance), leading to more myelosuppression, assessment of the kidney function before the treatment with topotecan starts is essential. Also dose/schedule adjustments should be based on the patient's treatment history with cytotoxic agents that have cumulative myelotoxicity (e.g., carboplatin) as well as the use of extensive prior radiotherapy [98]. Dose reductions have not shown to decrease response rates. Reducing the starting dose to 1.0 or 1.25 mg/m$^2$/day ×5 is recommended, and this may reduce the incidence of severe myelosuppression in such patients [99]. Hematopoietic growth factors, transfusion therapy, and schedule adjustments may also help manage myelosuppression [100]. Although the liver also contributes to the clearance of topotecan, no dose modifications are necessary in patients with impaired hepatic function [101]. As the thrombopenic effect of topotecan decreases with each next treatment cycle, even in patients who have been heavily pretreated, long-term use of topotecan as palliative therapy for the advanced ovarian cancer is feasible [102].

## Gemcitabine

Gemcitabine is a promising agent in combination with carboplatin in recurrent ovarian cancer [103]. Also, as a single agent in second-line treatment for advanced ovarian cancer, it is found to offer benefit. The response rates with single-agent gemcitabine range from 13 to 24 %, both in previously treated and untreated patients [104]. Doublets consisting of gemcitabine-cisplatin or gemcitabine-paclitaxel, in previously treated patients, induce responses in 53 and 40 % of the patients, respectively. Triplet combinations have also shown to be effective in early-stage trials, although dose-limiting myelosuppression occurs with gemcitabine plus paclitaxel plus carboplatin [105, 106].

Myelosuppression is the primary dose-limiting toxicity of gemcitabine, especially when given in combination with cisplatin or carboplatin because of their overlapping toxicity. Frequent monitoring of hematologic parameters and application of dose modifications, if needed to manage the anemia, leukopenia, and thrombocytopenia, is recommended [107, 108].

Other common adverse events are flu-like symptoms (fever, rigors, and malaise) and lethargia [109]. Less common is dyspnea, which must be distinguished from the symptoms of drug-induced pneumonitis and noncardiogenic pulmonary edema (NCPE), which are rare but life-threatening adverse events. Although the effects of NCPE are usually reversible with immediate intensive supportive therapy, gemcitabine should be stopped at the first sign of this complication [110, 111]. Other side effects of gemcitabine include grade 3 vomiting, manageable fever, peripheral edema, and alopecia; no cumulative hepatic or direct renal toxicities have been reported [109, 112].

After extended gemcitabine use, the development of thrombotic microangiopathy and a life-threatening hemolytic uremic syndrome can occur [113].

## Oral Etoposide

Etoposide is active in malignant ovarian germ cell tumors and gestational trophoblastic neoplasms. The commonly used chemotherapy regimen in these tumor types is BEP (bleomycin, etoposide, and cisplatin) [114].

The activity of prolonged oral administration of etoposide in second-line therapy for advanced ovarian cancer has been studied in a phase II trial by Rose et al. (GOG Group study). The same author studied this regimen in advanced recurrent LMS of the uterus and recurrent or advanced squamous cell carcinoma of the cervix but without success. In cervical cancer, prior radiation therapy limited the ability to deliver prolonged oral etoposide due to hematologic toxicity with grade 4 neutropenia and thrombocytopenia occurring in resp. 33.3 and 15 % of the patients [115–117].

Prolonged oral use of etoposide and higher cumulative doses in EOC have shown that there is an increased risk of developing secondary myelodysplasia and acute leukemias; therefore, this agent is mostly not used in the primary treatment setting. Severe hematologic toxicities are common during long-term etoposide therapy. Grade 3/4 neutropenia and leukopenia occur in 45 and 41 % of etoposide-treated patients, respectively. Deaths from neutropenic sepsis have been reported. Thrombocytopenia and anemia occur at a lower incidence compared with neutropenia and leukopenia. Myelosuppression from etoposide is generally reversible with no cumulative bone marrow toxicity [118]. Regular blood count and support with hematopoietic growth factors will be useful. The treatment of neutropenic fever and sepsis will be highlighted in another chapter.

Other manageable side effects are alopecia, nausea, vomiting, anaphylaxis, mucositis, and acute hypo- and hypertensive responses [119].

## Anthracyclines

Anthracyclines include doxorubicin and pegylated liposomal doxorubicin (PLD).

Doxorubicin is known to be an active agent in endometrial cancer and EOC, and it is often combined with a platinum compound [120–122]. Unfortunately, the clinical use of doxorubicin is limited by its dose-related cardiomyopathy, which becomes more prevalent with increasing cumulative doses. Doxorubicin therapy can be associated with irreversible cardiotoxicity, which may manifest as life-threatening arrhythmias during the acute phase of treatment and leads to a high risk of congestive heart failure [123]. The side effects of anthracyclines and their management are extensively described in Chap. 2.

PLD is a formulation of doxorubicin encapsulated in polyethylene glycol (PEG)-coated liposomes associated with a dramatic alteration in pharmacokinetics characterized by a prolonged circulation time and a small volume of distribution. Liposomes can eventually extravasate through abnormally permeable vessels, which are frequently associated with tumors, and can theoretically deliver high local levels of doxorubicin [124].

PLD is approved for the treatment of advanced ovarian cancer in women refractory to both platinum- and paclitaxel-based chemotherapy regimens. It has comparable efficacy with other second-line or salvage regimens and conventional doxorubicin but has a more favorable toxicity profile [125].

PLD is associated with a dose-limiting hand-foot syndrome (or palmar-plantar erythrodysesthesia syndrome) characterized by painful erythema, peeling, and occasional blistering, which can generally be managed by prolongation of the treatment interval to 4 weeks and/or dose reduction and ultimately drug withdrawal. Almost 50 % of all patients receiving PLD experience hand-foot syndrome (grade 3/4 in 23 % of the patients). There is no established pharmacologic treatment for the hand-foot syndrome, and the use of salves and behavior modification to prevent cracking of the skin can help to improve the pain [122].

The risk of cardiomyopathy with Doxil is reduced compared to free doxorubicin. Histologic examination of cardiac biopsies from patients who received cumulative doses of Doxil from 440 to 840 mg/m$^2$, without prior anthracycline exposure, revealed significantly less cardiac toxicity than in matched doxorubicin controls. However, the cumulative cardiotoxicity of the liposomal formulation has not been established; therefore, extended use of liposomal doxorubicin in patients with impaired myocardial function is contraindicated [126].

Other side effects of PLD are mucositis, hematologic toxicity, alopecia, acute nausea, and vomiting, all of which are manageable. In a phase III trial comparing carboplatin/PLD versus the standard TC regimen in patients with platinum-sensitive recurrent EOC, the combination with carboplatin/PLD was superior in terms of PFS and showed a better therapeutic index [121].

Unfortunately, PLD is currently unavailable for clinical use (as of October 2011). The supply of PLD has been limited because of production equipment failures at the contract manufacturing firm Ben Venue Laboratories (a unit of Germany-based Boehringer Ingelheim).

## Vincristine/Vinblastine

Vinca alkaloids are mainly used in ovarian germ cell tumors (OGCT). The first effective combination chemotherapy for patients with OGCT was the VAC regimen (vincristine, actinomycin D, and cyclophosphamide). Since a remarkable improvement of survival in male testicular cancer patients treated with PVB polychemotherapy (cisplatin, vinblastine, and bleomycin), this regimen was also introduced in OGCT. The PVB regimen proved to be active and more effective than the VAC regimen [127].

Despite the fact that there is only a small structural difference between vincristine and vinblastine, they have significantly different antitumor spectrums and toxicity patterns. Vinblastine has myelosuppression as its primary toxicity, whereas the dose-limiting toxicity for vincristine is the peripheral neuropathy. Toxicity first appears as loss of deep tendon reflexes with distal paresthesias. Cranial nerves can be affected, and the autonomic neuropathy can appear as a dynamic ileus, urinary bladder atony with retention, or hypotension. Older patients and patients who already have neuropathic symptoms due to diabetes mellitus, hereditary neuropathies, or earlier treatment with neurotoxic chemotherapy are thought to be more vulnerable for the development of chemotherapy-induced peripheral neuropathy. Vincristine-induced neuropathy usually starts after a cumulative dose of 5- to 6-mg vincristine (but autonomic neuropathy in particular can occur even after the first administration), and nearly all patients experience some degree of neuropathic signs or symptoms.

Management mainly consists of (cumulative) dose reduction or lower dose intensities, especially in patients who have a higher risk of developing neurotoxic side effects. Neuroprotective agents should ideally protect the nervous system without affecting the antitumor effect of the cytostatic agent. For many years now, potential neuroprotective agents (e.g., nerve growth factor, Org2766, glutamine, amifostine, glutamate, and vitamin E) have been studied, with different results. However, none of these agents can be recommended for standard use in daily clinical practice. Vincristine-induced neuropathy may persist for up to 40 months but in general has a good prognosis [128–130].

## Ifosfamide

Ifosfamide is one of the best-known alkylating agents. In gynecologic cancer, mostly it is used in association with cisplatin. In second-line therapy for ovarian cancer, it shows remarkable activity, even in patients refractory to cisplatin, with more severe, but always manageable toxicity [131].

In gynecologic sarcomas, ifosfamide is, together with doxo-rubicin, an important component in the regimen [132, 133]. The combination of cisplatin, ifosfamide, and doxorubicin (PIA) proved to be very active but too toxic [19].

The TIP (paclitaxel, ifosfamide, and cisplatinum) regimen is highly active (with response rates of 48 %) in locally advanced and relapsed/metastatic cervical cancer, although hematologic toxicity associated with this treatment is consid-erable and supportive measures (hematopoietic growth factors) are needed [134, 135].

The dose-limiting toxicities of ifosfamide are myelosup-pression (especially leukopenia) and hemorrhagic cystitis. Hemorrhagic cystitis is a diffuse inflammation of the bladder leading to dysuria, hematuria, and hemorrhage. Acrolein, a metabolite of ifosfamide and cyclophosphamide, is the main molecule responsible of this side effect. Hemorrhagic cystitis can be prevented by the use of aggressive hydration and the use of mesna (2-mercaptoethanesulfonic acid), which neu-tralizes the toxicity of the acrolein. Mesna binds acrolein and prevent its direct contact with uroepithelium [136].

Other side effects are nausea, vomiting, alopecia, neurologic disorders, and elevated serum creatinine levels. Neurologic symptoms include episodes of somnolence, lethargy, ataxia, disorientation, confusion, dizziness, malaise, depressive psy-chosis, and coma. These toxicities occur more frequently when ifosfamide is given over a 1-day period instead of 5 days. A total of 10–15 % of patients treated with ifosfamide develop an encephalopathy. The exact pathophysiologic mechanisms responsible for the development of ifosfamide-induced enceph-alopathy are not known. However, accumulation of chloroac-etaldehyde, toxic metabolite of ifosfamide, in the central nervous system is theorized to be the cause of the neurotoxic-ity. The intravenous use of methylene blue in a dosage of 6 × 50 mg/day for treatment and 4 × 50 mg/day, either intravenously or orally, for secondary prophylaxis of ifosfamide-induced encephalopathy is recommended [137].

Syndrome of inappropriate antidiuretic hormone secre-tion (SIADH) is characterized by hyponatremia and high urinary osmolality (>100 mOsm/kg) due to inappropriately high serum levels of arginine vasopressin in a clinically euvolemic patient. Hypouricemia urinary sodium level >40 mEq/L and low blood urea nitrogen (BUN) may also indicate diagnosis of SIADH. SIADH affects 1–2 % of all cancer patients and accounts for 30 % of hyponatremia in this population. Ifosfamide has been reported as a cause of SIADH. Hypertonic saline, loop diuretics, fluid restriction, and demeclocycline are mainstays of therapy for SIADH [138–140].

## Cyclophosphamide

Cyclophosphamide can be successfully used in ovarian cancer, soft-tissue sarcoma, and granulosa cell tumor. In ovarian cancer, the preferred regimen is the association with cisplatin. However, this regimen is less effective compared with the currently used TC standard regimen [141]. In soft-tissue sarcoma and granulosa cell tumors, it is preferably combined with Adriamycin and cisplatin [142, 143].

Side effects of cyclophosphamide include chemotherapy-induced nausea and vomiting, bone marrow suppression, stomach ache, diarrhea, darkening of the skin/nails, alopecia (hair loss) or thinning of hair, changes in color and texture of the hair, and lethargy. Hemorrhagic cystitis is a frequent complication that can be adequately prevented by sufficient fluid intake and mesna.

Cyclophosphamide is itself carcinogenic, potentially causing transitional cell carcinoma of the bladder as a long-term complication. Another serious side effect is acute myeloid leukemia, referred to as secondary AML. The risk of its development may be dependent on dose and a number of other factors, including the condition being treated, other agents or treatment modalities used (including radiotherapy), treatment intensity, and length of treatment. Cyclophosphamide-induced AML, when it happens, typically presents some years after treatment, with incidence peaking around 3–9 years. After 9 years, the risk has fallen to the level of the regular population. When AML occurs, it is often preceded by a myelodysplastic syndrome phase, before developing into overt acute leukemia. Cyclophosphamide-induced leukemia will often involve complex cytogenetics, which carries a worse prognosis than the de novo AML [144, 145].

## Bleomycin

Bleomycin, first isolated in 1966 by Umazawa and associates, is a cytotoxic antibiotic synthesized from *Streptomyces verticillus*. It is used primarily in the therapy of lymphomas, squamous cell carcinomas, and germ cell tumors and has little myelo-suppressive or immunosuppressive activity.

Bleomycin, etoposide, and cisplatin (BEP) regimen is a modified PVB regimen by substitution of etoposide for vin-blastine in ovarian germ cell tumors (OGCT), since the BEP regimen proved to be equally active but less toxic [146].

Bleomycin is an attractive addition to combination chemo-therapy regimens because of its broad activity and low myelotoxicity. However, pulmonary toxicity is the major complication limiting its use. Bleomycin is inactivated by a hydrolase enzyme that is relatively deficient in lung tissue. This probably contributes to the sensitivity of lung tissue to the effects of bleomycin. Pulmonary toxicity can present either as an interstitial pneumonitis with progressive fibrosis or, rarely, as an acute hypersensitivity reaction. In both syn-dromes, the most common symptoms are dyspnea and a non-productive cough. On examination of the chest, basal crepitations may be present, but often there are few abnor-mal physical signs. The hypersensitivity reaction may be asso-ciated with fever and eosinophilia. Several factors may contribute to the risk of development of bleomycin pulmo-nary damage. Above a total dose of 450–500 mg, the inci-dence of interstitial fibrosis rises from 35 to 40 %, and this is associated with a higher mortality. However, cases of pulmo-nary toxicity have been described in patients who have received less than 200 mg. The hypersensitivity reaction is not dose dependent. Concurrent or previous radiotherapy or therapy with other chemotherapeutic agents, especially cyclo-phosphamide, and oxygen therapy during or up to 6 months after the administration of bleomycin are additional risk factors. Renal failure may result in higher bleomycin serum levels. Concomitant cisplatin toxicity may contribute to the development of renal failure. Bleomycin should not be given to patients with creatinine clearances <30 mL/min because of the altered pharmacology of the drug in that situation.

There are some reports of symptomatic and radiographic improvement with corticosteroid therapy, especially in the acute situation. However, no controlled studies have been performed to test the role of steroids in treatment. In patients who seemed to improve on steroid therapy, the pulmonary function tests remained abnormal. As treatment of the progressive pulmonary involvement appears relatively unsuccessful, the emphasis should be placed on prevention. All patients who receive bleomycin should have serial pulmonary function tests. If any of the aforementioned risk factors are present, a high index of suspicion should be maintained. It is recommended that further bleomycin therapy should be withheld if the DLco falls below 40 % of the initial value, the FVC decreases by 20 %, or if any symptoms, signs, or chest radiograph features of toxicity appear [147–150].

## Methotrexate

As mentioned in the introduction, single-agent methotrexate (MTX) is the first choice for the treatment of low-risk GTN. However, actinomycin D (ACT-D) can be used as a first-line agent in patients with hepatic dysfunction or who have a known adverse reaction to MTX [45, 151]. In case of disease resistant to single agents, the preferred combination chemotherapy regimen is often MAC (MTX, ACT-D, and cyclophosphamide) or EMACO (etoposide, MTX, ACT-D, cyclophosphamide, and vincristine). MAC is preferred as the initial combination chemotherapy regimen since etoposide, which is a component of EMACO, is associated with an increased risk for secondary malignancies. Studies have shown that patients treated with more than 2 g/m$^2$ of etoposide had a relative risk of 16.6 for developing leukemia, 5.8 for breast cancer, 4.6 for colon cancer, and 3.4 for melanoma [152].

The most described side effects of MTX are mucositis (20–60 % rates) with mucosal ulcerations, myelosuppression, hepatotoxicity, allergic pneumonitis, and, in case of intrathecal use, meningeal irritation. High-dose MTX for doses ≥500 mg/m$^2$ is used in hematologic settings. These regimens deliver an otherwise lethal dose of MTX in a 4- to 36-h infusion, followed by a 2- to 3-day period of multiple leucovorin doses to terminate the toxic effect of MTX (leucovorin "rescue"). Successful rescue by leucovorin depends on rapid elimination of MTX by the kidneys, which requires aggressive pretreatment as well as posttreatment hydration and urinary alkalinization. The main toxicities of high-dose MTX are elevated serum transaminase levels and renal insufficiency, which can delay drug clearance. Doses between 50 and 500 mg/m$^2$, as used for malignant gestational trophoblastic disease, are considered intermediate-dose MTX. In general, these patients do not require aggressive hydration or urinary alkalinization. Leucovorin rescue is rarely needed with doses ≤250 mg/m$^2$ unless unexpected toxicity is encountered. When there is renal impairment, leucovorin should be repeated every 6 h until the serum level of MTX falls below 0.1 mmol/L. Alkalinization of urine helps in the excretion of MTX, as MTX and its metabolites are poorly soluble in acidic pH. An increase in the pH of urine from 6.0 to 7.0 increases the solubility of MTX and its metabolites by five to eight times. Aggressive hydration also helps with the renal excretion of MTX and its metabolites [153]. Attention has to be kept on concomitant medication, since many agents are known to prolong MTX elimination, including probenecid, salicylates, nonsteroidal anti-inflammatory drugs (NSAIDs), and weak organic acids [154].

## 5-Fluorouracil

The use of 5-fluorouracil (5-FU) has been studied in recurrent ovarian and cervical cancer, both in phase II trials [155, 156]. In both trials, the main side effects were myelosuppression and gastrointestinal toxicity.

The toxicity of 5-FU, which includes leukopenia, diarrhea, stomatitis, nausea, vomiting, and alopecia, differs with its schedule of administration. Dose-limiting toxicities of bolus 5-FU are diarrhea and myelosuppression. Hand-foot syndrome and stomatitis are also dose limiting with prolonged infusion. Coronary events induced by 5-FU are rare, but considering the potentially lethal nature of this toxicity, physicians should be aware of this possible side effect [157]. Overall, toxicities associated with fluorouracil are more common and more severe in patients with dihydropyrimidine dehydrogenase (DPD) deficiency. Individuals with complete or partial DPD deficiency have a strongly reduced capacity to metabolize 5-FU and therefore experience severe, and sometimes life-threatening, toxic effects from the increased levels of active drug. However, the screening of patients for the presence of DPD deficiency prior to the start of treatment with fluoropyrimidines is not routinely recommended [158].

Numerous approaches have been suggested for managing toxicities caused by 5-FU. The most obvious action would be to stop any further administration of 5-FU in case of severe gastrointestinal toxicity, this followed by aggressive supportive care. Antibiotic and antibacterial coverage may be used in treating potential bacterial and fungal infections resulting from the invasion of enteric organisms through the weakened gut lining. Dehydration and hypotension may be treated with appropriate fluid and electrolyte support. In the most severe cases, hospitalization in the intensive care unit may be necessary.

In case of mucositis, general approaches include effective oral care, dietary modifications, topical mucosal protectants (e.g., Caphosol), topical anesthetics, and systemic analgesics, if necessary. Chlorhexidine oral rinses, as a topical antimicrobial, may be an option to consider when treating an oral infection. Palifermin (keratinocyte growth factor-1) given intravenously has been studied in solid tumor cohorts but is currently not standard of care. One study suggested that palifermin may be useful in a dose of 40 (mu)μg/kg/day for 3 days for prevention of oral mucositis in patients receiving bolus 5-FU plus leucovorin.

Oral cryotherapy is recommended for prevention of oral mucositis in patients receiving bolus 5-FU chemotherapy [159].

## Trabectedin

Trabectedin is indicated in platinum-sensitive ovarian cancer (recurrence >6 months platinum-free interval) and sarcomas. Its main dose-limiting toxicity is hepatotoxicity and myelosuppression. Premedication with dexamethasone can strongly reduce drug-induced hepatotoxicity and myelosuppression [160]. In a phase II trial in relapsed platinum-sensitive ovarian cancer patients, both every-3-weeks trabectedin regimens, 1.5 mg/m$^2$ 24 h and 1.3 mg/m$^2$ 3 h, were active and reasonably well tolerated. The most common trabectedin-related adverse events were nausea, vomiting, and fatigue, most of them being grade 2 or 3, which were transient, noncumulative, and usually without clinical relevance [161]. However, apart from the advantage of a shorter infusion time, a slightly better safety profile was found for the 3-h schedule with respect to myelosuppression (neutropenia), fatigue, and vomiting. For management of myelosuppression and nausea/vomiting see previous section. The combination of PLD plus trabectedin (using the 3-h every-3-weeks regimen) has been evaluated versus PLD alone in patients with relapsed EOC in a recently finished randomized phase III trial. The results of this phase III trial have shown a statistically significant and clinically relevant patient benefit when trabectedin is combined with PLD [52].

## NKTR-102

NKTR-102 has been studied in an open label, phase II trial in a patient population with advanced platinum-refractory ovarian cancer (platinum-free interval <6 months). Median lines of prior therapy for women enrolled in the study were three, with 47 % of the women having failed prior treatment with pegylated liposomal doxorubicin. NKTR-102 was given either on a q14d or q21d regimen. Response rates were high, irrespective of the number of lines of prior therapy. Based on this highly promising data set, a phase III study is underway [54].

The most common grade 3 and 4 side effects were diarrhea, dehydration, hypokalemia, fatigue, nausea, and neutropenia, with most side effects being grade 3 in severity; all were manageable with supportive care. One patient in each dose regimen died due to neutropenic sepsis (q21d) and prerenal azotemia (q14d).

## Hormonal Therapy

Many gynecologic cancers, including epithelial and stromal ovarian cancers, endometrial carcinomas, and some gynecologic sarcomas, in particular ESS, express ER and/or PR receptors. Hormonal therapy is in many ways more attractive than chemotherapy in recurrent or metastatic gynecologic cancers, since the objective of treatment is palliation and prolongation of survival rather than cure.

Endocrine therapy is not associated with the more severe, acute toxicities of chemotherapy and can be administered for prolonged periods with relatively little cumulative toxicity.

There are numerous case reports, retrospective studies, and small phase 2 studies using a variety of hormonal therapies in this patient population. The most commonly used agents include progestogens, tamoxifen, and luteinizing hormone-releasing hormone (LHRH) agonists. More recently, aromatase inhibitors have also been prescribed [21, 162–164].

Although progestogens have been the mainstay of hormonal treatment in women with recurrent/metastatic endometrial cancer for many years, these agents can be associated with significant adverse effects, including weight gain, hypertension, fluid retention, increased blood sugar, insomnia, tremor, thrombosis, and pulmonary emboli. These can potentially worsen the quality of life and may be life-threatening [21].

Many side effects of endocrine therapy, such as hot flushes and mood disturbances, are related to estrogen deprivation and are common to tamoxifen and aromatase inhibitors (nonsteroidal: anastrozole and letrozole; steroidal: exemestane). Tamoxifen has estrogenic effects that are beneficial in some tissues; tamoxifen lowers serum cholesterol levels and protects against bone loss and cardiovascular disease but is also associated with potentially life-threatening side effects, such as thromboembolic disease (stroke or pulmonary embolism) and endometrial cancer [162]. Since aromatase inhibitors lack estrogenic activity, they are not associated with these serious adverse events. Aromatase inhibitors are also associated with a lower incidence of gynecologic symptoms (vaginal dryness, vaginal bleeding) and hot flushes than tamoxifen. However, AIs are associated with musculoskeletal side effects, such as arthralgia, myalgia, and bone loss, but these events are preventable or manageable [164]. In case of hot flushes nonpharmacological approaches such as avoidance of foods or situations that trigger hot flushes, wearing natural fabrics, and employing methods of rapid cooling, such as spray mists or moist wipes, can be effective. The potential benefits of vitamin E and therapies that contain isoflavones have failed to demonstrate any benefit. Data from placebo-controlled clinical trials indicate that the selective serotonin reuptake inhibitors or SSRIs (paroxetine, venlafaxine) are the most effective agents available for the prevention of hot flushes [165, 166].

Vaginal dryness occurs as a result of estrogen deprivation; it can cause pain during intercourse and, subsequently, contributes to loss of libido. Local lubricants can be used temporarily to alleviate symptoms. Topical vaginal estrogen preparations have been shown to relieve the symptoms of vaginal dryness [165, 166].

In postmenopausal women with early breast cancer, postoperative adjuvant AI therapy, which reduces circulating estrogen levels, has been associated with an increased incidence of arthralgia and myalgia compared with tamoxifen or placebo. Although muscular and joint pains are common side effects of AIs, affecting up to 35 % of patients, and can be troublesome in some individuals, symptoms are rarely severe enough to necessitate treatment discontinuation, and they usually improve with time. Where necessary, management options are available to help patients to cope with joint and/or muscle pains. Physical strategies, such as physiotherapy or massage, can help to relieve symptoms. Pharmaceutical intervention is limited to analgesics; nonsteroidal anti-inflammatory drugs, acetaminophen, or cyclooxygenase-2 inhibitors are effective in most patients, although stronger analgesics can be prescribed if necessary [167].

Loss of bone mass is a well-recognized consequence of estrogen deprivation. The recommended treatment depends on the extent of bone loss and includes reassurance, advice on lifestyle changes to slow or prevent further bone loss, such as increasing weight-bearing physical activity and taking dietary supplements (calcium and vitamin D), and drug therapy (e.g., with bisphosphonates in case of severe bone loss).

Hypercholesterolemia and cardiovascular disease have been reported more frequently in patients taking an aromatase inhibitor, but there is evidence to suggest that at least some of these effects reflect the absence of tamoxifen's beneficial estrogenic actions on these target tissues rather than a detrimental effect of the aromatase inhibitors. Patients taking an aromatase inhibitor should undergo regular screening for cardiovascular risk factors such as blood pressure monitoring and serum cholesterol measurements as part of routine health checks, but no specific management strategies are required [168].

## Other Cytotoxic Treatment Modalities

### Intraperitoneal Chemotherapy

The intraperitoneal (IP) delivery of cisplatin has been demonstrated in several evidence-based randomized phase 3 trials to improve overall survival when employed as first-line chemotherapy in patients with small-volume residual advanced ovarian cancer. Despite this fact, the use of IP chemotherapy is still today not accepted by all clinicians as the treatment of choice for optimally debulked EOC. The latter is due to a significantly reduced quality of life during treatment with IV/IP versus IV chemotherapy. In the GOG 172 study, patients in the IP/IV group experienced significantly more neurologic side effects and abdominal discomfort. Abdominal discomfort began to improve for both groups during treatment, and no differences in discomfort remained soon after the end of treatment. However, neurologic side effects remained worse in patients in the IP/IV group, even at 1 year after treatment [169].

Substantial local toxicity with abdominal pain and adhesion formation leading to bowel obstruction are of concern, as is the systemic toxicity associated with cisplatin, which remains an issue in case of IV/IP chemotherapy. The use of IP carboplatin is of particular interest, as it has been documented to have a more favorable toxicity profile compared to cisplatin. Another attractive property of IP carboplatin is that its use makes it easier to deliver in the setting of a busy oncology practice. Unfortunately, there are no comparison data of IP delivery of those two platinum agents showing their equivalence. Currently, phase I studies are ongoing with the IP delivery of carboplatin or paclitaxel [170–172].

## Hyperthermic Intraperitoneal Chemotherapy

For a discussion of hyperthermia in cervical cancer, see the introduction.

Locoregional treatments combining cytoreductive surgery and intraperitoneal chemohyperthermia (HIPEC) may improve survival for locoregional disease in recurrent ovarian cancer [173, 174]. However, morbidity and mortality of this treatment modality are substantial, and rates between 10 and 50 % have been reported in the literature. The most published results come from observational case series, and phase III trials are lacking [175]. The complications that occur are related to the cytoreductive surgery and the delivered chemotherapy. Postoperative complications can include respiratory failure, bacteremia, renal failure, pyelonephritis, pulmonary embolism, pneumonia, urinary infections, and pyrexia. Complications related to chemotherapy include toxicity of that particular drug (mainly cisplatin, oxaliplatin, mitomycin C). Iterative cytoreductive surgery with HIPEC can be performed; however, strict patient selection is essential, taking into consideration the origin of carcinomatosis, length of recurrence-free interval, age, comorbidity, and likelihood of achieving complete cytoreduction [176].

# Side Effects of Targeted Agents in Gynecologic Cancer

Important molecular pathways that regulate independency and insensitivity to signal transduction, angiogenesis, apoptosis, invasion, and metastatic potential of cancer cells have been described in development of gynecologic cancers. Medications that target these pathways are being developed and tested in the treatment of gynecologic cancers. Some of them have made their entry in clinical practice. In this section, the focus is on the side effects of targeted agents used in the treatment of early and recurrent gynecologic cancers.

## Ovarian Cancer

Several pathways have been identified in the genesis of ovarian cancer, and medication targeting the epidermal growth factor receptor (EGFR) and HER2 receptor, PARP repair mechanism, and angiogenesis are already in clinical testing or used in patients with ovarian cancer (Fig. 5.1). Most of these drugs are evaluated in recurrent or advanced disease, while one of them has been tested in adjuvant setting after primary debulking in combination with chemotherapy.

### Epidermal Growth Factor Receptor–Targeting Drugs

In ovarian cancer, the EGFR is overexpressed in 10–70 % with an average of 48 % of ovarian tumors [178]. The EGFR can be influenced by monoclonal antibodies (e.g., cetuximab) or small molecules (e.g., gefitinib, erlotinib, lapatinib), and they have been tested in several phase II studies with or without chemotherapy in patients with ovarian cancer [179].

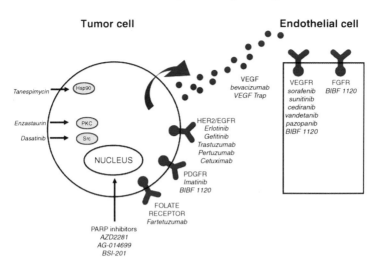

FIGURE 5.1 Targeted therapy agents under evaluation in phase II–III trials of epithelial ovarian cancer. *EGFR* epidermal growth factor receptor, *HER2* human epidermal growth factor receptor 2, *Hsp* heat shock protein, *PARP* poly(adenosine diphosphate-ribose) polymerase, *PDGFR* platelet-derived growth factor receptor, *PKC* protein kinase C, *VEGF* vascular endothelial growth factor, *VEGFR* VEGF receptor (Reprinted with permission from Banarjee and Gore [177])

## Monoclonal Antibodies

### Cetuximab

In several phase II studies, cetuximab scheduled as 400 mg/m$^2$/week followed by 250 mg/m$^2$/week was combined with chemotherapy in patients with ovarian cancer. In a study combining cetuximab with carboplatin (area under the curve [AUC] 6) in 28 evaluable patients with EGFR-positive ovarian cancer, the most commonly observed toxicities were grade 3 dermatologic toxicity (32 %), grade 3 thrombocytopenia (14 %), and metabolic toxicity (14 %). Hypersensitivity reactions occurred in 32 % of patients including 18 % grade 3/4 reactions partly due to cetuximab [180]. Another study combining cetuximab, carboplatin (AUC 6), and paclitaxel

(175 mg/m²) in 40 evaluable patients had as grade 3/4 treatment-related toxicities febrile neutropenia (12.5 %), rash (2.5 %), hypersensitivity reaction (7.5 %), and hypomagnesemia (12.5 %). Common grade 1/2 toxicities attributed to cetuximab included acneiform rash (82.5 %), hirsutism (7.5 %) or abnormal hair growth (25 %), and nail disorders (22.5 %) [181].

EGFR Tyrosine Kinase Inhibitors

*Gefitinib*

Gefitinib 500 mg/day was given to 30 women with recurrent or persistent epithelial ovarian or primary peritoneal carcinoma in a phase II study. The most commonly observed grade 3 toxicities in 27 evaluable patients were dermatologic toxicity (15 %) and diarrhea [182].

Gefitinib 500 mg/day was given to 24 patients with recurrent ovarian cancer in another phase II trial. Adverse events observed in this trial were generally mild, and the most common adverse events ≥2 grade were diarrhea (33 %), nausea (12 %) and vomiting (12 %), fatigue (17 %), rash (12 %), and hypoalbuminemia (21 %). Grade 4 hyponatremia was reported in one patient with short bowel syndrome and underlying adrenal insufficiency [183].

The combination of gefitinib and tamoxifen 40 mg/day was also studied in 56 patients with ovarian cancer refractory or resistant to platinum- and taxane-based therapy. The dosage of gefitinib had to be decreased from 500 to 250 mg/day in 14.9 % of patients, predominantly due to diarrhea (10.7 %). Most frequent drug-related adverse events were diarrhea and acne-like skin rash. Side effects were similar compared to gefitinib monotherapy, and the addition of tamoxifen did not increase toxicity [184].

*Erlotinib*

In a phase II study in 34 patients with ovarian cancer, rash and diarrhea were the main toxicities when erlotinib 150 mg/day was given as single agent [185]. When erlotinib 150 mg/day was combined with carboplatin (AUC 5 every 3 weeks), the toxicity profile did not change importantly in 20 patients with ovarian cancer treated with up to two prior chemotherapy regimens, and no excessive toxicity was noted [186]. However, when the combination of erlotinib and carboplatin with docetaxel followed by maintenance erlotinib was tested in patients with ovarian cancer, an unexpected high gastrointestinal toxicity was observed [187].

*Lapatinib*

Lapatinib, 1,500 mg/day orally, was tested as single agent in 25 evaluable patients with recurrent ovarian cancer. Toxicities reported were one grade 4 fatigue and some grade 3 toxicities [188].

The combination of oral lapatinib 1,250 mg/day with topotecan 3.2 mg/m$^2$ intravenously on days 1, 8, and 15 and lapatinib 1,250 mg PO daily, continuously in 28-day cycles, was tested in 18 patients with platinum-refractory or platinum-resistant ovarian cancer. This treatment resulted in significant grade 3/4 hematologic and nonhematologic toxicity with neutropenia (56 %), thrombocytopenia (28 %), and diarrhea (22 %) [189].

Drugs interfering with the EGFR seem not to be more toxic in patients with ovarian cancer. However, in combination with chemotherapeutic agents active in ovarian cancer such as topotecan, hematologic toxicity, although uncommon with this group of medication, may be a factor that should be taken into account.

## HER2-Receptor–Targeting Drugs

HER2-receptor expression in ovarian cancer has been variable and ranges from 1.8 to 35 % [179]. The HER2 receptor can be influenced by monoclonal antibodies or tyrosine kinase inhibitors, and some have been tested in patients with ovarian cancer (e.g., trastuzumab, pertuzumab, lapatinib) with limited effect, although in patients with HER2 overexpression tumors, the results may be better.

For trastuzumab, the most frequent side effects reported in these phase II studies when used as single agent were anemia, gastrointestinal issues, neuropathy, and fatigue [190]; for pertuzumab, diarrhea, abdominal pain, left ventricular ejection fraction (LVEF) decrease, atrial fibrillation, pericardial effusion, and pneumonia [191]; for lapatinib in combination with chemotherapy, hematologic toxicity and diarrhea have been reported [189].

## PARP Repair Mechanism–Interfering Drugs

Poly(ADP-ribose) polymerases (PARPs) are a family of nuclear enzymes that regulates the repair of DNA single-strand breaks through base excision repair [192]. It is an important mechanism in DNA damage repair together with the BRCA complex. In patients with inactivating mutations in the BRCA genes, PARP is the remaining repair mechanism for homologous recombination. Up to 50–60 % of epithelial ovarian cancers are defective in their ability to repair DNA damage using homologous recombination, and patients with these tumors might benefit from PARP inhibitors [193]. Several phase II studies with PARP inhibitors showed activity in recurrent platinum-sensitive ovarian cancer in combination with chemotherapy or as single-agent maintenance after chemotherapy [179].

### Olaparib

Olaparib is a competitive NAD + inhibitor that inhibits PARP activity. When used as single agent, olaparib 200 mg/day orally is generally well tolerated, and the most common drug-related toxicities are mild gastrointestinal symptoms (6 % grade 3 nausea; 2 % grade 3 vomiting and diarrhea) and fatigue (4 % grade 3). There were no obvious differences in the pattern of toxicities experienced by patients with BRCA1- or BRCA2-mutated ovarian cancer or between BRCA and non-BRCA mutation carriers [194].

Another phase II trial treated patients with BRCA1- or BRCA2-mutated ovarian cancer with single-agent olaparib in two different dosages (2× 100 mg daily and 2× 400 mg daily). In patients given olaparib 800 mg daily, the most frequent adverse events were nausea (42 % grade 1/2; 6 % grade 3/4), fatigue (30 % grade 1/2; 3 % grade 3/4), and anemia

(15 % grade 1/2; 3 % grade 3/4). The most frequent causally related adverse events in the cohort given 200 mg daily were nausea (29 % grade 1/2; 8 % grade 3/4) and fatigue (38 % grade 1/2) [195].

Two different dosages of olaparib (400 and 800 mg daily) were compared with pegylated liposomal doxorubicin (50 mg/m$^2$ intravenously every 28 days) in a randomized phase II trial in 97 patients with recurrent ovarian cancer with BRCA1 or BRCA2 deficiency. The most common adverse effects in the olaparib groups were grade 2 fatigue, gastrointestinal symptoms, anemia, and rash and were more commonly observed in the 800-mg olaparib group. The incidence of grade 3/4 events was low, although grade 3 anemia was seen more frequently in patients receiving olaparib 800 mg (13 %) [196].

PARP inhibitors are mostly well tolerated in patients with ovarian cancer, with gastrointestinal side effects and fatigue being the most frequently observed side effects.

## Angiogenesis Inhibition

Angiogenesis is a complex mechanism with different actors involved. Hypoxia is one of the main determinants of angiogenesis and is mediated by hypoxia-inducible factor (HIF). mTOR activates messenger RNA to produce HIF, which acts as a transcription factor that is influenced by the von Hippel-Lindau protein. On activation, HIF results in transcription of vascular endothelial growth factor (VEGF) which stimulates the endothelial cell to develop new sprouting vessels by activating the VEGF receptor (VEGFR). Molecules that act on all these factors have been tested in ovarian cancer.

### PI3K-PTEN-Akt-mTOR Pathway–Interfering Drugs

The mTOR inhibitors temsirolimus and everolimus are being tested as single agent or in combination with chemotherapy in ovarian cancer in several phase II trials. Behbakht et al. tested weekly 25-mg/m$^2$ temsirolimus in 54 heavily pretreated patients with persistent/recurrent epithelial ovarian cancer/primary peritoneal cancer, and grade 3/4 adverse events included metabolic (15 %) and gastrointestinal toxicities

(15 %), pain (11 %), and constitutional (9 %) and pulmonary (7 %) toxicities [197]. In six heavily pretreated Japanese patients with clear cell carcinoma, temsirolimus 10 mg/m$^2$/ week in a 3-weeks-on, 1-week-off schedule, no toxicities greater than grade 3 or toxicity requiring discontinuation were observed [198].

## Vascular Endothelial Growth Factor–Interfering Drugs

VEGF can be influenced by monoclonal antibodies against VEGF (bevacizumab) and VEGF trap (aflibercept), and both have been tested in patients with ovarian cancer.

### Bevacizumab

In a phase III trial, 1,528 patients with ovarian cancer were, after debulking, randomized to 6 cycles of carboplatin and paclitaxel with or without bevacizumab (7.5 mg/kg) for 5 or 6 cycles, and bevacizumab could continue for 12 additional cycles or until disease progression. Bevacizumab was associated with more grade 3, 4, and 5 toxic effects than chemotherapy alone (66 % vs. 55 %). Five deaths related to treatment or to treatment and disease were reported: one in the chemotherapy-alone group due to central nervous system ischemia and four in the bevacizumab group (one each from gastrointestinal perforation, intracerebral hemorrhage, recurrent bowel perforation and ovarian cancer, and neutropenic sepsis). Bevacizumab treatment was associated with an increase in any bleeding (40 % vs. 12 %), hypertension of ≥grade 2 (18 % vs. 2 %), thromboembolic events ≥grade 3 (7 % vs. 3 %), and gastrointestinal perforations (ten patients vs. three patients). In the bevacizumab group, the percentage of patients in whom abscesses, fistulas, or gastrointestinal perforations developed was similar in the group that received bevacizumab with their first cycle of chemotherapy and in the group that did not (3 % vs. 4 %) [15].

### Aflibercept

Aflibercept has been tested as single intravenous agent in patients with recurrent ovarian cancer in phase I and phase II studies [20, 199]. Most common toxicities included hypertension, proteinuria, headache, anorexia, and dysphonia; intestinal perforation was also reported. In a randomized phase II trial comparing the effect of aflibercept with placebo in patients with ascites, most common grade 3 or 4 adverse events were dyspnea (20 % vs. 8 %), fatigue or asthenia (13 % vs. 44 %), and dehydration (10 % vs. 12 %). The frequency of fatal intestinal perforation or intestinal fistula was higher with aflibercept (10 % vs. 4 %) [200].

Endothelial Receptor Kinase Inhibitors

Sunitinib is an oral platelet-derived growth factor (PDGF) and VEGF receptor inhibitor that interferes with endothelial proliferation and has been tested in patients with recurrent pretreated ovarian cancer in phase II studies.

Dose reductions from 50 mg/day, 4 weeks on, 2 weeks off, had to be done due to fluid accumulation (ascites, effusions) during off-treatment periods, and the recommended dose in patients with pretreated ovarian cancer according to Biagi et al. is 37.5 mg/day [201]. The most common reasons for missed doses were mucositis and hand-foot syndrome. Other reasons at the 50-mg dosing were nausea and at the 37.5-mg dosing, granulocytopenia, fatigue, anorexia, and hypertension.

Other adverse effects were uncommon, but low-grade fatigue, mucositis, nausea, taste alteration, hand-foot syndrome, diarrhea, hypertension, skin discoloration, and pain have been reported. Thyroid-stimulating hormone (TSH) elevations were observed in 43 % of patients. No gastrointestinal perforations were observed in this phase II study in 30 patients [201].

Another phase II study tested two different schedules of sunitinib (50 mg/day, 4 weeks on, 2 weeks off; and continuous 37.5 mg/day) in 73 patients with platinum-resistant ovarian cancer. There were no differences between both treatment arms in relation to toxicity. Grade 3/4 toxicities occurring in more than 1 % of the patients were thrombocytopenia (1.6 % vs. 4.3 %), leukopenia (1.9 % vs. 2.3 %), neutropenia (3.9 % vs. 3.3 %), hyponatremia (0.6 % vs. 1.6 %), liver test disturbances ((gamma)$\gamma$-GT

4.5 % vs. 6.1 %; ALT 1.0 % vs. 1.2 %), gastrointestinal syndrome (3 % vs. 1.5 %), and abdominal symptoms (1.1 % vs. 2.0 %) [202].

## Conclusion

Several targeted agents have been tested in patients with ovarian cancer in primary treatment and recurrent disease. In this patient population, similar side effects have been observed as in patients with other tumor types treated with these agents. Special attention should be given to their toxicity profile when used in adjuvant setting or in selected groups of patients with high risk factors for complications.

## *Cervical Cancer*

Although targeted therapies have been tested in cervical cancer, at the moment none of them made it into the clinic. Several monoclonal antibodies are tested in combination with chemotherapy or chemoradiation [203].

## Epidermal Growth Factor–Targeting Drugs

Since most cervical cancers are of spinocellular histology, combination of chemotherapy or radiotherapy with EGFR-interfering drugs seems a logical approach.

### Monoclonal Antibodies

Several monoclonal antibodies (cetuximab, panitumumab, nimotuzumab) are used in phase II studies in patients with locally advanced or recurrent/metastatic cervical cancer. Most studies are testing cetuximab in combination with cisplatin with or without radiotherapy.

When cetuximab (400 mg/m$^2$/week followed by 250 mg/m$^2$/week) was used as single agent in 35 evaluable heavily pretreated women, no grade 4 adverse events were reported, while the most common grade 3 adverse events were rash (14 %) and gastrointestinal problems (11 %) [204].

In the same setting, the combination of cetuximab with cisplatin (30 mg/m² on days 1 and 8 in a 21-day cycle) in 69 eligible and evaluable women induced grade 4 anemia (1 %), allergy (1 %), and metabolic (1 %) and vascular (1 %) toxicities. The most common grade 3 toxicities were metabolic (22 %), dermatologic (12 %), fatigue (9 %), and gastrointestinal (9 %) [205].

The testing of a triple combination of cetuximab with cisplatin (50 mg/m²/day day 1 q 3 weeks) and topotecan (0.75 mg/m²/day day 1–day 3 q 3 weeks) had to be stopped due to excessive toxicity. The most frequent adverse events in 19 evaluable patients were severe myelosuppression with grade 3/4 neutropenia (72 %), grade 3/4 thrombocytopenia (61 %), and grade 3 anemia (44.5 %). Main grade 3/4 nonhematologic toxicities were infection (39 %) and febrile neutropenia (28 %), skin reactions (22 %), renal toxicity (11 %), and pulmonary embolism (11 %). Five (28 %) patients died during the treatment, including three toxic deaths [206].

These data show that skin-related and gastrointestinal toxicities are the most common side effects of cetuximab in this patient population. The combination with cisplatin was feasible, while a triple combination with cisplatin and topotecan resulted in a too high toxicity profile.

When cetuximab (400 mg/m² loading dose followed by 250 mg/m²/week) was combined with weekly cisplatin (30 mg/m²) and pelvic or extended-field radiotherapy (EFRT) in a phase I study, the combination with pelvic irradiation was feasible, while EFRT resulted in a high incidence of gastrointestinal and hematologic toxicity. Cetuximab-related toxicities reported were hypersensitivity reactions and skin rash [207].

EGFR Tyrosine Kinase Inhibitors

*Lapatinib*

Single-agent lapatinib 1,500 mg/day ($n = 78$) was tested in a randomized phase II trial and compared to pazopanib 800 mg/day ($n = 74$) alone of the combination of both drugs (1,000-mg lapatinib + 400-mg pazopanib/day) ($n = 98$). In the lapatinib arm, the most common adverse events were diarrhea (58 %), nausea (33 %), and anorexia (32 %), compared with diarrhea (54 %), nausea (36 %), hypertension (30 %), and anorexia (28 %) in the pazopanib arm and diarrhea (76 %), vomiting (42 %), and anorexia (38 %) in the combination arm. The percentages of patients experiencing grade 3/4 adverse events were 41 % in the lapatinib-only arm, 54 % in the pazopanib arm, and 45 % in the combination arm. In addition, 14, 19, and 22 % of patients in the lapatinib, pazopanib, and combination arms, respectively, discontinued treatment due to adverse events, and the most common adverse events leading to discontinuation were dyspnea (5 %) and diarrhea (3 %) in the lapatinib arm, small bowel obstruction (3 %) and female genital fistula (3 %) in the pazopanib arm, and female genital fistula (3 %) in the combination arm.

In the lapatinib arm, 1 % of patients experienced absolute decreases in baseline LVEF compared with no patients in the pazopanib arm and 1 % of patients in the combination arm. Liver enzyme elevations from baseline were more frequent in patients receiving pazopanib than in patients receiving lapatinib or combination therapy [208].

## Angiogenesis Inhibition

### VEGF-Targeting Agents

Single-agent bevacizumab (15 mg/kg q 3 weeks) was tested in 46 women with recurrent cervical cancer. Five patients experienced a deep venous thrombosis, one with pulmonary embolus. There was one episode of grade 4 vaginal bleeding and one grade 4 urinary fistula. Other grade 3/4 events included hypertension (seven grade 3), cardiovascular (two grade 3), gastrointestinal (three grade 3; one grade 4), and genitourinary/renal (two grade 3; one grade 4 fistula). There was one toxic death due to infection [209].

The combination of bevacizumab with cisplatin and radiation was used as primary treatment for locally advanced cervical cancer [210]. In 49 evaluable patients, the most common adverse events were hematologic (80 %).

VEGFR-Targeting Agents

*Sunitinib*

Sunitinib (50 mg/day 4 weeks on, 2 weeks off) was tested in a phase II study in 19 women with locally advanced or metastatic cervical carcinoma who had received up to one prior line of chemotherapy for advanced disease. A higher rate of fistula formation (26.3 %) was observed and due to insufficient activity in cervical cancer development as a single agent was stopped [211].

*Pazopanib*

See paragraph on lapatinib.

These studies show that fistula development is a real concern in patients with cervical cancer who are treated with angiogenesis-targeting agents. This should be taken into account when incorporating these agents in combination therapy.

## Endometrial Cancer

Endometrial cancer comprises a heterogeneous group of tumors with distinct molecular characteristics. Two types of endometrial carcinoma (type I [endometrioid], type II [non-endometrioid]) have been determined based on molecular pathology, although they are not taken into account for the development and testing of targeted therapies.

The identification of activating mutations of kinases (e.g., PIK3CA, FGFR2) and loss of function of genes related to DNA repair (e.g., PTEN) may lead to more biology-driven clinical trials.

## Epidermal Growth Factor Receptor

Preliminary data did not show promising results in patients with endometrial cancer with EGFR tyrosine kinase inhibition.

Results of a phase II study with cetuximab in patients with endometrial cancer are awaited.

## EGFR Tyrosine Kinase Inhibitors

### Erlotinib

In a phase II study, patients with recurrent and or metastatic endometrial cancer were treated with erlotinib. The main toxicities were grade 1 or 2 rash (88 %), dry skin (61 %), and diarrhea (58 %), 13 % of which were of grade 3 severity. Other grade 3 toxicities included non-neutropenic infection and dyspnea, fatigue, arthralgia, keratitis/conjunctivitis, nausea, dehydration, and hypertension [212].

## HER2

HER2 amplification or overexpression has been demonstrated and linked to prognosis in endometrial cancer. Single-agent trastuzumab (4 mg/kg week 1, then 2 mg/kg weekly) was tested in 34 pretreated patients with HER2-positive endometrial carcinoma. Two deaths on treatment were considered possibly related to trastuzumab. One patient developed an infusion reaction and died from cardiac arrest 1 week after infusion, and the second patient suffered a myocardial infarction during her first course of therapy. Grade 3 toxicity consisted of gastrointestinal toxicity (three patients), anemia and pulmonary problems (two patients each), and metabolic disturbances and pain (one patient each) [213].

## Angiogenesis Inhibition

### PI3K-PTEN-Akt-mTOR Pathway

Temsirolimus has also been tested in patients with endometrial cancer. When given to 33 women with chemotherapy-naive or chemotherapy-treated endometrial cancer in a weekly schedule

(25-mg temsirolimus), the most common adverse events were fatigue, rash, mucositis, and pneumonitis. Asymptomatic pneumonitis was common (42 %) but was grade 3 in only 8 % of patients. Hematologic adverse events were generally mild in severity in both groups, with lymphopenia as the most common hematologic toxicity. Rash, anorexia, nausea, and diarrhea were more frequently reported in the previously treated cohort and mucositis in chemotherapy-naive patients [25].

The combination of weekly temsirolimus, 25 mg/day on days 1, 8, 15, and 22 every 4 weeks, and weekly topotecan, 1 mg/m$^2$ on days 1, 8, and 15 every 4 weeks, was tested in patients with gynecologic tumors, including endometrial cancer, and dose-limiting toxicities were asymptomatic neutropenia and thrombocytopenia [214].

Vascular Endothelial Growth Factor

*Bevacizumab*

Single-agent intravenous bevacizumab, 15 mg every 3 weeks, was tested in 52 evaluable patients with persistent or recurrent endometrial cancer after receiving one to two prior cytotoxic regimens. Adverse events were consistent with those expected with bevacizumab treatment. No gastrointestinal perforations or treatment-related deaths were reported. One patient had a grade 4 gastric hemorrhage, and another patient had a grade 3 rectal hemorrhage. Two patients had grade 3/4 thrombosis/embolism. Two patients had grade 3/4 proteinuria, and four patients had grade 3 hypertension [215].

*Aflibercept*

Patients with a recurrent or metastatic gynecologic carcinosarcoma and uterine leiomyosarcoma were treated with single-agent aflibercept without responses. Grade 3 or more toxicities were uncommon and included hypertension, fatigue, headache, and abdominal pain [216].

## Treatment

### EGFR-Targeting Agents

The side effects reported in patients with gynecologic cancers and treated with agents targeting the EGFR are similar to these described in other patient groups.

- Acneiform rash is one of the major skin toxicities with agents targeting the EGFR. Preventive measures are protecting the skin with sunscreens, avoiding dry skin, and enhancing skin hydration with tocopherol oil or gel and avoiding tight shoes. Treatment depends on the grade of toxicity; for grade 1 no specific measures are necessary, while for grade 2 topical antibiotic treatment with clindamycin 1 % gel, erythromycin 3 % gel/cream, or metronidazole 0.75–1 % cream/gel can be used. For pustules, oral semisynthetic tetracycline (minocycline 100 mg/day, doxycycline 100 mg/day) can be used for 4 weeks and until the rash is asymptomatic. For patients with grade 3, topical treatment together with systemic therapy with oral tetracycline and oral corticosteroids (methylprednisolone, 0.4 mg/kg; prednisone, 0.5 mg/kg) for up to 10 days can be combined. For highly symptomatic/nonresponsive patients, treatment with oral retinoids (isotretinoin 0.3–0.5 mg/kg), intravenous corticosteroids (methylprednisolone, dexamethasone), oral/intramuscular/intravenous antihistamines (e.g., chlorphenamine, cetirizine), intravenous antibiotics (amoxicillin/clavulanic acid, gentamicin), or hydration can be considered. In patients with grade 4 skin toxicity, topical treatment can be combined with systemic management with oral retinoids (isotretinoin, 0.3–0.5 mg/kg), intravenous corticosteroids (methylprednisolone, dexamethasone), oral/intramuscular/intravenous antihistamines (e.g., chlorphenamine, cetirizine), intravenous antibiotics (amoxicillin/clavulanic acid, gentamicin), and intravenous hydration [217].
- Diarrhea should be treated symptomatically with hydration and anticholinergic drugs (e.g., loperamide). However, anticholinergic drugs should be used with caution in patients with peritoneal metastasis because it can cause

and aggravate gastrointestinal obstruction.

- The addition of anti-EGFR monoclonal antibodies to standard anticancer therapy significantly increases the risk of hypomagnesemia [218]; with cisplatin pretreatment especially, this effect can be more pronounced. Asymptomatic hypomagnesemia can be treated with oral replacement therapy. Patients with clinical manifestations of hypomagnesemia should be treated with 50 mEq of intravenous magnesium given slowly over 8–24 h and repeated to maintain the plasma magnesium concentration above 1.0 mg/dL (0.4 mmol/L or 0.8 mEq/L).

- The combination with chemotherapy and the pretreatment in most patients with platinum compounds may lead to a higher hematologic toxicity than in non-platinum pretreated patients.

## Angiogenesis-Interfering Agents

Monoclonal Antibodies

- Hypertension (all grades) is one of the most common side effects of bevacizumab or aflibercept. It can be adequately controlled with oral antihypertensive drugs such as angiotensin-converting enzyme inhibitors, diuretics, and calcium channel blockers. The risk of bevacizumab- or aflibercept-associated hypertension does not correlate with the patients' baseline characteristics, underlying disease, or concomitant therapy. For patients with uncomplicated hypertension, the target blood pressure level is <140/90 mmHg. In cancer patients with comorbidities such as chronic kidney disease, a target blood pressure level of <135/85 mmHg should be recommended. Lifestyle modifications such as limiting intake of both saturated and unsaturated fats and salt (maximum 4 g/day) and increasing that of fruits, legumes, and vegetables without changing total caloric input should be encouraged. No clear recommendation for an antihypertensive agent can be made due to lack of studies addressing the subject. Antihypertensive medications that have been effectively used are angiotensin-converting enzyme inhibitors, diuretics, and calcium channel blockers or combinations of them [219].

- Proteinuria is also frequently observed in the treatment with bevacizumab against VEGF in other tumor types and was observed in 5 % of patients with ovarian cancer [15]. It is due to interference of bevacizumab with VEGF-dependent glomerular endothelial integrity and thrombotic microangiopathy. Monitoring by use of dipstick urinalyses should be considered in patients treated with bevacizumab, and in case of a positive result, a 24-h urine total-protein collection should be performed. Bevacizumab should be interrupted if urine protein secretion exceeds 2 g/24 h. After recovery, bevacizumab treatment may be restarted. There is no standard pharmacological treatment, but anti-angiotensin agents could be considered as first-line agents in the absence of renal failure, hyperkalemia, or renal artery stenosis [220].

- Venous and arterial thromboembolic events were seen in the phase III trial in 7 and 4 %, respectively, and were higher than in the control group [15]. Arterial thromboembolic events are a rare but serious complication and include myocardial or cerebrovascular events and peripheral vascular and mesenteric clots. Thrombotic prophylaxis, including low-molecular-weight heparin (LMWH), warfarin, or aspirin, may be considered in patients starting bevacizumab treatment. Both aspirin and LMWH have been used without increased bleeding complications, while warfarin translates in a higher bleeding complication rate compared to LMWH [220]. Patients with ≥grade 2 arterial thromboembolic events should discontinue bevacizumab while in venous thromboembolic events. Treatment can be temporarily held for grade 3 or asymptomatic grade 4 toxicities. Treatment consists of full anticoagulation, and bevacizumab treatment should be discontinued until stopping anticoagulation.

- Hemorrhage occurred in 40 % of patients treated with the chemotherapy-bevacizumab combination compared to 12 % in the chemotherapy-alone arm and has an important impact on complications depending on the location

(2 % central nervous hemorrhages) [15]. Bleeding is managed by standard supportive care, while bevacizumab treatment is discontinued [220].

- Gastrointestinal perforation has been described in 1–4 % of patients with other tumor types. In the phase III study, gastrointestinal perforations were reported somewhat more often in the bevacizumab arm. Also, the rate of intraabdominal abscess and fistula was higher, but when bevacizumab was given at the start of treatment, it did not lead to a higher complication rate [15]. In patients with recurrent ovarian cancer, risk factors for perforation were previous gastrointestinal surgery, carcinomatosis compromising overall bowel function, intermittent or chronic bowel obstruction, and poor nutrition. Nonsteroidal anti-inflammatory drugs should be avoided when considering bevacizumab treatment. Management of bowel complications after bevacizumab therapy is difficult, and an operative intervention versus conservative management should be carefully considered. The initial management may consist of intravenous antibiotics, bowel rest with nasogastric tube placement, and percutaneous intraperitoneal catheter placement. Increased risk of wound-healing complications is an important consideration when opting for an operative intervention. Bevacizumab treatment is stopped [220]. Similar precautions should be taken with aflibercept.

VEGFR Tyrosine Kinase Inhibitors

- While perforations are rarely seen with sunitinib, diarrhea has been reported as a frequent side effect (50 %), and 2–6 % of patients have grade 3/4 diarrhea. Oral hydration and antidiarrheal agents (e.g., loperamide) are the treatments for grade 1 or 2 diarrhea. In patients with grade 3/4 diarrhea, intravenous hydration and electrolyte correction are indicated, and treatment with sunitinib should be interrupted until the diarrhea resolves to ≤grade 1 [220].
- Hand-foot syndrome is a frequent reason for dose reduction in the treatment of sunitinib and appears during the first 6 weeks of treatment. Immediate intervention is

advised because early symptoms often resolve quickly with minimum effort, allowing continuation of therapy without dose reduction. Pharmacologic interventions such as systemic corticosteroids, vitamin E, pyridoxine, and topical steroids or 99 % dimethyl sulfoxide have been reported to be successful. Rapid symptom improvement is observed with temporary cessation of therapy, allowing reinstitution of the drug within 3–14 days [220].

- The incidence of hypothyroidism necessitating thyroid substitution is 12.1 per 100 person-years, and around 13.7 % of patients treated with sunitinib will receive thyroid substitution therapy [220]. Therefore, TSH should be checked regularly and is indicated in case of clinical suspicion of hypothyroidism [221].

## Summary

The activity of targeted agents in gynecologic cancers varies, while the toxicity profile seems similar to that observed in other tumor types. Nevertheless, some cautions should be used in patients that have previously received radiotherapy to the pelvic area, since fistula formation has been reported in patients with recurrent disease in this area (e.g., cervical cancer).

The treatment of toxicities due to targeted agent is similar to that in other tumor types.

## References

1. Boyle P, Ferlay J. Cancer incidence and mortality in Europe 2004. Ann Oncol. 2005;16:481–8.
2. Kurman RJ, Shih IEM. The origin and pathogenesis of epithelial ovarian cancer: a proposed unifying theory. Am J Surg Pathol. 2010;34:433–43.
3. Bast Jr RC. Molecular approaches to personalizing management of ovarian cancer. Ann Oncol. 2011;22 Suppl 8:viii5–15.
4. du Bois A, Quinn M, Thigpen T, Vermorken J, Avall-Lundqvist E, Bookman M, et al. 2004 consensus statements on the management of ovarian cancer: final document of the 3rd International Gynecologic

Cancer Intergroup Ovarian Cancer Consensus Conference (GCIG OCCC 2004). Ann Oncol. 2005;16 Suppl 8:viii7–12.

5. Colombo N, Peoretti M, Parma G, Lapresa M, Mancari R, Carinelli S, et al. Newly diagnosed and relapsed epithelial ovarian carcinoma: ESMO Clinical Practice Guidelines for diagnosis, treatment and follow-up. Ann Oncol. 2010;21 Suppl 5:v23–30.

6. Bell J, Brady MF, Young RC, Lage J, Walker JL, Look KY, et al. Randomized phase III trial of three versus six cycles of adjuvant carboplatin and paclitaxel in early stage epithelial ovarian carcinoma: a Gynecologic Oncology Group study. Gynecol Oncol. 2006; 102(3):432–9.

7. Bookman MA, Brady MF, McGuire W, Harper PG, Alberts DS, Friedlander M, et al. Evaluation of new platinum-based treatments in advanced-stage ovarian cancer: a phase III trial of thew Gynecologic Cancer Intergroup (GCIG). J Clin Oncol. 2009;27:1419–25.

8. Vasey PA, Jayson GC, Gordon A, Gabra H, Coleman R, Atkinson R, et al. Phase III randomized trial of docetaxel-carboplatin versus paclitaxel-carboplatin as first-line chemotherapy for ovarian carcinoma. J Natl Cancer Inst. 2004;96:1682–91.

9. Pignata S, Scambia G, Ferrandina G, Savarese A, Sorio R, Breda E, et al. Carboplatin plus paclitaxel versus carboplatin plus pegylated liposomal doxorubicin as first-line treatment for patients with ovarian cancer: the MITO-2 randomized phase III trial. J Clin Oncol. 2011;29(27):3628–35.

10. Katsumata N, Yasuda M, Takahashi F, Isonishi S, Jobo T, Aoki D, et al. Dose-dense paclitaxel once a week in combination with carboplatin every three weeks for advanced ovarian cancer: a phase 3, open-label, randomized controlled trial. Lancet. 2009;374:1331–8.

11. Vermorken JB. Intraperitoneal chemotherapy in first-line treatment for optimally debulked ovarian cancer: a new standard of care. In: Cervantes A, editor. International oncology update: new treatment of ovarian. Barcelona: Permanyer Publications; 2008. p. 1–12.

12. Pujade-Lauraine E, Alexandre J. Update of randomized trials in recurrent disease. Ann Oncol. 2011;22 Suppl 8:viii61–4.

13. Eric Pujade-Lauraine, Felix Hilpert, Béatrice Weber, Alexander Reuss, Andres Poveda, Gunnar Kristensen et al., AURELIA: A randomized phase III trial evaluating bevacizumab (BEV) plus chemotherapy (CT) for platinum (PT)-resistant recurrent ovarian cancer (OC). Journal of Clinical Oncology, 2012 ASCO Annual Meeting Proceedings (Post-Meeting Edition). Vol 30, No 18_suppl (June 20 Supplement), 2012: LBA5002.

14. Burger RB, Brady MF, Bookman MA, Fleming GF, Monk BJ, Huang H, et al. Incorporation of bevacizumab in the primary treatment of ovarian cancer. N Engl J Med. 2011;365:2473–83.

15. Perren TJ, Swart AM, Pfisterer J, Ledermann JA, Pujade-Lauraine E, Kristensen G, et al. A phase 3 trial of bevacizumab in ovarian cancer. N Engl J Med. 2011;365:2484–96.

230    S. Altintas et al.

16. Colombo N, Mangili G, Mammoliti S, Kalling M, Tholander B, Sternas L, et al. A phase II study of aflibercept in patients with advanced epithelial ovarian cancer and symptomatic malignant ascites. Gynecol Oncol. 2012;125(1):42–7.
17. Ledermann JA. Phase II randomized placebo controlled study of olaparib (AZD2281) in patients with platinum sensitive relapsed serous ovarian cancer (PSROC). J Clin Oncol. 2011;(Suppl):332s (abstr 5003).
18. Reed N, Millan D, Verheijen R, Castiglione M, ESMO Guidelines Working Group. Non-epithelial ovarian cancer: ESMO Clinical Practice Guidelines for diagnosis, treatment and follow-up. Ann Oncol. 2010;21 Suppl 5:v31–6.
19. Van Rijswijk RE, Vermorken JB, Reed N, Favalli G, Mendiola C, Zanaboni F, et al. Cisplatin, doxorubicin and ifosfamide in carcinosarcoma of the female genital tract: a phase II study of the European Organization for Research and Treatment of Cancer Gynaecological Cancer Group (EORTC 55923). Eur J Cancer. 2003;39(4):481–7.
20. Colombo N, Preti E, Landoni F, Carinelli S, Colombo A, Marini C, et al. Endometrial cancer: ESMO Clinical Practice Guidelines for diagnosis, treatment and follow-up. Ann Oncol. 2011;22 Suppl 6:vi35–9.
21. Lentz SS, Brady MF, Major FJ, Reid GC, Soper JT. High-dose megestrol acetate in advanced or recurrent endometrial carcinoma: a Gynecologic Oncology Group study. J Clin Oncol. 1966;14:357–61.
22. Thigpen JT, Brady MF, Alvarez RD, Adelson MD, Homesley HD, Manetta A, et al. Oral medroxyprogesterone acetate in the treatment of advanced or recurrent endometrial carcinoma: a dose–response study by the Gynecologic Oncology Group. J Clin Oncol. 1999;17(6):1736–44.
23. Garrett A, Quinn MA. Hormonal therapies and gynecologic cancers. Best Pract Res Clin Obstet Gynaecol. 2008;22:407–21.
24. Sjoquist KM, Martyn J, Edmondson RJ, Friedlander ML. The role of hormonal therapy in gynecologic cancer-current status and future directions. Int J Gynecol Cancer. 2011;21:1328–33.
25. Oza AM, Elit L, Tsao MS, Kamel-Reid S, Biagi J, Provencher DM, et al. Phase II study of temsirolimus in women with recurrent or metastatic endometrial cancer: a trial of the NCIC Clinical trials Group. J Clin Oncol. 2011;29(24):3278–85.
26. Sutton G, Kavanagh J, Wolfson A, et al. Corpus: mesenchymal tumors. In: Hoskins WJ, Perez CA, Young RC, et al., editors. Principles and practice of gynecologic oncology. Philadelphia: Lippincott Williams & Wilkins; 2005. p. 873–94.
27. Hensley ML. Role of chemotherapy and biomolecular therapy in the treatment of uterine sarcomas. Best Pract Res Clin Obstet Gynaecol. 2011;25(6):773–82.
28. Randall ME, Michael H, Vermorken J, et al. Uterine cervix. In: Hoskins WJ, Perez CA, Young RC, et al., editors. Principles and practice of gynecologic oncology. Philadelphia: Lippincott Williams & Wilkins; 2005. p. 743–823.

29. Haie-Meder C, Morico P, Castiglione M. Cervical cancer: ESMO Clinical Practice Guidelines for diagnosis, treatment and follow-up. Ann Oncol. 2010;21 Suppl 5:v37–40.
30. Movva S, Gold M, Grigsby P, et al. Challenges in the management of invasive cervical cancer. ASCO Educational Book 2009. Alexandria: American Society of Clinical Oncology. p. 295–300.
31. Green JA, Kirwan JM, Tierney JF. Survival and recurrence after concomitant chemotherapy and radiotherapy for cancer of the uterine cervix: a systematic review and meta-analysis. Lancet. 2001;358: 781–6.
32. Vale C, Tierney JF, Stewart LA, Brady M, Dinshaw K, Jakobsen A, et al. Reducing uncertainties about the effects of chemoradiotherapy for cervical cancer: a systematic review and meta-analysis of individual patient data from 18 randomized trials. J Clin Oncol. 2008;26: 5802–12.
33. Dueñas-González A, Zarba JJ, Patel F, et al. Phase III open label randomized study comparing concurrent gemcitabine plus cisplatin and radiation followed by adjuvant gemcitabine and cisplatin versus concurrent cisplatin and radiation in patients with stage IIB to IVA with carcinoma of the cervix. J Clin Oncol. 2011;29(13):1678–85.
34. Field SB. In vivo aspects of hyperthermic oncology. In: Field SB, Hand JW, editors. An introduction to the practical aspects of clinical hyperthermia. London: Taylor & Francis; 1990. p. 55–68.
35. Raaphorst GP. Fundamental aspects of hyperthermic biology. In: Field SB, Hand JW, editors. An introduction to the practical aspects of clinical hyperthermia. London: Taylor & Francis; 1990. p. 10–54.
36. Van der Zee J, González González D The Dutch Hyperthermia Trial: results in cervical cancer. Int J Hyperthermia. 2002;18(no.1):1–12.
37. Grogan M, Thomas GM, Melamed I, Wong FL, Pearcey RG, Joseph PK, et al. The importance of hemoglobin levels during radiotherapy for carcinoma of the cervix. Cancer. 1999;86(8):1528–36.
38. Moore DH, Blessing JA, McQuellon RP, Thaler HT, Cella D, Benda J, et al. Phase III study of cisplatin with or without paclitaxel in stage IVB, recurrent, or persistent squamous cell carcinoma of the cervix: a Gynecologic Oncology Group study. J Clin Oncol. 2004;22(15): 3113–9.
39. Monk BJ, Sill MW, McMeekin DS, Cohn DE, Ramondetta LM, Boardman CH, et al. Phase III trial of four cisplatin-containing doublet combinations in stage IVB, recurrent, or persistent cervical carcinoma: a Gynecologic Oncology Group study. J Clin Oncol. 2009; 27(28):4649–55.
40. Monk BJ, Willmott LJ, Sumner DA. Anti-angiogenesis agents in metastatic or recurrent cervical cancer. Gynecol Oncol. 2010;116(2):181–6.
41. Moore DH, Koh WJ, McGuire WP, et al. Vulva. In: Hoskins WJ, Perez CA, Young RC, et al., editors. Principles and practice of gynecologic oncology. Philadelphia: Lippincott Williams & Wilkins; 2005. p. 665–705.

42. Gadducci A, Cionini L, Romanini A, Fanucchi A, Genazzani AR. Old and new perspectives in the management of high-risk, locally advanced or recurrent, and metastatic vulvar cancer. Crit Rev Oncol Hematol. 2006;60(3):227–41.

43. Durrant KR, Mangioni C, Lacave AJ, George M, van der Burg ME, Guthrie D, et al. Bleomycin, methotrexate, and CCNU in advanced inoperable squamous cell carcinoma of the vulva: a phase II study of the EORTC Gynaecological Cancer Cooperative Group (GCCG). Gynecol Oncol. 1990;37(3):359–62.

44. Wagenaar HC, Colombo N, Vergote I, Hoctin-Boes G, Zanetta G, Pecorelli S, et al. Bleomycin, methotrexate, and CCNU in locally advanced or recurrent, inoperable, squamous-cell carcinoma of the vulva: an EORTC Gynaecological Cancer Cooperative Group Study. European Organization for Research and Treatment of Cancer. Gynecol Oncol. 2001;81(3):348–54.

45. May T, Goldstein DP, Berkowitz RS. Current chemotherapeutic management of patients with gestational trophoblastic neoplasia. Chemother Res Pract. 2011;2011:806256. Published online 2011 May 11. doi:10.1155/2011/806256.

46. Goldstein DP. Gestational trophoblastic neoplasia in the 1990s. Yale J Biol Med. 1991;64:639–51.

47. Kohorn EI. Negotiating a staging and risk factor scoring system for gestational trophoblastic neoplasia; a progress report. J Reprod Med. 2002;47(6):445–50.

48. Lurain JR, Nejad B. Secondary chemotherapy for high-risk gestational trophoblastic neoplasia. Gynecol Oncol. 2005;97(2):618–23.

49. Skeel RT. Handbook of cancer chemotherapy. 6th ed. Philadelphia: Lippincott Williams & Wilkins; 2003.

50. Chabner B, Longo DL. Cancer chemotherapy and biotherapy: principles and practice. 4th ed. Philadelphia: Lippincott Williams & Wilkins; 2005.

51. Takimoto CH, Calvo E. Principles of oncologic pharmacotherapy. In: Pazdur R, Wagman LD, Camphausen KA, Hoskins WJ, editors. Cancer management: a multidisciplinary approach. 11th ed. Lawrence: CMPMedica; 2008.

52. Monk BJ, Herzog TJ, Kaye SB, Krasner CN, Vermorken JB, Muggia FM, et al. Trabectedin plus pegylated liposomal Doxorubicin in recurrent ovarian cancer. Clin Oncol. 2010;28:3107–14.

53. Sanfilippo R, Grosso F, Jones RL, Banerjee S, Pilotti S, D'Incalci M, et al. Trabectedin in advanced uterine leiomyosarcomas: a retrospective case series analysis from two reference centers. Gynecol Oncol. 2011;123(3):553–6.

54. Vergote IB, Micha JP, Pippitt CH Jr, Rao GG, Spitz DL, Reed N, et al. Phase II study of NKTR-102 in women with platinum-resistant/refractory ovarian cancer. J Clin Oncol. 2010 ASCO annual meeting proceedings (Post-Meeting Edition). 28 (15 suppl) (May 20 Suppl), 2010:5013;28.

55. Kauffman D, et al. Clinical consequences and management of antineoplastic agents. In: Parrillo JE, Masur H, editors. The critically ill immunosuppressed patient: diagnosis and management. Rockville: Aspen Press; 1986.

56. Stampler KM, Holtz DO, Dunton CJ. Reducing excessive toxicity in ovarian cancer treatment: a personalized approach. Future Oncol. 2011;7:789–98.

57. Hensley ML, Hagerty KL, Kewalramani T, Green DM, Meropol NJ, Wasserman TH, et al. American Society of Clinical Oncology 2008 clinical practice guideline update: use of chemotherapy and radiation therapy protectants. J Clin Oncol. 2009;27(1):127–45.

58. Ozols RF, Young RC. High-dose cisplatin therapy in ovarian cancer. Semin Oncol. 1985;12 Suppl 6:21–30.

59. Verplanke AJ, Herber RF, de Wit R, Veenhof CH. Comparison of renal function parameters in the assessment of cis-platin induced nephrotoxicity. Nephron. 1994;66(3):267–72.

60. Mangioni C, Bolis G, Pecorelli S, Bragman K, Epis A, Favalli G, et al. Randomized trial in advanced ovarian cancer comparing cisplatin and carboplatin. J Natl Cancer Inst. 1989;81(19):1464–71.

61. Mansfield SH, Castillo M. MR of cis-platinum-induced optic neuritis. AJNR Am J Neuroradiol. 1994;15(6):1178–80.

62. Rao RD, Michalak JC, Sloan JA, Loprinzi CL, Soori GS, Nikcevich DA, et al. Efficacy of gabapentin in the management of chemotherapy-induced peripheral neuropathy: a phase 3 randomized, double-blind, placebo-controlled, crossover trial (N00C3). Cancer. 2007;110(9):2110–8.

63. Onoyama Y, Umezu T, Kuriaki Y, Honda N. Hypersensitivity reactions to cisplatin following multiple uncomplicated courses: a report on two cases. J Obstet Gynaecol Res. 1997;23(4):347–52.

64. Roila F, Herrstedt J, Aapro M, Gralla RJ, Einhorn LH, Ballatori E, et al. Guideline update for MASCC and ESMO in the prevention of chemotherapy- and radiotherapy-induced nausea and vomiting: results of the Perugia consensus conference. Ann Oncol. 2010;21 Suppl 5:v232–43.

65. Crawford J, Caserta C, Roila F, ESMO Guidelines Working Group. Hematopoietic growth factors: ESMO Clinical Practice Guidelines for the applications. Ann Oncol. 2010;21 Suppl 5:v248–51.

66. Rizzo JD, Brouwers M, Hurley P, Seidenfeld J, Arcasoy MO, Spivak JL, et al. American Society of Hematology/American Society of Clinical Oncology clinical practice guideline update on the use of epoetin and darbepoetin in adult patients with cancer. Blood. 2010;116(20):4045–59.

67. Piccart MJ, Lamb H, Vermorken JB. Current and future potential roles of the platinum drugs in the treatment of ovarian cancer. Ann Oncol. 2001;12(9):1195–203.

68. Parmar MK, Ledermann JA, Colombo N, du Bois A, Delaloye JF, Kristensen GB, et al. Paclitaxel plus platinum-based chemotherapy

versus conventional platinum-based chemotherapy in women with relapsed ovarian cancer: the ICON4/AGO-OVAR-2.2 trial. Lancet. 2003;361(9375):2099–106.

69. Ozols RF. Advanced ovarian cancer: a clinical update on first-line treatment, recurrent disease, and new agents. J Natl Compr Canc Netw. 2004;2 Suppl 2:S60–73.

70. Harper P. ICON 2 and ICON 3 data in previously untreated ovarian cancer: results to date. Semin Oncol. 1997;24(5 Suppl 15):S15-23–5.

71. Thigpen T, du Bois A, Mc Alpine J, DiSaia P, Fujiwara K, Hoskins W, et al. First line therapy in ovarian cancer trials. Int J Gynecol Cancer. 2011; 21:756–62.

72. Markman M, Kennedy A, Webster K. Clinical features of hypersensitivity reactions to carboplatin. J Clin Oncol. 1999;17(4):1141.

73. Jodrell DI, Egorin MJ, Canetta RM, Langenberg P, Goldbloom EP, Burroughs JN, et al. Relationships between carboplatin exposure and tumor response and toxicity in patients with ovarian cancer. J Clin Oncol. 1992;10(4):520–8.

74. Dizon DS, Sabbatini PJ, Aghajanian C, Hensley ML, Spriggs DR. Analysis of patients with epithelial ovarian cancer or fallopian tube carcinoma retreated with cisplatin after the development of a carboplatin allergy. Gynecol Oncol. 2002;84(3):378–82.

75. Katanyoo K, Tangjitgamol S, Chongthanakorn M, Tantivatana T, Manusirivithaya S, Rongsriyam K, et al. Treatment outcomes of concurrent weekly carboplatin with radiation therapy in locally advanced cervical cancer patients. Gynecol Oncol. 2011;123(3):571–6.

76. Keys HM, Bundy BN, Stehman FB, Muderspach LI, Chafe WE, Suggs 3rd CL, et al. Cisplatin, radiation and adjuvant hysterectomy for bulky stage IB cervical carcinoma. N Engl J Med. 1999;340: 1154–61.

77. Morris M, Eifel PJ, Lu J, Grigsby PW, Levenback C, Stevens RE, et al. Pelvic radiation with concurrent chemotherapy compared with pelvic and paraaortic radiation for high-risk cervical cancer. N Engl J Med. 1999;340:1137–43.

78. Peters 3rd WA, Liu PY, Barrett 2nd RJ, Stock RJ, Monk BJ, Berek JS, et al. Concurrent chemotherapy and pelvic radiation therapy compared with pelvic radiation therapy alone as adjuvant therapy after radical surgery in high-risk early stage cancer of the cervix. J Clin Oncol. 2000;18:1606–13.

79. Einstein MH, Parashar B, Sood B, Goldman N, Goldberg GL, Runowicz CD, et al. Long-term complications of concomitant chemoradiotherapy for locally advanced cervical cancer. Proc Am Soc Clin Oncol. 2002;21:abstr 2526.

80. Di Stefano M, Fagotti A, Ferrandina G, Francesco F, Daniela S, Giuseppe D, et al. Preoperative chemoradiotherapy in locally advanced cervical cancer: long-term outcome and complications. Gynecol Oncol. 2005;99:S166–70.

81. Bye A, Ose T, Kaasa S. Quality of life during pelvic radiotherapy. Acta Obstet Gynecol Scand. 1995;74:147–52.

82. Bookman MA, McGuire 3rd WP, Kilpatrick D, Keenan E, Hogan WM, Johnson SW, et al. Carboplatin and paclitaxel in ovarian carcinoma: a phase I study of the Gynecologic Oncology Group. J Clin Oncol. 1996;14(6):1895–902.

83. Cavaletti G, Bogliun G, Marzorati L, Zincone A, Marzola M, Colombo N, et al. Peripheral neurotoxicity of taxol in patients previously treated with cisplatin. Cancer. 1995;75(5):1141–50.

84. Vasey PA. Role of docetaxel in the treatment of newly diagnosed advanced ovarian cancer. J Clin Oncol. 2003;21:136s–44.

85. Vasey PA. Survival and longer term toxicity results of the SCOTROC study. Proc Am Soc Clin Oncol. 2002;21:804.

86. Markman M, Kennedy A, Webster K, Peterson G, Kulp B, Belinson J, et al. Combination chemotherapy with carboplatin and docetaxel in the treatment of cancers of the ovary and fallopian tube and primary carcinoma of the peritoneum. J Clin Oncol. 2001;19(7):1901–5.

87. Loprinzi CL, Reeves BN, Dakhil SR, Sloan JA, Wolf SL, Burger KN, et al. Natural history of paclitaxel-associated acute pain syndrome: prospective cohort study NCCTG N08C1. J Clin Oncol. 2011;29(11):1472–8.

88. Markman M, Kennedy A, Webster K, Kulp B, Peterson G, Belinson J. Use of low dose oral prednisone to prevent paclitaxel-induced myalgias and arthralgias. Gynecol Oncol. 1999;72:100–1.

89. Savarese D, Boucher J, Corey B. Glutamine treatment of paclitaxel induced myalgias and arthralgias. J Clin Oncol. 1998;16:3918–9.

90. Lenz HJ. Management and preparedness for infusion and hypersensitivity reactions. Oncologist. 2007;12(5):601–9.

91. Muggia FM, Braly PS, Brady MF, Sutton G, Niemann TH, Lentz SL, et al. Phase III randomized study of cisplatin versus paclitaxel versus cisplatin and paclitaxel in patients with suboptimal stage III or IV ovarian cancer: a gynecologic oncology group study. J Clin Oncol. 2000;18(1):106–15.

92. Eisenhauer EA, ten Bokkel Huinink WW, Swenerton KD, Gianni L, Myles J, van der Burg ME, et al. European-Canadian randomized trial of paclitaxel in relapsed ovarian cancer: high-dose versus low-dose and long versus short infusion. J Clin Oncol. 1994;12(12):2654–66.

93. Ostoros G, Pretz A, Fillinger J, Soltesz I, Dome B. Fatal pulmonary fibrosis induced by paclitaxel: a case report and review of the literature. Int J Gynecol Cancer. 2006;16 Suppl 1:391–3.

94. Sessa C, Marsoni S. Randomized single-agents trials in recurrent epithelial ovarian cancer. Int J Gynecol Cancer. 2005;15 Suppl 3:247–51.

95. Morris R, Munkarah A. Alternate dosing schedules for topotecan in the treatment of recurrent ovarian cancer. Oncologist. 2002;7 Suppl 5:29–35.

96. O'Reilly S, Fleming GF, Barker SD, Walczak JR, Bookman MA, McGuire 3rd WP, et al. Phase I trial and pharmacologic trial of sequences of paclitaxel and topotecan in previously treated ovarian epithelial malignancies: a Gynecologic Oncology Group study. J Clin Oncol. 1997;15(1):177–86.

97. Ten Bokkel Huinink W, Lane SR, Ross GA, International Topotecan Study Group. Long-term survival in a phase III, randomised study of topotecan versus paclitaxel in advanced epithelial ovarian carcinoma. Ann Oncol. 2004;15(1):100–3.

98. Armstrong D, O'Reilly S. Clinical guidelines for managing topotecan-related hematologic toxicity. Oncologist. 1998;3(1):4–10.

99. Rodriguez M, Rose PG. Improved therapeutic index of lower dose topotecan chemotherapy in recurrent ovarian cancer. Gynecol Oncol. 2001;83(2):257–62.

100. Armstrong DK. Topotecan dosing guidelines in ovarian cancer: reduction and management of hematologic toxicity. Oncologist. 2004;9(1):33–42.

101. O'Reilly S, Rowinsky E, Slichenmyer W, Donehower RC, Forastiere A, Ettinger D, et al. Phase I and pharmacologic studies of topotecan in patients with impaired hepatic function. J Natl Cancer Inst. 1996; 88(12):817–24.

102. Möbus V, Pfaff PN, Volm T, Kreienberg R, Kaubitzsch S. Long time therapy with topotecan in patients with recurrence of ovarian carcinoma. Anticancer Res. 2001;21(5):3551–6.

103. Pfisterer J, Plante M, Vergote I, du Bois A, Hirte H, Lacave AJ, et al. Gemcitabine plus carboplatin compared with carboplatin in patients with platinum-sensitive recurrent ovarian cancer: an inter-group trial of the AGO-OVAR, the NCIC CTG, and the EORTC GCG. J Clin Oncol. 2006;24(29):4699–707.

104. Hansen SW. Gemcitabine in the treatment of ovarian cancer. Int J Gynecol Cancer. 2001;11 Suppl 1:39–41.

105. Thigpen T. The role of gemcitabine in first-line treatment of advanced ovarian carcinoma. Semin Oncol. 2006;33(2 Suppl 6):S26–32.

106. Pfisterer J, Ledermann JA. Management of platinum-sensitive recurrent ovarian cancer. Semin Oncol. 2006;33(2 Suppl 6):S12–6.

107. Abbruzzese JL, Phase I. studies with the novel nucleoside analog gemcitabine. Semin Oncol. 1996;23(5 Suppl 10):25–31.

108. Lund B, Hansen OP, Neijt JP, Theilade K, Hansen M. Phase II study of gemcitabine in previously platinum-treated ovarian cancer patients. Anticancer Drugs. 1995;6 Suppl 6:61–2.

109. Sauer-Heilborn A, Kath R, Schneider CP, Höffken K. Severe non-haematological toxicity after treatment with gemcitabine. J Cancer Res Clin Oncol. 1999;125(11):637–40.

110. Briasoulis E, Pavlidis N. Noncardiogenic pulmonary edema: an unusual and serious complication of anticancer therapy. Oncologist. 2001;6(2):153–61.

111. Barlési F, Villani P, Doddoli C, Gimenez C, Kleisbauer JP. Gemcitabine-induced severe pulmonary toxicity. Fundam Clin Pharmacol. 2004;18(1):85–91.

112. Martin C, Lund B, Anderson H, Thatcher N. Gemcitabine: once-weekly schedule active and better tolerated than twice-weekly schedule. Anticancer Drugs. 1996;7(3):351–7.

113. Flombaum CD, Mouradian JA, Casper ES, Erlandson RA, Benedetti F. Thrombotic microangiopathy as a complication of long-term therapy with gemcitabine. Am J Kidney Dis. 1999;33(3):555–62.

114. Weinberg LE, Lurain JR, Singh DK, Schink JC. Survival and reproductive outcomes in women treated for malignant ovarian germ cell tumors. Gynecol Oncol. 2011;121(2):285–9.

115. Rose PG, Blessing JA, Mayer AR, Homesley HD. Prolonged oral etoposide as second-line therapy for platinum-resistant and platinum-sensitive ovarian carcinoma: a Gynecologic Oncology Group study. J Clin Oncol. 1998;16(2):405–10.

116. Rose PG, Blessing JA, Soper JT, Barter JF. Prolonged oral etoposide in recurrent or advanced leiomyosarcoma of the uterus: a gynecologic oncology group study. Gynecol Oncol. 1998;70(2):267–71.

117. Rose PG, Blessing JA, Van Le L, Waggoner S. Prolonged oral etoposide in recurrent or advanced squamous cell carcinoma of the cervix: a gynecologic oncology group study. Gynecol Oncol. 1998;70(2):263–6.

118. Fleming RA, Miller AA, Stewart CF. Etoposide: an update. Clin Pharm. 1989;8(4):274–93.

119. De Souza P, Friedlander M, Wilde C, Kirsten F, Ryan M. Hypersensitivity reactions to etoposide. A report of three cases and review of the literature. Am J Clin Oncol. 1994;17(5):387–9.

120. Fleming GF, Brunetto VL. Phase III trial of doxorubicin plus cisplatin with or without paclitaxel plus filgrastim in advanced endometrial carcinoma: a Gynecologic Oncology Group Study. J Clin Oncol. 2004;22:2159–66.

121. Pujade-Lauraine E, Wagner U, Aavall-Lundqvist E, Gebski V, Heywood M, Vasey PA, et al. Pegylated liposomal Doxorubicin and Carboplatin compared with Paclitaxel and Carboplatin for patients with platinum-sensitive ovarian cancer in late relapse. J Clin Oncol. 2010;28:3323–9.

122. Thigpen JT, Aghajanian CA, Alberts DS, Campos SM, Gordon AN, Markman M, et al. Role of pegylated liposomal doxorubicin in ovarian cancer. Gynecol Oncol. 2005;96(1):10–8.

123. Schwartz RG, McKenzie WB, Alexander J, Sager P, D'Souza A, Manatunga A, et al. Congestive heart failure and left ventricular dysfunction complicating doxorubicin therapy. Seven-year experience using serial radionuclide angiocardiography. Am J Med. 1987;82(6):1109–18.

124. Gabizon A, Catane R, Uziely R, Kaufman B, Safra T, Cohen R, et al. Prolonged circulation time and enhanced accumulation in malignant exudates of doxorubicin encapsulated in polyethylene-glycol coated liposomes. Cancer Res. 1994;54:987–92.

125. Alberts DS. Treatment of refractory and recurrent ovarian cancer. Semin Oncol. 1999;26(1 Suppl 1):8–14.

126. Berri G, Billingham M, Alderman E, Richardson P, Torti F, Lum B, et al. The use of cardiac biopsy to demonstrate reduced cardiotoxicity in AIDS Kaposi's sarcoma patients with pegylated liposomal doxorubicin. Ann Oncol. 1998;9:711–6.

127. Dimopoulos MA, Papadopoulou M, Andreopoulou E, Papadimitriou C, Pavlidis N, Aravantinos G, et al. Favorable outcome of ovarian germ cell malignancies treated with cisplatin or carboplatin-based chemotherapy: a Hellenic Cooperative Oncology Group study. Gynecol Oncol. 1998;70(1):70–4.

128. Tuxen MK, Hansen SW. Neurotoxicity secondary to antineoplastic drugs. Cancer Treat Rev. 1994;20:191–214.

129. Sahenk Z, Brady ST, Mendell JR. Studies on the pathogenesis of vincristine-induced neuropathy. Muscle Nerve. 1987;10:80–4.

130. Carlson K, Ocean AJ. Peripheral neuropathy with microtubule-targeting agents: occurrence and management approach. Clin Breast Cancer. 2011;11(2):73–81.

131. Markman M, Kennedy A, Sutton G, Hurteau J, Webster K, Peterson G, et al. Phase 2 trial of single agent ifosfamide/mesna in patients with platinum/paclitaxel refractory ovarian cancer who have not previously been treated with an alkylating agent. Gynecol Oncol. 1998;70(2):272–4.

132. Liu YL, Tsai SH, Chang FW, Yu MH. Ifosfamide-induced encephalopathy in patients with uterine sarcoma. Taiwan J Obstet Gynecol. 2010; 49(1):77–80.

133. Pearl ML, Inagami M, McCauley DL, Valea FA, Chalas E, Fischer M. Mesna, doxorubicin, ifosfamide, and dacarbazine (MAID) chemotherapy for gynecologic sarcomas. Int J Gynecol Cancer. 2002;12(6):745–8.

134. Kosmas C, Mylonakis N, Tsakonas G, Vorgias G, Karvounis N, Tsavaris N, et al. Evaluation of the paclitaxel–ifosfamide–cisplatin (TIP) combination in relapsed and/or metastatic cervical cancer. Br J Cancer. 2009;101:1059–65.

135. Buda A, Fossati R, Colombo N, Fei F, Floriani I, Gueli Alletti D, et al. Randomized trial of neoadjuvant chemotherapy comparing paclitaxel, ifosfamide, and cisplatin with ifosfamide and cisplatin followed by radical surgery in patients with locally advanced squamous cell cervical carcinoma: the SNAP01 (Studio Neo-Adjuvante Portio) Italian Collaborative Study. J Clin Oncol. 2005;23(18):4137–45.

136. Lissoni AA, Fei F, Rossi R, Fruscio R, Villa A, Zani G. Ifosfamide in the treatment of malignant epithelial ovarian tumors. Oncology. 2003;65 Suppl 2:59–62.

137. Pelgrims J, De Vos F, Van den Brande J. Methylene blue in the treatment and prevention of ifosfamide-induced encephalopathy: report of 12 cases and a review of the literature. Br J Cancer. 2000;82(2):291–4.
138. Ellison DH, Berl T. Clinical practice. The syndrome of inappropriate antidiuresis. N Engl J Med. 2007;356(20):2064–72.
139. Raftopoulos H. Diagnosis and management of hyponatremia in cancer patients. Support Care Cancer. 2007;15(12):1341–7.
140. Cantwell BM, Idle M, Millward MJ, Hall G, Lind MJ. Encephalopathy with hyponatremia and inappropriate arginine vasopressin secretion following an intravenous ifosfamide infusion. Ann Oncol. 1990;1(3):232.
141. Piccart MJ, Bertelsen K, James K. Randomized intergroup trial of cisplatin-paclitaxel versus cisplatin-cyclophosphamide in women with advanced epithelial ovarian cancer: three-year results. J Natl Cancer Inst. 2000;92(9):699–708.
142. Muntz HG, Goff BA, Fuller Jr AF. Recurrent ovarian granulosa cell tumor: role of combination chemotherapy with report of a long-term response to a cyclophosphamide, doxorubicin and cisplatin regimen. Eur J Gynaecol Oncol. 1990;11(4):263–8.
143. Signorelli M, Chiappa V, Minig L, Fruscio R, Perego P, Caspani G, et al. Platinum, anthracycline, and alkylating agent-based chemotherapy for ovarian carcinosarcoma. Int J Gynecol Cancer. 2009;19(6):1142–6.
144. Rochelle E, Curtis MA, Boice JD, Bernstein L, Greenberg RS, Flannery JT, et al. Risk of leukemia after chemotherapy and radiation treatment for breast cancer. N Engl J Med. 1992;326:1745–51.
145. Levine MN, Bramwell VH, Pritchard KI, Norris BD, Shepherd LE, Abu-Zahra H, et al. Randomized trial of intensive cyclophosphamide, epirubicin, and fluorouracil chemotherapy compared with cyclophosphamide, methotrexate, and fluorouracil in premenopausal women with node-positive breast cancer. National Cancer Institute of Canada Clinical Trials Group. J Clin Oncol. 1998;16(8):2651–8.
146. Williams S, Blessing JA, Liao SY, Ball H, Hanjani P. Adjuvant therapy of ovarian germ cell tumors with cisplatin, etoposide, and bleomycin: a trial of the Gynecologic Oncology Group. Clin Oncol. 1994;12(4):701–6.
147. Ginsberg SJ, Cornis RL. The pulmonary toxicity of neoplastic agents. Semin Oncol. 1982;9:34–7.
148. White DA, Stover DE. Severe bleomycin induced pneumonitis. Clinical features and response to corticosteroids. Chest. 1984;86:723–8.
149. O'Sullivan JM, Huddart RA, Norman AR, Nicholls J, Dearnaley DP, Horwich A, et al. Predicting the risk of bleomycin lung toxicity in patients with germ-cell tumours. Ann Oncol. 2003;14(1):91–6.
150. Carver JR, Shapiro CL, Ng A, Jacobs L, Schwartz C, Virgo KS, et al. American Society of Clinical Oncology clinical evidence review on

the ongoing care of adult cancer survivors: cardiac and pulmonary late effects. J Clin Oncol. 2007;25(25):3991–4008.

151. Osborne RJ, Filiaci V, Schink JC, Mannel RS, Alvarez Secord A, Kelley JL, et al. Phase III trial of weekly methotrexate or pulsed dactinomycin for low-risk gestational trophoblastic neoplasia: a gynecologic oncology group study. J Clin Oncol. 2011;29(7):825–31.

152. Rustin GJS, Newlands ES, Lutz JM, Holden L, Bagshawe KD, Hiscox JG, et al. Combination but not single-agent methotrexate chemotherapy for gestational trophoblastic tumors increases the incidence of second tumors. J Clin Oncol. 1996;14(10):2769–73.

153. Widemann BC, Adamson PC. Understanding and managing methotrexate nephrotoxicity. Oncologist. 2006;11:694–703.

154. De Miguel D, García-Suárez J, Martín Y, Gil-Fernández JJ, Burgaleta C. Severe acute renal failure following high-dose methotrexate therapy in adults with haematological malignancies: a significant number result from unrecognized co-administration of several drugs. Nephrol Dial Transplant. 2008;23(12):3762–6.

155. Look KY, Blessing JA, Valea FA, McGehee R, Manetta A, Webster KD, et al. Phase II trial of 5-fluorouracil and high-dose leucovorin in recurrent adenocarcinoma of the cervix: a Gynecologic Oncology Group study. Gynecol Oncol. 1997;67(3):255–8.

156. Look KY, Muss HB, Blessing JA, Morris M. A phase II trial of 5-fluorouracil and high-dose leucovorin in recurrent epithelial ovarian carcinoma. A Gynecologic Oncology Group Study. Am J Clin Oncol. 1995;18(1):19–22.

157. De Forni M, Malet-Martino MC, Jaillais P, Shubinski RE, Bachaud JM, Lemaire L, et al. Cardiotoxicity of high-dose continuous infusion fluorouracil: a prospective clinical study. J Clin Oncol. 1992;10:1795–801.

158. van Kuilenburg AB, Meinsma R, Zonnenberg BA, Zoetekouw L, Baas F, Matsuda K, et al. Dihydropyrimidinase deficiency and severe 5-fluorouracil toxicity. Clin Cancer Res. 2003;9:4363.

159. Peterson DE, Bensadoun RJ, Roila F, ESMO Guidelines Working Group. Management of oral and gastrointestinal mucositis: ESMO Clinical Practice Guidelines. Ann Oncol. 2011;22 Suppl 6:vi78–84.

160. Grosso F, Dileo P, Sanfilippo R, Stacchiotti S, Bertulli R, Piovesan C, et al. Steroid premedication markedly reduces liver and bone marrow toxicity of trabectedin in advanced sarcoma. Eur J Cancer. 2006;42(10):1484–90.

161. Del Campo JM, Roszak A, Bidzinski M, Ciuleanu TE, Hogberg T, Wojtukiewicz MZ, et al. Phase II randomized study of trabectedin given as two different every 3 weeks dose schedules (1.5 mg/m2 24 h or 1.3 mg/m2 3 h) to patients with relapsed, platinum-sensitive, advanced ovarian cancer. Ann Oncol. 2009;20(11):1794–802.

162. Karagol H, Saip P, Uygun K, Caloglu M, Eralp Y, Tas F, et al. The efficacy of tamoxifen in patients with advanced epithelial ovarian cancer. Med Oncol. 2007;24:39–43.

163. Fishman A, Kudelka AP, Tresukosol D, Edwards CL, Freedman RS, Kaplan AL, et al. Leuprolide acetate for treating refractory or persistent ovarian granulosa cell tumor. J Reprod Med. 1996;41:393–6.

164. Papadimitriou CA, Markaki S, Siapkaras J, Vlachos G, Efstathiou E, Grimani I, et al. Hormonal therapy with letrozole for relapsed epithelial ovarian cancer. Long-term results of a phase II study. Oncology (Williston). 2004;66:112–7.

165. Perez EA. Safety profiles of tamoxifen and the aromatase inhibitors in adjuvant therapy of hormone-responsive early breast cancer. Ann Oncol. 2007;18 Suppl 8:viii26–35.

166. Monnier A. Clinical management of adverse events in adjuvant therapy for hormone-responsive early breast cancer. Ann Oncol. 2007;18 Suppl 8:viii36–44.

167. Howell A, Cuzick J, Baum M, Buzdar A, Dowsett M, Forbes JF, et al. Results of the ATAC (arimidex, tamoxifen, alone or in combination) trial after completion of 5 years' adjuvant treatment for breast cancer. Lancet. 2005;365:60–2.

168. Breast International Group (BIG) 1–98 Collaborative Group, Thürlimann B, Keshaviah A, Coates AS, Mouridsen H, Mauriac L, Forbes JF, et al. A comparison of letrozole and tamoxifen in postmenopausal women with early breast cancer. N Engl J Med. 2005;353:2747–56.

169. Wenzel LB, Huang HQ, Armstrong DK, Walker JL, Cella D, Gynecologic Oncology Group. Health-related quality of life during and after intraperitoneal versus intravenous chemotherapy for optimally debulked ovarian cancer: a Gynecologic Oncology Group Study. J Clin Oncol. 2007;25(4):437–43.

170. Markman M. Intraperitoneal chemotherapy in the management of ovarian cancer: focus on carboplatin. Ther Clin Risk Manag. 2009;5(1):161–8.

171. Gould N, Sill MW, Mannel RS, Thaker PH, Disilvestro P, Waggoner S, et al. A phase I study with an expanded cohort to assess the feasibility of intravenous paclitaxel, intraperitoneal carboplatin and intraperitoneal paclitaxel in patients with untreated ovarian, fallopian tube or primary peritoneal carcinoma: a Gynecologic Oncology Group study. Gynecol Oncol. 2012;125(1):54–8.

172. Nagao S, Iwasa N, Kurosaki A, Nishikawa T, Ohishi R, Hasegawa K, et al. Intravenous/intraperitoneal paclitaxel and intraperitoneal carboplatin in patients with epithelial ovarian, fallopian tube, or peritoneal carcinoma: a feasibility study. Int J Gynecol Cancer. 2012;22(1):70–5.

173. Cotte E, Glehen O, Mohamed F, Lamy F, Falandry C, Golfier F, et al. Cytoreductive surgery and intraperitoneal chemo-hyperthermia for chemo-resistant and recurrent advanced epithelial ovarian cancer: prospective study of 81 patients. World J Surg. 2007;31(9):1813–20.

174. Helm CW, Randall-Whitis L, Martin RS, Metzinger DS, Gordinier ME, Parker LP, et al. Hyperthermic intraperitoneal chemotherapy in conjunction with surgery for the treatment of recurrent ovarian carcinoma. Gynecol Oncol. 2007;105(1):90–6.
175. Chua TC, Robertson G, Liauw W, Farrell R, Yan TD, Morris DL. Intraoperative hyperthermic intraperitoneal chemotherapy after cytoreductive surgery in ovarian cancer peritoneal carcinomatosis: systematic review of current results. J Cancer Res Clin Oncol. 2009;135(12):1637–45.
176. Golse N, Bakrin N, Passot G, Mohamed F, Vaudoyer D, Gilly FN, et al. Iterative procedures combining cytoreductive surgery with hyperthermic intraperitoneal chemotherapy for peritoneal recurrence: postoperative and long-term results. J Surg Oncol. 2012;106(2):197–203. Epub 2012 Feb 13.
177. Banarjee S, Gore M. The future of targeted therapies in ovarian cancer. Oncologist. 2009;14:706–16.
178. Hudson LG, Moss NM, Stack MS. EGF-receptor regulation of matrix metalloproteinases in epithelial ovarian carcinoma. Future Oncol. 2009;5(3):323–38.
179. Tagawa T, Morgan R, Yen Y, Mortimer J. Ovarian cancer: opportunity for targeted therapy. J Oncol. 2012;2012:682480.
180. Secord AA, Blessing JA, Armstrong DK, Rodgers WH, Miner Z, Barnes MN, Gynecologic Oncology Group, et al. Phase II trial of cetuximab and carboplatin in relapsed platinum-sensitive ovarian cancer and evaluation of epidermal growth factor receptor expression: a Gynecologic Oncology Group study. Gynecol Oncol. 2008;108(3):493–9.
181. Konner J, Schilder RJ, DeRosa FA, Gerst SR, Tew WP, Sabbatini PJ, et al. A phase II study of cetuximab/paclitaxel/carboplatin for the initial treatment of advanced-stage ovarian, primary peritoneal, or fallopian tube cancer. Gynecol Oncol. 2008;110(2):140–5.
182. Schilder RJ, Sill MW, Chen X, Darcy KM, Decesare SL, Lewandowski G, et al. Phase II study of gefitinib in patients with relapsed or persistent ovarian or primary peritoneal carcinoma and evaluation of epidermal growth factor receptor mutations and immunohistochemical expression: a Gynecologic Oncology Group Study. Clin Cancer Res. 2005;11(15):5539–48.
183. Posadas EM, Liel MS, Kwitkowski V, Minasian L, Godwin AK, Hussain MM, et al. A phase II and pharmacodynamic study of gefitinib in patients with refractory or recurrent epithelial ovarian cancer. Cancer. 2007;109(7):1323–30.
184. Wagner U, du Bois A, Pfisterer J, Huober J, Loibl S, Lück HJ, AGO Ovarian Cancer Study Group, et al. Gefitinib in combination with tamoxifen in patients with ovarian cancer refractory or resistant to platinum-taxane based therapy – a phase II trial of the AGO Ovarian Cancer Study Group (AGO-OVAR 2.6). Gynecol Oncol. 2007;105(1):132–7.

185. Gordon AN, Finkler N, Edwards RP, Garcia AA, Crozier M, Irwin DH, et al. Efficacy and safety of erlotinib HCl, an epidermal growth factor receptor (HER1/EGFR) tyrosine kinase inhibitor, in patients with advanced ovarian carcinoma: results from a phase II multicenter study. Int J Gynecol Cancer. 2005;15(5):785–92.

186. Hirte H, Oza A, Swenerton K, Ellard SL, Grimshaw R, Fisher B, et al. A phase II study of erlotinib (OSI-774) given in combination with carboplatin in patients with recurrent epithelial ovarian cancer (NCIC CTG IND.149). Gynecol Oncol. 2010;118(3):308–12.

187. Holmberg LA, Goff B, Veljovich D. Unexpected gastrointestinal toxicity from Docetaxel/Carboplatin/Erlotinib followed by maintenance Erlotinib treatment for newly diagnosed stage III/IV ovarian cancer, primary peritoneal, or fallopian tube cancer. Gynecol Oncol. 2011; 121(2):426.

188. Garcia AA, Sill MW, Lankes HA, Godwin AK, Mannel RS, Armstrong DK, et al. A phase II evaluation of lapatinib in the treatment of persistent or recurrent epithelial ovarian or primary peritoneal carcinoma: a gynecologic oncology group study. Gynecol Oncol. 2012;124(3):569–74.

189. Weroha SJ, Oberg AL, Ziegler KL, Dakhilm SR, Rowland KM, Hartmann LC, et al. Phase II trial of lapatinib and topotecan (LapTop) in patients with platinum-refractory/resistant ovarian and primary peritoneal carcinoma. Gynecol Oncol. 2011;122(1):116–20.

190. Bookman MA, Darcy KM, Clarke-Pearson D, Boothby RA, Horowitz IR. Evaluation of monoclonal humanized anti-HER2 antibody, trastuzumab, in patients with recurrent or refractory ovarian or primary peritoneal carcinoma with overexpression of HER2: a phase II trial of the Gynecologic Oncology Group. J Clin Oncol. 2003;21(2):283–90.

191. Gordon MS, Matei D, Aghajanian C, Matulonis UA, Brewer M, Fleming GF, et al. Clinical activity of pertuzumab (rhuMAb 2C4), a HER dimerization inhibitor, in advanced ovarian cancer: potential predictive relationship with tumor HER2 activation status. Oncology Group. J Clin Oncol. 2003;21(2):283–90.

192. Yuan Y, Liao YM, Hsueh CT, Mirshahidi HR. Novel targeted therapeutics: inhibitors of MDM2. ALK and PARP. J Hematol Oncol. 2011;4:16.

193. Mukhopadhyay A, Curtin N, Plummer R, Edmondson RJ. PARP inhibitors and epithelial ovarian cancer: an approach to targeted chemotherapy and personalised medicine. BJOG. 2011;118(4): 429–32.

194. Fong PC, Yap TA, Boss DS, Carden CP, Mergui-Roelvink M, Gourley C, et al. Poly(ADP)-ribose polymerase inhibition: frequent durable responses in BRCA carrier ovarian cancer correlating with platinum-free interval. J Clin Oncol. 2010;28(15):2512–9.

195. Audeh MW, Carmichael J, Penson RT, Friedlander M, Powell B, Bell-McGuinn KM, et al. Oral poly(ADP-ribose) polymerase

inhibitor olaparib in patients with BRCA1 or BRCA2 mutations and recurrent ovarian cancer: a proof-of-concept trial. Lancet. 2010;376(9737):245–51.

196. Kaye SB, Lubinski J, Matulonis U, Ang JE, Gourley C, Karlan BY, et al. Phase II, open-label, randomized, multicenter study comparing the efficacy and safety of olaparib, a poly (ADP-ribose) polymerase inhibitor, and pegylated liposomal doxorubicin in patients with BRCA1 or BRCA2 mutations and recurrent ovarian cancer. J Clin Oncol. 2012;30(4):372–9.

197. Behbakht K, Sill MW, Darcy KM, Rubin SC, Mannel RS, Waggoner S, et al. Phase II trial of the mTOR inhibitor, temsirolimus and evaluation of circulating tumor cells and tumor biomarkers in persistent and recurrent epithelial ovarian and primary peritoneal malignancies: a Gynecologic Oncology Group study. Gynecol Oncol. 2011;123(1):19–26.

198. Takano M, Kikuchi Y, Kudoh K, Goto T, Furuya K, Kikuchi R, et al. Weekly administration of temsirolimus for heavily pretreated patients with clear cell carcinoma of the ovary: a report of six cases. Int J Clin Oncol. 2011;16(5):605–9.

199. Coleman RL, Duska LR, Ramirez PT, Heymach JV, Kamat AA, Modesitt SC, et al. Phase 1–2 study of docetaxel plus aflibercept in patients with recurrent ovarian, primary peritoneal, or fallopian tube cancer. Lancet Oncol. 2011;12(12):1109–17.

200. Gotlieb WH, Amant F, Advani S, Goswami C, Hirte H, Provencher D, et al. Intravenous aflibercept for treatment of recurrent symptomatic malignant ascites in patients with advanced ovarian cancer: a phase 2, randomised, double-blind, placebo-controlled study. Lancet Oncol. 2012;13(2):154–62.

201. Biagi JJ, Oza AM, Chalchal HI, Grimshaw R, Ellard SL, Lee U, et al. A phase II study of sunitinib in patients with recurrent epithelial ovarian and primary peritoneal carcinoma: an NCIC Clinical Trials Group Study. Ann Oncol. 2011;22(2):335–40.

202. Baumann KH, du Bois A, Meier W, Rau J, Wimberger P, Sehouli J et al., A phase II trial (AGO 2.11) in platinum-resistant ovarian cancer: a randomized multicenter trial with sunitinib (SU11248) to evaluate dosage, schedule, tolerability, toxicity and effectiveness of a multitargeted receptor tyrosine kinase inhibitor monotherapy. Ann Oncol. 2012;23(9):2265–71.

203. Bellati F, Napoletano C, Gasparri ML, Visconti V, Zizzari IG, Ruscito I, et al. Monoclonal antibodies in gynecologic cancer: a critical point of view. Clin Dev Immunol. 2011;2011:890758.

204. Santin AD, Sill MW, McMeekin DS, Leitao Jr MM, Brown J, Sutton GP, et al. Phase II trial of cetuximab in the treatment of persistent or recurrent squamous or non-squamous cell carcinoma of the cervix: a Gynecologic Oncology Group study. Gynecol Oncol. 2011;122(3):495–500.

205. Farley J, Sill MW, Birrer M, Walker J, Schilder RJ, Thigpen JT, et al. Phase II study of cisplatin plus cetuximab in advanced, recurrent, and previously treated cancers of the cervix and evaluation of epidermal growth factor receptor immunohistochemical expression: a Gynecologic Oncology Group study. Gynecol Oncol. 2011;121(2): 303–8.

206. Kurtz JE, Hardy-Bessard AC, Deslandres M, Lavau-Denes S, Largillier R, Roemer-Becuwe C, et al. Cetuximab, topotecan and cisplatin for the treatment of advanced cervical cancer: a phase II GINECO trial. Gynecol Oncol. 2009;113(1):16–20.

207. Moore K, Sill M, Miller DS, et al. A phase I trial of concurrent cetuximab (CET), cisplatin (CDDP), and radiation therapy (RT) women with locally advanced cervical cancer (CXCA): a GOG study. J Clin Oncol. 29:2011(suppl; abstr 5032).

208. Monk BJ, Mas Lopez L, Zarba JJ, Oaknin A, Tarpin C, Termrungruanglert W, et al. Phase II, open-label study of pazopanib or lapatinib monotherapy compared with pazopanib plus lapatinib combination therapy in patients with advanced and recurrent cervical cancer. J Clin Oncol. 2010;28(22):3562–9.

209. Monk BJ, Sill MW, Burger RA, Gray HJ, Buekers TE, Roman LD. Phase II trial of bevacizumab in the treatment of persistent or recurrent squamous cell carcinoma of the cervix: a gynecologic oncology group study. J Clin Oncol. 2009;27(7):1069–74.

210. Schefter TE, Winter K, Kwon JS, Stuhr K, Balaraj K, Yaremko BP, et al. A phase II study of bevacizumab in combination with definitive radiotherapy and cisplatin chemotherapy in untreated patients with locally advanced cervical carcinoma: preliminary results of RTOG 0417. Int J Radiat Oncol Biol Phys. 2012;83(4):1179–84. Epub 2012 Feb 16.

211. Mackay HJ, Tinker A, Winquist E, Thomas G, Swenerton K, Oza A, et al. A phase II study of sunitinib in patients with locally advanced or metastatic cervical carcinoma: NCIC CTG Trial IND.184. Gynecol Oncol. 2010;116(2):163–7.

212. Oza AM, Eisenhauer EA, Elit L, Cutz JC, Sakurada A, Tsao MS, et al. Phase II study of erlotinib in recurrent or metastatic endometrial cancer: NCIC IND-148. J Clin Oncol. 2008;26(26):4319–25.

213. Fleming GF, Sill MW, Darcy KM, McMeekin DS, Thigpen JT, Adler LM, et al. Phase II trial of trastuzumab in women with advanced or recurrent, HER2-positive endometrial carcinoma: a Gynecologic Oncology Group study. Gynecol Oncol. 2010;116(1):15–20.

214. Temkin SM, Yamada SD, Fleming GF. A phase I study of weekly temsirolimus and topotecan in the treatment of advanced and/or recurrent gynecologic malignancies. Gynecol Oncol. 2010;117(3): 473–6.

215. Aghajanian C, Sill MW, Darcy KM, Greer B, McMeekin DS, Rose PG, et al. Phase II trial of bevacizumab in recurrent or persistent

endometrial cancer: a Gynecologic Oncology Group study. J Clin Oncol. 2011;29(16):2259–65.

216. Mackay HJ, Buckanovich RJ, Hirte H, Correa R, Hoskins P, Biagi J, et al. A phase II study single agent of aflibercept (VEGF Trap) in patients with recurrent or metastatic gynecologic carcinosarcomas and uterine leiomyosarcoma. A trial of the Princess Margaret Hospital, Chicago and California Cancer Phase II Consortia. Gynecol Oncol. 2012;125(1):136–40.

217. Pinto C, Barone CA, Girolomoni G, Russi EG, Merlano MC, Ferrari D, et al. Management of skin toxicity associated with cetuximab treatment in combination with chemotherapy or radiotherapy. Oncologist. 2011;16(2):228–38.

218. Petrelli F, Borgonovo K, Cabiddu M, Ghilardi M, Barni S. Risk of anti-EGFR monoclonal antibody-related hypomagnesemia: systematic review and pooled analysis of randomized studies. Expert Opin Drug Saf. 2012;11 suppl 1:S9–19.

219. Izzedine H, Ederhy S, Goldwasser F, Soria JC, Milano G, Cohen A, et al. Management of hypertension in angiogenesis inhibitor-treated patients. Ann Oncol. 2009;20(5):807–15.

220. Stone RL, Sood AK, Coleman RL. Collateral damage: toxic effects of targeted antiangiogenic therapies in ovarian cancer. Lancet Oncol. 2010;11(5):465–75.

221. Feldt S, Schüssel K, Quinzler R, Franzmann A, Czeche S, Ludwig WD, et al. Incidence of thyroid hormone therapy in patients treated with sunitinib or sorafenib: a cohort study. Eur J Cancer. 2012;48(7):974–81. Epub 2012 Feb 28.

# Chapter 6
## Genitourinary Cancer

**Bertrand F. Tombal**

**Abstract** Genitourinary cancers represent 12.8 % of cancer in both sexes and 21.5 % in men, accounting for 7 % of cancer deaths in both sexes and 10.5 % in men. Prostate cancer and renal cell carcinoma share the characteristic of being largely chemoresistant, with the relative exception of taxanes docetaxel and cabazitaxel, which modestly increase overall survival in late-stage prostate cancer. Prostate cancer is primarily treated by hormonal therapy, either by androgen deprivation or antiandrogens, and renal cell carcinoma is nowadays treated with agents targeting survival and angiogenesis pathways, including tyrosine kinase inhibitors (TKIs) sorafenib, sunitinib, and pazopanib; antivascular endothelial growth factor (VEGF) monoclonal antibody bevacizumab; and mammalian target of rapamycin (mTOR) inhibitors temsirolimus and everolimus. Neither hormone therapy nor targeted therapies eradicate prostate cancer and RCC but

B.F. Tombal, M.D., Ph.D.
Service d'Urologie, Cliniques Universitaires Saint Luc,
Université Catholique de Louvain,
Brussels, Belgium
e-mail: bertrand.tombal@uclouvain.be

M.A. Dicato (ed.), *Side Effects of Medical Cancer Therapy*,     247
DOI 10.1007/978-0-85729-787-7_6,
© Springer-Verlag London 2013

rather switch them to a more chronic state. This means that these treatments are prescribed chronically for an extended period of time. In such conditions, even the least bothersome side effect may profoundly alter the quality of life of patients. Ultimately, this is a threat to compliance and then to the chronic efficacy of these treatments. In addition, many of the side effects of these drugs often overlap with common chronic illnesses such as diabetes, hypertension, hypercholesterolemia, heart failure, and osteoporosis. An exhaustive knowledge of these side effects, proper monitoring, and in-depth education of patients are key elements to secure the efficacy of these treatments.

**Keywords**   Prostate cancer • Renal cell carcinoma • Androgen-deprivation therapy • Tyrosine kinase inhibitors • mTOR inhibitors • Side effects

# Introduction

Genitourinary cancers are the leading forms of cancer and cancer deaths. Based on data from GLOBOCAN 2008, 913,000 prostate cancers, 386,000 bladder cancers, 271,000 kidney cancers, and 52,000 testis cancers have been reported, accounting for 12.8 % of cancer in both sexes and 21.5 % in men. Owing mainly to major improvements in treatment modalities, which include surgery, radiotherapy, and innovative systemic treatments, genitourinary cancers account for only 7 % of cancer deaths in both sexes and 10.5 % of cancer deaths in men.

Two genitourinary malignancies, prostate cancer and renal cell carcinoma (RCC), are characterized by a limited usage of chemotherapy, in contrast to other cancer types. Prostate cancer is primarily treated by hormone therapy, mainly androgen-deprivation therapy (ADT). Metastatic castration-resistant prostate cancer (mCRCP) was considered a lethal disease until the publication of the results of two large trials with docetaxel. More than the benefit of docetaxel itself in mCRCP, which is limited anyway, these publications have moved the treatment of prostate cancer toward an era of multidisciplinary collaboration between specialties [1]. In contrast to many predictions, chemotherapy has never emerged as a major breakthrough treatment. It is only used in the late stages of the disease and with very modest overall survival benefit. Most studies assessing the combination of docetaxel with other classes of agent have failed to demonstrate significant benefit, and studies assessing earlier use are not conclusive. In contrast, a new twist is given to hormone therapy with the recent publication of the results with abiraterone acetate, an androgen synthesis inhibitor, and MDV3100, a novel antiandrogen. Both registration trials, conducted in a very late post-chemotherapy setting, have reported impressive benefit on overall survival. This demonstrates that prostate cancer is primarily a disease driven by the androgen receptor and that hormonal treatments, traditional and older, will remain the cornerstone strategy for years to come. Because of the particular importance of androgen-depriving therapies, a large part of this chapter will be devoted to the monitoring and prevention of side effects of hormone therapy.

Renal cell carcinoma, and especially its most frequent subtype clear cell carcinoma, is an even more peculiar disease, being both radio- and chemoresistant. Renal cell carcinoma was considered an immune-sensitive tumor as long as interferon-$\alpha$ (alpha)(IFN-$\alpha$) and high-dose interleukin (HD-IL2) were the only available treatments. The concomitant understanding of the importance of the VHL/HIF hypoxia pathways and the development of drug-targeting angiogenesis and survival pathways has revolutionized the approach to RCC. Today, six drugs have supplanted IFN-$\alpha$ (alpha) and IL2, including sorafenib, sunitinib, temsirolimus, everolimus, bevacizumab, and pazopanib. And more are yet to come. Although many of these drugs confer little or no benefit on overall survival, they have been widely accepted, and it is estimated that overall life span of patients is extended. But new modes of action have brought new types of side effects, to which physicians and patients need to become accustomed. These will be reviewed in the second part of this chapter.

Because several other chapters will address the toxicity of chemotherapy, we have chosen not to cover that topic and focus on hormone therapy of prostate cancer and targeted therapies of RCC.

# Side Effects of Hormonal Treatments in Prostate Cancer

Androgen-deprivation therapy by means of surgical castration or estrogens has been the standard treatment of advanced symptomatic prostate cancer since the seminal work of Charles Huggins in the late 40s [2]. Although there is only little or no benefit on overall survival when used alone, ADT is increasingly being used in asymptomatic patients in earlier disease stages who are not candidates for local treatment [3]. ADT is also used concomitantly and adjuvant to external beam radiation therapy (EBRT), a setup that has shown the most potential to improve overall survival.

As a result many patients are receiving ADT for a prolonged period of time and will be exposed much longer to side effects. ADT is traditionally recognized through its acute and more obnoxious side effects, which include loss of libido and erectile dysfunction, hot flushes, fatigue, and psychological side effects such as emotional instability, depression, or cognitive dysfunction [4–6]. Since patients are treated earlier, more attention has been given recently to long-term toxicity, including anemia, accelerated bone loss leading eventually to osteoporosis and fragility fractures, and sarcopenic obesity, which may lead to an increased risk of cardiovascular morbidity and mortality [7].

## Short-Term Adverse Events of ADT

### Hot Flushes

Hot flushes are described as sudden and uncomfortable heat sensations in the face, neck, upper chest, and back, lasting from seconds up to an hour. This side effect is one of the most common, described by up to 80 % of patients [5]. It is also one of the most bothersome side effects of ADT and may largely disrupt everyday life. Hot flushes are often triggered by stress, heat, sudden changes in body position, ingestion of warm or spicy food, or smoking [5].

Management of hot flushes includes informing patients to avoid triggering situations. If hot flushes are very bothersome for patients, medical therapy can be considered. Hormonal agents such as megestrol acetate, medroxyprogesterone acetate, cyproterone acetate, and low-dose diethylstilbestrol are very popular to treat bothersome hot flushes [4–6, 8]. Selective serotonin reuptake inhibitors (SSRIs) (i.e., venlafaxine or citalopram), (alpha) $\alpha$-adrenergic inhibitors (i.e., clonidine), and GABA analogue gabapentin are alternatives to hormonal agents, although their efficacy is usually lower [9–11]. Acupuncture and phytotherapy, especially sage extracts, can also be recommended to patients, despite lack of definitive robust scientific evidence [12, 13].

## Sexual Dysfunction

The negative impact of ADT on libido and sexual function is well known, including decrease of sexual desire and impotence [14]. Patients and their partners should be informed about this, as it can cause anxiety for both. It should be stressed, however, that the extent of sexual dysfunction vary widely from one patient to another and that a satisfying sexual and affective life is possible under ADT. From a historic review of the social and intellectual performances of eunuchs, Aucoin and Wassersug suggested that given the right cultural setting and individual motivation, ADT may actually enhance, rather than hinder, both social and sexual performance [15]. Traditional treatments of erectile dysfunction can be recommended in ADT-treated patients, including intra-cavernous injections of prostaglandins and/or phospodiesterase-5 inhibitors. Physicians should always remember that ADT induces first a libido problem and that patient and partner counseling may prove as effective as medications.

## Fatigue

Fatigue is one of the most common side effects of ADT. Although fatigue is very difficult to fight, lifestyle changes and especially physical exercise may help to alleviate fatigue and improve quality of life. A systematic review on 34 trials examining the effectiveness of physical exercise in improving the physical functioning and psychological well-being of prostate cancer patients during and after treatment suggested that cancer patients may indeed benefit from physical exercise [16]. The Fresh Start trial has randomized 543 subjects with newly diagnosed locoregional breast or prostate cancer to receive a 10-month-specific program promoting diet changes and physical exercise or nonspecific information. Although subjects in both arms significantly improved their lifestyle behavior, significantly greater improvement was observed in subjects receiving the diet- and exercise-specific information [17]. Physicians should try to convince patients to adopt a healthier lifestyle including a healthy diet and physical exercise. Fatigue may be further aggravated by the sarcopenia (loss of skeletal muscle mass) resulting from ADT, which directly impacts on muscle strength and reduces physical activity [18].

## Psychological Side Effects

Androgen-deprivation therapy may have psychological side effects such as reduced cognitive function (e.g., reduced concentration and memory problems) and emotional instability or even depression [5,6]. Patients and relatives should be informed about the likelihood of emotional changes and how to identify early signs of depression or decreased cognitive function in order to ensure rapid referral to a specialist. It is also important to explain these side effects to the patient's family so that they understand their nature and origin and can help the patient adapt to them. Depression can be severe, so that an increased risk of suicide in the months following diagnosis of advanced prostate cancer has been reported, probably as a mixed effect of the cancer diagnosis and the initiation of ADT [19].

## Adrenal Insufficiency

Abiraterone acetate is a newly developed and approved androgen synthesis inhibitor that increases overall survival in mCRPC [20]. Abiraterone's mode of action is different from LHRH agonists and antagonists since it targets CYP17, a key enzyme that mediates androgen synthesis in the testes and adrenal glands. Abiraterone not only inhibits the synthesis of androgens but also suppresses cortisol synthesis [21]. This induces a reciprocal increase in pituitary adrenocorticotrophic hormone (ACTH) and therefore an elevation of corticosterone. This may lead to fluid retention, hypokalemia, and hypertension. To prevent these side effects, abiraterone must be combined with corticosteroids, prednisolone, prednisone, or dexamethasone, or mineralocorticoids such as eplerenone.

## *Long-Term Adverse Events of ADT*

## Anemia

In at least 90 % of ADT patients, hemoglobin level will drop on average by 10 % [22]. Anemia associated with ADT is usually normocytic, normochromic, and due to the lack of androgen stimulation of erythroid precursors and a decrease in erythropoietin production. Anemia worsens fatigue [5]. Physicians should closely monitor hemoglobin levels in patients treated with ADT. Anemia may be aggravated by extensive invasion of the bone marrow, which occurs frequently in mCRPC patients. Subcutaneous administration of recombinant human erythropoietin and/or transfusion may be required in severe cases.

## Metabolic and Cardiovascular Side Effects

### Physiopathology of Cardiovascular Toxicity in ADT-Treated Patients

Androgen-deprivation therapy causes changes in the patient's body mass and composition [5, 18]. Suppression of testosterone level causes a situation known as sarcopenic obesity, combining muscular atrophy and an increase in fatty tissue [23,24]. By creating an imbalance between lean and fatty mass, sarcopenic obesity induces many of the phenotypic features of the metabolic syndrome, such as increased subcutaneous fat, increased total and high-density lipoprotein (HDL) cholesterol, and increased adiponectin levels [25,26]. The main cause of these metabolic changes is an increased peripheral resistance to insulin, leading to type 2 diabetes [27]. These metabolic changes may be facilitated by reduced physical activity resulting from fatigue and depression.

## Impact of Metabolic Changes on Cardiovascular Events

In a observational study on 37,443 men, Keating et al. reported that ADT significantly increases the risk of diabetes (hazard ratio [HR] 1.28; 95 % CI 1.19–1.38), coronary heart disease (CHD) (HR 1.19; 95 % CI 1.10–1.28), myocardial infarction (MI) (HR 1.28; 95 % CI 1.08–1.52), sudden death (HR 1.35; 95 % CI 1.18–1.54), and stroke (HR 1.22; 95 % CI 1.10–1.36). Combined androgen blockade and orchiectomy further increased all risks; in contrast, pure oral antiandrogen monotherapy had no detectable impact [28]. Another study on 73,196 men from Surveillance, Epidemiology, and End Results (SEER) Medicare data ($n = 73,196$) has confirmed these data. GnRH agonists were associated with increased risk of diabetes (HR 1.44; $p < 0.001$), CHD (HR 1.16; $p < 0.001$), MI (HR 1.11; $p = 0.03$), and sudden cardiac death (HR 1.16; $p = 0.004$) [29]. Saigal et al. have examined the risk of cardiovascular morbidity in 22,816 men ≥65 years with newly diagnosed prostate cancer on ADT also using the SEER Medicare data. They found that men who received ADT had a 20 % higher risk of cardiovascular morbidity compared with similar men who did not receive ADT (HR 1.20; $p < 0.05$) [30].

## Does ADT Increase the Risk of Death from Cardiovascular Disease?

Three retrospective cohort studies have suggested a significant increase in the risk of cardiovascular-related mortality from ADT, with HR of respectively 1.16, 1.35, and 2.6 [28, 31, 32].

The study by Tsai et al. included 4,892 patients from the Cancer of the Prostatic Urologic Research Endeavor (CAPSURE) database and suggested that ADT increases cardiovascular mortality in the subset of men undergoing radical prostatectomy for localized prostate cancer (HR = 2.6; $p = 0.002$) but not in a subset of men treated with external beam radiation therapy (EBRT) [32].

Not all published studies, however, have reported a relationship between ADT and greater risk of cardiovascular death. Secondary analyses of four randomized controlled studies from the Radiation Therapy Oncology Group (RTOG) or European Organization for Research and Treatment of Cancer (EORTC) have found no association between neo-adjuvant or adjuvant ADT and cardiovascular-related mortality [33–36]. It has to be noted that these studies were not primarily designed to specifically assess cardiovascular mortality. A recent EORTC randomized study comparing EBRT plus 6 months or 3 years of ADT in patients with locally advanced prostate cancer showed no significant difference in the incidence of fatal cardiac events at 5-year follow-up in patients receiving ADT of longer duration (4.0 % vs. 3.0 %, respectively) [37].

Whether there is a causal relationship between ADT and cardiovascular morbidity and mortality remains controversial and continues to be studied. However, at this point in time, experts believe that it is reasonable to state that there may be an association between ADT and cardiovascular events and death because of the adverse effect of ADT on risk factors for cardiovascular disease [38]. On October 20, 2010, the US Food and Drug Administration (FDA) notified the manufacturers of the GnRH agonists of the need to add new safety information to the warnings and precautions section of the drug labels [39]. This new information warns about increased risk of diabetes and certain cardiovascular diseases (heart attack, sudden cardiac death, stroke) in men receiving these medications for the treatment of prostate cancer.

Risk Factors for Cardiovascular Events

The risk of cardiovascular disease is not correlated with the duration of hormone therapy. Previous longitudinal studies have shown that 6 months of ADT was enough to induce metabolic changes causing the increase in cardiovascular risk [25, 26]. In the study reported by Keating et al., the increased cardiovascular risk was observed within the initial 12 months of ADT [28]. Age seems to be an important predictive factor. In the epidemiological survey by Tsai et al., the impact of ADT on cardiovascular risk was much higher for men >65 years old than for younger men [32]. The 5-year cumulative incidence of cardiovascular mortality was 5.5 % for patients ≥65 years who received ADT and 2 % for non-ADT controls. For younger patients, the 5-year cumulative incidence of CV mortality was 3.6 % for those who received ADT and 2 % in those not treated with ADT.

In addition to age, preexisting comorbidities are very important. Nanda et al. reported the results of a retrospective study including 5,077 men with localized or locally advanced prostate cancer who were treated by EBRT with or without a median of 4 months of neo-adjuvant ADT [40]. They found that the use of neo-adjuvant ADT was associated with an increased risk of all-cause mortality among men with a history of coronary artery disease (CAD)-induced congestive heart failure (CHF) or myocardial infarction (MI) but not among men with no comorbidity or a single CAD risk factor. In the subgroup of patients with CAD-induced CHF or MI, 26.3 % deaths were reported in ADT-treated patients and 11.2 % deaths in non-ADT-treated controls (HR 1.96; 95 % CI 1.04–3.71; $p = 0.04$) [40]. D'Amico et al. have analyzed post-hoc pooled data on 1,372 patients from three randomized trials of EBRT with or without ADT for localized prostate cancer [41]. They found a shorter time to fatal MI in men aged ≥65 years who received 6 months of ADT compared with men in this age group with no ADT use $(p = 0.017)$. Additional evidence to support this result is needed.

## Monitoring and Prevention of Cardiovascular Events

Physicians should carefully monitor the metabolic and cardiovascular parameters of patients treated with ADT, including blood pressure, serum lipid level, and hemoglobin and fasting serum glucose levels [4–6, 42, 43]. Physicians should encourage patients to adopt a healthier lifestyle, including an appropriate low-fat diet and regular physical exercise. Nobes et al. have investigated the effects of metformin and lifestyle changes on the development of ADT-related metabolic changes [44]. In total, 40 men scheduled to receive 6 months ADT have been randomized between standard care and 6 months of metformin, a low glycemic index diet, and an exercise program. After 6 months, significant improvements in abdominal perimeter, weight, body mass index, and systolic blood pressure were seen in the intervention arm compared to controls.

Resistance training is a form of strength training in which each effort is performed against a specific opposing force generated by resistance. Resistance exercise is used to develop the strength and size of skeletal muscles. Properly performed, resistance training can provide significant functional benefits and improvement in overall health and well-being. A study conducted by Galvão et al. demonstrated that 20 weeks of progressive resistance exercise performed in a rehabilitation clinic increased muscle strength and endurance and preserved whole-body lean mass with no change in fat mass [45]. Segal et al. demonstrated that men assigned to resistance exercise had less interference from fatigue on activities of daily living and a better quality of life than untrained men [46]. The same group demonstrated that a combination of both resistance and aerobic exercise mitigates fatigue in patients treated by EBRT with or without ADT [47]. Resistance exercise generated longer-term improvements and additional benefits for quality of life, strength, triglyceride levels, and body fat. Baumann et al. have performed a meta-analysis of 25 randomized controlled trials regarding physical activities in prostate cancer patients, including 21 investigating exercise interventions during the phase of medical treatment and 4 during the aftercare [48]. This meta-analysis suggests that incontinence, fitness, fatigue, body constitution, and also quality of life can be improved by clinical exercise in patients during and after prostate cancer treatment. Only four studies, all conducted during medical treatment, reached the level "1b" and concluded that "supervised" exercise is more effective than "non-supervised" exercise.

TABLE 6.1 Prospective studies measuring bone loss associated with ADT

| Study | Treatment | BMD decrease at 12 months (%) |
|---|---|---|
| Eriksson et al. (1995) [49] | Orchiectomy | Hip: 9.6 |
| | | Radius: 4.5 |
| Maillefert et al. (1999) [53] | GnRH agonist | Hip: 3.9 |
| | | Lumbar spine: 4.6 |
| Daniell (1997) [54] | Orchiectomy | Hip: 2.4 |
| | GnRH agonist | |
| Daniell et al. (2000) [55] | GnRH agonist | Hip: 0.6 |
| | | Lumbar spine: 2.3 |
| Higano et al. (2004) [56] | LHRH agonist + antiandrogen | Hip: 2.7 |
| | | Lumbar spine: 4.7 |
| Mittan et al. (2002) [57] | GnRH agonist | Hip: 3.3 |
| | | Radius: 5.3 |

## Skeletal Complications of ADT

### Cancer Treatment–Induced Bone Loss (CTIBL) and ADT

The association between surgical castration and accelerated bone loss, and the fact that administration of estrogens does not prevent this, was first described more than 15 years ago [49]. Longitudinal studies suggest that bone loss accelerates after the age of 70 years in men, probably related to the decrease in testosterone and estradiol levels observed in aging males [50–52]. Prospective studies measuring bone loss associated with ADT have been performed for more than 10 years and have consistently observed a significant deterioration of bone mineral density (BMD) over time (Table 6.1). Substantial bone loss begins very early in the course of treatment with ADT. Mittan et al. reported that, in comparison to 15 age-matched untreated controls, the concentration of urinary N-telopeptide (uNtx, a biomarker for bone resorption) in patients receiving ADT was significantly higher after 6 months of treatment, indicative of early bone loss [57].

## ADT and Fragility Fractures

Several epidemiologic studies have confirmed that CTIBL increases the risk of fragility fractures (Table 6.2), which in turn may decrease survival. Several risk factors for fragility fractures have been identified, the most important being the duration of ADT. In a Cox proportional hazards analysis of Shahinian's epidemiologic survey, there was a statistically significant relation between the duration of ADT and the subsequent risk of fracture [58]. The relative risk of any fracture was 1.07 for patients receiving 1–4 doses of trimonthly GnRH agonists, 1.22 for 5–8 doses, 1.45 for ≥9 doses, and 1.54 for patients treated by orchiectomy. In addition to ADT duration, other risk factors for fracture include race and low body mass index ($<25$ kg/m$^2$) [61]. In Alibhai's survey, independent predictors of fragility and any fracture were increasing age, prior bone thinning medications, chronic kidney disease, prior dementia, prior fragility fracture, and prior osteoporosis diagnosis or treatment ($p < 0.05$) [60].

## Monitoring and Prevention of CTIBL in ADT-Treated Patients

Since bone loss occurs rapidly during ADT, physicians should inform patients and take all appropriate measures to monitor and minimize bone loss as early as possible during treatment. Early diagnosis of bone loss and treatment to improve bone health are important to protect patients from fractures, which are difficult to heal in mature adults.

Dual-energy x-ray absorptiometry (DXA) should be used to monitor spine, hip, or total body BMD. The spine is the preferred site of densitometry for serial measurement of bone mass to monitor changes in BMD [62]. When spine measurements are technically invalid, especially in the presence of bone metastases, total hip BMD should be assessed [62]. Status of bone health is typically based on the T-score measurement that compares a patient's BMD to that of a 30-year-old healthy person (baseline).

TABLE 6.2 Reported fracture risk in patients receiving hormone therapy[a]

| Study | Patients n. | ADT duration (years) | Fracture risk (%) | | | | | |
| | | | All sites | | Hip | | Hospitalization | |
| | | | ADT | No ADT | ADT | No ADT | ADT | No ADT |
| --- | --- | --- | --- | --- | --- | --- | --- | --- |
| Shahinian et al. (2005) [58] | 50,613 | 1–5 | 19.6 | 12.6 | 4.06 | 2.06 | 5.19 | 2.37 |
| Smith et al. (2005) [59] | 11,661 | >12 | 7.88* | 6.51* | 1.26* | 0.98* | | |
| Alibhai et al. (2010) [60] | 19,079 | 6.7 | 17.2 | 12.7 | 2.6 | 2 | 8 | 5.7 |

*Abbreviation: ADT* androgen-deprivation therapy

*p<0.05

[a]Rate (%) per person per year

TABLE 6.3 Risk ratio for hip fracture according to risk factors adjusted for age and bone mineral density in men and women

| Risk factor for hip fracture | Adjusted risk ratio (95 % CI) |
|---|---|
| *Low or high BMI* | |
| 20 vs. 25 | 1.42 (1.23–1.65) |
| 30 vs. 25 | 1.00 (0.82–1.21) |
| Prior fracture at >50 years of age | 1.62 (1.30–2.01) |
| Parental history of hip fracture | 2.28 (1.48–3.51) |
| Current smoking | 1.60 (1.27–2.02) |
| Use of systemic corticosteroids for >3 months | 2.25 (1.60–3.15) |
| Excessive alcohol use | 1.70 (1.20–2.42) |
| Rheumatoid arthritis | 1.73 (0.94–3.20) |
| *Low testosterone* | |
| Hip fracture | 1.88 (1.24–2.82) |
| Other non-vertebral fracture | 1.32 (1.03–1.68) |

Adapted from [63]

For every standard deviation below this baseline, the relative risk of fracture increases from 1.5- to 2.5-fold. A patient with a T-score above −1 is considered to have healthy bone, a score of −1 to −2.5 is osteopenic, below −2.5 is osteoporotic, and a score below −2.5 with any associated fracture is considered severely osteoporotic [63]. A patient with a T-score below −2.5 has approximately an 11-fold increase in the risk of developing a fracture than a patient with normal BMD [64]. There is no uniform recommendation about when to perform the first DXA scan in patients treated with ADT. The European Association of Urology (EAU) guidelines recommend performing the first DXA scan before long-term ADT is initiated, but there is no cut-off duration defining long-term ADT and no recommendation on scheduling of subsequent DXA scans [65]. Similarly, physicians should be attentive to the presence of additional risk factors, as highlighted by Ebeling (Table 6.3) [63].

In terms of prevention, patients should be encouraged to make specific lifestyle changes: cessation of smoking, moderate alcohol and caffeine consumption, and regular weight-bearing exercises [5]. Patients should also be encouraged to consume a healthy diet of foods and beverages containing calcium (dairy) and vitamin D (fatty fish). The recommended daily intake of calcium should be 1,200–1,500 mg, and serum levels of hydroxyvitamin D should be maintained at ≥30 ng/mL [63, 66]. If necessary, supplementation with cholecalciferol at doses of 800–2,000 IU/day should be given. A systematic review of around 64,000 men and women showed that a daily intake of calcium (≥1,200 mg) or calcium with vitamin D (≥800 IU daily) reduced the frequency of osteoporotic fractures by 12 % in men and women aged ≥50 years [67]. Physical exercise is also a very important part of preventing bone loss. Resistance exercise is particularly favorable for maintaining or improving bone mass and architecture while also being safe for older people [68].

### Pharmacologic Prevention and Treatment of CTIBL in ADT-Treated Patients

The EAU guidelines acknowledge that patients with osteoporosis or severe osteoporosis should be treated with a bisphosphonates even though these agents are not approved for this indication [65]. The last posted version of the National Comprehensive Cancer Network (NCCN) guidelines on prostate cancer advises pharmacologic treatment for men when the 10-year probability of hip fracture is ≥3 % or major osteoporosis-related fracture is ≥20 % [69]. The NCCN guidelines recommend assessing fracture risk using the FRAX algorithm (www.shef.ac.uk/FRAX/index.htm) by considering CTIBL as "secondary osteoporosis." The FRAX algorithm, however, has never been prospectively validated on a cohort of ADT-treated men.

## Bisphosphonates

Pamidronate (at a dose of 60 mg IV every 12 weeks) was the first bisphosphonate to be studied for the prevention of CTIBL in prostate cancer in a randomized controlled trial [70].

After 1 year, BMD decreased by 3.3 % at the lumbar spine ($p < 0.001$) and by 1.8 % at the hip ($p > 0.005$) in untreated patients. No change in BMD occurred in patients receiving pamidronate. Fracture rate was not reported.

Two double-blind, randomized, placebo-controlled clinical trials have evaluated the effect of zoledronic acid on BMD in ADT-treated patients with non-metastatic prostate cancer. In the first trial, patients received zoledronic acid, 4 mg, or placebo IV every 3 months for 1 year [71]. Mean lumbar spine BMD increased by 5.6 % in men receiving the bisphosphonate ($n = 42$) but decreased by 2.2 % in the placebo group ($n = 37$) ($p < 0.001$). The second trial evaluated the efficacy of a 4-mg annual zoledronic acid infusion [72]. Mean BMD of the lumbar spine increased by 4.0 % with the bisphosphonate and decreased by 3.1 % with the placebo ($p < 0.001$); the total hip BMD increased by 0.7 % with the bisphosphonate and decreased by 1.9 % with placebo and ($p = 0.004$). To date, none of the studies with zoledronic acid have demonstrated a benefit on fractures.

The oral bisphosphonate, alendronate, at the weekly dosage of 70 mg, has also been tested in 44 men, of whom 39 % had osteoporosis and 52 % had low BMD at baseline [73]. In men treated with alendronate, BMD increased over 1 year by 3.7 % ($p < 0.001$) at the spine and 1.6 % ($p = 0.008$) at the femoral neck. Among men in the placebo group, there were reductions in BMD of 1.4 % ($p = 0.045$) at the spine and 0.7 % ($p = 0.081$) at the femoral neck.

## Low-Dose Denosumab

Denosumab is a fully human monoclonal antibody that specifically inhibits RANKL, a critical mediator of osteoblast-to-osteoclast crosstalk. Injection of denosumab results in a prolonged inhibition of bone remodeling in postmenopausal women [74]. The prospective, randomized, placebo-controlled hormonal ablation therapy (HALT) study has investigated the benefit of denosumab in the prevention of CTIBL and fractures in 1,400 patients with non-metastatic prostate cancer receiving

ADT [75]. To be eligible for the study, patients had to be 70 years of age or older or alternatively had either a low BMD (T-score at the lumbar spine, total hip, or femoral neck of less than −1.0) at baseline or history of an osteoporotic fracture. Denosumab was administered every 6 months subcutaneously at a dose of 60 mg. After 24 months, BMD at the lumbar spine had increased by 5.6 % in the denosumab group as compared with a loss of 1.0 % in the placebo group ($p < 0.001$). Patients who received denosumab had a decreased incidence of new vertebral fractures at 36 months (1.5 % vs. 3.9 % with placebo) (relative risk: 0.38; 95 % CI 0.19–0.78; $p = 0.006$). The rates of adverse events were similar between the two groups. Recently, denosumab was approved for the management of bone loss associated with treatment of prostate cancer [76].

## Checklist for Monitoring Patients Receiving ADT

Before initiating treatment:

- Inform the patient about the occurrence of hot flushes and provide lifestyle recommendations to avoid excessive triggering.
- Inform the patient and his partner about libido, mood, and cognitive changes.
- Encourage maintaining and even increasing social activities and networking, possibly referring to patient support groups.
- Inform in due time the patient's general practitioner, cardiologist, and endocrinologist about initiation of ADT. Advise the patient to schedule a follow-up visit with these specialists within 6 months.
- Provide dietetic counseling and recommend resistance exercise. This will be done optimally by referring the patient to a dietician and physical therapist or by administrating a specifically designed coaching program.
- Search for risk factors of bone loss, and perform an immediate DXA scan, if they are present.

During treatment:

- In addition to PSA and testosterone measurements and imaging studies that are required for oncologic follow-up, it is recommended to measure weight and abdominal perimeter (or preferably body fatty tissue content by impedance technique), blood pressure, and dose hemoglobin, fasting cholesterol (total and HDL), triglyceride, and glucose levels. In case of abnormalities, refer the patient to a specialist.
- Advise a DXA scan after 1–2 years of ADT.

# Side Effects of Targeted Therapies for Renal Cell Carcinoma

The treatment of RCC has been revolutionized by the development in the early 2000s of six therapies targeting the VHL/HIF pathways. These belong to three different classes of drug: the tyrosine kinase inhibitors (TKIs), including sunitinib and pazopanib, and also the multikinase inhibitor sorafenib; the antivascular endothelial growth factor (VEGF) monoclonal antibody bevacizumab; and the mammalian target of rapamycin (mTOR) inhibitors temsirolimus and everolimus [77–87]. Although most of these drugs have individually demonstrated little benefit on overall survival, the prognosis for advanced RCC is shifting progressively toward that of a chronic treatable disease (Table 6.4). A result of this is that patients are nowadays treated for increasingly longer periods of time with these agents.

Because these drugs belong to new therapeutic classes, they cause class side effects that are new for physicians and have raised new challenges related to their management. Most of these side effects are not life-threatening but can severely hamper the quality of life of patients on the long run. Because it is very important to secure long-term compliance to oral drugs, it is critical that side effects are managed preemptively and that patients are correctly informed and educated

TABLE 6.4 Summary of benefit of new targeted agents used in RCC

| Agent | N | ORR (%) | Median PFS (months) | Median OS (months) |
|---|---|---|---|---|
| *First-line therapy* | | | | |
| Sunitinib vs. IFN-α [83, 84] | 750 | 47 vs. 12<br>p < 0.001 | 11.0 vs. 5<br>p < 0.001 | 26.4 vs. 21.8<br>p = 0.051 |
| Temsirolimus vs. IFN-α (alpha) [81] | 626 | 8.6 vs. 4.8<br>NS | 5.5 vs. 3.1<br>p < 0.0001 | 10.9 vs. 7.1<br>p = 0.008 |
| Bevacizumab + IFN-α(alpha) vs. IFN-α (alpha) [79] | 649 | 31 vs. 13<br>p = 0.0001 | 10.2 vs. 5.4<br>p = 0.0001 | IFN-α(alpha) 19.8<br>B/IFN-α (alpha) NR<br>p = 0.0267 |
| Bevacizumab + IFN-α (alpha) vs. IFN-α (alpha) [86] | 732 | 26 vs. 13<br>p < 0.0001 | 8.5 vs. 5.2<br>p < 0.0001 | NR |
| Sorafenib vs. IFN-α (alpha) [80] | 189 | 5 vs. 9 | 5.7 vs. 5.6<br>p = 0.504 | NR |

| | | | | | | |
| --- | --- | --- | --- | --- | --- | --- |
| Pazopanib vs. placebo [87] | 435 | 30 vs. 3 $p<0.001$ | | 9.2 vs. 4.2 $p<0.001$ | | 21.1 vs. 18.7 $p=0.02$ |
| *Second-line therapy* | | | | | | |
| Sorafenib vs. placebo [77] | 750 | 10 vs. 2 $p<0.001$ | | 5.5 vs. 2.8 $p<0.001$ | | 17.8 vs. 15.2 |
| Everolimus vs. placebo [82] | 410 | 5 vs. 0 NS | | 4.9 vs. 1.9 $p<0.0001$ | | 14.8 vs. 14.4 |
| Axitinib vs. sorafenib [85] | 723 | | | 6.7 vs. 4.7 $p<0.001$ | | |

about the preventive measures. There are many generic side effects associated with TKIs and mTOR inhibitors, including fatigue, hypertension, and diarrhea. In addition, there are several agent-specific side effects: proteinuria, with bevacizumab plus IFN; hypothyroidism, with sunitinib; hand-foot skin reaction (HFSR), most often seen with sorafenib; hepatotoxicity, most often seen with pazopanib; and hyperlipidemia, most often seen with the mTOR inhibitors [77–79, 87–93]. These side effects and their respective frequencies are summarized in Table 6.5.

The impact of side effects can be greatly limited if the patient is well informed and one encourages activating preventive measures. Even mild side effects may have a great impact on a patient's quality of life and require temporary dose reduction or treatment discontinuation. Physicians should be aware of comorbidities such as diabetes and hypertension that may also increase the risk of certain side effects. To ensure early detection and optimal management of side effects and to maximize patient benefits and compliance, it is important that the physician be aware of the range of manageable side effects associated with each agent and that this information is effectively communicated to the patients.

## Life-Threatening Side Effects

In addition to these frequent side effects, potentially life-threatening or lethal adverse events have been reported in the Summary of Product Characteristics of the European Medicines Agency.

*Sorafenib* has been reported to cause reversible posterior leukoencephalopathy, hypertensive crisis, cardiac ischemia and myocardial infarction, gastrointestinal perforation, and hemorrhage [88]. Pre-neoplasic skin lesions such as actinic keratosis and keratoacanthomas, but also squamous cell carcinoma, have been reported.

*Sunitinib* has been reported to cause life-threatening hematologic, cardiovascular, and venous thromboembolic events, pancreatic and hepatobiliary complications, gastrointestinal perforation, and hemorrhage [89].

TABLE 6.5  Most commonly reported side effects in Summary of Product Characteristics European Medicines Agency for sorafenib [88], sunitinib [89], pazopanib [93], bevacizumab [91], temsirolimus [90], and everolimus [92]

| Side effect | TKIs | | Anti-VEGF | | mTOR inhibitor | |
|---|---|---|---|---|---|---|
| | Sorafenib | Sunitinib | Pazopanib | Bevacizumab | Temsirolimus | Everolimus |
| *Gastrointestinal disorders* | | | | | | |
| Constipation | C | VC | | VC | | |
| Diarrhea | VC | VC | VC | VC | VC | VC |
| Dyspepsia | C | VC | | | | |
| Dry mouth | C | VC | | | | C |
| Flatulence | | C | C | | C | |
| Glossodynia | | VC | | | | C |
| Nausea | | VC | VC | VC | VC | VC |
| Oral pain | | C | | | VC | C |
| Stomatitis | C | VC | C | VC | VC | VC |
| Vomiting | VC | VC | VC | VC | VC | VC |
| Abdominal pain | | | VC | C | C | |

B.F. Tombal

TABLE 6.5 (continued)

| Side effect | TKIs | | Anti-VEGF | | mTOR inhibitor | |
| --- | --- | --- | --- | --- | --- | --- |
| | Sorafenib | Sunitinib | Pazopanib | Bevacizumab | Temsirolimus | Everolimus |
| Gastrointestinal perforation | UC | | | C | UC | |
| *Dermatologic side effects* | | | | | | |
| Acne | C | C | | | VC | C |
| Alopecia | VC | C | C | | | C |
| Dry skin | C | VC | | VC | | VC |
| Erythema | VC | C | C | | | C |
| Hair color changes | | VC | VC | | | |
| HFSR | VC | VC | | C | | C |
| Nail disorder | C | C | | | VC | VC |
| Pruritus | VC | C | C | | VC | |
| Rash | VC | VC | C | | VC | VC |
| Skin discoloration | | VC | | VC | | |
| Bacterial and viral infections | UC | | UC | C | VC | VC |

*Respiratory disorders*

| | | | | | | |
|---|---|---|---|---|---|---|
| Cough | C | C | C | | VC | VC |
| Dyspnea | | C | | C | VC | VC |
| Epistaxis | | VC | C | C | VC | VC |
| Pneumonitis | UC | C | | | C | VC |
| Pleural effusion | | | | | C | |
| *Cardiovascular disorders* | | | | | | |
| Ejection fraction decreased | C | C | UC | | | |
| Hemorrhage | VC | | | | VC | VC |
| Hypertension | C | VC | UC | VC | C | VC |
| Deep vein thrombosis | | | | C | | |
| Thromboembolism | | | | C | C | C |
| Supraventricular tachycardia | | | | C | | |
| Pulmonary embolism | | | UC | C | C | |

(continued)

TABLE 6.5 (continued)

| Side effect | TKIs | Anti-VEGF | | | mTOR inhibitor | |
| --- | --- | --- | --- | --- | --- | --- |
| | Sorafenib | Sunitinib | Pazopanib | Bevacizumab | Temsirolimus | Everolimus |
| *Metabolic disorders* | | | | | | |
| Anorexia | C | VC | C | VC | VC | VC |
| Hypokalemia | | | | | VC | C |
| Hyperglycemia | | | | | VC | VC |
| Hypercholesterolemia | | | | | VC | VC |
| Hyperlipidemia | | | | | VC | VC |
| Hypophosphatemia | VC | | C | | VC | C |
| *Hematologic disorders* | | | | | | |
| Neutropenia | C | VC | C | VC | C | C |
| Thrombocytopenia | C | VC | C | VC | VC | VC |
| Anemia | C | VC | | C | VC | VC |
| Leucopenia | C | C | C | VC | C | C |
| Lymphopenia | VC | C | | | C | C |
| *Laboratory abnormalities* | | | | | | |
| Creatinine increase | C | C | | | VC | C |

| | | | | | | |
|---|---|---|---|---|---|---|
| Increase liver enzyme | UC | UC | VC | | C | C |
| Proteinuria | | UC | C | VC | C | C |
| *Central nervous system disorders* | | | | | | |
| Headache | VC | VC | C | C | VC | |
| Peripheral sensory neuropathy | C | C | UC | VC | | |
| Depression | C | C | | C | C | |
| Intracerebral bleeding | | | | | C | |
| Taste disturbance | | VC | VC | VC | VC | |
| *Musculoskeletal disorders* | | | | | | |
| Arthralgia–myalgia | C | VC | C | VC | VC | C |
| *Ophthalmologic side effects* | | | | | | |
| Lacrimation increased | | C | | VC | | |
| Eyelid edema | | C | | VC | | VC |
| Conjunctivitis | | | | C | | VC |
| Eyelash decoloration | | | UC | | | |

(continued)

TABLE 6.5 (continued)

| Side effect | TKIs | | Anti-VEGF | | mTOR inhibitor | |
| --- | --- | --- | --- | --- | --- | --- |
| | Sorafenib | Sunitinib | Pazopanib | Bevacizumab | Temsirolimus | Everolimus |
| *Others* | | | | | | |
| Allergic reactions | UC | UC | | C | | |
| Fatigue | VC | VC | VC | VC | VC | VC |
| Hypothyroidism | UC | C | C | | | |
| Hyperthyroidism | UC | UC | | VC | | |
| Insomnia | | C | | VC | VC | VC |
| Mucosal inflammation | VC | VC | C | C | | |
| Edema | | VC | C | | VC | VC |
| Pyrexia | | | | | VC | VC |

Adapted from [94]

Frequencies are reported as very common (VC; ≥1/10 patients), common (C; ≥1/100 to <1/10 patients), or uncommon (UC; ≥1/1,000 to <1/100 patients). Cases are empty if the incidence of the side effect is not reported in Eu SmPC or cannot be estimated from the data available

The association of *bevacizumab + IFN-α* has been reported to cause hypertensive encephalopathy, cardiac failure, thromboembolic events, gastrointestinal perforation, and hemorrhage [91].

*Pazopanib* has been reported to cause gastrointestinal perforation and gastrointestinal fistula, arterial thrombotic events, hemorrhage, and severe hepatotoxicity [93].

*Temsirolimus* has been reported to cause hypersensitivity/infusion reactions, intracerebral bleeding, bowel perforation, pericardial effusion, pneumonitis, renal failure, and delay wound healing [90].

*Everolimus* has been reported to cause noninfectious pneumonitis and infections [92].

## Prevention and Management of Most Common Side Effects

### Dermatologic Side Effects

Early recognition of dermatologic complications is critical, and patients should be taught to report the development of any new skin lesions.

*Rash* and *hand-foot skin reaction* (*HFSR*) are among the most troubling and common side effect of TKIs. Hand-foot skin reaction occurs in 30–60 % of patients receiving sorafenib and 15–20 % of patients treated with sunitinib. Hand-foot skin reaction appears usually after 2–4 weeks of treatment. The onset and severity of HFSR appear to be dose-dependent and often disappear rapidly upon treatment discontinuation. The physiopathology of HFSR is unclear, although it is relatively infrequent with pazopanib. The severity of HFSR can range from minimal skin changes (grade 1) to painful ulcerative dermatitis (grade 3) and often results in dose reduction.

There are no dedicated studies defining the degree of benefit of commonly reported measures for the management of HFSR. Preventive measures for HFSR include removal of any existing hyperkeratosic areas and calluses beforehand [95]. It is important that pressure areas are protected and treated with moisturizing creams or ointments. During treatment, care should be taken to reduce exposure of the hands and feet to hot water and to avoid constrictive footwear, friction, and trauma arising from exercise. Shoes with padded insoles (and possibly also gloves) can be worn. There may be benefit in sparingly applying moisturizing cream to the hands and feet and educating patients on the first signs of HFSR [96]. Wearing soft and not constrictive shoes and even gloves is recommended. Once it is present, HSFR should be managed with topical application of corticoids-containing cream. Dose reduction, interruption, and event discontinuation may be required for grade 2/3 toxicities.

Management strategies for rash require first differentiating nonserious rash, which is usually moderate and not associated with systemic symptoms, from more severe hypersensitivity reactions such as drug reaction with eosinophilia and systemic symptoms (DRESS) syndrome or Stevens–Johnson syndrome. These are usually associated with mucosal involvement, bullous lesions, and systemic and biological signs. Meticulous skin care, moisturizing cream, and urea-containing lotion are key preventive and therapeutic measures. They require immediate drug discontinuation and specialized dermatologic support.

## Infections

Everolimus and temsirolimus have dose-dependent immunosuppressive properties and can therefore predispose patients to infections. In the temsirolimus phase III study, infections were reported in 27 % of patients (grade 3/4 in 5 %) receiving temsirolimus versus 14 % in the control arm [81]. In the everolimus phase III study, infections were reported in 13 % of patients (grade 3/4 in 4 %) versus 2 % (grade 3/4 in 0 %) in the control arm [82]. Physicians should be aware of this increased risk and should ensure that any preexisting infections are adequately treated before initiation of mTOR inhibitors. It is particularly important that patients with pulmonary infiltrates or pulmonary symptoms, which are also frequent with mTOR inhibitors, are rigorously assessed for signs of infection, owing to the potential overlap between pulmonary infections and noninfectious pneumonitis.

## Gastrointestinal Side Effects

### Diarrhea

Diarrhea is one of the most common side effects of anticancer therapy. It is not only inconvenient but also potentially life-threatening if not sufficiently managed. There are a number of published clinical guidelines for the management of diarrhea in cancer patients that apply also to targeted therapies in RCC [97]. Patients must be advised to avoid foods that may aggravate diarrhea and favor foods that increase the consistency of stools. In case of persistent diarrhea, it is important to maintain abundant liquid and salt intake by using, for example, a WHO solution containing 30 mL (6 level teaspoon) of sugar and 2.5 mL (1/2 level teaspoon) of salt, dissolved into 1 L of water. Loperamide is widely prescribed for anticancer therapy-related diarrhea. For grade 3 or 4 diarrhea, dose adjustments or even discontinuation may be required.

### Oral or Upper Gastrointestinal Complications

Oral and upper tract gastrointestinal complications of targeted therapies are very common and include mucositis, stomatitis, dry mouth, and taste loss or disturbance [88–93]. Mucositis is characterized by painful inflammation and ulceration of the mucous membranes lining the digestive tract, whereas stomatitis more specifically refers to painful inflammation of the mucous lining of the mouth. A meta-analysis by Worthington et al. has evaluated the effectiveness of prophylactic agents for preventing stomatitis in patients receiving chemotherapy [98]. Results from their analysis suggest that amifostine, a Chinese medicine (that involved mixtures of 5 or 11 herbs, including honeysuckle flower, licorice root, and magnolia bark), hydrolytic enzymes (pepsin, trypsin, and chymotrypsin, or Wobe-Mugos preparation of enzymes), and ice chips may be beneficial in preventing or reducing the severity of stomatitis. There is consistent evidence from small high-quality studies that red and infrared low-level laser therapy (LLLT) can partly prevent development of cancer therapy-induced oral mucositis. LLLT also significantly reduced pain, severity, and duration of symptoms in patients with cancer therapy-induced oral mucositis [99].

## Anorexia and Weight Loss

Anorexia may result as much from a loss of appetite caused by cancer as from treatment-related nausea, vomiting, oral pain, diarrhea, and loss or disturbance of taste. Anorexia-related symptoms, which include weakness, fatigue, depression, tooth loss, and organ damage, can have a negative impact on health-related quality of life, can affect a patient's ability to perform daily tasks, and can result in death in severe cases. Pharmacologic intervention may be required in case of severe cachexia; these include megestrol acetate [100], eicosapentaenoic acid diester [101], medroxyprogesterone acetate [102], and mixtures of beta-hydroxyl beta-methyl butyrate, glutamine, and arginine [103].

## Gastrointestinal Perforation

Gastrointestinal perforation is a rare but potentially fatal complication that has been reported in association with all the targeted agents except (to date) everolimus [88–91, 93]. The highest rate is seen with bevacizumab as demonstrated in a meta-analysis of 17 randomized studies, including more than 12,000 patients with various cancers, that reported an overall incidence of gastrointestinal perforation of 0.9 % [104]. Risk factors for gastrointestinal perforation include history of past diverticulitis or ulcers, radiation exposure, recent sigmoidoscopy or colonoscopy, gastrointestinal obstruction, and multiple previous surgeries. Gastrointestinal perforation is an indication for immediate discontinuation of anticancer therapy and appropriate treatment of the perforation.

# Metabolic Toxicities

## Fatigue

Fatigue is a persistent, subjective sense of emotional, physical, and/or cognitive tiredness or exhaustion. Fatigue often results from multiple causes. It can be a cancer-related side effect, an adverse event of the treatment, as well as the symptom of other conditions, including hypothyroidism, anemia, depression, sleep disturbances, or pain, that are often seen with targeted therapies [105]. Therefore, any underlying cause of fatigue should first be ruled out before making specific recommendation to the patient. Patients should be encouraged to conserve energy, to reschedule activities to periods of peak energy, and to stay active in order to promote sleep. Alternative approaches such as stress management, relaxation techniques, and nutritional support may be useful [106].

## Hypothyroidism

Hypothyroidism is a very common side effect of sunitinib [89]. Preexisting hypothyroidism should be detected and treated before starting sunitinib treatment, as recommended in the EU SmPC [89]. There is no consensus on the frequency of thyroid function monitoring under treatment, although initially monthly TSH dosage are advisable [107]. There is no clear recommendation whether these recommendations for thyroid function monitoring should be extended to all patients treated with TKIs.

## Hyperglycemia

Hyperglycemia is a very common side effect of the mTOR inhibitors temsirolimus and everolimus [92, 93]. It is recommended to monitor fasting serum glucose before initiating treatment with everolimus or temsirolimus and periodically thereafter. Hyperglycemia should be treated with dietary modifications and an increase in the dose or initiation of insulin and/or hypoglycemic agent therapy.

## Cardiovascular Side Effects

### Hypertension

Arterial hypertension is a common side effect of inhibitors of the VEGF pathway, reported at a frequency of between 12 and 41 % in patients treated with sorafenib, sunitinib, bevacizumab + IFN-α (alpha), or pazopanib [88–91]. Management of angiogenesis inhibitor-related hypertension should follow the recommendations of the European Society of Hypertension.

Blood pressure (BP) monitoring is mandatory before and during therapy; however, there is general disagreement about when and how BP should be measured [94, 108, 109]. The routine use of home BP monitoring may be valuable in standard care for early detection and accurate assessment of BP changes [108, 109]. Home monitoring can be recommended, but then patients need to be provided with individualized thresholds for contacting their physician. When diagnosed, hypertension should be treated with standard antihypertensive therapy with a preference for angiotensin-converting enzyme (ACE) and inhibitors and angiotensin II receptor blockers (ARBs).

## Cardiovascular Events

Initiation of TKIs and inhibitor of the VEGF pathway requires careful monitoring of cardiac effects. Generally, VEGF-targeted agents should be used with caution in any patients with clinically significant cardiovascular disease or preexisting congestive heart failure, and these patients should be closely monitored for clinical signs of heart failure. Periodic measurements of LVEF using echocardiography or magnetic resonance imaging are the recommended methods for monitoring cardiac function during cancer treatment [110–112]. Since cardiac dysfunction can be hampered by other side effects such as hypothyroidism or hypertension, these conditions should be carefully monitored and managed. Except for few anecdotal cases, if is not known whether left ventricular dysfunction is reversible upon treatment cessation.

## Venous and Arterial Thromboembolism

Venous thromboembolism (VTE) is a common complication in cancer patients [113, 114]. Risk factors include age older than 65 years, previous VTE events, and surgery. It is not clear whether targeted agents increased the risk of VTE. Although the EU

SmPC for bevacizumab does not mention VTE as a side effect, a meta-analysis of 15 studies investigating the treatment of various solid tumors with bevacizumab suggested an increased incidence of VTE, 12 % for all grades and 6 % for high grade [115]. General recommendations on the prophylaxis and treatment of thrombosis in cancer patients have been produced by ASCO and the American College of Chest Physician [116]. Anticoagulation prophylaxis is not recommended for ambulatory patients with cancer receiving systemic treatment, whether the increased risk of thrombotic events with some targeted agents warrants prophylaxis in ambulatory patients remains unclear. Especially, acetylsalicylic acid or other antiplatelet drugs should be used with caution in association with anti-VEGF agents because of the increased risk of bleeding.

## Wound Healing and Hemorrhage

Wound healing is one the most important challenge that surgeons face when confronted with RCC patients treated with targeted therapies. This has been well documented with bevacizumab so that the EU SmPC includes a black box warning recommending treatment discontinuation for at least 28 days in case of surgery. In case of elective surgery, treatment should be discontinued at least 3 weeks before [91]. Signs of wound dehiscence or infection should be regularly monitored. TKIs and mTOR inhibitors may also impair wound healing, although clear data and recommendations on the minimal duration of treatment interruption before or after surgery are still lacking, with suggestions ranging from 7 to 14 days. Of note, one study with TKIs found that in RCC patients undergoing cytoreductive nephrectomy or resection of retroperitoneal recurrence, rates of incision-related complications were similar between patients treated with preoperative sorafenib, sunitinib, or bevacizumab and those who underwent up-front surgery [117].

Minor hemorrhagic events such as epistaxis are common in patients treated with bevacizumab, sunitinib, temsirolimus, and everolimus [89–92]. The impact of minor bleeding events can be limited by good patient education. In contrast, severe life-threatening events are more exceptional, mostly occurring with bevacizumab. However, it has raised the concern of treating patients' metastases of the central nervous system (CNS) with bevacizumab + IFN-α (alpha). These patients were excluded from the registration trial. TKIs sorafenib and sunitinib can be safely administered to patients with CNS metastases that have been irradiated. One of the primary measures against bleeding is an optimal control of blood pressure to avoid hypertension.

## Summary

The unique sensitivity of prostate cancer to hormone therapy and of kidney cancer to therapies targeting the VHL/HIF pathways is creating a unique therapeutic portfolio, which does not include chemotherapy. These classes of drugs share the particularities of having to be prescribed for extended periods of time because they do not eradicate the disease but rather switch it to a more chronic state. Emerging therapies generate the hope of multiple sequential treatments that will effectively prolong the duration of life. Most of their side effects are more bothersome than really morbid, but because these drugs are administered chronically, it may result in profound alteration of the patients' quality of life. Ultimately, this is a threat to compliance and a danger hampering the chronic efficacy of these treatments. In addition, the side effects of many of these drugs often overlap with common, widespread chronic illnesses such as diabetes, hypertension, hypercholesterolemia, and heart failure. Therefore, the management of these side effects is of utmost complexity so that only a multidisciplinary preventive approach involving physicians, nurses, and properly educated patients will guarantee an optimal efficacy.

## References

1. Sternberg CN. Novel treatments for castration-resistant prostate cancer. Eur J Cancer. 2011;47 Suppl 3:S195–9. doi:10.1016/S0959-8049(11)70165-4.
2. Huggins C, Hodges CV. The effect of estrogens and androgen injection on serum phosphatases in metastatic carcinoma of the prostate. Cancer Res. 1941;1:1941.

3. Shahinian VB, Kuo YF, Freeman JL, Orihuela E, Goodwin JS. Increasing use of gonadotropin-releasing hormone agonists for the treatment of localized prostate carcinoma. Cancer. 2005;103(8):1615–24. doi:10.1002/cncr.20955.

4. Gomella LG. Contemporary use of hormonal therapy in prostate cancer: managing complications and addressing quality-of-life issues. BJU Int. 2007;99 Suppl 1:25–9; discussion 30.

5. Holzbeierlein JM. Managing complications of androgen deprivation therapy for prostate cancer. Urol Clin North Am. 2006;33(2):181–90, vi.

6. Mottet N, Prayer-Galetti T, Hammerer P, Kattan MW, Tunn U. Optimizing outcomes and quality of life in the hormonal treatment of prostate cancer. BJU Int. 2006;98(1):20–7.

7. Van Poppel H, Tombal B. Cardiovascular risk during hormonal treatment in patients with prostate cancer. Cancer Manag Res. 2011;3:49–55. doi:10.2147/CMR.S16893.

8. Moyad MA, Merrick GS. Statins and cholesterol lowering after a cancer diagnosis: why not? Urol Oncol. 2005;23(1):49–55.

9. Barton D, LaVasseur B, Sloan JA, Stella PJ, Flynn K, Dyar M, et al. A phase III trial evaluating three doses of citalopram for hot flashes: NCCTG trial N05C9. J Clin Oncol. 2008;26:A9538.

10. Loprinzi CL, Goldberg RM, O'Fallon JR, Quella SK, Miser AW, Mynderse LA, et al. Transdermal clonidine for ameliorating post-orchiectomy hot flashes. J Urol. 1994;151(3):634–6.

11. Loprinzi CL, Khoyratty BS, Dueck A, Barton DL, Jafar S, Rowland KM, et al. Gabapentin for hot flashes in men: NCCTG trial N00CB. J Clin Oncol. 2007;25(18S):A9005.

12. Spetz Holm AC, Frisk J, Hammar ML. Acupuncture as treatment of hot flashes and the possible role of calcitonin gene-related peptide. Evid Based Complement Alternat Med. 2012;579321. doi:10.1155/2012/579321.

13. Vandecasteele K, Ost P, Oosterlinck W, Fonteyne V, Neve WD, Meerleer GD. Evaluation of the efficacy and safety of Salvia officinalis in controlling hot flashes in prostate cancer patients treated with androgen deprivation. Phytother Res. 2012;26(2):208–13. doi:10.1002/ptr.3528.

14. Potosky AL, Reeve BB, Clegg LX, Hoffman RM, Stephenson RA, Albertsen PC, et al. Quality of life following localized prostate cancer treated initially with androgen deprivation therapy or no therapy. J Natl Cancer Inst. 2002;94(6):430–7.

15. Aucoin MW, Wassersug RJ. The sexuality and social performance of androgen-deprived (castrated) men throughout history: implications for modern day cancer patients. Soc Sci Med. 2006;63(12):3162–73.

16. Knols R, Aaronson NK, Uebelhart D, Fransen J, Aufdemkampe G. Physical exercise in cancer patients during and after medical treatment: a systematic review of randomized and controlled clinical trials. J Clin Oncol. 2005;23(16):3830–42.

17. Demark-Wahnefried W, Clipp EC, Lipkus IM, Lobach D, Snyder DC, Sloane R, et al. Main outcomes of the FRESH START trial:

a sequentially tailored, diet and exercise mailed print intervention among breast and prostate cancer survivors. J Clin Oncol. 2007;25(19):2709–18.

18. Higano CS. Side effects of androgen deprivation therapy: monitoring and minimizing toxicity. Urology. 2003;61(2 Suppl 1):32–8.

19. Fang F, Keating NL, Mucci LA, Adami HO, Stampfer MJ, Valdimarsdottir U, et al. Immediate risk of suicide and cardiovascular death after a prostate cancer diagnosis: cohort study in the United States. J Natl Cancer Inst. 2010;102(5):307–14. doi:10.1093/jnci/djp537.

20. de Bono JS, Logothetis CJ, Molina A, Fizazi K, North S, Chu L, et al. Abiraterone and increased survival in metastatic prostate cancer. N Engl J Med. 2011;364(21):1995–2005. doi:10.1056/NEJMoa1014618.

21. Attard G, Reid AH, Auchus RJ, Hughes BA, Cassidy AM, Thompson E, et al. Clinical and biochemical consequences of CYP17A1 inhibition with abiraterone given with and without exogenous glucocorticoids in castrate men with advanced prostate cancer. J Clin Endocrinol Metab. 2012;97(2):507–16. doi:10.1210/jc.2011-2189.

22. Strum SB, McDermed JE, Scholz MC, Johnson H, Tisman G. Anaemia associated with androgen deprivation in patients with prostate cancer receiving combined hormone blockade. Br J Urol. 1997;79(6): 933–41.

23. Galvao DA, Spry NA, Taaffe DR, Newton RU, Stanley J, Shannon T, et al. Changes in muscle, fat and bone mass after 36 weeks of maximal androgen blockade for prostate cancer. BJU Int. 2008; 102(1):44–7.

24. Galvao DA, Taaffe DR, Spry N, Joseph D, Turner D, Newton RU. Reduced muscle strength and functional performance in men with prostate cancer undergoing androgen suppression: a comprehensive cross-sectional investigation. Prostate Cancer Prostatic Dis. 2008;12(2):198–203.

25. Braga-Basaria M, Dobs AS, Muller DC, Carducci MA, John M, Egan J, et al. Metabolic syndrome in men with prostate cancer undergoing long-term androgen-deprivation therapy. J Clin Oncol. 2006;24(24): 3979–83.

26. Smith MR, Lee H, McGovern F, Fallon MA, Goode M, Zietman AL, et al. Metabolic changes during gonadotropin-releasing hormone agonist therapy for prostate cancer: differences from the classic metabolic syndrome. Cancer. 2008;112(10):2188–94.

27. Smith MR, Lee H, Nathan DM. Insulin sensitivity during combined androgen blockade for prostate cancer. J Clin Endocrinol Metab. 2006;91(4):1305–8.

28. Keating NL, O'Malley AJ, Freedland SJ, Smith MR. Diabetes and cardiovascular disease during androgen deprivation therapy: observational study of veterans with prostate cancer. J Natl Cancer Inst. 2010;102(1):39–46.

29. Keating NL, O'Malley AJ, Smith MR. Diabetes and cardiovascular disease during androgen deprivation therapy for prostate cancer. J Clin Oncol. 2006;24(27):4448–56.
30. Saigal CS, Gore JL, Krupski TL, Hanley J, Schonlau M, Litwin MS. Androgen deprivation therapy increases cardiovascular morbidity in men with prostate cancer. Cancer. 2007;110(7):1493–500.
31. Keating GM. Triptorelin embonate (6-month formulation). Drugs. 2010;70(3):347–53.
32. Tsai HK, D'Amico AV, Sadetsky N, Chen MH, Carroll PR. Androgen deprivation therapy for localized prostate cancer and the risk of cardiovascular mortality. J Natl Cancer Inst. 2007;99(20):1516–24.
33. Efstathiou JA, Bae K, Shipley WU, Hanks GE, Pilepich MV, Sandler HM, et al. Cardiovascular mortality and duration of androgen deprivation for locally advanced prostate cancer: analysis of RTOG 92–02. Eur Urol. 2008;54(4):816–24.
34. Efstathiou JA, Bae K, Shipley WU, Hanks GE, Pilepich MV, Sandler HM, et al. Cardiovascular mortality after androgen deprivation therapy for locally advanced prostate cancer: RTOG 85–31. J Clin Oncol. 2009;27(1):92–9.
35. Roach 3rd M, Bae K, Speight J, Wolkov HB, Rubin P, Lee RJ, et al. Short-term neoadjuvant androgen deprivation therapy and external-beam radiotherapy for locally advanced prostate cancer: long-term results of RTOG 8610. J Clin Oncol. 2008;26(4):585–91.
36. Studer UE, Whelan P, Albrecht W, Casselman J, de Reijke T, Hauri D, et al. Immediate or deferred androgen deprivation for patients with prostate cancer not suitable for local treatment with curative intent: European Organisation for Research and Treatment of Cancer (EORTC) Trial 30891. J Clin Oncol. 2006;24(12):1868–76.
37. Bolla M, de Reijke TM, Van Tienhoven G, Van den Bergh AC, Oddens J, Poortmans PM, et al. Duration of androgen suppression in the treatment of prostate cancer. N Engl J Med. 2009;360(24):2516–27. doi:10.1056/NEJMoa0810095.
38. Levine GN, D'Amico AV, Berger P, Clark PE, Eckel RH, Keating NL, et al. Androgen-deprivation therapy in prostate cancer and cardiovascular risk: a science advisory from the American Heart Association, American Cancer Society, and American Urological Association: endorsed by the American Society for Radiation Oncology. Circulation. 2010;121(6):833–40. doi:10.1161/CIRCULATIONAHA.109.192695.
39. Food and Drug Administration. 2010. FDA Drug Safety Communication: Update to ongoing safety review of GnRH agonists and notification to manufacturers of GnRH agonists to add new safety information to labeling regarding increased risk of diabetes and certain cardiovascular diseases. http://www.fda.gov/Drugs/DrugSafety/ucm229986.htm.
40. Nanda A, Chen MH, Braccioforte MH, Moran BJ, D'Amico AV. Hormonal therapy use for prostate cancer and mortality in men with

coronary artery disease-induced congestive heart failure or myocardial infarction. JAMA. 2009;302(8):866–73. doi:10.1001/jama.2009.1137.

41. D'Amico AV, Denham JW, Crook J, Chen MH, Goldhaber SZ, Lamb DS, et al. Influence of androgen suppression therapy for prostate cancer on the frequency and timing of fatal myocardial infarctions. J Clin Oncol. 2007;25(17):2420–5.

42. Moyad MA. Promoting general health during androgen deprivation therapy (ADT): a rapid 10-step review for your patients. Urol Oncol. 2005;23(1):56–64.

43. Schow DA, Renfer LG, Rozanski TA, Thompson IM. Prevalence of hot flushes during and after neoadjuvant hormonal therapy for localized prostate cancer. South Med J. 1998;91(9):855–7.

44. Nobes JP, Langley SE, Klopper T, Russell-Jones D, Laing RW. A prospective, randomized pilot study evaluating the effects of metformin and lifestyle intervention on patients with prostate cancer receiving androgen deprivation therapy. BJU Int. 2012;109(10):1495–502. doi:10.1111/j.1464-410X.2011.10555.x. Epub 2011 Sep 20.

45. Galvao DA, Nosaka K, Taaffe DR, Spry N, Kristjanson LJ, McGuigan MR, et al. Resistance training and reduction of treatment side effects in prostate cancer patients. Med Sci Sports Exerc. 2006;38(12):2045–52.

46. Segal RJ, Reid RD, Courneya KS, Malone SC, Parliament MB, Scott CG, et al. Resistance exercise in men receiving androgen deprivation therapy for prostate cancer. J Clin Oncol. 2003;21(9):1653–9.

47. Segal RJ, Reid RD, Courneya KS, Sigal RJ, Kenny GP, Prud'Homme DG, et al. Randomized controlled trial of resistance or aerobic exercise in men receiving radiation therapy for prostate cancer. J Clin Oncol. 2009;27(3):344–51.

48. Baumann FT, Zopf EM, Bloch W. Clinical exercise interventions in prostate cancer patients – a systematic review of randomized controlled trials. Support Care Cancer. 2012;20(2):221–33. doi:10.1007/s00520-011-1271-0.

49. Eriksson S, Eriksson A, Stege R, Carlstrom K. Bone mineral density in patients with prostatic cancer treated with orchidectomy and with estrogens. Calcif Tissue Int. 1995;57(2):97–9.

50. Szulc P, Delmas PD. Biochemical markers of bone turnover in men. Calcif Tissue Int. 2001;69(4):229–34.

51. Fink HA, Ewing SK, Ensrud KE, Barrett-Connor E, Taylor BC, Cauley JA, et al. Association of testosterone and estradiol deficiency with osteoporosis and rapid bone loss in older men. J Clin Endocrinol Metab. 2006;91(10):3908–15. doi:10.1210/jc.2006-0173.

52. Murphy S, Khaw KT, Cassidy A, Compston JE. Sex hormones and bone mineral density in elderly men. Bone Miner. 1993;20(2):133–40.

53. Maillefert JF, Sibilia J, Michel F, Saussine C, Javier RM, Tavernier C. Bone mineral density in men treated with synthetic gonadotropin-releasing hormone agonists for prostatic carcinoma. J Urol. 1999;161(4): 1219–22.

54. Daniell HW. Osteoporosis after orchiectomy for prostate cancer [see comments]. J Urol. 1997;157(2):439–44.
55. Daniell HW, Dunn SR, Ferguson DW, Lomas G, Niazi Z, Stratte PT. Progressive osteoporosis during androgen deprivation therapy for prostate cancer. J Urol. 2000;163(1):181–6.
56. Higano C, Shields A, Wood N, Brown J, Tangen C. Bone mineral density in patients with prostate cancer without bone metastases treated with intermittent androgen suppression. Urology. 2004;64(6): 1182–6.
57. Mittan D, Lee S, Miller E, Perez RC, Basler JW, Bruder JM. Bone loss following hypogonadism in men with prostate cancer treated with GnRH analogs. J Clin Endocrinol Metab. 2002;87(8):3656–61.
58. Shahinian VB, Kuo YF, Freeman JL, Goodwin JS. Risk of fracture after androgen deprivation for prostate cancer. N Engl J Med. 2005;352(2):154–64.
59. Smith MR, Lee WC, Brandman J, Wang Q, Botteman M, Pashos CL. Gonadotropin-releasing hormone agonists and fracture risk: a claims-based cohort study of men with nonmetastatic prostate cancer. J Clin Oncol. 2005;23(31):7897–903.
60. Alibhai SM, Duong-Hua M, Cheung AM, Sutradhar R, Warde P, Fleshner NE, et al. Fracture types and risk factors in men with prostate cancer on androgen deprivation therapy: a matched cohort study of 19,079 men. J Urol. 2010;184(3):918–23. doi:10.1016/j.juro.2010.04.068.
61. Oefelein MG, Ricchuiti V, Conrad W, Seftel A, Bodner D, Goldman H, et al. Skeletal fracture associated with androgen suppression induced osteoporosis: the clinical incidence and risk factors for patients with prostate cancer. J Urol. 2001;166(5):1724–8.
62. Lenchik L, Kiebzak GM, Blunt BA. What is the role of serial bone mineral density measurements in patient management? J Clin Densitom. 2002;5 Suppl:S29–38.
63. Ebeling PR. Clinical practice. Osteoporosis in men. N Engl J Med. 2008;358(14):1474–82.
64. Cummings SR, Black DM, Nevitt MC, Browner W, Cauley J, Ensrud K, et al. Bone density at various sites for prediction of hip fractures. The Study of Osteoporotic Fractures Research Group. Lancet. 1993;341(8837):72–5.
65. Heidenreich A, Bolla M, Joniau S, Mason M, Matveev V, Mottet N, et al. 2010. Guidelines on prostate cancer. Eur Assoc Urol. http://www.uroweb.org/?id=218&gid=3.
66. Tinetti ME. Clinical practice. Preventing falls in elderly persons. N Engl J Med. 2003;348(1):42–9.
67. Tang BM, Eslick GD, Nowson C, Smith C, Bensoussan A. Use of calcium or calcium in combination with vitamin D supplementation to prevent fractures and bone loss in people aged 50 years and older: a meta-analysis. Lancet. 2007;370(9588):657–66.

68. Benton MJ, White A. Osteoporosis: recommendations for resistance exercise and supplementation with calcium and vitamin D to promote bone health. J Community Health Nurs. 2006;23(4):201–11.

69. Clinical practice guidelines in oncology. Prostate cancer. V.1. 2011. http://www.nccn.org/professionals/physician_gls/PDF/prostate.pdf. Accessed 1 June 2010.

70. Smith MR, McGovern FJ, Zietman AL, Fallon MA, Hayden DL, Schoenfeld DA, et al. Pamidronate to prevent bone loss during androgen-deprivation therapy for prostate cancer. N Engl J Med. 2001;345(13):948–55.

71. Smith MR, Eastham J, Gleason DM, Shasha D, Tchekmedyian S, Zinner N. Randomized controlled trial of zoledronic acid to prevent bone loss in men receiving androgen deprivation therapy for non-metastatic prostate cancer. J Urol. 2003;169(6):2008–12.

72. Michaelson MD, Kaufman DS, Lee H, McGovern FJ, Kantoff PW, Fallon MA, et al. Randomized controlled trial of annual zoledronic acid to prevent gonadotropin-releasing hormone agonist-induced bone loss in men with prostate cancer. J Clin Oncol. 2007;25(9):1038–42.

73. Greenspan SL, Nelson JB, Trump DL, Resnick NM. Effect of once-weekly oral alendronate on bone loss in men receiving androgen deprivation therapy for prostate cancer: a randomized trial. Ann Intern Med. 2007;146(6):416–24.

74. Bekker PJ, Holloway DL, Rasmussen AS, Murphy R, Martin SW, Leese PT, et al. A single-dose placebo-controlled study of AMG 162, a fully human monoclonal antibody to RANKL, in postmenopausal women. J Bone Miner Res. 2004;19(7):1059–66. doi:10.1359/JBMR.040305.

75. Smith MR, Egerdie B, Hernandez Toriz N, Feldman R, Tammela TL, Saad F, et al. Denosumab in men receiving androgen-deprivation therapy for prostate cancer. N Engl J Med. 2009;361(8):745–55.

76. European Medicines Agency Prolia -EMEA/H/C/001120 -N/0003. http://www.ema.europa.eu/docs/en_GB/document_library/EPAR_-_Product_Information/human/001120/WC500093526.pdf. Accessed 31 Jan 2011.

77. Escudier B, Eisen T, Stadler WM, Szczylik C, Oudard S, Siebels M, et al. Sorafenib in advanced clear-cell renal-cell carcinoma. N Engl J Med. 2007;356(2):125–34. doi:10.1056/NEJMoa060655.

78. Escudier B, Eisen T, Stadler WM, Szczylik C, Oudard S, Staehler M, et al. Sorafenib for treatment of renal cell carcinoma: final efficacy and safety results of the phase III treatment approaches in renal cancer global evaluation trial. J Clin Oncol. 2009;27(20):3312–8. doi:10.1200/JCO.2008.19.5511.

79. Escudier B, Pluzanska A, Koralewski P, Ravaud A, Bracarda S, Szczylik C, et al. Bevacizumab plus interferon alfa-2a for treatment of metastatic renal cell carcinoma: a randomised, double-blind phase III trial. Lancet. 2007;370(9605):2103–11. doi:10.1016/S0140-6736(07)61904-7.

80. Escudier B, Szczylik C, Hutson TE, Demkow T, Staehler M, Rolland F, et al. Randomized phase II trial of first-line treatment with sorafenib versus interferon Alfa-2a in patients with metastatic renal cell carcinoma. J Clin Oncol. 2009;27(8):1280–9. doi:10.1200/JCO.2008.19.3342.
81. Hudes G, Carducci M, Tomczak P, Dutcher J, Figlin R, Kapoor A, et al. Temsirolimus, interferon alfa, or both for advanced renal-cell carcinoma. N Engl J Med. 2007;356(22):2271–81. doi:10.1056/NEJMoa066838.
82. Motzer RJ, Escudier B, Oudard S, Hutson TE, Porta C, Bracarda S, et al. Efficacy of everolimus in advanced renal cell carcinoma: a double-blind, randomised, placebo-controlled phase III trial. Lancet. 2008;72(9637):449–56. doi:10.1016/S0140-6736(08)61039-9.
83. Motzer RJ, Hutson TE, Tomczak P, Michaelson MD, Bukowski RM, Oudard S, et al. Overall survival and updated results for sunitinib compared with interferon alfa in patients with metastatic renal cell carcinoma. J Clin Oncol. 2009;27(22):3584–90. doi:10.1200/JCO.2008.20.1293.
84. Motzer RJ, Hutson TE, Tomczak P, Michaelson MD, Bukowski RM, Rixe O, et al. Sunitinib versus interferon alfa in metastatic renal-cell carcinoma. N Engl J Med. 2007;356(2):115–24. doi:10.1056/NEJMoa065044.
85. Rini BI, Escudier B, Tomczak P, Kaprin A, Szczylik C, Hutson TE, et al. Comparative effectiveness of axitinib versus sorafenib in advanced renal cell carcinoma (AXIS): a randomised phase 3 trial. Lancet. 2011;378(9807):1931–9. doi:10.1016/S0140-6736(11)61613-9.
86. Rini BI, Halabi S, Rosenberg JE, Stadler WM, Vaena DA, Ou SS, et al. Bevacizumab plus interferon alfa compared with interferon alfa monotherapy in patients with metastatic renal cell carcinoma: CALGB 90206. J Clin Oncol. 2008;26(33):5422–8. doi:10.1200/JCO.2008.16.9847.
87. Sternberg CN, Davis ID, Mardiak J, Szczylik C, Lee E, Wagstaff J, et al. Pazopanib in locally advanced or metastatic renal cell carcinoma: results of a randomized phase III trial. J Clin Oncol. 2010;28(6):1061–8. doi:10.1200/JCO.2009.23.9764.
88. European Medicines Agency EU SmPC 06/01/2012 Nexavar -EMEA/H/C/000690 -IB/0031/G. http://www.ema.europa.eu/docs/en_GB/document_library/EPAR_-_Product_Information/human/000690/WC500027704.pdf. Accessed 23 Mar 2012.
89. European Medicines Agency EU SmPC 16/03/2012 Sutent -EMEA/H/C/000687 -IB/0034. http://www.ema.europa.eu/docs/en_GB/document_library/EPAR_-_Product_Information/human/000687/WC500057737.pdf. Accessed 23 Mar 2012.
90. European Medicines Agency Eu SmPC 02/09/2011 Torisel -EMEA/H/C/000799 -T/0039. http://www.ema.europa.eu/docs/en_GB/document_library/EPAR_-_Product_Information/human/000799/WC500039912.pdf. Accessed 23 Dec 2012.

91. European Medicines Agency EU SmPC 06/02/2012 Avastin -EMEA/H/C/000582 -II/0048. http://www.emea.europa.eu/docs/en_GB/document_library/EPAR_-_Product_Information/human/000582/WC500029271.pdf. Accessed 23 Dec 2012.

92. European Medicines Agency EU SmPC 22/11/2011 Afinitor -EMEA/H/C/001038 -II/0014. http://www.ema.europa.eu/docs/en_GB/document_library/EPAR_-_Product_Information/human/001038/WC500022814.pdf. Accessed 22 Mar 2012.

93. European Medicines Agency EU SmPC 24/10/2011 Votrient -EMEA/H/C/001141 -II/0005, II/0006, II0008. http://www.emea.europa.eu/docs/en_GB/document_library/EPAR_-_Product_Information/human/001141/WC500094272.pdf. Accessed 23 Dec 2012.

94. Eisen T, Sternberg CN, Robert C, Mulders P, Pyle L, Zbinden S, et al. Targeted therapies for renal cell carcinoma: review of adverse event management strategies. J Natl Cancer Inst. 2012;104(2):93–113. doi:10.1093/jnci/djr511.

95. Lacouture ME, Wu S, Robert C, Atkins MB, Kong HH, Guitart J, et al. Evolving strategies for the management of hand-foot skin reaction associated with the multitargeted kinase inhibitors sorafenib and sunitinib. Oncologist. 2008;13(9):1001–11. doi:10.1634/theoncologist.2008-0131.

96. Negrier S, Ravaud A. Optimisation of sunitinib therapy in metastatic renal cell carcinoma: adverse-event management. Eur J Cancer. 2007;Suppl 5(7):12–9.

97. Benson 3rd AB, Ajani JA, Catalano RB, Engelking C, Kornblau SM, Martenson Jr JA, et al. Recommended guidelines for the treatment of cancer treatment-induced diarrhea. J Clin Oncol. 2004;22(14):2918–26. doi:10.1200/JCO.2004.04.132.

98. Worthington HV, Clarkson JE, Eden OB. Interventions for preventing oral mucositis for patients with cancer receiving treatment. Cochrane Database Syst Rev. 2007;(4):CD000978. doi:10.1002/14651858.CD000978.pub3.

99. Bjordal JM, Bensadoun RJ, Tuner J, Frigo L, Gjerde K, Lopes-Martins RA. A systematic review with meta-analysis of the effect of low-level laser therapy (LLLT) in cancer therapy-induced oral mucositis. Support Care Cancer. 2011;19(8):1069–77. doi:10.1007/s00520-011-1202-0.

100. Loprinzi CL, Ellison NM, Schaid DJ, Krook JE, Athmann LM, Dose AM, et al. Controlled trial of megestrol acetate for the treatment of cancer anorexia and cachexia. J Natl Cancer Inst. 1990;82(13):1127–32.

101. Fearon KC, Barber MD, Moses AG, Ahmedzai SH, Taylor GS, Tisdale MJ, et al. Double-blind, placebo-controlled, randomized study of eicosapentaenoic acid diester in patients with cancer cachexia. J Clin Oncol. 2006;24(21):3401–7. doi:10.1200/JCO.2005.04.5724.

102. Madeddu C, Maccio A, Panzone F, Tanca FM, Mantovani G. Medroxyprogesterone acetate in the management of cancer cachexia. Expert Opin Pharmacother. 2009;10(8):1359–66. doi:10.1517/14656560902960162.

103. Berk L, James J, Schwartz A, Hug E, Mahadevan A, Samuels M, et al. A randomized, double-blind, placebo-controlled trial of a beta-hydroxyl beta-methyl butyrate, glutamine, and arginine mixture for the treatment of cancer cachexia (RTOG 0122). Support Care Cancer. 2008;16(10):1179–88. doi:10.1007/s00520-008-0403-7.

104. Hapani S, Chu D, Wu S. Risk of gastrointestinal perforation in patients with cancer treated with bevacizumab: a meta-analysis. Lancet Oncol. 2009;10(6):559–68. doi:10.1016/S1470-2045(09)70112-3.

105. Network. NCC NCCN clinical practice guidelines in oncology: cancer-related fatigue. http://www.nccn.org/. Accessed 17 Feb 2010.

106. Turner JS, Cheung EM, George J, Quinn DI. Pain management, supportive and palliative care in patients with renal cell carcinoma. BJU Int. 2007;99(5 Pt B):1305–12.

107. Wolter P, Stefan C, Decallonne B, Dumez H, Bex M, Carmeliet P, et al. The clinical implications of sunitinib-induced hypothyroidism: a prospective evaluation. Br J Cancer. 2008;99(3):448–54. doi:10.1038/sj.bjc.6604497.

108. Bamias A, Lainakis G, Manios E, Koroboki E, Karadimou A, Zakopoulos N, et al. Could rigorous diagnosis and management of hypertension reduce cardiac events in patients with renal cell carcinoma treated with tyrosine kinase inhibitors? J Clin Oncol. 2009;27(15):2567–9. doi:10.1200/JCO.2008.21.6028; author reply 2569–70.

109. Bamias A, Lainakis G, Manios E, Koroboki E, Gyftaki R, Zakopoulos N, et al. Diagnosis and management of hypertension in advanced renal cell carcinoma: prospective evaluation of an algorithm in patients treated with sunitinib. J Chemother. 2009;21(3):347–50.

110. Altena R, Perik PJ, van Veldhuisen DJ, de Vries EG, Gietema JA. Cardiovascular toxicity caused by cancer treatment: strategies for early detection. Lancet Oncol. 2009;10(4):391–9. doi:10.1016/S1470-2045(09)70042-7.

111. Force T, Kerkela R. Cardiotoxicity of the new cancer therapeutics – mechanisms of, and approaches to, the problem. Drug Discov Today. 2008;13(17–18):778–84. doi:10.1016/j.drudis.2008.05.011.

112. Telli ML, Witteles RM, Fisher GA, Srinivas S. Cardiotoxicity associated with the cancer therapeutic agent sunitinib malate. Ann Oncol. 2008;19(9):1613–8. doi:10.1093/annonc/mdn168.

113. Elice F, Rodeghiero F, Falanga A, Rickles FR. Thrombosis associated with angiogenesis inhibitors. Best Pract Res Clin Haematol. 2009;22(1):115–28. doi:10.1016/j.beha.2009.01.001.

114. Zangari M, Fink LM, Elice F, Zhan F, Adcock DM, Tricot GJ. Thrombotic events in patients with cancer receiving antiangiogenesis

agents. J Clin Oncol. 2009;27(29):4865–73. doi:10.1200/JCO.2009.22.3875.

115. Nalluri SR, Chu D, Keresztes R, Zhu X, Wu S. Risk of venous thromboembolism with the angiogenesis inhibitor bevacizumab in cancer patients: a meta-analysis. JAMA. 2008;300(19):2277–85. doi:10.1001/jama.2008.656.

116. Geerts WH, Bergqvist D, Pineo GF, Heit JA, Samama CM, Lassen MR, et al. Prevention of venous thromboembolism: American College of Chest Physicians Evidence-Based Clinical Practice Guidelines. 8th ed. Chest. 2008;133(6 Suppl):381S–453. doi:10.1378/chest.08-0656.

117. Margulis V, Matin SF, Tannir N, Tamboli P, Swanson DA, Jonasch E, et al. Surgical morbidity associated with administration of targeted molecular therapies before cytoreductive nephrectomy or resection of locally recurrent renal cell carcinoma. J Urol. 2008;180(1):94–8. doi:10.1016/j.juro.2008.03.047.

# Chapter 7
## Central Nervous System

**Miriame Mino, Krisztian Homicsko, and Roger Stupp**

**Abstract** Tumors of the central nervous system (CNS) differ in many ways from other tumors. First, these tumors are separated by an important natural barrier, the blood–brain barrier, with the aim of defending the CNS from external noxa but, in the case of cancer, limiting the efficacy of therapy. Second, the tumors of the CNS are malignant not only because of their biological behavior but because of their localization. Even very small and slow-growing tumors localized at important regions of the brain, like the brainstem, can have serious, deleterious, and fatal impact. Finally, tumors of the CNS have a very important impact on the quality of life of patients, with long-term disabling effects on everyday

M. Mino, M.D.
Internal Medicine, Centre Médico-Chirugical de la Broye,
Payerne, Switzerland

K. Homicsko, M.D., Ph.D.
Medical Oncology, Department of Oncology, Centre Hospitalier
Universitaire Vaudois, Lausanne, Switzerland

R. Stupp, M.D. (✉)
Departments of Neurosurgery and Clinical Neurosciences,
Centre Hospitalier Universitaire Vaudois and University of Lausanne,
Lausanne, Switzerland
e-mail: roger.stupp@chuv.ch

M.A. Dicato (ed.), *Side Effects of Medical Cancer Therapy,*
DOI 10.1007/978-0-85729-787-7_7,
© Springer-Verlag London 2013

293

life. Therefore, tumors of the CNS require early diagnosis and a rapid multidisciplinary approach to choose optimal treatment. In these cases, special attention must be taken to select chemotherapies and targeting agents that do cross the blood–brain barrier.

The focus of this chapter is side effects from chemotherapies used to treat a wide variety of tumors, from gliomas to metastatic (meningeal disease) lesions from other organs. This chapter will discuss the main complications from the treatment of CNS disease (glioma, medulloblastoma, and carcinomatous meningitis), specifically from radiotherapy, from cytotoxic and targeted anticancer therapy, and from supportive care measures.

**Keywords**    CNS • glioblastoma • Temozolomide • Bevacizumab Intrathechal chemotherapy • Blood–brain barrier

# Introduction

The focus of this chapter is on side effects of treatment of primary tumors of the central nervous system (CNS) and particularities of supportive care with tumor manifestations in the CNS. For the management of secondary (metastatic) tumor manifestations in the CNS, the reader should also refer to the respective chapters of the primary tumor of origin. As a general rule, brain metastases will respond in a similar manner to chemotherapy than other systemic disease, provided the agent crosses the blood–brain barrier and sufficient drug concentrations in the CNS can be achieved. This chapter will briefly discuss the main complications from the treatment of CNS disease, specifically for radiotherapy, from cytotoxic and targeted anticancer therapy, and from supportive care measures.

Classification of primary brain tumors according to the World Health Organization is based on their cell of origin. The most common malignant tumors in adults are glioma, which account for approximately 2 % of all cancers; in children and young adults, embryonic tumors in the CNS are among the

TABLE 7.1  The most commonly used agents in CNS tumors

Temozolomide

Nitrosoureas

   Carmustine (BCNU)

   Lomustine (CCNU)

   Fotemustine

   Nimustine (ACNU)

Procarbazine

Vincristine

Bevacizumab

Irinotecan (CPT11)

Ifosfamide

Carboplatin

Etoposide

Cytarabine

Methotrexate

Thiotepa

most frequent tumor manifestations. Primary CNS lymphoma is often (but not exclusively) associated with chronic immunodeficiency (e.g., AIDS, after organ transplant).

Due to their infiltrative nature and their localization in the CNS, a complete resection of gliomas and other brain tumors is often not achievable. Even after macroscopic gross total resection, gliomas virtually always recur. Thus, additional therapy with radiation and/or chemotherapy is indicated. The blood–brain barrier, although often partially disrupted at the site of the tumor, is an obstacle to delivery of adequate concentrations of chemotherapy to the brain. The most commonly used agents in the treatment of primary CNS tumors are summarized in Table 7.1.

# Radiotherapy

Historically, radiotherapy has been the sole treatment of malignancies in the brain. The radiation fields, the dose, and the fractionation vary from precise stereotaxic irradiation (radiosurgery) to focal or whole brain radiotherapy. The primary determinants of toxicity are the administered cumulative dose, the dose of individual fractions, and the irradiated volume. Vulnerability and radiosensitivity differ between the various structures of the CNS. In high-grade glioma, focal radiotherapy to the tumor with a safety margin of 1.5–2 cm up to a total dose of approximately 60 Gy in 1.8- to 2-Gy fractions is commonly delivered. At doses above 60 Gy, the risk of long-term damage to the normal brain tissue increases exponentially, with no increase in efficacy. For low-grade glioma doses of 50 Gy suffice. For brain metastases with overall poor prognosis, a simpler hypofractionated regime of $10 \times 3$ Gy is frequently prescribed. The main side effects can be divided into reversible short-term and irreversible long-term toxicity (Table 7.2). Acute side effects are hair loss (may persist), fatigue, somnolence, and nausea and vomiting. Since radiotherapy induces inflammation, the tumor- and mass effect-related symptoms like headaches, nausea and vomiting, and neurologic symptoms may temporarily increase during radiotherapy. The practice of routine prophylactic steroid administration during cranial irradiation has been abandoned, and steroids should be introduced in case of symptoms only. The major long-term side effect of irradiation of the brain is leukoencephalopathy, which is due to destruction of the myelin sheaths covering nerve fibers. The symptoms are greatly variable, from a frequent pure radiologic finding without clinical symptoms to mild confusion and cognitive impairment to progressive invalidating dementia and functional deficits. Factors that contribute to the development of neurocognitive deficiency include volume of irradiation, patient's age (brains of older patients are more vulnerable), tumor volume and localization, and genetic factors [1]. Because of the developing brain, children below the age of 3 years are particularly sensitive to radiotherapy. In adults, 26 % of patients develop leukoencephalopathy as early as 3 months after the

TABLE 7.2 Side effects of radiotherapy after brain or spinal cord irradiation

| Time after irradiation | Symptoms |
|---|---|
| *Brain* | |
| Acute (days) | Increased ICP, nausea and vomiting |
| Early delayed (weeks) | Somnolence syndrome, fatigue, hair loss, symptoms of tumor recurrence |
| Delayed (months–years) | |
| (a) Necrosis | Dementia, symptoms of tumor recurrence |
| (b) Leukoencephalopathy | Dementia or asymptomatic |
| *Spinal cord* | |
| Early delayed (weeks) | Lhermitte's sign |
| Delayed (months–years) | |
| (a) Necrosis | Transverse myelopathy |
| (b) Hemorrhage | Acute myelopathy |
| (c) Motor neuron disease | Flaccid paraparesis, amyotrophy |
| (d) Arachnoiditis | Asymptomatic |
| (e) SMART syndrome | SMART syndrome: stroke-like migraine attacks after radiation therapy |

end of whole brain radiotherapy. After 3 months of whole brain radiotherapy. Preexisting leukoaraiosis seems to be a major determinant of long-term damage [2].

# Chemotherapy

Drug therapy is used alone, as single agents, or in combination regimens and concomitant with radiotherapy. In the following sections, the most commonly used agents are discussed, with specific focus on dosing and toxicity when used for the treatment of brain tumors and CNS disease.

## Agents Commonly Used Against Glioma

### Temozolomide (EU, Temodal; USA, Temodar)

Temozolomide (TMZ), an alkylating cytotoxic agent, is nowadays the most commonly used drug in the treatment of malignant glioma [3]. It is used in a variety of different dosages and regimens, usually either as a single agent or in combination with concomitant radiotherapy (Table 7.3 and Fig. 7.1) [9]. Since it is rapidly absorbed in the gut with almost 100 % bioavailability, oral formulation is possible and permits ease of administration and dosing. It readily crosses the blood–brain barrier, allowing for cytotoxic tumor tissue concentrations [10].

TMZ is usually well tolerated. Gastrointestinal intolerance is the most common side effect, while myelosuppression is dose limiting. The severity of the observed toxicities is variable, and the incidence depends on the dosing regimen. For the scheme of intermittent, once a day for 5 consecutive days administration, antiemetic prophylaxis is almost always required. Continuous low-dose and metronomic regimens often do not require any antiemetic drug beyond the first 2–3 days of administration. Profound lymphocytopenia, on the other hand, is commonly observed with continuous dosing, while late thrombocytopenia is more frequent with the intermittent regimen.

Table 7.4 presents the common side effects of TMZ, all grades, compared to radiotherapy.

### Hematologic

Myelosuppression, in particular late occurrence (>21 days after treatment start) thrombocytopenia, is a side effect of TMZ.

During chemoradiotherapy, TMZ is given at a daily (7/7d) dose of 75 mg/m$^2$, approximately, 1–2 h before irradiation (including weekends and days without radiotherapy), starting simultaneously with the first day of radiotherapy until the last day of irradiation, which is usually 30 fractions over 40–49 days max [5]. Although myelosuppression is rarely observed before

TABLE 7.3 Dosing regimens of TMZ

| Schedule | Dose (mg/m²) | Dose intensity (mg/m²/week) | References |
|---|---|---|---|
| Daily for 5 days, repeat every 28 days | 150–200 | 250 | Initially an approved standard dosing |
| Daily for 42–49 days | 75 | 315 | Brock et al. [4] approved in conjunction with radiotherapy (Stupp et al. [5]) |
| Daily continuously nonstop (metronomic) | 50 | 350 | Perry et al. [6] |
| Daily for 7 days, repeat every 14 days | 100–150 | 525 | Tolcher et al. [7] |
| Daily for 21 days, every 28 days | 75–100 | 525 | Tolcher et al. [7] |
| Daily for 3 days, every 14 days | 300 | 450 | Vera et al. [8] |

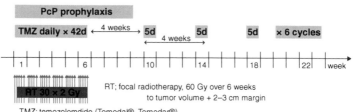

FIGURE 7.1 Standard-of-care radiochemotherapy regimen. *TMZ* temozolomide (Temodal®, Temodar®)

week 3, complete blood counts are to be performed weekly. Low blood counts may occur several weeks after the end of chemoradiotherapy (continue to monitor CBC!). When the platelet count drops below $75 \times 10^9$/L (grade 2) or the neutrophil count is $<1 \times 10^9$/L (grade 3), chemotherapy should be temporarily suspended. It can be restarted once the values have recovered (neutrophils > 1.5, thrombocytes > 100, or toxicity grade < 2). Occurrence of toxicity during concomitant chemoradiotherapy is not a reason for not proceeding with standard adjuvant/maintenance chemotherapy after the end of the chemoradiotherapy.

With the standard 5-day, daily dosing regimen, the nadir commonly occurs after 3 weeks (days 21–28). During initial treatment cycles, blood counts should be checked on day 22 and day 29 (= day 1 of the subsequent cycle). Occasionally, patients require an additional delay of 3–14 days until blood counts recover. In case of severe myelosuppression (e.g., ≥ grade 3 or delayed recovery), dose reduction by 50 mg/m$^2$ is recommended. In case of hematologic toxicity during chemoradiotherapy, prudence is advised when dosing the initial cycle of subsequent adjuvant therapy (dose for cycle 1: 150 mg/m$^2$/day for 5 days, to be escalated in the absence of significant hematologic toxicity to 200 mg/m$^2$).

Profound lymphocytopenia occurs frequently with the continuous TMZ regimen (e.g., during concomitant chemoradiotherapy) and may be further enhanced by the frequent administration of corticosteroids. These patients are at risk for *Pneumocystis jirovecii* pneumonia (PCP, formerly known as *Pneumocystis carinii*), and primary prophylaxis should be

TABLE 7.4  Common side effects of temozolomide (TMZ), all grades, compared to radiotherapy (RT) only

| | RT alone (%) | RT+TMZ (%) | Comment/treatment/ prevention |
|---|---|---|---|
| Nausea | 16 | 36 | 5-HT3 agonist, domperidone, or metoclopramide, 30 min before TMZ. Take caps on an empty stomach. Eat small, frequent meals |
| Vomiting | 6 | 20 | See above |
| Constipation | 6 | 18 | Laxatives; drink well; exercise, if possible |
| Headache | 17 | 19 | Painkillers |
| Fatigue | 49 | 54 | Rest |
| Convulsions | 7 | 6 | Optimize antiepileptic treatment. Interactions with TMZ and some antiepileptic drugs |
| Anorexia | 9 | 19 | |
| Skin rash | 15 | 19 | Avoid sun exposure, especially when undergoing RT |
| Alopecia | 63 | 69 | RT, not TMZ, will induce alopecia |
| Infection | 5 | 9 | |
| Leukopenia/ neutropenia | 6 | 9 | See paragraph on hematotoxicity |
| Thrombocytopenia | 1 | 4 | See paragraph on hematotoxicity |

Table created with data from Cohen et al. [11] and [5]

considered (Table 7.5). Other complications associated with an immunosuppressed state are reactivation of herpes zoster infection, exacerbation of chronic hepatitis, and Kaposi sarcoma.

TABLE 7.5  Prophylaxis of Pneumocystis pneumonia

A high frequency of opportunistic infections was observed in the
first trials using the continuous low-dose TMZ regimen [12, 13], and
a primary prophylaxis was introduced for subsequent clinical trials.
The manufacturer's recommendation is primary prophylaxis during
TMZ/RT (see Temodal/Temodar package insert). Alternatively, some
institutions follow on a regular basis the total lymphocyte and CD4-
positive lymphocyte count, and prophylaxis is proposed if the CD4 value
is less than 200–250/mm$^3$ or the total lymphocyte count is <500 mm$^3$.
Commonly recommended prophylactic regimens are as follows:

| Agent | Dose and frequency | Remarks |
| --- | --- | --- |
| Pentacarinat (pentamidine) | 300-mg inhalation, every 4 weeks | In the authors' experience the preferred regimen |
| Trimethoprim-sulfamethoxazole (Bactrim, Septra) | 1 double-strength (160/800 mg) tablet 3×/week (Monday, Wednesday, Friday) | Cave myelosuppression with sulfa drugs |
| Dapsone (Dapsone) | 100 mg 1×/day | If intolerance to TMP-SMX |

Gastrointestinal

One of the most common side effects of TMZ is mild to moderate
nausea and occasional vomiting that can be prevented by a
low-dose prophylactic administration of 5-HT3 inhibitors
(e.g., lower-dose ondansetron, 4 mg; granisetron, 1 mg) or
metoclopramide in almost all patients. Because 5-HT3 antagonists are associated with their own toxicity, like constipation
and headache, chronic repeated dosing is to be avoided. In the
authors' experience, a low dosage of the 5-HT3 antagonist
during the first 2–5 days of a cycle is usually sufficient. With
the continuous TMZ dosing regimens, a simple antiemetic
prophylaxis with metoclopramide or domperidone will commonly

suffice, and up to half of the patients may not need any anti-emetic treatment beyond the first days of treatment.

Alopecia

TMZ does not induce alopecia; however, radiotherapy will. It can be partial or complete and is seen in up to 63 % of patients after radiochemotherapy.

Infection (Oral Thrush, Wound Infection, Herpes Simplex)

Immunosuppression (e.g., lymphocytopenia) induced by chronic TMZ administration (and often exacerbated by concomitant corticosteroids) will lead to oral candidemia, herpes reactivation, or wound infection. Other than consideration of PCP prophylaxis (as described earlier), prophylactic antibiotic therapy is not recommended.

Neurologic and Psychiatric

Side effects such as anxiety, sleeping disorder, emotional instability, drowsiness, dizziness, confusion, memory loss, blurred vision, and concentration difficulties have been observed. These side effects may be partly caused by TMZ, but they have also been observed in patients treated by radiotherapy only and may be explained by the tumor itself or the frequent corticosteroid administration.

Before the widespread utilization of TMZ alone and concomitant with radiotherapy, the combination of procarbazine, lomustine (CCNU), and vincristine (known as the PCV regimen) has been used since the 1980s [14]. Due to ease of administration and overall excellent tolerance, TMZ has largely replaced the PCV regimen; superiority of either treatment has never been formally investigated. The PCV regimen requires intravenous administration of vincristine, and the regimen is associated with a high incidence of myelosuppression, occasional infections, and frequent treatment delays.

# Nitrosoureas (Lomustine, Carmustine, Nimustine, and Fotemustine)

Lomustine (CCNU), carmustine (BCNU), nimustine (ACNU), and fotemustine are alkylating nitrosourea anticancer cytotoxic drugs [15]. They produce DNA and RNA alkylation. They are greatly soluble in lipids, which allows their passage through the blood–brain barrier. The main toxicities are hematologic and gastrointestinal. Myelosuppression is the dose-limiting side effect. Lomustine is the drug most commonly used for glioma therapy and is one of the components of the PCV regimen (Table 7.6). ACNU and fotemustine are used occasionally in some countries such as Germany and Japan (ACNU) and France and Italy (fotemustine). Carmustine was for long the standard of care in the United States [17]. As a single agent the standard dose of lomustine is 130 mg/m²; however, in combination and in patients having received prior chemotherapy, only a reduced dose of 90–110 mg/m² can be tolerated. In many countries, lomustine comes only in capsules of 40 mg, thus limiting dose titration. It is given by mouth once every 6–8 weeks.

## Myelosuppression

The myelosuppression is dose dependent and cumulative and occurs late in the treatment cycle (nadir fifth week, occasionally even later). Thrombocytopenia observed around day 28 is often followed by neutropenia occurring after day 35. The leukopenia can persist up to 2–3 months after the end of the treatment.

## Gastrointestinal System

Frequency of side effects is variable. Nausea and vomiting most often appears 4–6 h after administration and may persist for 24–48 h, associated with anorexia for 2–3 days. Antiemetic treatment usually has a good effect on nausea. Mild and clinically nonsignificant elevation of liver function tests is often observed. Stomatitis and diarrhea are often seen.

TABLE 7.6 The PCV regimen

The PCV regimen was developed in the late 1970s [16], aiming at a non-cross-resistant combination of three agents with activity against brain tumors. For vincristine, antitumor activity was assumed based on the neurologic toxicity induced by this agent. For over 20 years, this regimen was considered the most active treatment against malignant glioma and used in many large clinical trials. Unfortunately, a sufficient antitumor activity as adjuvant treatment in newly diagnosed glioma patients could never be established, albeit that antitumor activity was demonstrated in subgroup analyses. One reason for failure may have been the substantial toxicity, in particular the overlapping hematotoxicity induced by these agents, which led to frequent delays, early treatment discontinuations, or fatal complications. Several modifications and variations of the regimen exist.

| Agent | Dose (mg/m$^2$) | Days of administration |
|---|---|---|
| Modified PCV | | |
| Procarbazine | 60 | 8–21 |
| CCNU | 110 | 1 |
| Vincristine | 1.4 | 8, 29 |
| British PCV | | |
| Procarbazine | 100 | 1–10 |
| CCNU | 110 | 1 |
| Vincristine | 1.5 | 1 |

## Neurologic System

When combining lomustine with other drugs, neurologic side effects such as apathy, confusion, stuttering, and disorientation have, in rare cases, been described.

## Respiratory System

One of the limitations of nitrosourea therapy is idiopathic pulmonary fibrosis, most commonly seen with carmustine. Moderate to severe respiratory insufficiency is thus a relative contraindication to the treatment with nitrosoureas. If pulmonary symptoms occur, presenting often with a diffuse infiltrate, and once other causes have been ruled out, treatment is a prolonged course of corticosteroids [18].

## Procarbazine

Procarbazine is another alkylating agent causing DNA crosslinks followed by DNA breaks. Myelosuppression is the main side effect, with neutropenia and thrombocytopenia being dose limiting. Nausea and vomiting are common. Within the PCV regimen, the dosage is 60 mg/m$^2$ daily PO for 14 days (day 8–day 21); as a single agent, doses of 100–150 mg/m$^2$ for 14 days are usually well tolerated. Procarbazine comes as capsules of 50 mg each.

### Hematologic

Toxicity (neutropenia, thrombocytopenia) may commence 1 week after the beginning of the treatment, and it can persist up to 2 weeks after withdrawal.

### Gastrointestinal

Nausea and vomiting can usually be prevented by standard antiemetic treatment.

### Immunologic and Skin Rash

Hypersensitivity reactions with eosinophilia and fever are common. The reactions can be IgE-mediated but are also associated with a type III reaction manifested by pulmonary toxicity and cutaneous reactions [19]. The higher frequency of hypersensitivity reactions in brain tumor patients has been associated with the concomitant administration of antiepileptic drugs [20]. A diffuse, pruritic, erythematous maculopapular rash has been reported in 12–35 % of glioma patients. Note that procarbazine inhibits alcohol dehydrogenase and may cause disulfiram-like reactions when a patient consumes alcohol.

### Neurologic

Drowsiness and peripheral neuropathy are regularly seen.

Respiratory

Rare cases of pneumonitis (see immunologic) have been reported; it may be severe and irreversible. The treatment is procarbazine withdrawal and corticosteroid therapy [21].

Hypertensive Crisis

Food containing high levels of tyramine (e.g., red wine, overripe bananas, mature cheese) may cause hypertensive crisis, since procarbazine is a monoamine oxidase (MAO) inhibitor.

# Vincristine

Vincristine is a vinca alkaloid that binds to tubulin dimers, inhibiting microtubule assembly and in turn blocking cell division during the mitotic phase [22]. The side effects of vincristine are dependent on the total dose given. The dose-limiting side effect is neurotoxicity. Recent studies have questioned whether vincristine sufficiently penetrates through the blood–brain barrier, and it may not be an effective agent against brain tumors [23]. The standard weekly dose is 1.4 mg/m$^2$ (usually capped at a maximum dose of 2 mg), as part of the PCV regimen given on days 8 and 29.

The most common side effect is alopecia, while the most troublesome is neuromuscular adverse reactions. Leukopenia and severe myelosuppression are rare. Vincristine is metabolized in the liver via the CYP3A4-mediated enzymes; it may thus increase metabolism of CYP3A4-dependent antiepileptic drugs. Caution is advised in patients with hepatic insufficiency.

Alopecia

This is the most common side effect. Regrowth of hair usually happens 6 weeks after the interruption of treatment.

Neuromuscular

Frequently, a sequence in the development of the neuromuscular side effects can be observed with the treatment continuation. The initial sensory impairment and paresthesia are followed by neuropathic pain, and finally motor difficulties occur. No treatment that could reverse the neuromuscular manifestations has so far been reported.

### Gastrointestinal

Constipation with or without pain has been regularly seen; therefore, prophylactic laxatives should be proposed. Rarely, paralytic ileus can be seen, especially in young and elderly patients, which upon withdrawal of vincristine can regress spontaneously.

### Ocular

Rarely, visual side effects such as transient cortical blindness, optic nerve atrophy with blindness, and nystagmus can occur.

### Neurotoxicity

Inadvertent intrathecal administration of vincristine can cause ascending radiculomyeloencephalopathy, which in most cases is fatal. Immediate cerebrospinal fluid aspiration must be followed by intrathecal irrigation, including intrathecal administration of fresh-frozen plasma that can eventually bind vincristine. A few cases of patients who received rapid supportive care and survived intrathecal vincristine have been reported [24–26].

### Pulmonary

In rare cases administration of vincristine has led to bronchospasm, especially when combined with mitomycin C. This can occur immediately after the administration or several hours later. In these cases vincristine should not be readministered.

### Accidental Extravasation

It can cause severe local reaction and tissue necrosis. Hyaluronidase injection at the site of extravasation must be considered, since vincristine breaks down hyaluronic acid in the connective/soft tissue, allowing the further dispersion of vincristine. Heat packs applied for 20 min QID during 3 days are recommended because this can lead to vasodilatation and consequently to diffusion and elimination of the drug from the site of injection [27].

## Bevacizumab (Avastin)

Bevacizumab is a monoclonal neutralizing antibody inhibiting the growth factor VEGF-A, the ligand to the VEGF receptor, highly expressed on tumor-associated endothelial cells [28]. This is an attractive treatment target in patients with glioblastoma because this tumor is highly vascular and expresses high levels of VEGF-A. The commonly used dose of bevacizumab is 10 mg/kg every 2 weeks, although lower doses might be equally effective. Formal dose-finding studies in brain tumors were not conducted. Bevacizumab is approved in recurrent/relapsed glioblastoma in the United States and Switzerland. In many European countries, it is used regularly, although the extension of the indication to brain tumors was rejected by the European Medicines Agency due to the absence of any controlled efficacy data. Definitive phase III trials are finally ongoing.

While bevacizumab clearly allows the reduction of corticosteroid therapy and will lead to temporary neurologic improvement, particularly in patients with severe peritumoral edema, its effect on survival is less evident and contested. The possible modest benefit of bevacizumab has to be balanced against potential risks and toxicity and, ultimately, cost [29].

The most common side effects are hypertension, asthenia, fatigue, vomiting, diarrhea, and abdominal pain, while the most serious side effects are gastrointestinal perforation, hemorrhage, and both arterial and venous thromboembolic events. There is no myelosuppression when used as a single agent.

It should be noted that administration of bevacizumab leads to a reduction in contrast enhancement, the standard metric of objective response, making the radiologic follow-up difficult. Contrast-enhanced magnetic resonance imaging has revealed a significant reduction of the vascular supply, as evidenced by a decrease in intratumoral blood flow and volume. The vascular remodeling induced by anti-VEGF-A treatment leads to a more hypoxic tumor microenvironment. Concerns have been raised that the tumor's remodeling may lead to a more aggressive tumor phenotype. A metabolic change in the tumor cells toward glycolysis leads to enhanced tumor cell invasion of the normal brain tissue [30, 31].

Hypertension

Bevacizumab is thought to induce hypertension by decreasing nitric oxide production, resulting in vasoconstriction [32]. This also leads to increased sodium reabsorption in the kidney. Hypertension is a dose-dependent side effect; the frequency increases exponentially with increased doses [33]. With the commonly used high doses of bevacizumab (10 mg/kg), hypertension of any degree has been observed in up to one-third of the patients; however, it was considered severe ($\geq$ grade 3, i.e., systolic blood pressure >180 mmHg and diastolic blood pressure >110 mmHg) in only 5 % [34]. Preexisting hypertension should be treated before initiation of bevacizumab. Hypertensive exacerbation will further increase the risk for intracranial hemorrhage.

Figure 7.2 shows the management of hypertension and proteinuria. The management of bevacizumab-induced hypertension follows the general principles of hypertension treatment [35]. In patients with cardiovascular risk factors, the treatment goal is 130/80; in others, 140/90. The antiangiogenic treatment should be withdrawn if clinically significant hypertension persists despite proper management or in case of a hypertensive crisis or symptomatic hypertensive encephalopathy (headaches, attention disorder, confusion, or coma).

Patients with previous hypertension are, like all hypertensive patients, at higher risk of developing proteinuria. A potential mechanism for proteinuria is by the inhibition of VEGF on the podocytes leading to renal damage [36]. Urinary dipstick analysis should be performed before initiating and during the treatment.

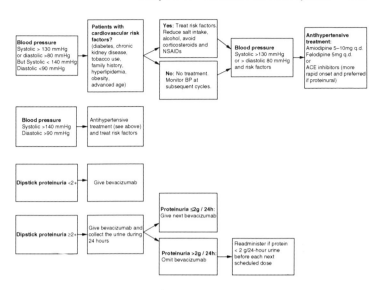

FIGURE 7.2 Management of hypertension and proteinuria

As long as proteinuria over 24 h is not less than 2 g, bevacizumab should not be given. Nephrotic syndrome occurs in 0.5 % of patients, and treatment must be withdrawn. Proteinuria is seen less commonly in patients with CNS tumors than in other cancer types, likely explained by the shorter exposure to bevacizumab due to tumor progression occurring at a median of 4 months. Similar to patients with hypertension and proteinuria, agents such as angiotensin-converting enzyme (ACE) inhibitors or angiotensin II receptor blockers (ARBs) are the first choice.

Arterial and Venous Thromboembolism

Patients with gliomas are at higher risk of venous thrombotic events [37], while the incidence of arterial thromboembolism is not known to be increased. Patients treated with bevacizumab are at higher risk of developing arterial and/or venous thromboembolism [38]. This includes stroke, transient ischemic attacks, myocardial infarction, deep venous thrombosis, and pulmonary embolism. Patients with a previous history of arterial thromboembolism or age older than 65 are at higher risk of developing thromboembolic complications and must be carefully monitored. Bevacizumab therapy should be definitively discontinued in patients having presented with an arterial thrombotic event. The presence of a venous thromboembolic event is a relative contraindication to continuation of bevacizumab therapy; risks and benefits need to be evaluated individually. The requirement of systemic anticoagulation may slightly increase the risk for an intracranial hemorrhage, a risk that is already more pronounced owing to the presence of recurrent tumor in the brain (high vascularization of recurrent glioblastoma may lead to spontaneous bleeding) and further exacerbated by bevacizumab therapy. Nevertheless, current, albeit limited, experience indicates no substantial increase of serious intracranial hemorrhage when patients are treated simultaneously by systemic anticoagulation and bevacizumab [39]. Low molecular weight heparins (LMWH) are more often used than oral anticoagulants, since fewer drug interactions are expected with potentially improved efficacy [40].

Bleeding

Patients treated with bevacizumab have an increased risk of bleeding, especially at the tumor site [41]. Higher doses of bevacizumab increase the risk of bleeding. The mechanism of the bleeding is thought to be via inhibition of the endothelial cell survival and proliferation leading to damaged blood vessels. The most common type of bleeding is epistaxis, but more serious bleeding like intracerebral, gastrointestinal, or pulmonary can also be seen. If any grade 3 or 4 bleeding occurs, the treatment must be withdrawn. The risk of intracranial hemorrhage does not seem to be more elevated in patients with glioblastoma than in other patients treated with bevacizumab. Intracranial bleeding more frequently occurs during progression, regardless of bevacizumab use.

## Surgical Complications After Prior Bevacizumab Therapy

### Wound Healing

Antiangiogenic therapy interferes with wound healing [42]. Vascular endothelial growth factor is essential for neovascularization, and bevacizumab interferes with this mechanism. The long biological half-life of bevacizumab (median, 20 days; range, 11–50 days) has led to the recommendation not to administer bevacizumab 4 weeks before and 4 weeks after undergoing major surgery or before complete healing of the wound. One study showed that bevacizumab interferes more with wound healing if it is given preoperatively than postoperatively [43].

### Gastrointestinal Perforation

In a large meta-analysis with 12, 294 patients, perforation was seen in 1 % of patients [44]. Most relevant risk factors in brain tumor patients are constipation, diverticular disease, peptic ulcers, and concomitant use of corticosteroids. In any case of gastrointestinal perforation, the treatment must be immediately withdrawn.

### Heart Failure

In clinical trials, congestive heart failure has been seen in patients receiving bevacizumab. The symptoms are from asymptomatic reduction of left ventricle ejection fraction on cardiac ultrasound to symptomatic heart failure needing inpatient care. Many of these studies included breast cancer patients after prior exposure to anthracyclines and/or trastuzumab. One study suggests that the toxicity may be spontaneously reversible [45].

### Perfusion Reactions

Patients may develop hypersensitivity and infusion reactions. This is seen in less than 5 % of patients. The majority of reactions are mild to moderate. More severe reactions were noted in 0.2 % of patients. Premedication is not warranted. If a reaction occurs, the infusion shall be stopped and symptoms treated. Rechallenging patients can be discussed, but it must be based on the goals of the therapy and the severity of the reaction.

Posterior Reversible Encephalopathy Syndrome

One of the infrequent but very serious side effects is posterior reversible leukoencephalopathy (PRLE) [46]. The differential diagnosis between PRLE and hypertensive encephalopathy can be difficult. The main symptoms are headache, seizures, altered mental status, nausea, troubled vision, or cortical blindness; most patients are markedly hypertensive. At CT/MR imaging the brain typically demonstrates focal regions of symmetric hemispheric edema. It is thought that the causes of PRLE can be failure of cerebral vasomotor autoregulation due to hypertension or primary endothelial damage. The mechanisms resemble preeclampsia. The symptoms usually resolve with efficient treatment of hypertension and with withdrawal of bevacizumab.

## Irinotecan (CPT11)

Irinotecan is a semisynthetic derivative of camptothecin, which acts as a DNA topoisomerase I inhibitor [47]. It easily crosses the blood–brain barrier. Topoisomerase I is localized in the cell nucleus and regulates DNA topology, facilitating nuclear processes such as DNA replication, recombination, and repair. The active metabolite of irinotecan, SN-38, binds to the topoisomerase I-DNA complex. Topoisomerase I and II activities are significantly increased in malignant tumors due to DNA damage, thus making irinotecan an interesting drug for the treatment of gliomas. Irinotecan and its metabolites are secreted via the liver and depend on the P450 enzyme complex [48]. As brain tumor patients commonly receive antiepileptic drugs, drug-drug interactions may occur. Notable are phenytoin, carbamazepine and derived substances, and the nowadays rarely used phenobarbital, which will induce cytochrome P450 CYP3A4 enzymes, leading to faster clearance of irinotecan and thus diminishing or eliminating its activity [49].

Different dosing regimens of irinotecan have been established, initially for gastrointestinal cancer [50]. In brain tumors, irinotecan has been given as a weekly ×4 administration every 6 weeks at a dose of 125 mg/m$^2$ or in combination with bevacizumab every 2 weeks at a 125-mg/m$^2$ dose. In our experience we commonly increase the dose up to 180 mg/m$^2$, similar to the established gastrointestinal dose. Higher doses of up to 340 mg/m$^2$ have been suggested for patients taking enzyme-inducing antiepileptic drugs; however, it is much safer to switch patients to the well-established non-enzyme-inducing antiepileptic agents [51].

The main side effects of irinotecan are diarrhea and hematotoxicity.

Gastrointestinal

Profound and delayed diarrhea is the dose-limiting toxicity of irinotecan. Diarrhea will occur in the majority of patients, being severe in up to 20 %. Diarrhea typically occurs in two phases: early, within the first 24 h, and late, after 5–7 days. Early diarrhea is due to the cholinergic toxic syndrome (see later section) and self-limiting. Patients having received radiotherapy on the pelvic region, patients with leukocytosis, performance status of two or more, and women are at a higher risk of developing diarrhea. Late diarrhea occurs several days after irinotecan administration. Most common is the appearance of diarrhea on the fifth day in the case of a schedule of every 2 weeks (high dosage) and on the eleventh day in case of the weekly treatment. Patients must be informed of this side effect; in case of diarrhea adequate oral rehydration is imperative. Loperamide, 4 mg as an initial dose and 2 mg with every loose stool, shall be given at the first signs of diarrhea, up to eight or more doses/24 h. Repeated loperamide administration every 2 h is recommended for another 12 h after the last episode of diarrhea, but total exposure should not exceed 48 h, thus avoiding consecutive paralytic ileus.

Delayed diarrhea often coincides with myelosuppression; thus, patients at this stage are particularly vulnerable. Forced rehydration, if needed intravenous, should be considered, with low threshold to hospitalization in case of prolonged diarrhea, dehydration, or fever.

In patients with hyperbilirubinemia (1.5–3 times higher than the normal level), liver function tests must be surveyed weekly. Irinotecan is to be withdrawn if bilirubin is three times higher than normal. Prophylactic antiemetic drugs are to be given before each cycle to avoid nausea and vomiting, which are a common side effects.

## Hematologic

Neutropenia has been seen in almost 80 % of patients treated by irinotecan monotherapy; severe neutropenia ($<0.5 \times 10^6$ G/L) has been seen in 22 % of patients. The hematotoxicity is reversible, with a nadir around the eighth day and subsequent rapid recovery. The neutropenia is not cumulative. Anemia is seen in 58 % of patients. Thrombocytopenia is seen less frequently; approximately 10 % of patients will be seen with thrombocytes less than $100 \times 10^6$ G/L.

## Dermatologic

Reversible alopecia is very common.

## The Cholinergic Toxic Syndrome

This syndrome is specific to irinotecan and can be seen in up to 42 % of patients treated with irinotecan; it can be severe in one-fourth of patients [52]. The main symptoms are diarrhea, abdominal pain, hypotension, shivering, dizziness, blurred vision, miosis, transpiration, and hypersalivation while receiving the chemotherapy or within the following 24 h. The symptoms can be relieved by premedication with 0.25–0.5 mg of atropine given subcutaneously.

## Other Commonly Used Agents in CNS Malignancies

For the treatment of germ cell tumors, primitive neuroectodermal tumors (PNET), and medulloblastoma, combination regimens including ifosfamide, cisplatin or carboplatin, and etoposide are frequently administered [53, 54]. The backbone of treatment of primary CNS lymphoma is high-dose methotrexate, either alone or in combination with cytarabine or ifosfamide (± the monoclonal antibody rituximab) [55, 56]. We briefly discuss ifosfamide; cytarabine and methotrexate are reviewed in the section on leptomeningeal disease. For the other agents the reader should refer to other sections of this book.

### Ifosfamide

Ifosfamide is a nitrogen mustard alkylating agent and an analogue of cyclophosphamide. First, ifosfamide is activated to 4-hydroxyifosfamide in the liver, which is then transformed into the active compound isoaldophosphamide. In addition to myelosuppression, characteristic toxicities of this agent include hemorrhagic cystitis, renal insufficiency, and ill-defined diffuse cognitive and cerebellar symptoms. Common dosing is 750–1,000 mg/m$^2$/day as a continuous several-hour infusion for 4–5 days. The usual dose for medulloblastoma is 900 mg/m$^2$/day in a continuous infusion over 5 days [57].

#### Gastrointestinal

Nausea and vomiting is seen in approximately half of patients. Usual antiemetic prophylaxis by 5-HT3 antagonists is recommended.

#### Dermatologic

Reversible alopecia is very common.

## Neurologic

Ten to twenty percent of patients will have symptoms of encephalopathy such as hallucinations, drowsiness, confusion, and depressive psychosis. Drowsiness is the most common symptom, and it can rapidly progress to coma. These symptoms are seen from a couple of hours to up to a couple of days after the administration of the drug. In any case, the drug should be immediately suspended. After halting the administration, the median duration of the symptoms is 3 days. Interactions with other CNS-depressing drugs must be considered and the drugs withdrawn. High doses of ifosfamide illogical truncation administered over a short time, preexisting neurologic or renal dysfunction, and low serum albumin appear to be significant risk factors. In patients with grade 3–4 encephalopathy, IV administration of methylene blue (50 mg every 4 h until symptoms resolve) may be considered. The pathophysiology of this encephalopathy is poorly understood, but the cause seems to be due to chloroacetaldehyde accumulation in the nervous system. It can be (1) directly neurotoxic, (2) deplete CNS glutathione, and (3) inhibit mitochondrial oxidative phosphorylation, leading to impaired fatty acid metabolism. Methylene blue has a redox potential and restores mitochondrial respiratory chain function; it prevents transformation of chloroethylamine into chloroacetaldehyde and restores hepatic gluconeogenesis [58]. Little evidence exists for the prophylactic use of methylene blue in combination with ifosfamide.

## Kidneys and Bladder

Micro- or macrohematuria is seen very commonly. It is dose dependent and can be prevented and/or alleviated by simultaneous administration of mesna. Mesna is an organosulfur compound. It is converted to an inactivated form in the blood and filtered by the kidneys, where it is reactivated. Ifosfamide and cyclophosphamide, when given in high doses, produce the metabolite acrolein, which is toxic to the bladder. Mesna binds to and inactivates acrolein, consequently reducing local side effects in bladder. If cystitis develops during ifosfamide administration despite correct mesna dosing, the treatment should be suspended until micro- or macrohematuria disappears. During ifosfamide infusion correct hydration is important, and the bladder must be emptied on a regular basis. Tubular damage has been proposed to be the cause of renal failure seen in some patients. Mesna does not protect against renal toxicity.

Hematologic

Patients pretreated with other chemotherapy regimens or radiotherapy and with preexisting renal insufficiency are at increased risk of myelotoxicity, which can sometimes be very important. Leukopenia is seen more often than thrombocytopenia. The nadir is at 8–10 days and is usually normalized at 3–4 weeks.

## Treatment of Leptomeningeal Carcinomatosis (Carcinomatous Meningitis)

Melanoma, breast and lung cancer, and hematologic and lymphoid malignancies are the most common origins of leptomeningeal dissemination [59]. Localized metastases may be treated by focal irradiation, while diffuse meningeal involvement requires intrathecal or high-dose systemic chemotherapy. Efficacy of intrathecal therapy may be limited by perturbed cerebrospinal fluid flow. Occasionally, direct intraventricular injection or access over a surgically implanted reservoir (Ommaya or Rickham) is preferred over administration by lumbar puncture, thus allowing a more homogenous distribution of the chemotherapeutic agent. The objective is to relieve and control symptoms, while often additional systemic therapy for adequate antitumor control is needed. In patients with high-risk hematologic malignancies, prophylactic intrathecal chemotherapy is often recommended [60]. Nevertheless, literature on the value of intrathecal therapy remains scarce and lacks controlled trials.

Three agents are used for intrathecal chemotherapy: cytarabine, methotrexate, and thiotepa. Adverse reactions are not uncommon. When administered intrathecally, chemical aseptic meningitis is the most common side effect seen in 20–40 % of patients and is characterized by fever, nausea and vomiting, headache, back pain radiating to the extremities, and photophobia. This can be reduced by using preservative-free diluent (saline) and preservative-free chemotherapy preparations. Late adverse events occurring more than 4–6 months after treatment, such as leukoencephalopathy with symptoms such as dementia and ataxia, must not be forgotten. The incidence is probably underestimated; it is probably higher than 20 % in patients surviving more than 4 months.

## Cytarabine

Cytarabine (araC) is an antimetabolic agent that damages DNA formation during the S phase of the cell cycle. The liposomal formulation of cytarabine [...] is lipophilic and has a long half-life. Liposomal cytarabine (DepoC  -> DepoCyte) is lipophilic long half-life. The liposomal formula maintains a therapeutic concentration in the CSF for 28 days, while the conventional form is entirely eliminated within 1–2 days [61]. Conventional intrathecal dose is 50 mg; with a short half-life, this should be repeated two times a week. In contrast, a liposomal formulation of cytarabine for prolonged cytotoxic exposure exists, thus requiring one administration (50 mg) every 2 weeks only. Liposomal cytarabine is approved for leptomeningeal metastases of hematologic malignancies [62].

### Systemic Doses of Cytarabine

Cytarabine is the most frequently used agent against acute leukemia. For more detailed information the reader is referred to the chapter on hematologic malignancies.

### Neurologic

In approximately 10 % of patients treated with high doses ($\geq 3$ g/m$^2$) administered intravenously every 12 h, an acute cerebellar syndrome develops [63]. The initial symptom is somnolence. Cerebellar signs are then noted on neurologic examination, and patients may not be able to ambulate. In many patients the symptoms usually resolve after the withdrawal of cytarabine, although prolonged and persistent symptoms have been observed. There is no specific therapy other than suspending chemotherapy.

Hematologic

High doses of cytarabine will induce profound myelosuppression.

Gastrointestinal

Diarrhea, mucositis, intestinal ulceration, and ileus can be seen. The gastrointestinal side effects are often dose limiting.

## Methotrexate

Methotrexate (MTX) is a folate antimetabolite, thus interfering with DNA synthesis, repair, and cellular replication. Methotrexate has been used for a wide variety of cancers (sarcomas, lymphomas, breast cancer) and also for autoimmune disorders. Methotrexate has a very good distribution in all tissues [64]. While passage through the blood–brain barrier requires administration of high systemic doses to obtain adequate drug concentrations in the central nervous system, intrathecal administration will allow the use of lower doses for the control of leptomeningeal disease with less systemic toxicity. However, drug penetration is limited to the distribution of the cerebrospinal fluid. The dose of MTX varies greatly from oral weekly 10 mg/m$^2$ for rheumatoid arthritis [65] to high-dose chemotherapy of ≥3 g/m$^2$ in primary brain lymphomas or up to 12 g/m$^2$ for osteosarcoma patients [66]. The commonly used dose for intrathecal administration is 12.5–15 mg/dose, which is to be repeated once or twice per week until the CSF clears and then once a week or once a month for maintenance treatment. A more intensive regimen proposed is 15 mg/day for 5 consecutive days every 2 weeks [67]; its relative efficacy has not been formally investigated.

## Hematologic

Myelosuppression can be seen when administered intrathecally.

## Transverse Myelopathy

An isolated spinal cord dysfunction develops rarely hours to days after the administration of MTX without compressive lesion. Patients develop back or leg pain followed by paraplegia, sensory loss, and sphincter dysfunction. The majority of patients recover, but further administration is contraindicated.

## Acute Encephalopathy

Somnolence, confusion, and seizures are seen within 24 h after treatment; they usually resolve spontaneously.

## Subacute Encephalopathy

After repeated injections of MTX, motor function impairments such as paraparesis/paraplegia, tetraplegia, cerebellar dysfunction, cranial nerve paralysis, and seizures can occur.

## Methotrexate Administered in High Doses Intravenously

Intravenous administration of high doses ($>3$ g/m$^2$) of MTX may also be used in the treatment of meningeal disease to achieve cytotoxic doses in the CNS. The incidence and severity of acute side effects are related to dose and frequency of administration. In primary lymphoma of the central nervous system, high-dose IV MTX is the backbone of therapy. Methotrexate is also an active agent in systemic breast cancer and may allow the control of leptomeningeal disease.

Younger patients seem to better tolerate the high-dose MTX therapy, presumably due to better end-organ function and rapid elimination. Caution is to be used in patients with renal and hepatic insufficiency. The common side effects of high-dose MTX are alopecia, neutropenia, renal toxicity (more commonly in older patients), nausea, diarrhea, and stomatitis. Hepatic toxicity with transaminitis is seen.

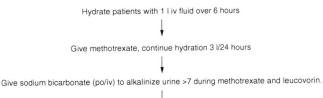

Hydrate patients with 1 l iv fluid over 6 hours

Give methotrexate, continue hydration 3 l/24 hours

Give sodium bicarbonate (po/iv) to alkalinize urine >7 during methotrexate and leucovorin.

At least 24h after beginning of high-dose methotrexate, start rescue with leucovorin.

24 hours after initiating the treatment with methotrexate: measure S-methotrexate, continue 1×/24h. Adapt doses of leucovorin according to concentration of methotrexate: higher concentration: higher dose. Control kidney and liver functions closely.

Give leucovorin at least 72h after initiation of methotrexate. Only stop when methotrexate concentration is below 0.1μmol/l.

FIGURE 7.3 Administration of high-dose methotrexate with leuco-vorin rescue

The presence of third-space fluids is a contraindication to the administration of high-dose MTX. High concentrations of MTX can accumulate in these spaces, leading to a prolonged MTX exposure and increased toxicity. Drainage of ascites or pleural effusion must be done before introducing the drug.

The use of high-dose IV MTX has been associated with the development of chronic delayed leukoencephalopathy in patients with or without a history of craniospinal irradiation.

High-dose MTX is a potential lethal dose, and before leucovorin rescue was initiated as a standard part of the regimen, 6 % drug-related death was noted, most frequently due to the immunosuppression. Therefore, high-dose MTX administration is followed by leucovorin rescue to inhibit the toxicity of MTX on the normal cells (Fig. 7.3). The timing of the rescue is important, since introducing too early the rescue leads to a diminished effect on the tumor cells. The administration of leucovorin can be delayed up to 24–36 h without, in general, important MTX toxicity. Several schedules of leucovorin rescue exist. If the concentration of MTX is higher than 1 μmol/L at 48 h, increasing the dose of leucovorin must be considered.

The rescue must continue for at least 72 h and until the concentration of MTX is at a nontoxic level (0.01–0.1 μmol/L).

Methotrexate is principally excreted by the kidneys. A glomerular filtration rate of 60 mL/min is in general considered as a minimum for high-dose MTX administration. It should be noted that the presence of a normal serum creatinine does not predict MTX toxicity [68]. A high urine flow and an alkaline pH must be ensured to prevent precipitation of MTX in the urine, causing nephrotoxicity.

## Thiotepa

Thiotepa is an alkylating agent. It crosses the blood–brain barrier well, achieving high concentrations and resulting in high levels of the active metabolite, TEPA. When administered intrathecally, thiotepa is cleared from CSF within minutes and completely eliminated within 4 h. The initial dose is 10 mg twice weekly for 4 weeks followed by one injection per week for another 4 weeks, with maintenance with one injection per month. Due to its important hematotoxicity, intrathecal administration is preferred, because it is generally well tolerated [69].

### Hematologic

Systemic myelosuppression has been seen even with intrathecal administration. Systemic administration of thiotepa causes profound bone marrow suppression, especially thrombocytopenia.

# Supportive Care

## Corticosteroids

The use of corticosteroids is the cornerstone for symptom relief in CNS tumors [70]. Primary or secondary malignancies arising in the brain perturb the normal vasculature and induce inflammation, with water extravasation leading to an increase of the intracranial pressure (ICP). The most important symptoms of increased ICP are fatigue, headaches, nausea and vomiting, bradycardia, and bradypnea. If untreated, increased ICP will result in brain herniation and ultimately death. The rapid initiation of corticosteroids could potentially reduce edema and also the symptoms. The most frequently used corticosteroid is dexamethasone, which has less pronounced mineralocorticoid effects than other steroids. The initial dose of dexamethasone is a 10-mg IV bolus followed by 4 mg every 6 h (16 mg/day). Since this scheme does not follow the normal diurnal changes of blood corticoids, we prefer the scheme of 8 mg twice a day in the morning and at noon. This administration reduces insomnia induced by dexamethasone. In dose-finding studies dexamethasone had been increased up to 40 mg, but there was no evidence for improved effectiveness. Once the desired acute effect has been achieved, the dose of dexamethasone should be rapidly tapered in order to avoid long-term perturbation of the hypothalamic-pituitary-adrenocortical (HPA) axis and toxicity from prolonged corticosteroid administration. Tapering consists in empiric reduction of 2–4 mg every 2–3 days. While the initial reduction in doses – empiric reduction of 2–4 mg every 2–3 days – can be rapid, the final tapering before definitive cessation of the treatment should be done more slowly, with decrements of 0.5–1 mg every 3–7 days, depending on the duration of prior steroid exposure. Common side effects are hyperglycemia, gastritis, gastrointestinal bleeding, osteoporosis, immunosuppression, skin fragility and striae, obesity, psychosis and euphoria, or myopathy with weakness of the lower extremities and neck. Steroid-induced myopathy and secondary diabetes may be misleading of disease progression and need to be excluded. Restrictive steroid prescription and appropriate surveillance may prevent these frequent complications.

## Antiepileptics

The most common side effects of antiepileptic drugs (AEDs) are gastrointestinal toxicity in the form of nausea, vomiting, and diarrhea, and skin rash. Further common side effects of

AEDs are sleepiness and unsteadiness. Carbamazepine, phenobarbital, phenytoin, and sodium valproate could induce osteoporosis or osteomalacia. Furthermore, AEDs can influence memory, especially when high doses are applied. In case side effects are detected, either dose reduction should be tried or a rotation should be proposed with an AED with a different class of effect. Antiepileptic drugs such as phenytoin, phenobarbital, and carbamazepine induce the hepatic enzyme P450 (enzyme-inducing antiepileptic drugs, EIADs). Several chemotherapeutic agents, including, irinotecan, lomustine, vincristine, and procarbazine, are metabolized by the cytochrome P450. While patients with malignant gliomas are treated with these therapies, their metabolism can be increased and thus can lead to diminished efficacy. Brain tumor patients treated with EIAEDs are recommended to change to third-generation antiepileptic drugs like levetiracetam.

# References

1. Soussain C, Ricard D, Fike JR, Mazeron JJ, Psimaras D, Delattre JY. CNS complications of radiotherapy and chemotherapy. Lancet. 2009;374(9701):1639–51. Epub 10 Nov 2009.
2. Conill C, Berenguer J, Vargas M, Lopez-Soriano A, Valduvieco I, Marruecos J, et al. Incidence of radiation-induced leukoencephalopathy after whole brain radiotherapy in patients with brain metastases. Clin Transl Oncol. 2007;9(9):590–5. Epub 9 Oct 2007.
3. Dresemann G. Temozolomide in malignant glioma. Onco Targets Ther. 2010;3:139–46. Epub 22 Sept 2010.
4. Brock CS, Newlands ES, Wedge SR, Bower M, Evans H, Colquhoun I, et al. Phase I trial of temozolomide using an extended continuous oral schedule. Cancer Res. 1998;58(19):4363–7.
5. Stupp R, Mason WP, van den Bent MJ, Weller M, Fisher B, Taphoorn MJ, et al. Radiotherapy plus concomitant and adjuvant temozolomide for glioblastoma. N Engl J Med. 2005;352(10):987–96. Epub 11 Mar 2005.
6. Perry JR, Belanger K, Mason WP, Fulton D, Kavan P, Easaw J, et al. Phase II trial of continuous dose-intense temozolomide in recurrent malignant glioma: RESCUE study. J Clin Oncol. 2010;28(12):2051–7.
7. Tolcher AW, Gerson SL, Denis L, Geyer C, Hammond LA, Patnaik A, et al. Marked inactivation of O6-alkylguanine-DNA alkyltransferase activity with protracted temozolomide schedules. Br J Cancer. 2003;88(7):1004–11.

8. Vera K, Djafari L, Faivre S, Guillamo JS, Djazouli K, Osorio M, et al. Dose-dense regimen of temozolomide given every other week in patients with primary central nervous system tumors. Ann Oncol. 2004;15(1):161–71.

9. Stupp R, van den Bent MJ, Hegi ME. Optimal role of temozolomide in the treatment of malignant gliomas. Curr Neurol Neurosci Rep. 2005;5(3):198–206. Epub 4 May 2005.

10. Abrey LE, Christodoulou C. Temozolomide for treating brain metastases. Semin Oncol. 2001;28(4 Suppl 13):34–42. Epub 11 Sept 2001.

11. Cohen MH, Johnson JR, Pazdur R. Food and Drug Administration drug approval summary: temozolomide plus radiation therapy for the treatment of newly diagnosed glioblastoma multiforme. Clin Cancer Res. 2005;11(19 Pt 1):6767–71.

12. Stupp R, Dietrich PY, Ostermann Kraljevic S, Pica A, Maillard I, Maeder P, et al. Promising survival for patients with newly diagnosed glioblastoma multiforme treated with concomitant radiation plus temozolomide followed by adjuvant temozolomide. J Clin Oncol. 2002;20(5):1375–82. Epub 1 Mar 2002.

13. Su YB, Sohn S, Krown SE, Livingston PO, Wolchok JD, Quinn C, et al. Selective CD4+ lymphopenia in melanoma patients treated with temozolomide: a toxicity with therapeutic implications. J Clin Oncol. 2004;22(4):610–6. Epub 17 Jan 2004.

14. Levin VA, Wara WM, Davis RL, Vestnys P, Resser KJ, Yatsko K, et al. Phase III comparison of BCNU and the combination of procarbazine, CCNU, and vincristine administered after radiotherapy with hydroxyurea for malignant gliomas. J Neurosurg. 1985;63(2):218–23. Epub 1 Aug 1985.

15. Katz ME, Glick JH. Nitrosoureas: a reappraisal of clinical trials. Cancer Clin Trials. 1979;2(4):297–316. Epub 1 Jan 1979.

16. Gutin PH, Wilson CB, Kumar AR, Boldrey EB, Levin V, Powell M, et al. Phase II study of procarbazine, CCNU, and vincristine combination chemotherapy in the treatment of malignant brain tumors. Cancer. 1975;35(5):1398–404. Epub 1 May 1975.

17. Reithmeier T, Graf E, Piroth T, Trippel M, Pinsker MO, Nikkhah G. BCNU for recurrent glioblastoma multiforme: efficacy, toxicity and prognostic factors. BMC Cancer. 2010;10:30. Epub 4 Feb 2010.

18. Block M, Lachowiez RM, Rios C, Hirschl S. Pulmonary fibrosis associated with low-dose adjuvant methyl-CCNU. Med Pediatr Oncol. 1990;18(3):256–60. Epub 1 Jan 1990.

19. Lee C, Gianos M, Klaustermeyer WB. Diagnosis and management of hypersensitivity reactions related to common cancer chemotherapy agents. Ann Allergy Asthma Immunol. 2009;102(3):179–87; quiz 87–9, 222. Epub 10 Apr 2009.

20. Lehmann DF, Hurteau TE, Newman N, Coyle TE. Anticonvulsant usage is associated with an increased risk of procarbazine hypersensitivity reactions in patients with brain tumors. Clin Pharmacol Ther. 1997;62(2):225–9. Epub 1 Aug 1997.

21. Mahmood T, Mudad R. Pulmonary toxicity secondary to procarbazine. Am J Clin Oncol. 2002;25(2):187–8. Epub 11 Apr 2002.
22. Aydin B, Patil M, Bekele N, Wolff JE. Vincristine in high-grade glioma. Anticancer Res. 2010;30(6):2303–10. Epub 24 July 2010.
23. Boyle FM, Eller SL, Grossman SA. Penetration of intra-arterially administered vincristine in experimental brain tumor. Neuro Oncol. 2004;6(4):300–5. Epub 21 Oct 2004.
24. Qweider M, Gilsbach JM, Rohde V. Inadvertent intrathecal vincristine administration: a neurosurgical emergency. Case report. J Neurosurg Spine. 2007;6(3):280–3. Epub 16 Mar 2007.
25. Al Ferayan A, Russell NA, Al Wohaibi M, Awada A, Scherman B. Cerebrospinal fluid lavage in the treatment of inadvertent intrathecal vincristine injection. Childs Nerv Syst. 1999;15(2–3):87–9. Epub 7 May 1999.
26. Michelagnoli MP, Bailey CC, Wilson I, Livingston J, Kinsey SE. Potential salvage therapy for inadvertent intrathecal administration of vincristine. Br J Haematol. 1997;99(2):364–7. Epub 31 Dec 1997.
27. Thakur JS, Chauhan CG, Diwana VK, Chauhan DC, Thakur A. Extravasational side effects of cytotoxic drugs: a preventable catastrophe. Indian J Plast Surg. 2008;41(2):145–50. Epub 1 July 2008.
28. Glade-Bender J, Kandel JJ, Yamashiro DJ. VEGF blocking therapy in the treatment of cancer. Expert Opin Biol Ther. 2003;3(2):263–76. Epub 29 Mar 2003.
29. Garfield DH, Hercbergs A. Fewer dollars, more sense. J Clin Oncol. 2008;26(32):5304–5; author reply 5. Epub 16 Oct 2008.
30. Keunen O, Johansson M, Oudin A, Sanzey M, Rahim SA, Fack F, et al. Anti-VEGF treatment reduces blood supply and increases tumor cell invasion in glioblastoma. Proc Natl Acad Sci USA. 2011;108(9):3749–54. Epub 16 Feb 2011.
31. Paez-Ribes M, Allen E, Hudock J, Takeda T, Okuyama H, Vinals F, et al. Antiangiogenic therapy elicits malignant progression of tumors to increased local invasion and distant metastasis. Cancer Cell. 2009;15(3):220–31. Epub 3 Mar 2009.
32. Robinson ES, Khankin EV, Choueiri TK, Dhawan MS, Rogers MJ, Karumanchi SA, et al. Suppression of the nitric oxide pathway in metastatic renal cell carcinoma patients receiving vascular endothelial growth factor-signaling inhibitors. Hypertension. 2010;56(6):1131–6. Epub 20 Oct 2010.
33. Nazer B, Humphreys BD, Moslehi J. Effects of novel angiogenesis inhibitors for the treatment of cancer on the cardiovascular system: focus on hypertension. Circulation. 2011;124(15):1687–91. Epub 12 Oct 2011.
34. Friedman HS, Prados MD, Wen PY, Mikkelsen T, Schiff D, Abrey LE, et al. Bevacizumab alone and in combination with irinotecan in recurrent glioblastoma. J Clin Oncol. 2009;27(28):4733–40. Epub 2 Sept 2009.

35. Copur MS, Obermiller A. An algorithm for the management of hypertension in the setting of vascular endothelial growth factor signaling inhibition. Clin Colorectal Cancer. 2011;10(3):151–6. Epub 23 Aug 2011.
36. Izzedine H, Massard C, Spano JP, Goldwasser F, Khayat D, Soria JC. VEGF signalling inhibition-induced proteinuria: mechanisms, significance and management. Eur J Cancer. 2010;46(2):439–48. Epub 17 Dec 2009.
37. Semrad TJ, O'Donnell R, Wun T, Chew H, Harvey D, Zhou H, et al. Epidemiology of venous thromboembolism in 9489 patients with malignant glioma. J Neurosurg. 2007;106(4):601–8. Epub 17 Apr 2007.
38. Hurwitz HI, Saltz LB, Van Cutsem E, Cassidy J, Wiedemann J, Sirzen F, et al. Venous thromboembolic events with chemotherapy plus bevacizumab: a pooled analysis of patients in randomized phase II and III studies. J Clin Oncol. 2011;29(13):1757–64. Epub 23 Mar 2011.
39. Norden AD, Bartolomeo J, Tanaka S, Drappatz J, Ciampa AS, Doherty LM, et al. Safety of concurrent bevacizumab therapy and anticoagulation in glioma patients. J Neurooncol. 2012;106(1):121–5. Epub 28 June 2011.
40. Agnelli G, George DJ, Kakkar AK, Fisher W, Lassen MR, Mismetti P, et al. Semuloparin for thromboprophylaxis in patients receiving chemotherapy for cancer. N Engl J Med. 2012;366(7):601–9. Epub 18 Feb 2012.
41. Ranpura V, Hapani S, Wu S. Treatment-related mortality with bevacizumab in cancer patients: a meta-analysis. JAMA. 2011;305(5):487–94. Epub 3 Feb 2011.
42. Hompes D, Ruers T. Review: incidence and clinical significance of Bevacizumab-related non-surgical and surgical serious adverse events in metastatic colorectal cancer. Eur J Surg Oncol. 2011;37(9):737–46. Epub 19 July 2011.
43. Clark AJ, Butowski NA, Chang SM, Prados MD, Clarke J, Polley MY, et al. Impact of bevacizumab chemotherapy on craniotomy wound healing. J Neurosurg. 2011;114(6):1609–16. Epub 15 Dec 2010.
44. Hapani S, Chu D, Wu S. Risk of gastrointestinal perforation in patients with cancer treated with bevacizumab: a meta-analysis. Lancet Oncol. 2009;10(6):559–68. Epub 2 June 2009.
45. Hawkes EA, Okines AF, Plummer C, Cunningham D. Cardiotoxicity in patients treated with bevacizumab is potentially reversible. J Clin Oncol. 2011;29(18):e560–2. Epub 25 May 2011.
46. Lou E, Turner S, Sumrall A, Reardon DA, Desjardins A, Peters KB, et al. Bevacizumab-induced reversible posterior leukoencephalopathy syndrome and successful retreatment in a patient with glioblastoma. J Clin Oncol. 2011;29(28):e739–42. Epub 9 Sept 2011.
47. Ohno R, Okada K, Masaoka T, Kuramoto A, Arima T, Yoshida Y, et al. An early phase II study of CPT-11: a new derivative of camptothecin, for the treatment of leukemia and lymphoma. J Clin Oncol. 1990;8(11):1907–12. Epub 1 Nov 1990.

48. Chu XY, Kato Y, Sugiyama Y. Multiplicity of biliary excretion mechanisms for irinotecan, CPT-11, and its metabolites in rats. Cancer Res. 1997;57(10):1934–8. Epub 15 May 1997.
49. Vredenburgh JJ, Desjardins A, Reardon DA, Friedman HS. Experience with irinotecan for the treatment of malignant glioma. Neuro Oncol. 2009;11(1):80–91. Epub 12 Sept 2008.
50. Douillard JY, Cunningham D, Roth AD, Navarro M, James RD, Karasek P, et al. Irinotecan combined with fluorouracil compared with fluorouracil alone as first-line treatment for metastatic colorectal cancer: a multicentre randomised trial. Lancet. 2000;355(9209):1041–7. Epub 1 Apr 2000.
51. Vredenburgh JJ, Desjardins A, Herndon 2nd JE, Marcello J, Reardon DA, Quinn JA, et al. Bevacizumab plus irinotecan in recurrent glioblastoma multiforme. J Clin Oncol. 2007;25(30):4722–9. Epub 20 Oct 2007.
52. Abigerges D, Chabot GG, Armand JP, Herait P, Gouyette A, Gandia D. Phase I and pharmacologic studies of the camptothecin analog irinotecan administered every 3 weeks in cancer patients. J Clin Oncol. 1995;13(1):210–21. Epub 1 Jan 1995.
53. Kaye SB, Mead GM, Fossa S, Cullen M, de Wit R, Bodrogi I, et al. Intensive induction-sequential chemotherapy with BOP/VIP-B compared with treatment with BEP/EP for poor-prognosis metastatic nonseminomatous germ cell tumor: a randomized Medical Research Council/European Organization for Research and Treatment of Cancer study. J Clin Oncol. 1998;16(2):692–701. Epub 20 Feb 1998.
54. Geyer JR, Sposto R, Jennings M, Boyett JM, Axtell RA, Breiger D, et al. Multiagent chemotherapy and deferred radiotherapy in infants with malignant brain tumors: a report from the Children's Cancer Group. J Clin Oncol. 2005;23(30):7621–31. Epub 20 Oct 2005.
55. Kiefer T, Hirt C, Spath C, Schuler F, Al-Ali HK, Wolf HH, et al. Long-term follow-up of high-dose chemotherapy with autologous stem-cell transplantation and response-adapted whole-brain radiotherapy for newly diagnosed primary CNS lymphoma: results of the multicenter Ostdeutsche Studiengruppe Hamatologie und Onkologie OSHO-53 phase II study. Ann Oncol. 2012;23(7):1809–12. Epub 24 Nov 2011.
56. Graber JJ, Omuro A. Pharmacotherapy for primary CNS lymphoma: progress beyond methotrexate? CNS Drugs. 2011;25(6):447–57. Epub 9 June 2011.
57. Yasuda K, Taguchi H, Sawamura Y, Ikeda J, Aoyama H, Fujieda K, et al. Low-dose craniospinal irradiation and ifosfamide, cisplatin and etoposide for non-metastatic embryonal tumors in the central nervous system. Jpn J Clin Oncol. 2008;38(7):486–92. Epub 25 June 2008.
58. Ajithkumar T, Parkinson C, Shamshad F, Murray P. Ifosfamide encephalopathy. Clin Oncol (R Coll Radiol). 2007;19(2):108–14. Epub 16 Mar 2007.

59. Groves MD. Leptomeningeal disease. Neurosurg Clin N Am. 2011;22(1):67–78, vii. Epub 27 Nov 2010.

60. Boogerd W, van den Bent MJ, Koehler PJ, Heimans JJ, van der Sande JJ, Aaronson NK, et al. The relevance of intraventricular chemotherapy for leptomeningeal metastasis in breast cancer: a randomised study. Eur J Cancer. 2004;40(18):2726–33. Epub 2 Dec 2004.

61. Chamberlain MC, Khatibi S, Kim JC, Howell SB, Chatelut E, Kim S. Treatment of leptomeningeal metastasis with intraventricular administration of depot cytarabine (DTC 101). A phase I study. Arch Neurol. 1993;50(3):261–4. Epub 1 Mar 1993.

62. Dunton SF, Nitschke R, Spruce WE, Bodensteiner J, Krous HF. Progressive ascending paralysis following administration of intrathecal and intravenous cytosine arabinoside. A Pediatric Oncology Group study. Cancer. 1986;57(6):1083–8. Epub 15 Mar 1986.

63. Rubin EH, Andersen JW, Berg DT, Schiffer CA, Mayer RJ, Stone RM. Risk factors for high-dose cytarabine neurotoxicity: an analysis of a cancer and leukemia group B trial in patients with acute myeloid leukemia. J Clin Oncol. 1992;10(6):948–53. Epub 1 June 1992.

64. Bleyer WA. The clinical pharmacology of methotrexate: new applications of an old drug. Cancer. 1978;41(1):36–51. Epub 1 Jan 1978.

65. Maini R, St. Clair EW, Breedveld F, Furst D, Kalden J, Weisman M, et al. Infliximab (chimeric anti-tumour necrosis factor alpha monoclonal antibody) versus placebo in rheumatoid arthritis patients receiving concomitant methotrexate: a randomised phase III trial. ATTRACT Study Group. Lancet. 1999;354(9194):1932–9. Epub 6 Jan 2000.

66. Bramwell VH, Burgers M, Sneath R, Souhami R, van Oosterom AT, Voute PA, et al. A comparison of two short intensive adjuvant chemotherapy regimens in operable osteosarcoma of limbs in children and young adults: the first study of the European Osteosarcoma Intergroup. J Clin Oncol. 1992;10(10):1579–91. Epub 1 Jan 1992.

67. Gauthier H, Guilhaume MN, Bidard FC, Pierga JY, Girre V, Cottu PH, et al. Survival of breast cancer patients with meningeal carcinomatosis. Ann Oncol. 2010;21(11):2183–7. Epub 1 May 2010.

68. Kerr IG, Jolivet J, Collins JM, Drake JC, Chabner BA. Test dose for predicting high-dose methotrexate infusions. Clin Pharmacol Ther. 1983;33(1):44–51. Epub 1 Jan 1983.

69. Berg SL, Poplack DG. Advances in the treatment of meningeal cancers. Crit Rev Oncol Hematol. 1995;20(1–2):87–98. Epub 1 Aug 1995.

70. Dietrich J, Rao K, Pastorino S, Kesari S. Corticosteroids in brain cancer patients: benefits and pitfalls. Expert Rev Clin Pharmacol. 2011;4(2):233–42. Epub 15 June 2011.

# Chapter 8
# Bone Marrow Toxicity: Red Blood Cells

**Pere Gascon**

**Abstract**  Anemia is a common manifestation in patients with cancer. Its cause can be multifactorial: the cancer itself, chemotherapy treatments, infiltration of bone marrow by cancer cells, hemolysis, nutritional deficiencies, blood loss, inflammation, and so forth. A major consequence of anemia is fatigue, a symptom that impacts the quality of life of cancer patients, and it can also compromise patients' compliance with their treatments. A new generation of anticancer agents, antitargeted therapies, is widely used in oncology. Some of these new agents are associated with anemia, although their mechanism is not yet understood.

We now have different options to correct chemotherapy- or cancer treatment–induced anemia: red blood cell (RBC) transfusions, iron, and erythropoiesis-stimulating agents (ESAs). Their safety profile is good if we know when and how to administer them.

Red blood cell transfusions are reserved for critical situations, when the patient presents with symptomatic severe

P. Gascon, M.D., Ph.D.
Division of Medical Oncology, Department of Hematology-Oncology,
Institut Clinic de Malalties Hemato-Oncologiques,
Barcelona, Spain
e-mail: gascon@clinic.ub.es

M.A. Dicato (ed.), *Side Effects of Medical Cancer Therapy*,       333
DOI 10.1007/978-0-85729-787-7_8,
© Springer-Verlag London 2013

anemia. In addition to the possibility that the RBCs carry viruses and other pathogens, some new alarm signals associated with their use have been raised over the last few years and are currently being investigated. Of particular concern are RBCs that have been stored for more than 2 weeks in the blood banks. Apparently, they lose some of their oxygen-carrying capacity and their ability to cross the capillaries.

Iron has long been an agent used to correct the anemia of blood loss. Recently, however, the administration of intravenous iron has become more popular, because the new preparations do not provoke the allergic and anaphylactic reactions seen with the old preparations. Intravenous iron is now being used in combination with ESAs to produce faster and more robust corrections of anemia in the so-called functional iron deficiency, a type of anemia associated with chronic diseases and inflammation. In this condition there is a need for soluble iron, because one of the factors released during inflammation is hepcidin, a peptide that blocks the absorption of oral iron in the duodenum.

Finally, oncologists can utilize ESAs (recombinant human erythropoietin) for chemotherapy-induced anemia. Although, they have been used for more than 20 years, over the last 5 years, several alarm signals have been associated with them. Their safety has been questioned after few clinical trial publications reported a poor outcome in patients receiving these agents in comparison to the control arm without ESAs. Many hypotheses have been suggested: ESAs would promote tumor growth via the presence of EPO receptors in cancer cells, a fact seriously questioned by recent publications; ESAs induce thromboembolic events; and so on. Another adverse event associated with the use of ESAs is pure red cell aplasia, in which the ESA molecule undergoes some structural changes due to physical or chemical conditions, causing the development of anti-EPO antibodies. This situation has been described only in patients with chronic renal failure receiving ESAs. The latest meta-analysis on ESAs regarding adverse events concludes that as long as ESAs are being used according to registry specifications in the setting of chemotherapy-induced anemia and the level of hemoglobin does not go beyond 12 g/dL, their use is safe.

**Keywords**  Anemia • Red blood cell transfusions • Iron Erythropoiesis-stimulating agents • Adverse events • Pure red cell aplasia • Erythropoietin • Thromboembolic events

# Frequency and Causes of Anemia in Oncology

Anemia is a common manifestation in patients with cancer. More than 80 % of cancer patients undergoing chemotherapy develop anemia (hemoglobin [Hb] level <12 g/dL) [1]. Information on the prevalence and effects of anemia can be found in the literature from clinical trials of anemia treatments or chemotherapy [2–7]. The data generated by these studies came from well-designed and selected populations of patients. However, little was known about what happens day to day in doctors' offices or hospitals until the European Cancer Anemia Survey (ECAS) study was published [1]. This study, in which 15,367 patients were evaluated, is probably the best ever performed to understand the incidence and prevalence of anemia in cancer patients. This prospective study demonstrated a prevalence of anemia at enrollment of 39.3 % (Hb < 10.0 g/dL, 10 %) and 67.0 % during the survey (Hb < 10.0 g/dL, 39.3 %). Low Hb levels were found to correlate with poor performance status. Incidence of anemia was 53.7 % (Hb < 19 g/dL, 15.2 %).

Anemia in the cancer patient can be caused by a variety of conditions in what constitutes the so-called anemic syndrome, either caused by the same tumor or by the effects or complications of cancer treatments [1]. The causes of anemia are multifactorial: (1) bone marrow infiltration by cancer cells; (2) nutritional deficits such as vitamin B12, folic acid, or iron; (3) hemolysis; (4) myelosupression secondary to chemotherapy or radiotherapy; (5) toxicity induced by the new antitargeted therapies; (6) low endogenous erythropoietin levels; and (7) anemia of chronic disease, also known as functional iron deficiency (Fig. 8.1). The unexpected finding of low erythropoietin levels in cancer patients by Miller et al. in 1990 [8], together with the toxicity induced by chemotherapy, sets

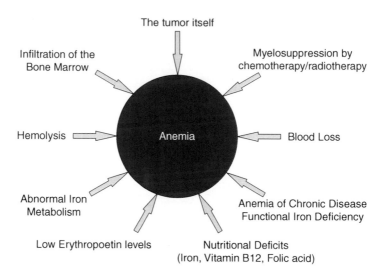

The tumor itself

Infiltration of the
Bone Marrow

Myelosuppression by
chemotherapy/radiotherapy

Hemolysis

Anemia

Blood Loss

Abnormal Iron
Metabolism

Anemia of Chronic Disease
Functional Iron Deficiency

Low Erythropoetin levels

Nutritional Deficits
(Iron, Vitamin B12, Folic acid)

FIGURE 8.1 Causes of anemia in the patient with cancer (Adapted from [2, 8, 9])

the basis for the use of this agent in cancer patients. Vitamin B12, folic acid, and iron are necessary factors for red blood cell production. Blood loss can be a common association, particularly in colorectal cancer, endometrial cancer (bleeding), or lung cancer (hemoptysis). Anemia can be seen occasionally in cancer patients due to hemolysis secondary to particular chemotherapeutic agents. A short red blood cell half-life has also been reported [9].

Anemia in cancer can also be caused indirectly by the same inflammatory process associated with the disease. In this case, cytokines are produced, with some of them having relevant biological effects with regard to anemia. Two of them, interleukin-1 (IL-1$\alpha$ [alpha], $\beta$ [beta]) and tumor necrosis factor (TNF-$\alpha$ [alpha]), are known to inhibit the production of erythropoietin by the kidneys. Another important cytokine is IL-6, a proinflammatory factor that acts on the liver to induce the production of hepcidin, a small peptide that has an important role in iron metabolism [10, 11]. It is considered the most important factor in the anemia of chronic disease, also known as functional iron deficiency.

Hepcidin induces the degradation of ferroportin, the iron transport protein from the gastrointestinal tract cells or from iron-storage pools in reticuloendothelial cells, mainly macrophages. In other words, hepcidin works in the duodenum, inhibiting the oral absorption of iron, and in the bone marrow, blocking the release of the iron contained in the macrophages. It is understandable that with this scenario, the red blood cells' progenitors lack the two major sources of iron for new red blood cell formation: the gastrointestinal tract, where the enterocytes are unable to absorb either nutritional or therapeutic iron, and the bone marrow, where the macrophages, scavenger cells, do not release the sequestrated iron obtained from the senescent red blood cells [12].

The fact that chemotherapy agents induce anemia is well known. Because dividing cells are targets for these agents, we observed cytotoxicity on cancer cells as well as toxicity in bone marrow cells (myelotoxicity), since most of these cells are in a constant proliferative state. However, we are now facing a quite different scenario in treating cancer since the arrival to our hospital pharmacies of the new targeted agents (tyrosine kinase inhibitors, mTOR inhibitors, monoclonal antibodies, antiangiogenics, etc.). Interestingly, some reports recently published show some of these new agents causing grade 1–2 anemia (range: 15–30 %). Among the monoclonal antibodies, trastuzumab has been associated with mild anemia, and bevacizumab has a reduced risk of anemia effect [13–17]. The mechanism(s) of anemia are still unknown for all new targeted agents. Some recent publications established that many of these agents induce by themselves various degrees of fatigue, in some cases quite important, and independently of the level of Hb of the patient.

# The Therapy of Anemia

## Red Blood Cell Transfusions

Prior to the introduction of human recombinant epoetins, there were no other treatment options for the correction of anemia than red blood cell transfusions or iron; in many cases, the option was not to give anything. The AIDS epidemic puts blood transfusions under the magnifying glass, and although the safety of our modern blood banks has never been so good, still blood transfusions are associated with unwanted effects. A transfusion of red blood cells causes a sharp increase in Hb level as well as an increase in blood viscosity that varies with the number of units transfused. Interestingly, there has been no large clinical trial to demonstrate an improvement in quality of life after blood transfusions, as has been the case for epoetins.

## Erythropoiesis-Stimulating Agents

Human recombinant epoetins were introduced in the early 1990s. Initially there were epoetin alfa and epoetin beta. Both agents are similar to the endogenous molecule, erythropoietin. Ten years later, a new modified erythropoietin molecule was introduced in our pharmacies, darbepoetin alfa. Since the three molecules stimulate erythropoiesis, they are currently called erythropoiesis-stimulating agents (ESAs) (Table 8.1). Over the last 20 years, more than 15,000 cancer patients with anemia have been enrolled in multiple clinical trials of ESAs to assess the efficacy, side effects, and quality of life. This massive clinical experience with ESAs has demonstrated that they are well tolerated and can effectively increase Hb levels and decrease transfusion use [3–7, 9, 18, 19]. Initially, epoetins were administrated three times weekly following the pattern used for dialysis in chronic renal failure patients. Lately, once-a-week administration has become the most popular schedule. In addition, darbepoetin alfa has an administration schedule of every 3 weeks, besides the once-a-week presentation [20]. In general, ESAs produce significant decreases in transfusion requirements and significant increases in Hb level (around 1 g/dL in 4 weeks), with hematopoietic response rates ranging from 55 to 74 % [3–7, 9, 18, 19]. In addition, correction of the anemia by ESAs has been correlated, in a significant way, with improvement in the quality of life of cancer-anemic patients. Fatigue is a major symptom of anemia. Cancer-related fatigue

TABLE 8.1   Erythropoiesis-stimulating agents

| | Darbepoetin alfa (Aranesp) | Epoetin alfa (Eprex/Epogen) | Epoetin beta (NeoRecormon) |
|---|---|---|---|
| Indication | Chemotherapy-induced anemia in solid tumors | Chemotherapy-induced anemia in solid tumors, lymphoma, or multiple myeloma | Treatment and prevention of anemia in platinum-based chemotherapy in solid tumors, multiple myeloma, low-grade myeloma, non-Hodgkin, and chronic lymphocytic leukemia |
| Bioequivalence | 1 μg | 200 U | 200 U |
| Preparations/schedule | 150 μg/sc QW = 30,000 U[a] | 10,000 U sc/TIW | 10,000 U sc/TIW |
| | 500 μg/sc QTW = 100,000 U[a] | 30,000 U sc/QW | 30,000 U sc/QW |
| | | 40,000 U sc/QW | |

[a] Approved dose/regimen

has a profound effect on patient quality of life, affecting physical and emotional well-being, as well as relationships with family and friends. The greatest incremental improvement in quality of life occurs when the Hb level increases from 11 to 12 g/dL (range: 11–13 g/dL) [21].

As a result of so many social and medical changes in attitude, anemia management practices have changed over the years. This is reflected by the guidelines for anemia treatment issued first by the American Society of Hematology (ASH) jointly with the American Society of Clinical Oncology (ASCO) [22], by the National Comprehensive Cancer Network (NCCN) [23] and, more recently, by the European Organisation for Research and Treatment of Cancer [24]. The three guidelines strongly recommended ESA treatment for cancer patients with anemia receiving chemotherapy who have a Hb level <10 g/dL. However, the three guidelines differ somewhat regarding recommendations for treatment of patients with Hb levels of 10–12 g/dL. The correction of anemia should not go over 12 g/dL (Table 8.2) [28].

Recently, a new generation of ESA-like agents has been approved by the European Regulatory Agency (EMA). The loss of the patent of the originals has produced a new generation of similar but not identical agents. These are called biosimilars in Europe or follow-on biologics in the United States [29]. Among the biosimilars for anemia, there are already three approved agents: HX575, XM01 (in reality, this agent is an original if one follows its clinical development), and SB309. All these agents receive different trade names in occasions with the same agent. For instance, HX575 has been registered with three different names: Binocrit (Sandoz, Princeton, NJ, USA), Epoetina Hexal (Hexal Biotech, Germany), and Abseamed (Medice Arzneimittel Putter, Germany). Another biosimilar, SB309, has been registered as epoetin zeta and its trade names, Silapo (STADA, Bad Vilbel, Germany) and Retacrit (Hospira, Warwickshire, UK). The third biosimilar for anemia is epoetin theta. In fact, this agent is an original but generally is included in the biosimilar list, probably owing to the timing of its introduction to the market, the same as the real biosimilars. Its trade name is Eporatio (Ratiopharm-TEVA, Ulm, Germany) [29].

TABLE 8.2 Summary of international evidence-based guidelines for treating cancer-induced anemia

| Recommendation | ASCO/ASH | NCCN | EORTC [10] | ESMO [25] |
|---|---|---|---|---|
| Initiate ESA therapy | Hb ≤10 g/dL (clinical decision if Hb 10 to ≤12 g/dL) | Hb ≤11 g/dL | Hb 9–11 g/dL (clinical decision if Hb ≤11.9 g/dL) | Hb ≤10 g/dL |
| Goal of treatment | The lowest Hb concentration needed to avoid transfusions | Maintain Hb between 10 and 12 g/dL | Target Hb should be around 12 g/dL | Hb should not exceed 12 g/dL |

Rizzo et al. [26]
NCCN Clinical Practice Guidelines in Oncology [27]

ESAs should be given to patients with chemotherapy-induced anemia to reduce blood transfusions and to increase quality of life. ESAs should not be given when there are other treatable causes of anemia, such as iron deficiency anemia or vitamin deficiencies. ESAs should not be given in radiotherapy when this treatment option is the only anticancer treatment or in anemia associated with cancer in the absence of any active anticancer treatment.

## Iron

It is well known that ESAs have a response rate that is suboptimal, ranging from 55 to 74 % in most published clinical trials [30]. Several explanations have been found, but in general it is accepted mostly due to functional iron deficiency. The remarkable improvement in the response rate observed with the concomitant administration of intravenous iron to ESAs strongly suggests this possibility. Functional iron deficiency (i.e., lack of bioavailable iron) is a clinical entity where erythropoiesis is impaired owing in part to the sequestration of iron [31] by the macrophages and a blockage of enteral iron absorption mostly mediated by hepcidin [31]. In other words, oral iron is poorly absorbed or not absorbed at all, and bone marrow iron, although present in the bone marrow, is not available to the making of red blood cells. Parenteral iron therapy has subsequently become an important adjunct to obtaining and maintaining adequate Hb levels in patients with cancer who are receiving chemotherapy. However, despite the good results observed with parenteral iron, many oncologists are still reluctant to use it because of the poor safety profile observed in the past with the old iron preparations, particularly high molecular weight dextran (HMWD). The new intravenous preparations (ferric gluconate, ferric carboxymaltose, iron isomaltoside, iron sucrose) show not only a much better safety profile but a much easier administration.

Over the last few years, seven studies on the use of intravenous iron supplementation have been conducted and their results published. In all cases, intravenous iron was delivered concomitantly with ESAs in the treatment of anemia secondary to chemotherapy [32–37]. Except in one study, the study by Steensma et al. [38], all others were favorable to the arm of intravenous iron. In this study, the authors compared parenteral, oral, or no iron supplementation in patients with chemotherapy-associated anemia treated with darbepoetin alfa [38]. Interestingly, the results contrast with the other six other publications [32–37] and two reported clinical trials [39,40] on the benefits of supplementing iron intravenously in patients receiving a concomitant ESA. It is tempting to posit some potential explanations. The first likely explanation is that the total administered dose of iron seems to be low, approximately 650 mg total [41], compared to the Bastit study [35], which is very similar in design to the Steensma study [38]. In the former, the total iron dose delivered was 400 mg higher [41]. This fact has to do with the design of this study, which planned a total iron dose of 937.5 mg iron, which represents the second lowest dose of iron among the published trials (750–3,000 mg). Furthermore, it would be the lowest dose when calculated on a weekly basis (62.5 mg/week). This, by itself, may have limited the potential benefit of intravenous iron supplementation in this particular study.

According to some authors [41, 42], the lack of response to intravenous ferric gluconate in the Steensma study [38] may be attributed to a suboptimal dosing regime (i.e., a very low average dose but too high single doses) and a high proportion of dropouts rather than a lack of intravenous iron efficacy. In this regard, it is interesting to analyze the results from two recent meta-analyses that confirm the superiority of parenteral intravenous iron over oral or no iron supplementation in terms of better hematopoietic responses and a reduction in blood transfusions [43, 44]. These two meta-analyses had already included data of this trial as presented by Steensma et al. at the 2009 American Society of Hematology (ASH) Congress [45].

Many physicians are still reluctant to incorporate routine use of intravenous iron, largely because of poor understanding and misconceptions of the clinical nature of adverse events reportedly in the past. All of these adverse events were associated with the administration of HMW intravenous iron dextran. Because of that, parenteral iron is therefore underused in oncology patients with anemia. A large body of clinical evidence, with more than 1,000 patients evaluated in clinical trials involving the use of intravenous iron, demonstrates an excellent safety profile and a substantial benefit with the new intravenous iron preparations. Interestingly, recently a few publications have reported that intravenous iron sucrose alone was given to patients with gynecological cancer who were receiving chemotherapy; these patients achieved a higher Hb and hematocrit than the control group [46] and had less transfusions requirements [47] and achieved correction of the anemia with ferric carboxymaltose alone [48]. Further research is required to elucidate a future role for intravenous iron in the management of chemotherapy-induced anemia in cancer patients.

# Side Effects of the Treatments of Anemia

## Red Blood Cell Transfusions

Red blood cell transfusions are safer than ever. However, complications from blood transfusions still remain a major concern: infections (viral, bacterial contamination), acute and delayed hemolytic reactions, and acute lung injury are among the most frequent complications. Therefore, blood transfusions are reserved for critical situations but not for mild to moderate degrees of anemia [49]. Recently, some alarm signals have appeared with the use of red blood cell transfusions related to their storage time at the blood bank. Several publications, mainly in the fields of intensive care, cardiology, and trauma, have reported on these complications [50–52]. Most results imply the development of severe complications when blood is older than 2 weeks (see Table 8.3) [55, 56].

TABLE 8.3  Red blood cell transfusions: risks of complications

| Risk factor | Estimated frequency | | No. deaths per million units |
| --- | --- | --- | --- |
| | Per million units | Per actual unit | |
| Infection | | | |
| HIV | | | – |
| Viral | 0.4–0.7 | 1/1,400,000–1/2,400,000 | |
| Hepatitis A | 1 | 1/1,000,000 | 0 |
| Hepatitis B | 7–32 | 1/30,000–1/250,000 | 0–0.14 |
| Hepatitis C | 0.6–1.2 | 1/872,000–1/1,700,000 | – |
| HTLV types I/II | 0.5–4 | 1/250,000–1/2,000,000 | 0 |
| Parvovirus B19 | 100 | 1/10,000 | 0 |
| Bacterial contamination | | | |
| Red cells | 2 | 1/500,000 | 0.1–0.25 |
| | | | – |

(continued)

TABLE 8.3  (continued)

| Risk factor | Estimated frequency | No. deaths per million units |
|---|---|---|
| Acute hemolytic reactions | 1–4 | 1/250,000–1/1,000,000 | 0.67 |
| Delayed hemolytic reactions | 1,000 | 1/1000 | 0.4 |
| Transfusion-related acute lung injury | 200 | 1/5000 | 0.2 |
| Incorrect transfusions (human error) | | 1/14,000–19,000 | |
| Red blood cell storage | (1) | (1) | (1) |

Modified from Goodnough et al. [53] and Klein et al. [54]
References [49–51]

## Erythropoiesis-Stimulating Agents

Over the last 10 years, more than 15,000 patients have participated in clinical trials with different ESAs. The massive clinical experience with these agents has demonstrated that they are well tolerated and safe if used according to registry. Efficacy has been proven in several randomized, placebo-controlled trials [57–61]. These agents decrease the number of blood transfusions and improve the quality of life. All data have been collected and summarized in meta-analysis [62, 63].

## Pure Red Cell Anemia

A potential adverse event in the administration of biopharmaceuticals, due to their molecular complexity and their laborious fabrication, is immunogenicity, the possibility of inducing antibody formation. This was the case with epoetin alfa (during the years 1998 and 2003). Only chronic renal patients receiving epoetin alfa were affected [64]. No oncology patients were reported. The condition is called pure red cell anemia (PRCA), and it is caused by antibodies against endogenous erythropoietin. As expected, this medical condition results in no available erythropoietin, associated with severe anemia. The clinical course of antibody-mediated anemia is characterized by a sudden fall in hemoglobin concentration despite ESA therapy, with reticulocyte counts declining to very low levels $< 20 \times 10^9$/L. Affected patients, due to the severity of the anemia, rapidly become transfusion dependent. A bone marrow aspiration shows the absence or near absence of erythroid progenitor cells. The confirmation of PRCA is the detection in the serum of these patients of neutralizing antibodies that not only neutralize the biological activity of the exogenous ESA but also endogenous erythropoietin, thus preventing red cell production in the bone marrow.

PRCA related to ESA therapy is a very rare medical entity, with an exposure-adjusted incidence of 0.02–0.03 per 10,000 patient-years [65]. The peak incidence of PRCA related to ESA therapy occurred during 2002 and 2003, following the report of few cases of chronic renal patients [66]. The cause of this disease has remained elusive, although several factors are believed to have been implicated [64]. The initial most obvious cause was the removal of human serum albumin (HSA) from the epoetin alfa preparation (Eprex, Janssen-Ortho, Toronto, Canada), which was a requirement by the European authorities due to the concern about the transmission of Creutzfeldt-Jakob disease (prions). HSA was replaced by polysorbate 80, and it was initially thought that this vehicle itself might be involved in PRCA development. Another hypothesis is the so-called rubber leachates. The company had introduced a preloaded syringe with a rubber stop. It was not until after the company replaced the rubber stop with one made of Teflon that the cases began to decrease. A third hypothesis, very plausible at the time, was that it was due to a break in the cold storage chain, which rendered the protein molecule less stable. This fact leads to conformational changes in the tertiary structure of the molecule that was the ultimate cause for its immunogenicity. In total more than 200 cases were reported.

## Thromboembolic Events

The use of ESAs has been associated with a higher incidence of thromboembolic events (TEs). In general there is an increased risk of around 1.5–3 % [67,68]. A recent meta-analysis of all randomized, controlled studies of epoetin beta ($n=12$) [69] evaluated the impact of therapy at different hemoglobin-initiation levels and to different target Hb levels on overall survival, tumor progression, and TEs. An analysis of risk factors predisposing patients to TEs under epoetin beta therapy was also performed. A total of 2,297 patients were included in the analysis. The study showed a significantly increased TE rate with epoetin beta compared with control (0.22 events/patient-year vs. 0.14 events/patient-year) and an increased risk of TEs with this agent. These results are consistent with those reported by the meta-analyses of the Cochrane Collaboration [67, 68]. Subgroup analyses based on hemoglobin-initiation level indicate a correlation between hemoglobin-initiation level and risk of TE. This increased TE risk is seen in all of these agents, and it is adequately reflected in the product labeling for all approved ESAs. Among the several risk factors shown for TEs, the most relevant include increasing age (>65), prolonged immobility, malignant disease, multiple trauma, major surgery, previous venous TE, and chronic heart failure [70]. Another meta-analysis to evaluate venous TEs associated with ESA administration reviewed 38 trials including 8,172 patients and found a risk rate of 1.57 (CI 95 % of 1.31–1.87) [68]. A study-level and patient-level meta-analysis on the benefits and risks of using ESAs in lung cancer patients reported a 10.5 % for darbepoetin alfa versus 7.2 % for the placebo arm. The study evaluated nine ($n = 9$) trials with a total of 2,342 patients [69]. A recent publication reported an association between RBC and platelet transfusions and an increased risk of TEs and mortality in cancer patients [71]. Interestingly, another recent publication by Fujisaka et al. [72], treating 186 patients with cancer receiving epoetin beta 36,000 IU or placebo weekly for 12 weeks according to the European regulation, showed no significant differences in adverse events; the incidence of TE was 1.1 % in both groups. One has to be careful with these data owing to the low number of patients included in this study. A provocative explanation for the high risk for thrombocytosis and venous thromboembolism in cancer patients with chemotherapy-induced anemia has been given recently by Henry et al. [73]. These authors suggest that these events may be related to ESA-induced iron-restricted erythropoiesis, which, interestingly, is reversed by intravenous administration of iron.

Finally, it is worth noting the results of a prospective, multicenter observational study of venous TE in cancer patients receiving chemotherapy. It was observed that those patients with platelet counts $\geq 350,000/mm^3$ were associated with a higher incidence of thrombosis independent of recombinant EPO therapy [74]. These results suggest that a high prechemotherapy platelet count could be a marker to identify patients at risk for venous thrombosis (Table 8.4) [74].

Table 8.4 Adverse effects associated with erythropoiesis-stimulating agents

Thromboembolic events[a]

Arterial hypertension[b]

Pure red cell aplasia [c]

Increased mortality[d]

Stroke, [a] seizures[e]

Pain and swelling at the site of administration[f]

[a]RR:1.67 (1.35–2.06)
[b]0.02–0.03/10,000 patient-years (exposure-adjusted incidence)
[c]Overall survival (OS) HR: 1.08 (CI 95 %: 0.99–1.18) [68] and OS HR:1.04 (95 % CI:0.97–1.11) and 1.10 (95 % CI:0.98–1.24) for on-study mortality [62]
[d]$\geq 1/100$ to $< 1/10$
[e]$\geq 1/1000$ to $< 1/100$
[f]$\geq 1/10$

## Increased Mortality

In the early 2000s, two publications reported positive clinical outcomes in cancer patients receiving epoetins treated with chemotherapy. One clinical trial used epoetin alfa and the other used darbepoetin alfa; both were compared to a placebo arm [3, 60]. Although both trials did not have survival as an end point, both were highly favorable to the ESA arm in terms of survival. This fact reinforced many old theoretical arguments of the past that suggested that ESAs, by correcting the anemia, would improve tissue oxygenation. As a consequence, tumor tissues would be rendered more sensitive to cancer treatments: radiotherapy and chemotherapy. The follow-up of this rationale was that by maintaining higher Hb levels (higher oxygenation) during the course of the cancer treatment, one should expect better outcomes. This situation led to a series of clinical trials aimed not only at the correction of the anemia but to its prevention. Unfortunately, many of the trials were poorly designed, and soon some of these newly designed clinical trials were showing, unexpectedly, better outcomes in the placebo arm. In particular, the results of two of them showed, for the first time, an association between erythropoietin treatment and increased mortality [75, 76]. The results raised concerns about the safety of ESAs when targeting high Hb levels (13–14 g/dL or higher). A critical analysis of these publications [75, 76] presents serious methodological limitations. The first was an off-label use of epoetin beta using only radiotherapy for head and neck cancer achieving Hb levels of 14–15.5 g/dL and higher, and the second was an anemia-prevention study, also an off-label use, with epoetin alfa in breast cancer patients. The design of these two clinical trials could have confounded the results and probably influenced the conclusions [77, 78]. In addition, three more studies have been recently published that report a detrimental impact of ESA treatment on survival [79–81]. Many interpretations of these unexpected findings [82, 83] suggest that increased mortality may be because of a higher risk of TEs with the use of ESA therapy. These agents used off label may have caused blood hyperviscosity due to the high hematocrits achieved. Another explanation, very popular until recently, has been that ESAs may promote tumor growth through erythropoietin receptor (EpoR) activation and/or stimulation of angiogenesis [84–87]. This issue has been and still is very controversial due to the detection by some authors [85] of EpoRs on the surface of cancer cells using an anti-EpoR polyclonal antibody (A-20). Some recent publications argue against the validity of these data. One report suggested that the polyclonal antibody (A-20) recognizes heat shock protein-70 (HSP-70) and not the real EpoR. The same authors have identified some genetic homologies between the two molecules [88]. The same authors have published the results on a KO mouse for EpoR shows staining with the polyclonal antibody A-20 in both the KO mouse and in the control, which clearly suggests nonspecific binding of A-20 [88]. More recently, a monoclonal antibody against the EpoR (A82) [89] has failed to identify any EpoR in 67 human cell lines of different tumor pathologies [90] and in 182 fresh human tissue samples from different patients with different types of cancer [91].

In the last 7 years, there have been an important number of trials on ESAs in cancer patients with a variety of outcomes. As a consequence, several meta-analyses have been performed to bring some light to the field. A meta-analysis published by Bohlius et al. [68] collected the data of 57 trials and 9,353 cancer patients. The analysis included randomized, controlled clinical trials on treatment as well as on prophylaxis (off-label) and in cancer patients with anemia without concurrent anticancer treatment (off-label). The effect on overall survival gave an HR of 1.08 (95 % CI: 0.99–1.18). In 2009, an individual patient-based meta-analysis was published by Bohlius et al. [62]. The number of patients analyzed was 13,933 from 53 trials. The final results on overall survival resulted in a worse outcome for the patients enrolled in the ESA group (HR: 1.06; 95 % CI: 1.00–1.12). On-study mortality HR for the total group of patients was 1.17 (95 % CI: 1.06–1.30). Interestingly, for the 10,441 patients who received only chemotherapy, the HR for overall survival was 1.04 (95 % CI: 0.97–1.11). In their publication, the authors state that ESAs are safe for chemotherapy-induced anemia. Six other meta-analyses have been performed: five showing a neutral effect of the ESA group (no significant effect on overall survival) [63, 92–95] and one [96] showing a worse overall survival in the group who received ESA.

Ross et al. analyzed 21,378 patients from 49 studies and found no differences in TEs or mortality between the ESA arm and the control arm [92]. Aapro et al. [93] analyzed 1,413 patients from eight studies (epoetin beta, $n=800$; control, $n=613$). There was a significantly reduced risk of rapidly progressive disease for epoetin beta (RR 0.78; 95 % CI: 0.62, 0.99; $P=0.042$). Glaspy et al. [63] evaluated 15,323 cancer patients with anemia receiving chemotherapy/radiotherapy, radiotherapy-only treatment or anemia of cancer receiving no treatment from 60 studies. Results indicated that ESA use did not significantly affect mortality (60 studies: OR=1.06; 95 % CI: 0.97–1.15) or disease progression (26 studies: OR=1.01; 95 % CI: 0.90–1.14).

In a pooled analysis of individual patient-level data from all randomized, double-blind, placebo-controlled trials of darbepoetin alfa, Ludwig et al. [94] found that this agent did not increase mortality and affected neither progression-free survival nor disease progression. Overall survival and progression-free survival seemed to be better in those patients who achieved Hb >12 or >13 g/dL as compared with those who did not [94]. The same authors investigated the effect of blood transfusions on rates of Hb increase. In the absence of transfusions, the percentage of patients with >1 g/dL in 14 days or >2 g/dL in 28 days increase in Hb was 68.8 % for darbepoetin alfa and 52.3 % for placebo or 39.1 % for darbepoetin alfa and 19.2 % for placebo, respectively. Interestingly, the results show that an increase of 1 or 2 g/dL in Hb levels resulting from blood transfusions was associated with an increased risk of death and disease progression. Furthermore, when blood transfusions were excluded from the analysis, the increase in Hb rates was not associated with an increased risk for disease progression or death. In summary, blood transfusions were associated with a greater risk for disease progression and death in both treatment arms and with a greater risk for embolism/thrombosis in the darbepoetin-alfa arm.

More recently, Aapro et al. reported results of an updated meta-analysis of 12 randomized, controlled studies of epoetin beta conducted in 2,301 patients undergoing cancer therapy [95], including three recently completed trials with longer-term follow-up in patients with head and neck cancer [75], patients with metastatic breast cancer [97], and patients with cervical cancer [98]. The results of this meta-analysis based on individual patient-level data showed no statistically significant difference between patients receiving epoetin beta and standard treatment in terms of overall survival. In fact, the authors describe a favorable trend with respect to the risk of disease progression for patients receiving this agent [95]. Bennett et al. [96] reported a meta-analysis of phase 3 trials comparing ESAs with placebo or standard of care for the treatment of anemia among patients with cancer. A total of 13,611 patients included in 51 clinical trials were evaluated for survival. Patients with cancer who received ESAs had increased mortality risks (HR = 1.10; 95 % CI: 1.01–1.20) than the placebo or the standard of care arm.

Interestingly, over the last couple of years, several studies have been reported with a major aim being the safety of ESAs. Results show either a neutral clinical outcome or a beneficial one [19, 72, 99–104].

In any event, a major consequence of the safety concerns raised by some studies on ESAs in the treatment of cancer-induced anemia has been the requirement, by the European regulatory authorities, to introduce a warning on the product labels for marketed ESAs to be restricted to a hemoglobin-initiation level <10 g/dL and a Hb target not to exceed 12 g/dL. However, the updated EORTC treatment guidelines recommend the initiation of ESA therapy at Hb levels between 9 and 11 g/dL and the target for treatment with ESAs to achieve a Hb level of ~12 g/dL [105]. ASCO guidelines recommend the initiation of ESA therapy at Hb level <10 g/dL and to use ESA to achieve the lowest Hb concentration needed to avoid transfusions [22]. ESMO guidelines also recommend starting ESAs at Hb ≤ 10 g/dL and Hb target not to exceed 12 g/dL (see Table 8.4) [25].

Further research is required to elucidate these still unanswered issues regarding the safety of ESAs for correction of chemotherapy-induced anemia. Two large, multicenter, ongoing clinical trials with a major aim in survival, one in breast cancer using epoetin alfa and the other on lung cancer using darbepoetin alfa, will bring, hopefully, the right answers.

## Iron

The old preparations of intravenous iron, particularly high molecular weight dextran (HMWD), presented serious adverse effects ranging from allergies to anaphylactic reactions. This is the reason why many oncologists currently are reluctant to use it. The poor safety profile observed in the past with the old iron preparations was well documented. The new intravenous preparations (ferric gluconate, ferric carboxymaltose, iron isomaltoside, iron sucrose) show not only a much better safety profile but a much easier administration. Adverse effects are related to non-transferrin-bound iron (NTBI): toxicity occurs from the release of weakly bound iron. This is what occurred with the old preparations such as HMWD; the new preparations have a very strong iron-binding capacity that translates into much less free iron, the critical point for the serious events of the past, in particular anaphylaxis. The most common adverse effects of the new preparations are back pain, dyspnea, and hypotension [38]. Other adverse effects associated with intravenous iron in the past (e.g., myalgia, pruritus, rash) were not more common than with oral iron or placebo.

In seven published randomized trials, there was no difference in adverse events in the intravenous iron group compared with the no iron or oral iron groups [32–38]. There was no evidence for (1) increased risk of infection, (2) increase in cardiovascular morbidity, or (3) increase in tumor incidence or progression. The incidence of life-threatening adverse events with intravenous iron was <1:700,000 when high MW iron dextran was avoided [106].

# References

1. Ludwig H, Van Belle S, Barrett-Lee P, Birgegård G, Bokemeyer C, Gascón P, et al. The European Cancer Anaemia Survey (ECAS): a large, multinational, prospective survey defining the prevalence, incidence and treatment of anaemia in cancer patients. Eur J Cancer. 2004;40(15):2293–307.
2. Ludwig H, Strasser K. Symptomatology of anemia. Semin Oncol. 2001;28 Suppl 8:7–14.
3. Littlewood TJ, Bajetta E, Nortier JW, Vercammen E, Rapoport B, Epoetin Alfa Study Group. Effects of epoetin alfa on hematologic parameters and quality of life in cancer patients receiving non platinum chemotherapy: results of a randomized, double-blind, placebo-controlled trial. J Clin Oncol. 2001;19:2865–74.
4. Glaser CM, Millesi W, Kornek GV, Lang S, Schüll B, Watzinger F, et al. Impact of hemoglobin level and use of recombinant erythropoietin on efficacy of preoperative chemoradiation therapy for squamous cell carcinoma of the oral cavity and oropharynx. Int J Radiat Oncol Biol Phys. 2001;50:705–15.

5. Glaspy F, Bukowski R, Steinberg D, Taylor C, Tchekmedyian S, Vadhan-Raj S, for the Procrit Study Group. Impact of therapy with epoetin alfa on clinical outcomes in patients with nonmyeloid malignancies during cancer chemotherapy in community oncology practice. J Clin Oncol. 1997;15:1218–34.

6. Demetri GD, Kris M, Wade J, Degos L, Cella D. Quality-of-life benefit in chemotherapy patients treated with epoetin alfa is independent of disease response or tumor type: results from a prospective community oncology study. J Clin Oncol. 1998;16:3412–25.

7. Gabrilove JL, Cleeland CS, Livingston RB, Sarokhan B, Winer E, Einhorn LH. Clinical evaluation of once-weekly dosing of epoetin alfa in chemotherapy patients: improvements in hemoglobin and quality of life are similar to three-times-weekly dosing. J Clin Oncol. 2001;19:2875–82.

8. Miller CB, Jones RJ, Piantadosi S, Abeloff MD, Spivak JL. Decreased erythropoietin response in patients with the anemia of cancer. N Engl J Med. 1990;322(24):1689–92.

9. Glaspy J. Erythropoietin in cancer patients. Annu Rev Med. 2009;60:181–92.

10. Haurani FI. Hepcidin and the anemia of chronic disease. Ann Clin Lab Sci. 2006;36(1):3–6.

11. Nemeth E, Ganz T. The role of hepcidin in iron metabolism. Acta Haematol. 2009;122(2–3):78–86.

12. Rivera S, Liu L, Nemeth F, Gabayan V, Sorensen OE, Ganz T. Hepcidin excess induces the sequestration of iron and exacerbates tumor-associated anemia. Blood. 2005;105:1797–802.

13. Johnson DH, Fehrenbacher L, Novotny WF, Herbst RS, Nemunaitis JJ, Jablons DM, et al. Randomized phase II trial comparing bevacizumab plus carboplatin and paclitaxel with carboplatin and paclitaxel alone in previously untreated locally advanced or metastatic non-small-cell lung cancer. J Clin Oncol. 2004;22(11):2184–91.

14. Miller KD, Chap LI, Holmes FA, Cobleigh MA, Marcom PK, Fehrenbacher L, et al. Randomized phase III trial of capecitabine compared with bevacizumab plus capecitabine in patients with previously treated metastatic breast cancer. J Clin Oncol. 2005;23(4): 792–9.

15. Sher AF. Effect of bevacizumab on the risk of chemotherapy-associated anemia in cancer patients. A meta-analysis. J Clin Oncol. 2010;28(suppl: abstract 9136):15a.

16. Eisen T, Sternberg CN, Robert C, Mulders P, Pyle L, Zbinden S, et al. Targeted therapies for renal cell carcinoma: review of adverse event management strategies. J Natl Cancer Inst. 2012;104(2):93–113.

17. Keefe DM, Bateman EH. Tumor control versus adverse events with targeted anticancer therapies. Nat Rev Clin Oncol. 2011;9(2):98–109.

18. Henry D. The evolving role of epoetin alfa in cancer therapy. Oncologist. 2004;9:97–107.

19. Blohmer JU, Paepke S, Sehouli J, Boehmer D, Kolben M, Würschmidt F, et al. Randomized phase III trial of sequential adjuvant chemoradiotherapy with or without erythropoietin Alfa in patients with high-risk cervical cancer: results of the NOGGO-AGO intergroup study. J Clin Oncol. 2011;29(28):3791–7.

20. Wauters I, Vansteenkiste J. Darbepoetin alfa in the treatment of chemotherapy-induced anaemia. Expert Opin Biol Ther. 2009;9(2): 221–30.

21. Crawford J, Cella D, Cleeland CS, Cremieux PY, Demetri GD, Sarokhan BJ, et al. Relationship between changes in hemoglobin level and quality of life during chemotherapy in anemic cancer patients receiving epoetin alfa therapy. Cancer. 2002;95:888–95.

22. Rizzo JD, Somerfield MR, Hagerty KL, Seidenfeld J, Bohlius J, Bennett CL, et al. Use of epoetin and darbepoetin in patients with cancer: 2007 American Society of Clinical Oncology/American Society of Hematology clinical practice guideline update. J Clin Oncol. 2008;26(1):132–49.

23. National Comprehensive Cancer Network. Practice guidelines in oncology. Cancer and treatment-related anemia. vol.1. National Comprehensive Cancer Network, Inc., Fort Washington, Philadelfia 2008. www.nccn.org.

24. Aapro MS, Link H. September 2007 update on EORTC guidelines and anemia management with erythropoiesis-stimulating agents. Oncologist. 2008;13 Suppl 3:33–6.

25. Schrijvers D, De Samblanx H, Roila F, ESMO Guidelines Working Group. Erythropoiesis-stimulating agents in the treatment of anaemia in cancer patients: ESMO Clinical Practice Guidelines for use. Ann Oncol. 2010;21 Suppl 5:v244–7.

26. Rizzo JD, Brouwers M, Hurley P, Seidenfeld J, Arcasoy MO, Spivak JL, et al. American Society of Hematology/American Society of Clinical Oncology clinical practice guideline update on the use of epoetin and darbepoetin in adult patients with cancer. Blood. 2010;116(20):4045–59. Epub 2010 Oct 25.

27. NCCN Clinical Practice Guidelines in Oncology 2012. Available at: http://www.nccn.org.

28. Lichtin AE. Clinical practice guidelines for the use of erythroid-stimulating agents: ASCO, EORTC, NCCN. Cancer Treat Res. 2011;157:239–48.

29. Kamioner D. Erythropoietin biosimilars currently available in hematology-oncology. Target Oncol. 2012;7 Suppl 1:25–8. Epub 2012 Jan 18.

30. Bohlius J, Weingart O, Trelle S, Engert A. Cancer-related anemia and recombinant human erythropoietin – an updated overview. Nat Clin Pract Oncol. 2006;3:152–64.

31. Goodnough LT. Erythropoietin and iron-restricted erythropoiesis. Exp Hematol. 2007;35:167–72.

32. Auerbach M, Ballard H, Trout JR, McIlwain M, Ackerman A, Bahrain H, et al. Intravenous iron optimizes the response to recombinant human erythropoietin in cancer patients with chemotherapy-related

anemia: a multicenter, open-label, randomized trial. J Clin Oncol. 2004;22:1301–7.

33. Henry DH, Dahl NV, Auerbach M, Tchekmedyian S, Laufman LR. Intravenous ferric gluconate significantly improves response to epo-etin alfa versus oral iron or no iron in anemic patients with cancer receiving chemotherapy. Oncologist. 2007;12:231–42.

34. Hedenus M, Birgegard G, Nasman P, Ahlberg L, Karlsson T, Lauri B, et al. Addition of intravenous iron to epoetin beta increases hemo-globin response and decreases epoetin dose requirement in anemic patients with lymphoproliferative malignancies: a randomized mul-ticenter study. Leukemia. 2007;21:627–32.

35. Bastit L, Vandebroek A, Altintas S, Gaede B, Pintér T, Suto TS, et al. Randomized, multicenter, controlled trial comparing the efficacy and safety of darbepoetin alpha administered every 3 weeks with or without intravenous iron in patients with chemotherapy-induced anemia. J Clin Oncol. 2008;26:1611–8.

36. Pedrazzoli P, Farris A, Del PS, Del Gaizo F, Ferrari D, Bianchessi C, et al. Randomized trial of intravenous iron supplementation in patients with chemotherapy-related anemia without iron deficiency treated with darbepoetin alpha. J Clin Oncol. 2008;26:1619–25.

37. Auerbach M, Silberstein PT, Webb RT, Averyanova S, Ciuleanu TE, Shao J, et al. Darbepoetin alfa 300 or 500 ug once every 3 weeks with or without intravenous iron in patients with chemotherapy-induced anemia. Am J Hematol. 2010;85(9):655–93.

38. Steensma DP, Sloan JA, Dakhil SR, Dalton R, Kahanic SP, Prager DJ, et al. Phase III, randomized study of the effects of parenteral iron, oral iron, or no iron supplementation on the erythropoietic response to darbepoetin alfa for patients with chemotherapy-associ-ated anemia. J Clin Oncol. 2011;29:97–105.

39. Beguin Y, Maertens J, De Prijck B, Schots R, Frere P, Bonnet C, et al. Darbepoetin-alfa and I.V. iron administration after autologous hematopoietic stem cell transplantation: a prospective randomized multicenter trial. Blood. 2008;112(11). Abstract 54.

40. Bellet RE, Ghazal H, Flam M, Drelichman A, Gabrail N, Woytowitz D, et al. A phase III randomized controlled study comparing iron sucrose intravenously (IV) to no iron treatment of anemia in cancer patients undergoing chemotherapy and erythropoietin stimulating agent (ESA) therapy. J Clin Oncol. 2007;25(18s). Abstract 9109.

41. Auerbach M. Intravenous iron failed to improve erythropoietic response in patients with chemotherapy-induced anemia. 2010, http://www.hemonctoday.com/article.aspx?rid=78461.

42. Aapro M, Beguin Y, Birgegärd G, Gascón P, Hedenus M, Osterborg A. Too low iron doses and too many dropouts in negative iron trials? J Clin Oncol. 2011;29(17):e525–6.

43. Gafter-Gvili A, Rozen-Zvi B, Vidal L, Gafter U, Vansteenkiste JF, Shpilberg O. Intravenous iron supplementation for the treatment of

cancer-related anemia – systematic review and meta-analysis. Blood. 2010;116:21. Abstract 4249.

44. Mhaskar R, Wao H, Kumar A, Miladinovic B, Djulbegovic B. Role of iron supplementation to erythropoiesis stimulating agents in the management of chemotherapy-induced anemia in cancer patients: a systematic review and meta-analysis. Blood. 2010;116:21. Abstract 2055.

45. Steensma D, Dakhil SR, Novotny PJ, Kahanic SP, Kugler JW, Stella PJ, et al. A phase III, randomized study of the effects of parenteral iron, oral iron, or no iron supplementation on the erythropoietic response to darbepoetin alfa for patients with chemotherapy-associated anemia: a study of the Mayo Clinic Cancer Research Consortium (MCCRC). Blood. 2009;114:22. Abstract 3008.

46. Dangsuwan P, Manchana T. Blood transfusion reduction with intravenous iron in gynecologic cancer patients receiving chemotherapy. Gynecol Oncol. 2010;116(3):522–5.

47. Kim YT, Kim SW, Yoon BS, Cho HJ, Nahm EJ, Kim SH, et al. Effect of intravenously administered iron sucrose on the prevention of anemia in the cervical cancer patients treated with concurrent chemoradiotherapy. Gynecol Oncol. 2007;105(1):199–204.

48. Steinmetz T, Tschechne B, Virgin G, et al. Ferric carboxymaltose for the correction of cancer- and chemotherapy-associated anemia in clinical practice. Eur J Cancer. 2011;47(S1):221–2. Abstract 3000.

49. Hebert PC, Wells G, Blajchman MA, Marshall J, Martin C, Pagliarello G, et al. A Multicenter, randomized, controlled clinical trial of transfusion requirements in critical care. N Engl J Med. 1999;340:409–17.

50. Taylor RW, O'Brien J, Trottier SJ, Manganaro L, Cytron M, Lesko MF, et al. Red blood transfusions and nosocomial infections in critically ill patients. Crit Care Med. 2006;34:2302–8.

51. Bernard AC, Davenport DL, Chang PK, Vaughan TB, Zwischenberger JB. Intraoperative transfusion of 1U to 2U packed red blood cells is associated with increased 30-day mortality, surgical-site infection, pneumonia and sepsis in general surgery patients. J Am Coll Surg. 2009;208:931–7.

52. Gorman Koch C, Li L, Sessler DI, Figueroa P, Hoeltge GA, Mihaljevic T, et al. Duration of red-cell storage and complications after cardiac surgery. N Engl J Med. 2008;358:1229–39.

53. Goodnough LT, Brecher ME, Kanter MH, AuBuchon JP. Transfusion medicine. N Engl J Med. 1999;340(6):438–47.

54. Klein HG, Spahn DR, Carson JL. Red blood cell transfusion in clinical practice. Lancet. 2007;370(9585):415–26.

55. Yazdanbakhsh K, Bao W, Zhong H. Immunomodulatory effects of stored red blood cells in transfusion medicine: adverse complications of stored blood. Hematology Am Soc Hematol Educ Program. 2011;2011:466–9.

56. Roback JD. Vascular effects of red blood cell storage lesion in transfusion medicine: adverse complications of stored blood. Hematology Am Soc Hematol Educ Program. 2011;2011:475–9.

57. Cascinu S, Fedeli A, Del Ferro E, Luzi Fedeli S, Catalano G. Recombinant human erythropoietin treatment in cisplatin-associated anemia: a randomized, double-blind trial with placebo. J Clin Oncol. 1994;12:1058–62.

58. Cazzola M, Messinger D, Battistel V, Bron D, Cimino R, Enller-Ziegler L, et al. Recombinant human erythropoietin in the anemia associated with multiple myeloma or non-Hodgkin's lymphoma: dose finding and identification of predictors of response. Blood. 1995;86(12):4446–53.

59. Witzig TE, Silberstein PT, Loprinzi CL, Sloan JA, Novotny PJ, Mailliard JA, et al. Phase III, randomized, double-blind study of epoetin alfa compared with placebo in anemic patients receiving chemotherapy. J Clin Oncol. 2005;23(12):2606–17.

60. Vansteenkiste J, Pirker R, Massuti B, Barata F, Font A, Fiegl M, et al. Double-blind, placebo-controlled, randomized phase III trial of darbepoetin alfa in lung cancer patients receiving chemotherapy. J Natl Cancer Inst. 2002;94(16):1211–20.

61. Hedenus M, Adriansson M, San Miguel J, Kramer MH, Schipperus MR, Juvonen E, et al. Efficacy and safety of darbepoetin alfa in anaemic patients with lymphoproliferative malignancies: a randomized, double-blind, placebo-controlled study. Br J Haematol. 2003;122(3):394–403.

62. Bohlius J, Schmidlin K, Brillant C, Schwarzer G, Trelle S, Seidenfeld J, et al. Recombinant human erythropoiesis-stimulating agents and mortality in patients with cancer: a meta-analysis of randomised trials. Lancet. 2009;373(9674):1532–42.

63. Glaspy J, Crawford J, Vansteenkiste J, Henry D, Rao S, Bowers P, et al. Erythropoiesis-stimulating agents in oncology: a study-level meta-analysis of survival and other safety outcomes. Br J Cancer. 2010;102(2):301–15.

64. Macdougall IC, Roger SD, de Francisco A, Goldsmith DJ, Schellekens H, Ebbers H, et al. Antibody-mediated pure red cell aplasia in chronic kidney disease patients receiving erythropoiesis-stimulating agents: new insights. Kidney Int. 2012;81(8):727–32. doi:10.1038/ki.2011.500. Epub 2012 Feb 15.

65. McKoy JM, Stonecash RE, Cournoyer D, Rossert J, Nissenson AR, Raisch DW, et al. Epoetin-associated pure red cell aplasia: past, present, and future considerations. Transfusion. 2008;48:1754–62.

66. Casadevall N, Nataf J, Viron B, Kolta A, Kiladjian JJ, Martin-Dupont P, et al. Pure red-cell aplasia and antierythropoietin antibodies in patients treated with recombinant erythropoietin. N Engl J Med. 2002;346:469–75.

67. Bohlius J, Langensiepen S, Schwarzer G, Seidenfeld J, Piper M, Bennett C, et al. Recombinant human erythropoietin and overall survival in cancer patients: results of a comprehensive meta-analysis. J Natl Cancer Inst. 2005;97:489–98.

68. Bohlius J, Wilson J, Seidenfeld J, Piper M, Schwarzer G, Sandercock J, et al. Erythropoietin or darbepoetin for patients with cancer. Cochrane Database Syst Rev. 2006 Jul 19;(3):CD003407.

69. Aapro M, Osterwalder B, Scherhag A, Burger HU. Epoetin-beta treatment in patients with cancer chemotherapy-induced anaemia: the impact of initial haemoglobin and target haemoglobin levels on survival, tumour progression and thromboembolic events. Br J Cancer. 2009;101(12):1961–71.

70. Anderson FA, Spencer FA. Risk factors for venous thromboembolism. Circulation. 2003;107:I-9–16.

71. Khorana AA, Francis CW, Blumberg N, Culakova E, Refaai MA, Lyman GH, et al. Blood transfusions, thrombosis, and mortality in hospitalized patients with cancer. Arch Intern Med. 2008;168(21):2377–81.

72. Fujisaka Y, Sugiyama T, Saito H, Nagase S, Kudoh S, Endo M, et al. Randomised, phase III trial of epoetin-β to treat chemotherapy-induced anaemia according to the EU regulation. Br J Cancer. 2011;105(9):1267–72.

73. Henry DH, Dahl NV, Auerbach MA. Thrombocytosis and venous thromboembolism in cancer patients with chemotherapy induced anemia may be related to ESA induced iron restricted erythropoiesis and reversed by administration of IV iron. Am J Hematol. 2012;87(3):308–10.

74. Khorana AA, Francis CW, Culakova E, Lyman GH. Risk factors for chemotherapy-associated venous thromboembolism in a prospective observational study. Cancer. 2005;104:2822–9.

75. Henke M, Laszig R, Rube C, Schäfer U, Haase KD, Schilcher B, et al. Erythropoietin to treat head and neck cancer patients with anaemia undergoing radiotherapy: randomised, double-blind, placebo-controlled, trial. Lancet. 2003;362:1255–60.

76. Leyland-Jones B, Semiglazov V, Pawlicki M. Maintaining normal hemoglobin levels with epoetin alfa in mainly nonanemic patients with metastatic breast cancer receiving first-line chemotherapy: a survival study. J Clin Oncol. 2005;23:5960–72.

77. Leyland-Jones B, Mahmud S. Erythropoietin to treat anaemia in patients with head and neck cancer [letter]. Lancet. 2004;363:80.

78. Vaupel P, Mayer A. Erythropoietin to treat anaemia in patients with head and neck cancer [letter]. Lancet. 2004;363:992.

79. Overgaard J, Hoff C, Sand Hansen H, et al. Randomized study of the importance of novel erythropoiesis stimulating protein (Aranesp) for the effect of radiotherapy in patients with primary squamous cell carcinoma of the head and neck (HNSCC) – the Danish Head and Neck Cancer Group DAHANCA 10. Eur J Cancer (Suppl). 2007;5(6):7.

80. Smith Jr RE, Aapro MS, Ludwig H, Pintér T, Smakal M, Ciuleanu TE, et al. Darbepoetin alpha for the treatment of anemia in patients with active cancer not receiving chemotherapy or radiotherapy:

results of a phase III, multicenter, randomized, double-blind, placebo-controlled study. J Clin Oncol. 2008;26(7):1040–50.

81. Wright JR, Ung YC, Julian JA, Pritchard KI, Whelan TJ, Smith C, et al. Randomized, double-blind, placebo-controlled trial of erythropoietin in non-small-cell lung cancer with disease-related anemia. J Clin Oncol. 2007;25(9):1021–3.

82. Besarab A, Bolton WK, Browne JK, Egrie JC, Nissenson AR, Okamoto DM, et al. The effects of normal as compared with low hematocrit values in patients with cardiac disease who are receiving hemodialysis and epoetin. N Engl J Med. 1998;339:584–90.

83. Luksenburg H, Weir A, Wager R. FDA Briefing Document: Safety Concerns Associated with Aranesp (darbepoetin alfa) Amgen, Inc. and Procrit (epoetin alfa) Ortho Biotech, L.P., for the Treatment of Anemia Associated with Cancer Chemotherapy. 2004. http://www.fda.gov/ohrms/dockets/ac/cder04.html#oncologic.

84. Kelleher DK, Thews O, Vaupel P. Can erythropoietin improve tumor oxygenation? Strahlenther Onkol. 1998;174(Suppl IV):20–3.

85. Acs G, Acs P, Beckwith SM, Pitts RL, Clements E, Wong K, et al. Erythropoietin and erythropoietin receptor expression in human cancer. Cancer Res. 2001;61:3561–5.

86. Arcasoy MO, Amin K, Karayal AF, Chou SC, Raleigh JA, Varia MA, et al. Functional significance of erythropoietin receptor expression in breast cancer. Lab Invest. 2002;82(7):911–8.

87. Yasuda Y, Fujita Y, Matsuo T, Koinuma S, Hara S, Tazaki A, et al. Erythropoietin regulates tumour growth of human malignancies. Carcinogenesis. 2003;24:1021–9.

88. Elliott S, Busse L, Bass MB, Lu H, Sarosi I, Sinclair AM, et al. Anti-Epo receptor antibodies do not predict Epo receptor expression. Blood. 2006;107(5):1892–5.

89. Elliott S, Busse L, McCaffery I, Rossi J, Sinclair A, Spahr C, et al. Identification of a sensitive anti-erythropoietin receptor monoclonal antibody allows detection of low levels of EpoR in cells. J Immunol Methods. 2010;352(1–2):126–39.

90. Swift S, Ellison AR, Kassner P, McCaffery I, Rossi J, Sinclair AM, et al. Absence of functional EpoR expression in human tumor cell lines. Absence of functional EpoR expression in human tumor cell lines. Blood. 2010;115(21):4254–63.

91. McCaffery I, Rossi J, Paweletz K, Tudor Y, Elliot S, Fitzpatrick VD, et al. Analysis of cell surface erythropoietin receptor (EpoR) expression and function in human epithelial tumor tissues reveals no detectable expression or function. J Clin Oncol. 2009;27(suppl):15s and poster. Abstract 11104.

92. Ross SD, Allen IE, Henry DH, Seaman C, Sercus B, Goodnough LT, et al. Clinical benefits and risks associated with epoetin and darbepoetin in patients with chemotherapy-induced anemia: a systematic review of the literature. Clin Ther. 2006;28(6):801–31.

93. Aapro M, Coiffier B, Dunst J, Osterborg A, Burger HU, et al. Effect of treatment with epoetin beta on short-term tumour progression and survival in anaemic patients with cancer: a meta-analysis. Br J Cancer. 2006;95(11):1467–73.

94. Ludwig H, Crawford J, Osterborg A, Vansteenkiste J, Henry DH, Fleishman A, et al. Pooled analysis of individual patient-level data from all randomized, double-blind, placebo-controlled trials of darbepoetin alfa in the treatment of patients with chemotherapy-induced anemia. J Clin Oncol. 2009;27(17):2838–47.

95. Aapro M, Scherhag A, Burger HU. Effect of treatment with epoetin beta on survival, tumour progression and thromboembolic events in patients with metastatic cancer: an updated meta-analysis of 12 randomized controlled studies including 2301 patients. Br J Cancer. 2008;99(1):14–22.

96. Bennett CL, Silver SM, Djulbegovic B, Samaras AT, Blau CA, Gleason KJ, et al. Venous thromboembolism and mortality associated with recombinant erythropoietin and darbepoetin administration for the treatment of cancer-associated anemia. JAMA. 2008;299(8):914–24.

97. Aapro M, Leonard RC, Barnadas A, Marangolo M, Untch M, Malamos N, et al. Effect of once weekly epoetin beta on survival in patients with metastatic breast cancer receiving anthracycline- and/or taxane-based chemotherapy – results of the BRAVE study. J Clin Oncol. 2008;26:592–8.

98. Strauss HG, Haensgen G, Dunst J. Effects of anemia correction with epoetin beta in patients receiving radiochemotherapy for advanced cervical cancer. Int J Gynecol Cancer. 2008;18(3):515–24.

99. Cantrell LA, Westin SN, Van Le L. The use of recombinant erythropoietin for the treatment of chemotherapy-induced anemia in patients with ovarian cancer does not affect progression-free or overall survival. Cancer. 2011;117(6):1220–6.

100. Pronzato P, Cortesi E, van der Rijt CC, Bols A, Moreno-Nogueira JA, de Oliveira CF, et al. Epoetin alfa improves anemia and anemia-related, patient-reported outcomes in patients with breast cancer receiving myelotoxic chemotherapy: results of a European, multicenter, randomized, controlled trial. Oncologist. 2010;15(9):935–43. Epub 2010 Aug 26.

101. Moebus V, Jackish C, Lueck H-J, du Bois A, Thomssen C, Kurbacher C, et al. Intense dose-dense sequential chemotherapy with epirubicin, paclitaxel, and cyclophosphamide compared with conventional scheduled chemotherapy in high-risk primary breast cancer: mature results of an AGO phase III study. J Clin Oncol. 2010;28(17):2874–80.

102. Untch M, von Minckwitz G, Konecny G, Conrad U, Fett W, Kurzeder C, et al. PREPARE trial. A randomized phase III trial comparing preoperative, dose-dense, dose intensified chemotherapy with epirubicin, paclitaxel and CMF versus a standard dosed

epirubicin/cyclophosphamide followed by paclitaxel ± darbepoetin alfa in primary breast cancer – long-term results. Ann Oncol. 2011;22:1999–2006.

103. Nitz U, Gluz O, Oberhoff C, Reimer T, Schumacher C, Hackmann J, et al. Adjuvant chemotherapy with or without darbepoetin alfa in node-positive breast cancer: survival and quality of life analysis from the prospective randomized WSG ARA Plus trial. San Antonio Breast Cancer symposium. Cancer Res. 2011;71(s24):PD07-63s.

104. Delarue R. Survival effect of darbepoetin alfa in patients with diffuse large B-cell lymphoma (DLBCL) treated with immunochemotherapy. The LNH03-6B study. J Clin Oncol. 2011;29:561s. Abstract 9048.

105. Bokemeyer C, Aapro MS, Courdi A, Foubert J, Link H, Osterborg A, et al. EORTC guidelines for the use of erythropoietic proteins in anaemic patients with cancer: 2006 update. Eur J Cancer. 2007;43(2):258–70.

106. Chertow GM, Mason PD, Vaage-Nilsen O, Ahlmén J. Update on adverse drug events associated with parenteral iron. Nephrol Dial Transplant. 2006;21(2):378–82.

107. Vansteenkiste J, Glaspy J, Henry D, Ludwig H, Pirker R, Tomita D, et al. Benefits and risks of using erythropoiesis-stimulating agents (ESAs) in lung cancer patients: study-level and patient-level meta-analyses. Lung Cancer. 2012;76(3):478–85.

# Chapter 9
## Bone Marrow Toxicity: White Blood Cells

**Matti S. Aapro**

**Abstract** Chemotherapy-induced febrile neutropenia (FN) may lead to dose reductions and/or delays that may decrease the chances of curative or life-prolonging treatment and is related to increased patient mortality. While often associated with a need for hospitalization, this complication can also be treated in an outpatient setting in low-risk patients. Prophylactic treatment with granulocyte colony-stimulating factors (G-CSFs), such as filgrastim (including approved biosimilars), lenograstim, or pegfilgrastim, is available to reduce the risk of chemotherapy-induced neutropenia and its consequences, according to the European Organisation for Research and Treatment of Cancer (EORTC) and other guidelines. Prophylactic G-CSF is recommended in patients receiving a chemotherapy regimen with a risk of FN above 20 %. Patient-related risk factors (in particular, elderly age [≥65 years]) may increase the overall risk of FN and need to be evaluated to decide the use of prophylaxis for regimens with intermediate (10–20 %) risk of FN.

M.S. Aapro, M.D.
Department of Medical Oncology,
Institut Multidisciplinaire d'Oncologie,
Clinique de Genolier, Genolier, Switzerland
e-mail: maapro@genolier.net

M.A. Dicato (ed.), *Side Effects of Medical Cancer Therapy,*     365
DOI 10.1007/978-0-85729-787-7_9,
© Springer-Verlag London 2013

**Keywords**   Granulocyte colony-stimulating factor • Filgrastim • Lenograstim • Pegfilgrastim • Biosimilars • Neutropenia Febrile neutropenia • Chemotherapy • Guidelines • EORTC

## Introduction

Chemotherapy-induced febrile neutropenia (FN) with infection may increase patient mortality, and both FN and mortality risk can be prevented with appropriate use of granulocyte colony-stimulating factors (G-CSFs) [1]. Febrile neutropenia is seen most often during the first cycle of myelosuppressive therapy and has been documented to occur in 287/2,692 (10.7 %) of adult cancer patients during the first three cycles of chemotherapy [2]. Prevention of FN reduces hospital admissions, antibiotic usage, and the need for dose reductions or delays in chemotherapy administration, which are associated with a poorer cancer outcome, at least in curative settings [3].

In 2010, a guidelines working party of the European Organisation for Research and Treatment of Cancer (EORTC) systematically reviewed available published data and derived evidence-based recommendations on the appropriate use of G-CSF in adult patients receiving chemotherapy [4]. These recommendations are very similar to those of other groups like the American Society of Clinical Oncology (ASCO) [5] and the European Society for Medical Oncology (ESMO) [6].

This chapter will discuss the six recommendations put forward by the EORTC guidelines [4].

## Definition of Febrile Neutropenia and Complication Risk Assessment

Febrile neutropenia is defined as an absolute neutrophil count (ANC) of $<0.5 \times 10^9/L$, or $<1.0 \times 10^9/L$ predicted to fall below $0.5 \times 10^9/L$ within 48 h, with fever or clinical signs of sepsis. Currently, the ESMO defines fever in this setting as a rise in axillary temperature to $>38.5$ °C sustained for at least 1 h. It is suggested that therapy be initiated if a temperature

TABLE 9.1 Score derived from the logistic equation of the Multinational Association of Supportive Care in Cancer (MASCC) predictive model (1,386 patients with FN)

| Determinant | Points |
|---|---|
| Burden of illness | |
| No or mild symptoms | 5 |
| Moderate symptoms | 3 |
| No hypotension | 5 |
| No chronic obstructive pulmonary disease | 4 |
| Solid tumor or no previous fungal infection in hematologic cancer | 4 |
| Outpatient status | 3 |
| No dehydration | 3 |
| Age <60 years | 2 |
| Threshold: score ≥21 (maximum 26) predicting less than 5 % of severe complications | |

Adapted from [7]

of >38.0 °C is present for at least 1 h or a reading of >38.5 °C is obtained on a single occasion [6].

Recognizing patients at risk for complications of FN is of major importance in that it determines the possibility of outpatient versus inpatient management of the event. This can be achieved using risk indices, and one of these has been developed by the Multinational Association of Supportive Care in Cancer (MASCC) (Table 9.1) [7]. According to the MASCC score, patients with a score of 21 or more points are considered at low risk, while all other patients are considered at high risk of infectious complications.

# Side Effects and Precautions for Use of G-CSF

Bone, joint, or muscle pain is a common (20 % incidence) adverse event associated with G-CSF treatment, occurring with the same frequency whether the agent is pegylated or not.

It is generally easy to manage with standard analgesics. Leukocytosis (white blood cell count $>100 \times 10^9$/L) after G-CSF administration has been rarely observed and does not occur more frequently with pegfilgrastim. G-CSFs can induce elevation of cancer antigen 15–3, which is used for monitoring breast cancers [8].

G-CSF usage is contraindicated during chemoradiotherapy to the chest owing to an increased risk of complications and death, and there is also a risk of worsening thrombocytopenia when such agents are given immediately before or simultaneously with chemotherapy [6].

# Is There a Risk of Leukemia Related to G-CSF Usage?

Since the development of G-CSF, there has been a debate about the potential leukemogenic risk of the product. The Surveillance, Epidemiology, and End Results (SEER) analysis of patients with breast cancer aged ≥65 years reported an incidence of myelodysplastic syndrome (MDS)/acute myeloid leukemia (AML) of 1.77 % among 906 patients receiving growth factor support compared with 1.04 % among the 4,604 patients not receiving colony-stimulating factors. One has to note that patients receiving growth factor tended to have positive lymph nodes and received either more intense radiation therapy or high-dose cyclophosphamide treatment [9]. These findings did raise concern that G-CSF use in a high-dose setting among breast cancer patients could be associated with a high risk of secondary MDS or AML. The report of a US registry data analysis has shown that the overall risk is small, even among elderly patients [10].

A meta-analysis of randomized, controlled trials has shown that there is a modestly increased risk of AML/MDS (approximately 4 per 1,000 cases) associated with the use of particular chemotherapy schedules in combination with G-CSF support. Notably a significant increase in risk of AML/MDS was observed where G-CSF support was associated with a greater total dose of chemotherapy (Mantel-Haenszel relative risk [RR] = 2.334, $P$ = 0.009) but not when the planned total dose of chemotherapy with G-CSF was the same in each study arm, such as dose-dense schedules. Furthermore, all-cause mortality was decreased in patients receiving chemotherapy with G-CSF support. Greater reductions in mortality were observed with greater chemotherapy dose intensity [1].

Finally, one should mention the long-term observation of healthy donors whose progenitor cells were stimulated by G-CSF. The report concerns 2,408 unrelated PBSC donors prospectively evaluated by the National Marrow Donor Program (NMDP) between 1999 and 2004. Six percent of donors experienced grade III-IV CALGB toxicities, and 0.6 % experienced toxicities that were considered serious and unexpected. Complete recovery was universal, however, and no late adverse events (AEs) attributable to donation have been identified. The authors concluded that peripheral blood stem cell collection in unrelated donors is generally safe, but nearly all donors will experience bone pain, one in four will have significant headache, nausea, or citrate toxicity, and a small percentage will experience serious short-term AEs [11].

# Why Not to Use Antibiotics to Prevent Febrile Neutropenia

The use of antibiotic prophylaxis to prevent infection and infection-related complications in cancer patients at risk of neutropenia is not recommended by the EORTC guidelines. There was some suggestion of benefit in some analyses [12, 13], but other groups discuss that the presently available evidence is too limited to allow conclusions to be drawn regarding the relative merits of antibiotic versus CSF primary prophylaxis [14–16].

In one study the ciprofloxacin antibiotic prophylaxis was without efficacy against FN in patients with breast cancer treated with docetaxel-based therapy, but some benefit is observed when it is added to pegfilgrastim [17]. This recommendation 1 of the EORTC working party takes into account the finding that, in randomized controlled trials in patients receiving chemotherapy, routine fluoroquinolone prophylaxis has been shown to lead to an increase in resistance among gram-positive and gram-negative isolates compared with non-prophylaxed controls in randomized controlled trials in patients receiving chemotherapy [13]. The clinical consequences of resistance development are a major concern nowadays, and it is important to avoid unwarranted use of antibiotics to lower the risk of drug resistance.

Finally, one may mention the potential benefit of G-CSF, which may help prevent or treat mucositis and stomatitis and decrease diarrhea in some studies [17–19].

## EORTC Recommendation 1: Patient-Related Risk Factors for Increased Incidence of FN

> Patient-related risk factors should be evaluated in the overall assessment of FN risk before administering each cycle of chemotherapy. Particular consideration should be given to the elevated risk of FN for elderly patients (aged 65 and over). Other adverse risk factors that may influence FN risk include advanced stage of disease, experience of previous episode(s) of FN, lack of G-CSF use, and absence of antibiotic prophylaxis. However, please note that the indiscriminate use of antibiotic prophylaxis for patients undergoing treatment for solid tumors or lymphoma is not recommended, either by this working party or the EORTC Infectious Disease Group. *Recommendation grade: B.* [4]

## Discussing EORTC Recommendation 1: Patient-Related Risk Factors for Increased Incidence of FN and Complications of FN

Older age (particularly $\geq 65$ years) is the patient-related factor most consistently associated with an increase in FN risk, and this patient group consistently benefits from G-CSF prophylaxis [20].

Several investigators have developed models for predicting neutropenia based on the current risk factors. Such models may prove to be invaluable clinical tools. A study has been

performed to develop and validate a risk model for neutropenic complications in cancer patients receiving chemotherapy. The study population consisted of 3,760 patients with
common solid tumors or malignant lymphoma who were
beginning a new chemotherapy regimen. The risk of neutropenic complications was confirmed to be greatest in cycle 1.
After adjustment for cancer type and age, major independent
risk factors in multivariate analysis included prior chemotherapy, abnormal hepatic and renal function, low white
blood count, chemotherapy, and planned delivery greater
than 85 % [21].

## EORTC Recommendation 2: Chemotherapy Regimens Associated with Increased Risk of FN

> Consideration should be given to the elevated risk of FN when
> using certain chemotherapy regimens, summarized in Table 5.
> *Recommendation grade: A/B* (depending on the evidence for each
> chemotherapy regimen). It should be noted that this list is not
> comprehensive and there may be other drugs or regimens associ-
> ated with an increased risk of FN. [4]

### Discussing EORTC Recommendation 2: Chemotherapy Regimens Associated with Increased Risk of FN

The literature review by the EORTC committee provides a
listing of chemotherapy regimens, which helps clinicians
when evaluating the need for prophylactic intervention. An
important consideration is that targeted agents may exacerbate the risk of myelosuppression. One has to consider that
for many regimens the reporting of FN has been done with
different definitions of FN and in many cases may be underestimated. It is also important to realize that patients admit-
ted to protocols are subject to screening and various inclusion/
exclusion criteria and therefore often in a better general status
than usual patients. Thus, the risk of FN is probably higher

than that observed in the study report. Finally, very often the use of prophylactic antibiotics or even G-CSF is not mentioned in the published papers.

## EORTC Recommendation 3: G-CSF to Support Chemotherapy

In situations where dose-dense or dose-intense chemotherapy strategies have survival benefits, prophylactic G-CSF should be used as a supportive treatment. *Recommendation grade: A.*

If reductions in chemotherapy dose intensity or density are known to be associated with a poor prognosis, primary G-CSF prophylaxis should be used to maintain chemotherapy. Examples of this could be when the patient is receiving adjuvant or potentially curative treatment, or when the treatment intent is to prolong survival. *Recommendation grade A.* Where treatment intent is palliative, use of less myelosuppressive chemotherapy or dose/schedule modification should be considered. *Recommendation grade: B.* [4]

## Discussing EORTC Recommendation 3: G-CSF to Support Intensive Chemotherapy Regimens

Intensification of chemotherapy regimens with dose-dense (increased frequency) or dose-intense (increased dose) chemotherapy is increasingly used and has been shown in some situations to improve long-term clinical outcomes. Multiple studies have indicated that, because the time to neutrophil recovery is around 12 days, pegfilgrastim can be safely administered after chemotherapy in patients receiving treatment at 14-day intervals, as demonstrated in a breast cancer study [22].

Benefits of growth factor administration to maintain intended dose frequency and intensity have been confirmed by a level I meta-analysis of nine randomized controlled trials (seven with G-CSF) in the setting of malignant lymphoma. Eight of the trials showed better dose intensity in the growth factor arm than in the control arm [23].

In another meta-analysis by Kuderer et al., ten trials were identified that used relative dose intensity (RDI) as an outcome. The average RDI among control patients ranged from 71.0 to 95.0 %, with a mean of 86.7 %. Among G-CSF-treated patients, the average RDI ranged from 91.0 to 99.0 %, with a mean of 95.1 %. None of the 10G-CSF treatment arms reported a mean RDI of <90 %, whereas six of ten control groups reported a mean RDI of <90 %, with four control arms averaging an RDI of ≤85 %. This represents an 8.4 % increase in dose intensity. Average RDI was significantly higher in patients who received G-CSF compared with control patients ($P<0.001$) [24].

The lack of evidence that dose modifications decrease the benefit of palliative treatments has lead the EORTC group not to recommend use of growth factors to sustain such regimens.

## EORTC Recommendation 4: Impact of the Overall FN Risk on G-CSF Use

The risk of complications related to FN should be assessed individually for each patient *at the beginning of each cycle*. When assessing FN risk, the clinician should take into account patient-related risk factors (recommendation 1), the chemotherapy regimen and associated complications (recommendations 2 and 3), and treatment intent (recommendation 3). Prophylactic G-CSF is recommended when there is ≥20 % overall risk of FN. When chemotherapy regimens associated with an FN risk of 10 %–20 %, particular attention should be given to the assessment of patient characteristics that may increase the overall risk of FN. *Recommendation grade: A.* [4]

## Discussing EORTC Recommendation 4: Impact of the Overall FN Risk on G-CSF Use

There is strong evidence supporting the use of G-CSF to prevent FN coming from three level I meta-analyses. It should, however, be noted that while the meta-analyses support the use of G-CSF to reduce FN, some individual studies included in these publications did not [23–25].

In the lymphoma meta-analysis, with four studies analyzed, the underlying risk of FN (neutrophils below $1.0 \times 10^9/L$) was at least 36 % and RR reduction with G-CSF was approximately 26 % (RR 0.74; 95 % CI 0.62, 0.89). In a review of solid tumors, the underlying FN risk was approximately 50 % and RR reduction with G-CSF was approximately 50 %. In the largest comprehensive meta-analysis of patients with lymphoma or solid tumors across 15 randomized controlled trials (nine trials with filgrastim, five with lenograstim, and one with pegfilgrastim), in which the overall underlying risk of FN was 37 %, the RR reduction with G-CSF was 46 % (RR 0.54; 95 % CI 0.43, 0.67; $P = <0.001$) [24].

In summary, recommendations 1–3 of the EORTC identify a number of factors that should influence the clinician when considering primary prophylactic G-CSF for patients scheduled to receive chemotherapy. Each of these factors should be incorporated into an assessment of the overall risk of FN for each patient on an individual, case-by-case basis.

## EORTC Recommendation 5: G-CSF in Patients with Existing FN

> Treatment with G-CSF for patients with solid tumours and malignant lymphoma and ongoing FN is indicated only in special situations. These are limited to those patients who are not responding to appropriate antibiotic management and who are developing life-threatening infectious complications (such as severe sepsis or septic shock). *Recommendation grade*: *B*. [4]

## Discussing EORTC Recommendation 5: G-CSF in Patients with Existing FN

There are no large randomized studies about the use of growth factors in patients with existing FN. One meta-analysis has presented evidence that when G-CSF or GM-CSF is used therapeutically in conjunction with standard therapy (intravenous antibiotics and other supportive care) for patients with ongoing FN, there is a marginal but statistically significant improvement in FN-related events compared with standard treatment alone [26]. The authors of this meta-analysis do, however, indicate that this result requires further investigation as the analysis was not adequately powered to observe the impact of CSF use in patients with ongoing FN.

The EORTC recommendations are similar to those of ASCO and err on the side of caution, as it is clearly preferable to administer a drug that can enhance the activity and production of leukocytes in a situation of high risk for the patient.

## EORTC Recommendation 6: Choice of Formulation

Filgrastim, lenograstim and pegfilgrastim have clinical efficacy and we recommend the use of any of these agents, according to current administration guidelines, to prevent FN and FN-related complications, where indicated. Filgrastim biosimilars are now also a treatment option in Europe. *Recommendation grade: A.* [4]

## Discussing EORTC Recommendation 6: Choice of Formulation

The EORTC guidelines do not suggest a preference for the type of G-CSF. Two biosimilars to daily filgrastim have been approved in Europe and are marketed by various companies using different trade names: Ratiograstim (filgrastim; XM02), Filgrastim Ratiopharm, Ratiopharm GmbH; Biograstim (filgrastim; XM02), CT Arzneimittel GmbH; Tevagrastim (filgrastim; XM02), Teva Generics GmbH; filgrastim Zarzio (EP2006), Sandoz GmbH; and filgrastim Hexal (EP2006), Hexal Biotech Forschungs GmbH.

The guidelines indicate that because biosimilar products are not generic products, a switch from filgrastim to a biosimilar is considered a change in clinical management. To ensure traceability and thus robust pharmacovigilance, clinicians are encouraged to identify a product by brand name and ensure that no changes in treatment are made without informing both physician and patient. We have discussed in a recent position paper on biosimilars [27] the stringent criteria under which the products recognized by the European Medicines Agency are produced and alluded to the lower cost of biosimilars that should allow clinicians to adhere to international guidelines [28].

Unlike daily G-CSF, pegfilgrastim is not eliminated rapidly, and rates of turnover are regulated by neutrophil level. Active levels of pegfilgrastim persist for approximately 14 days or until neutrophil recovery is achieved. Several studies suggest that pegfilgrastim might achieve a better protection from febrile neutropenia than filgrastim, and meta-analyses confirm this impression [29]. Certainly the once-per-cycle administration of pegfilgrastim can be of importance in many clinical settings. The EORTC guidelines group has, however, commented that except for one study the superiority of pegfilgrastim was seen when filgrastim was used for a relatively short 5- to 7-day period, which does not comply with current guidelines. ESMO recommendations state that administration of daily G-CSF should start 24–72 h after chemotherapy and continue until ANC recovery, which typically takes 10–11 days [6].

# Summary

In conclusion, the EORTC working party has produced up-to-date recommendations for G-CSF use that are relevant to current European clinical practice, as summarized in Fig. 9.1. Such guidance should improve patient management strategies in oncology across Europe. There are, however, still many areas where guidelines committees lack sufficient level I supportive evidence to clarify some recommendations, as discussed in this chapter.

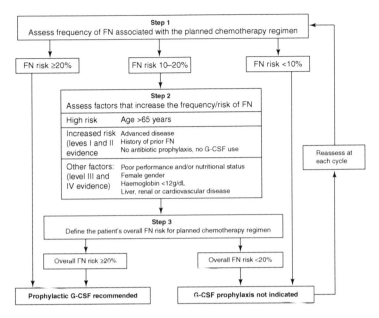

FIGURE 9.1 EORTC patient assessment algorithm to decide primary prophylactic G-CSF usage. *FN* febrile neutropenia, *G-CSF* granulocyte colony-stimulating factor (Adapted from Aapro et al. [4], Copyright 2011. with permission from Pergamon)

# References

1. Lyman G, Dale D, Wolff DA, Culakova E, Poniewierski MS, Kuderer NM, et al. Acute myeloid leukemia or myelodysplastic syndrome in randomized controlled clinical trials of cancer chemotherapy with granulocyte colony-stimulating factor: a systematic review. J Clin Oncol. 2010;28:2914–24.
2. Crawford J, Dale DC, Kuderer NM, Culakova E, Poniewierski MS, Wolff D, et al. Risk and timing of neutropenic events in adult cancer patients receiving chemotherapy: the results of a prospective nationwide study of oncology practice. J Natl Compr Canc Netw. 2008;6:109–18.
3. Krell D, Jones AL. Impact of effective prevention and management of febrile neutropenia. Br J Cancer. 2009;101 Suppl 1:S23–6.
4. Aapro MS, Bohlius J, Cameron DA, Dal Lago L, Donnelly JP, Kearney N, et al. 2010 update of EORTC guidelines for the use of

granulocyte-colony stimulating factor to reduce the incidence of chemotherapy-induced febrile neutropenia in adult patients with lymphoproliferative disorders and solid tumours. Eur J Cancer. 2011;47:8–32.

5. Smith TJ, Khatcheressian J, Lyman GH, Ozer H, Armitage JO, Balducci L, et al. 2006 update of recommendations for the use of white blood cell growth factors: an evidence-based clinical practice guideline. J Clin Oncol. 2006;24:3187–205.

6. Crawford J, Caserta C, Roila F. ESMO Guidelines Working Group. Hematopoietic growth factors: ESMO Clinical Practice Guidelines for the applications. Ann Oncol. 2010;21 Suppl 5:v248–51.

7. Klastersky J, Paesmans M, Rubenstein EB, Boyer M, Elting L, Feld R, et al. The Multinational Association for Supportive Care in Cancer risk index: a multinational scoring system for identifying low-risk febrile neutropenic cancer patients. J Clin Oncol. 2000;18:|3038–51.

8. Aapro M, Crawford J, Kamioner D. Prophylaxis of chemotherapy-induced febrile neutropenia with granulocyte colony-stimulating factors: where are we now? Support Care Cancer. 2010;18(5):529–41.

9. Hershman D, Neugut AI, Jacobson JS, Wang J, Tsai WY, McBride R, et al. Acute myeloid leukemia or myelodysplastic syndrome following use of granulocyte colony-stimulating factors during breast cancer adjuvant chemotherapy. J Natl Cancer Inst. 2007;99:196–205.

10. Touw IP, Bontenbal M. Granulocyte colony-stimulating factor: key (f)actor or innocent bystander in the development of secondary myeloid malignancy? J Natl Cancer Inst. 2007;99:183–6.

11. Pulsipher MA, Chitphakdithai P, Miller JP, Logan BR, King RJ, Rizzo JD, et al. Adverse events among 2408 unrelated donors of peripheral blood stem cells: results of a prospective trial from the National Marrow Donor Program. Blood. 2009;113:3604–11.

12. Cullen M, Steven N, Billingham L, Gaunt C, Hastings M, Simmonds P, et al. Antibacterial prophylaxis after chemotherapy for solid tumors and lymphomas. N Engl J Med. 2005;353:988–98.

13. Bucaneve G, Micozzi A, Menichetti F, Martino P, Dionisi MS, Martinelli G, et al. Levofloxacin to prevent bacterial infection in patients with cancer and neutropenia. N Engl J Med. 2005;353:977–87.

14. Gafter-Gvili A, Fraser A, Paul M, Leibovici L. Meta-analysis: antibiotic prophylaxis reduces mortality in neutropenic patients. Ann Intern Med. 2005;142:979–95.

15. Herbst C, Naumann F, Kruse EB, Monsef I, Bohlius J, Schulz H, et al. Prophylactic antibiotics or G-CSF for the prevention of infections and improvement of survival in cancer patients undergoing chemotherapy. Cochrane Database Syst Rev. 2009;(1):CD007107.

16. van de Wetering MD, de Witte MA, Kremer LC, Offringa M, Scholten RJ, Caron HN. Efficacy of oral prophylactic antibiotics in neutropenic afebrile oncology patients: a systematic review of randomised controlled trials. Eur J Cancer. 2005;41:1372–82.

17. von Minckwitz G, Kummel S, du Bois A, Eiermann W, Eidtmann H, Gerber B, et al. Pegfilgrastim +/− ciprofloxacin for primary prophylaxis with TAC (docetaxel/doxorubicin/cyclophosphamide) chemotherapy for breast cancer. Results from the GEPARTRIO study. Ann Oncol. 2008;19:292–8.

18. Sternberg CN, de Mulder PH, Schornagel JH, Théodore C, Fossa SD, van Oosterom AT, et al. Randomized phase III trial of high-dose intensity methotrexate, vinblastine, doxorubicin, and cisplatin (MVAC) chemotherapy and recombinant human granulocyte colony-stimulating factor versus classic MVAC in advanced urothelial tract tumors: European Organization for Research and Treatment of Cancer Protocol no. 30924. J Clin Oncol. 2001;19:2638–46.

19. Martin M, Lluch A, Segui MA, Ruiz A, Ramos M, Adrover E, et al. Toxicity and health-related quality of life in breast cancer patients receiving adjuvant docetaxel, doxorubicin, cyclophosphamide (TAC) or 5–fluorouracil, doxorubicin and cyclophosphamide (FAC): impact of adding primary prophylactic granulocyte-colony stimulating factor to the TAC regimen. Ann Oncol. 2006;17:1205–12.

20. Aapro M, Schwenkglenks M, Lyman GH, Lopez Pousa A, Lawrinson S, Skacel T, et al. Pegfilgrastim primary prophylaxis vs. current practice neutropenia management in elderly breast cancer patients receiving chemotherapy. Crit Rev Oncol Hematol. 2010;74:203–10.

21. Lyman G, Kuderer N, Crawford J, Wolff DA, Culakova E, Poniewierski MS, et al. Predicting individual risk of neutropenic complications in patients receiving cancer chemotherapy. Cancer. 2011;117:1917–27.

22. Piedbois P, Serin D, Priou F, et al. Dose-dense adjuvant chemotherapy in node-positive breast cancer: docetaxel followed by epirubicin/cyclophosphamide (T/EC), or the reverse sequence (EC/T), every 2 weeks, versus docetaxel, epirubicin and cyclophosphamide (TEC) every 3 weeks. AERO B03 randomized phase II study. Ann Oncol. 2007;18:52–7.

23. Bohlius J, Herbst C, Reiser M, Schwarzer G, Engert A. Granulopoiesis-stimulating factors to prevent adverse effects in the treatment of malignant lymphoma (review). Cochrane Database Syst Rev. 2008;(4):CD003189. doi:10.1002/14651858.CD003189.pub4.

24. Kuderer NM, Dale DC, Crawford J, Lyman GH. Impact of primary prophylaxis with granulocyte colony-stimulating factor on febrile neutropenia and mortality in adult cancer patients receiving chemotherapy: a systematic review. J Clin Oncol. 2007;25:3158–67.

25. Lyman GH, Kuderer NM, Djulbegovic B. Prophylactic granulocyte colony-stimulating factor in patients receiving dose-intensive cancer chemotherapy: a meta-analysis. Am J Med. 2002;112:406–11.

26. Clark OA, Lyman GH, Castro AA, Clark LG, Djulbegovic B. Colony-stimulating factors for chemotherapy-induced febrile neutropenia: a meta-analysis of randomized controlled trials. J Clin Oncol. 2005;23:4198–214.

27. Aapro MS. What do prescribers think of biosimilars? Target Oncol. 2012;7 Suppl 1:S51–5.
28. Aapro M, Cornes P, Abraham I. Comparative cost-efficiency across the European G5 countries of various regimens of filgrastim, biosimilar filgrastim, and pegfilgrastim to reduce the incidence of chemotherapy-induced febrile neutropenia. J Oncol Pharm Pract. 2012;18(2): 171–9.
29. Cooper KL, Madan J, Whyte S, Stevenson MD, Akehurst RL. Granulocyte colony-stimulating factors for febrile neutropenia prophylaxis following chemotherapy: systematic review and meta-analysis. BMC Cancer. 2011;23:404–11.

# Chapter 10
# Dermatologic Side Effects of Systemic Anticancer Therapy

**Caroline Robert, Christina Mateus,
and Alexander M.M. Eggermont**

**Abstract**  Skin, hair, and nails are almost always modified by systemic cancer therapies. These changes can sometimes result in severe adverse events, but most of the patients present with light and moderate skin side effects. Nevertheless, these dermatologic manifestations can significantly impact patients' quality of life, especially in the case of new targeted agents that are sometimes prescribed continuously over long periods of time.

Patients have to be informed in advance about the skin symptoms that might occur during the course of their treatments. Preventive and symptomatic measures can be advised or prescribed that might optimize treatment compliance and improve quality of life.

C. Robert, M.D., Ph.D. (✉)
Department of Dermatology and U INSERM U981,
Institute Gustave Roussy, Villejuif, France
e-mail: caroline.robert@igr.fr

C. Mateus, M.D.
Department of Dermatology, Institute Gustave Roussy,
Villejuif, France

A.M.M. Eggermont, M.D., Ph.D.
Department of Surgical and Medical Oncology,
Institut de Cancérologie Gustave Roussy, Villejuif- Paris, France

M.A. Dicato (ed.), *Side Effects of Medical Cancer Therapy*,
DOI 10.1007/978-0-85729-787-7_10,
© Springer-Verlag London 2013

381

Close interaction between oncologists and dermatologist is warranted in order to describe, characterize, and manage the numerous and sometimes new and original skin manifestations of new cancer therapies. In this chapter, we will focus on the side effects associated with new targeted anticancer agents since oncologists and physicians are less informed about this field than they are about skin side effects of classical chemotherapeutic agents.

**Keywords**   Cancer treatment • Skin adverse events • Targeted agents • Hand-foot skin reaction • Folliculitis • Keratoacanthomas • Skin squamous cell carcinoma • Hair changes • Paronychia

# Introduction

Abnormalities leading to cell transformation and unrestrained proliferation are usually linked to a deregulation of the normal signaling pathways that control cell differentiation and/or proliferation. New drugs targeting these pathways are being developed. They block more or less specifically one or several enzymes, usually kinases, that are sequentially activated following a chain reaction, from the surface of the cell membrane after binding of a ligand to the corresponding cell surface receptor to the inside of the cell cytoplasm.

Targeted therapies that rely on the specific inhibition of biological events implicated in oncogenic or proliferative processes are now commonly used and still actively being developed. Two types of molecules can be used to inhibit a protein kinase: (1) small molecules designed to inhibit the enzymatic activity of specific kinases (the suffix "–ib" is usually used to name these molecules) and (2) larger molecules, monoclonal antibodies (mAb, suffix "–ab") that bind to ligand or receptors to prevent their interaction and the subsequent pathway activation.

When a skin modification occurs during the course of a cancer treatment, the first question to address is whether this symptom is related to therapy or not. Indeed, infectious, inflammatory, and specific skin lesions as well as graft-versus-host disease-related rash can also be observed in these patients and have to be identified. Sometimes, the patients are treated with multiple drugs, and it is not easy to know which one is responsible for the skin changes observed.

Second, it is critical to identify the serious hypersensitivity skin reactions that require treatment discontinuation and/or specific management. The signs that suggest the possibility of a DRESS (drug reaction with eosinophilia and systemic symptom), Stevens-Johnson syndrome, or a TEN (toxic epidermal necrolysis) include mucosal involvement, bullous lesions, and the association with clinical or biological systemic symptoms such as elevated temperature, transaminase elevation, or hypereosinophilia.

In this chapter, we will review the skin side effects of anti-EGFR agents, anti-vascular endothelial growth factor (VEGFR), anti-kit, platelet-derived growth factor receptor (PDGFR) and bcr-abl inhibitors, RAF inhibitors, as well as the ones induced by mammalian target of rapamycin (mTOR) inhibitors.

Management of these numerous and various side effects associated with targeted agents will also be addressed, although they are still mostly empirical and rely on expert advices and consensus.

# EGFR Inhibitors

The epidermal growth factor receptor (EGFR) belongs to the family of HER receptors, which comprises four members: HER1 to HER4. HER1/EGFR is expressed by 30–100 % of solid tumors, in which increased activity of this receptor is a poor prognostic factor. Several compounds, small molecule inhibitors or monoclonal antibodies, can specifically block HER1 or HER2 or both. All agents targeting EGFR produce the same spectrum of skin side effects with a direct dose effect.

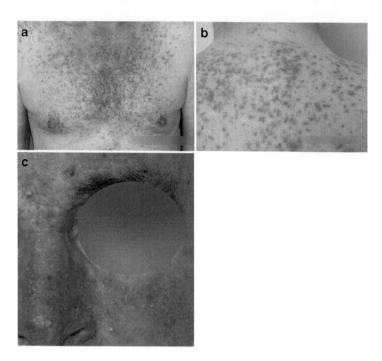

FIGURE 10.1 Papulopustular rash in a patient treated with EGFR inhibitor on the seborrheic areas of the trunk (**a, b**) and face (**c**)

## Papulopustular Rash/Folliculitis of the Seborrheic Areas

Papulopustular rash/folliculitis of the seborrheic areas (Fig. 10.1a–c) is the most common, the earliest, and the most impressive skin side effect of anti-EGFR agents, occurring in more than 75 % of patients after 1–2 weeks of therapy [1]. It is often described as acneiform, but in reality differs from an acne because although the lesions are follicular papulopustules located in the seborrheic areas (face, scalp, trunk), no retentional lesions or comedones are present. The severity varies from a few lesions to a profuse eruption that is described as uncomfortable and sometimes even painful by the patients. Durable pigmented postinflammatory maculae can be observed, especially in patients with pigmented skin.

Pathology shows nonspecific aseptic suppurative folliculitis, but mononuclear cells are recruited at the early stages, before neutrophils are recruited.

The most commonly used classification is the CTCAE (common terminology criteria for adverse events) grading system version 4. Another classification, more adapted to the side effects of anti-EGFR, has been proposed.

Severe rashes (grade 3) occur in less than 10 % of patients [1, 2]. They require local and systemic treatment and sometimes a dose reduction and even temporary treatment discontinuation. A progressive attenuation of the folliculitis is usually observed after several months [3].

The mechanism underlying this folliculitis is related to the critical role of the EGF receptor in epidermal and pilosebaceous follicle homeostasis [4, 5] involving primary cytokines like IL-1$\alpha$ (alpha) and TNF$\alpha$ (alpha) [6].

Interestingly, the occurrence and intensity of this eruption are associated with a better tumor response and overall survival of patients [7]. Several hypotheses can be formulated to explain this correlation. It has been suggested that some polymorphisms of EGFR might be associated with both the appearance of cutaneous signs and better antitumor responses [8]. This toxicity/efficacy correlation could also be explained by better bioavailability of the drug in the skin and the tumor. However, other hypotheses cannot be excluded, such as that of a beneficial effect of the inflammatory/immune reaction in the skin and perhaps also in the tumor.

Management of this eruption relies, as usual, on a good information from the patient prior to treatment initiation as well as on symptomatic topical and/or systemic treatments, depending on the severity of the rash and the impact on the patient [1, 9–11].

Topical treatment, relying on local antibiotics (erythromycin, clindamycin, metronidazole) and copper- and zinc-based antiseptic creams, is usually sufficient in the case of a grade 1 eruption. Patients are allowed and advised to camouflage the lesions with appropriate nonocclusive makeup (tested as noncomedogenic). Topical corticosteroids are usually effective when antibiotics are not sufficient [12].

Systemic treatment is used when the lesions are extensive, profuse, or poorly tolerated by the patient (grades 2 and 3). Cyclines (doxycycline, 100–200 mg/day) are used as first-line therapy for 4–8 weeks and for longer periods of time, if needed. Cyclines are probably active in this indication through their anti-inflammatory action. Preventive treatment with tetracyclines has been evaluated in some prospective studies. These studies have shown that tetracyclines reduced both the intensity and impact of the eruption, but not the incidence of the rash [13, 14]. Patients should be advised to avoid sun exposure during tetracycline treatment because of the phototoxicity of this class of antibiotics.

Psychological management of patients should not be neglected, and it is critical to regularly tackle questions about the impact of the eruption on their socio-occupational and emotional lives.

Doses of anti-EGFR should be reduced if the skin reaction is severe or if the treatment is poorly tolerated by the patient (grade 3). The folliculitis is dose dependent and rapidly attenuates after the reduction or interruption of treatment. It does not necessarily recur upon resumption of therapy.

## Paronychia

Paronychia (Fig. 10.2) is probably the most concerning side effect of EGFR inhibitors since it frequently has functional consequences and its treatment is difficult. It presents as an inflammation of the periungual folds that resembles an ingrowing nail. In fact, it is a pyogenic granuloma that grows on top of the lateral fold of the nail. It more often affects the toes than the fingers, and more specifically the large toes, probably because it is the most frequently traumatized. Paronychia occurs later in the course of the treatment, after at least a month of treatment, and is less frequently observed than the folliculitis. It occurs in 10–25 % of patients [15]. The

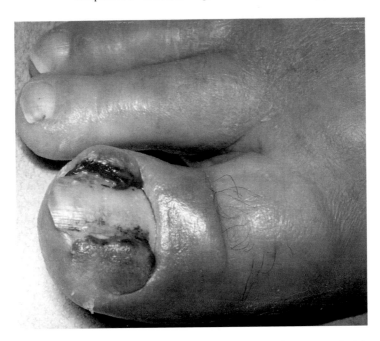

FIGURE 10.2 Paronychia of the right big toe in a patient treated with EGFR inhibitor

impact on daily life can be major, as these lesions are painful and can prevent the patient from wearing shoes and interfere with their walking. As with folliculitis, the lesions are aseptic, but superinfections are common. Management is difficult, and the aim is to reduce the extent of the granulation tissue or even destroy it completely by using either topical corticosteroids that can also be injected in the pyogenic granuloma (close monitoring is important as steroids promote superinfections) or by chemical cautery with liquid nitrogen, silver nitrate, or trichloroacetic acid. Surgical excision followed by the application of phenol can be necessary and is an effective treatment, but it must be performed by experienced physicians. Indeed, it can induce periosteitis if phenol is too vigorously applied. Prophylactic measures such as avoiding friction, traumas, and manipulations and wearing wide, open shoes minimize aggravating factors.

## Xerosis

Dry skin is reported in about one-third of the patients after 1–3 months of treatment. It is, in reality, observed in almost all the patients treated with EGFR inhibitors. Xerosis is usually diffuse and easily controlled by emollients. They are more effective if applied after showering, on skin that is still humid. Long, hot baths should be avoided. Xerosis can also predominate on the extremities, where it can result in painful, fissured dermatitis of the finger pulp or heels that can have painful and functional impacts. Vitamin A- or urea-based ointments can help patients.

## Hair Modification

Alopecia and a change in hair texture are observed after 2–3 months of treatment in almost all of the patients treated (Fig. 10.3a, b). Alopecia with hair loss in the temporal recesses and the frontal region resembling androgenic alopecia occurs frequently, as does modification of the hair texture, which becomes "straw-like," dry, and fine [1].

Facial hypertrichosis is common, as is eyelash trichomegaly, with fine and wavy eyelashes, after several months of treatment. The eyelashes can curve back toward the conjunctiva and cause keratitis. All these hair side effects are more readily apparent in women, who are inconvenienced more than men by these side effects [16].

Patients can be advised to use hair conditioners, to wax their facial hair, and to regularly trim their eyelashes to prevent conjunctive complications.

# kit and bcr-abl Inhibitors: Imatinib, Nilotinib, and Dasatinib

Imatinib (Gleevec, Novartis, New York, NY, USA), nilotinib (Tasigna, Novartis, New York, NY, USA), and dasatinib (Sprycel, Bristol-Myers Squibb, New York, NY, USA) inhibit c-kit,

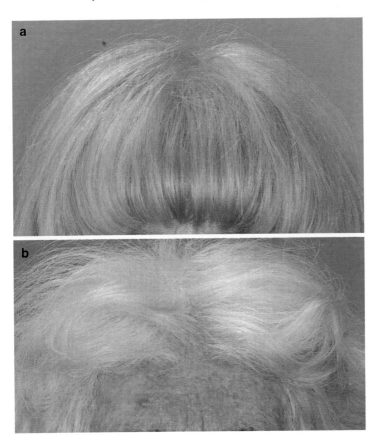

FIGURE 10.3 Hair modification. Photo taken before (**a**) and 3 months after (**b**) initiation of treatment with anti-EGFR therapy

PDGFR, and the bcr-abl fusion protein, characteristic for chronic myeloid leukemia (CML). The c-kit receptor (CD117) is activated by mutation in the majority of gastrointestinal stromal tumors (GIST), and the bcr-abl protein is the product of the translocation between chromosomes 9 and 22 found in chronic myeloid leukemia (CML). PDGFRα (alpha) is involved in hypereosinophilic syndrome, and TEL-PDGFRβ (beta) is involved in chronic myelomonocytic leukemia (CMMoL). The loop, PDGFR/PDGFR, is involved in dermatofibrosarcoma.

Overall, these three drugs are well tolerated, and although skin manifestations are the most frequent nonhematologic AEs, they are rarely severe and usually do not require treatment interruption.

## Imatinib (Gleevec)

More information is available for imatinib than for other, more recent drugs targeting kit or PDGFR. Dermatologic manifestations of imatinib are common but rarely severe, with a prevalence ranging from 9.5 to 69 % [17–23].

Edema, predominating on the face and more visible on the periorbital areas in the morning and inferior parts of the body in the evening, is reported in 63–84 % of cases and appears, on average, 6 weeks after initiation of treatment [19–24]. It can be severe, with substantial weight gain and even pleural and/or peritoneal effusions or cerebral edema [25]. The pathophysiology is unclear and is thought to be due to a modification of interstitial fluid homeostasis linked to PDGFR inhibition [1].

Maculopapular eruptions are described in up to 50 % of the patients and appear, on average, 9 weeks after the initiation of therapy [19, 24]. They are usually mild to moderate, self-limiting, or easily manageable with antihistamines or topical steroids [23]. Pathological studies demonstrate nonspecific perivascular mononuclear cell infiltrates [19, 24]. More severe eruptions (grades 3 and 4) have rarely been reported [19].

Several well-documented cases of Stevens-Johnson syndrome have been published [26–31] as well as several cases of acute generalized exanthematous pustulosis [32, 33] and a case of DRESS (drug reaction with eosinophilia and systemic symptoms) [34].

Nilotinib-associated rash is reported in 17–35 % of the patients, pruritus in 13–24 %, alopecia in 10 %, and xerosis in 13–17 %. The majority of the cases are mild to moderate and dose dependent [35, 36].

The most frequently reported dermatologic side effects reported with dasatinib are localized or diffuse maculo-papular rashes (13–27 %) that are often associated with pruritus (11 %) [15].

Exacerbations of psoriasis or psoriasiform eruptions have also been described [19, 37] as well as follicular pustular eruptions similar to pustular psoriasis [37] or eruptions resembling pityriasis rosea [38, 39].

Several cases of palmoplantar hyperkeratoses and nail dystrophies have also been reported [40].

Lichenoid eruptions, sometimes associated with mucosal erosive or lichenoid intrabuccal lesions, have been reported [41–47]. They usually present as red-purple papular lesions localized symmetrically on the trunk and limb.

Pigmentary changes (Fig. 10.4) – localized or diffuse pigmentation modifications – have been frequently reported with imatinib, and rare cases have been reported with dasatinib and nilotinib. Homogeneous depigmentation has been observed, particularly in patients with pigmented black or tanned skin (phototypes 5–6), with a reported prevalence of 16–40 % [19, 48, 49]. Conversely, cases of hyperpigmentation or even repigmentation of the skin and hair have been reported [19, 50, 51]. These pigmentary changes are reversible upon treatment discontinuation and might be due to the inhibition of c-kit, whose involvement in melanogenesis via the transcription factor MITF is well established [52, 53].

Several other various skin manifestations have been reported such as urticaria, neutrophilic dermatosis, vascular purpura [54], pseudolymphoma [55], and photosensitive eruptions [19, 56].

Eruptions and edema seem to be dose dependent. Indeed, the prevalence of drug eruptions increases with the daily dosage [19, 21]. This suggests pharmacologic and not immunologic mechanisms in the development of this type of manifestation [57].

With dasatinib, mucosal involvement has also been reported with mucositis and stomatitis in 16 % of the patients [58, 59].

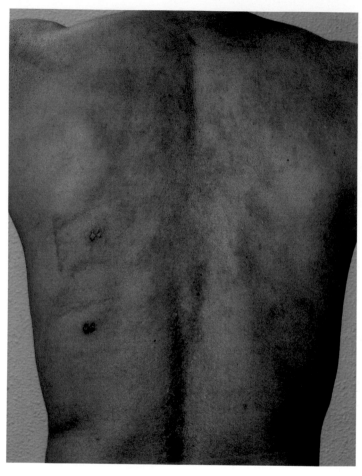

FIGURE 10.4 Hyperpigmented maculae in a patient treated with imatinib

## Management

Moderate periorbital edema does not require any treatment. Diffuse and/or severe edema can be alleviated by electrolyte monitoring and diuretics.

The majority of eruptions are easily managed with antihistamines and topical treatments, emollients, and/or corticosteroids and do not require treatment discontinuation. However, since most of the reported side effects are dose dependent, in the case of severe or persistent manifestations uncontrolled by symptomatic treatments, a dose reduction can be done. Obviously, in cases of severe and potentially life-threatening dermatologic adverse effects, treatment should be discontinued and not reintroduced.

## Antiangiogenic Agents: Sorafenib, Sunitinib, and Pazopanib

Small molecule kinase inhibitors like sorafenib (Nexavar, Bayer, Wayne, NJ, USA), sunitinib (Sutent, Pfizer, New York, NY, USA), and pazopanib (Votrient, GlaxoSmithKline, Philadelphia, PA, USA) are antiangiogenic agents targeting VEGF receptors (VEGFR) as well as additional receptors like PDGF receptors, kit, Flt3, and RAF (for sorafenib). They are indicated in the treatment of renal cell cancer, hepatocellular carcinoma, or GIST. Antiangiogenic small molecule inhibitors have various and numerous adverse effects; however, mucocutaneous manifestations are usually the most preeminent of them and frequently impact quality of life of the patients, often threatening compliance to treatment [1, 60, 61]. On the other hand, another antiangiogenic agent, bevacizumab (Avastin, Genentech, South San Francisco, CA, USA), which is a monoclonal antibody binding VEGF and preventing its binding to its receptors, has few cutaneous side effects.

Some adverse effects, like hand-foot skin reaction, genital rash, and subungual splinter hemorrhages, are common to the three compounds sorafenib, sunitinib, and pazopanib. Some other manifestations are more specifically observed with one or two of these drugs, as is the case for keratoacanthomas and squamous cell carcinoma of the skin, which occurs only in association of sorafenib and not with sunitinib or pazopanib.

## Hand-Foot Skin Reaction

Hand-foot skin reaction (HFSR) is frequent and usually occurs during the first weeks of treatment. It affects 10–63 % of patients treated with sorafenib (with 2–36 % of grade 3 severity) [62–68], 10–28 % of patients treated with sunitinib (4–12 % of grade 3) [69–71], and 11 % with pazopanib (2 % grade 3) [72–74].

It is different from the hand-foot syndrome seen with classical chemotherapies like capecitabine, 5-fluorouracil (5-FU) (Fig. 10.5), pegylated doxorubicin, or cytarabine chemotherapy [75–77]. With VEGFR inhibitors, the lesions are predominantly located on pressure or friction areas (metatarsal heads, heels, sides of the feet, metacarpophalangeal joints) and rapidly become hyperkeratotic (Fig. 10.6). With classical chemotherapies, hand-foot lesions are not limited to pressure areas and the lesions are inflammatory, erythematous, and possibly desquamative for several weeks. Hyperkeratosis can also occur but later after the beginning of the treatment. Hand and feet inflammation can also be seen with antiangiogenic agents, with erythema, desquamation, and even bullous lesions. An erythematous ring surrounding the hyperkeratotic lesions is also quite common [1, 60, 78]. The HFSR is classically bilateral and symmetrical [79]. Areas of preexisting hyperkeratotic lesions seem to confer a predisposition for painful sole involvement [79, 80]. While not life-threatening, HFSR can be very painful, interfering with everyday activities such as walking or holding objects. Prodromal subjective symptoms with mild tingling and numbness of the hands and feet are frequent [78].

The main pathological abnormalities observed in HFSR are keratinocyte degeneration with a perivascular lymphocytic infiltrate and sometimes eccrine squamous syringometaplasia [79, 81, 82]. Sequential pathological modifications found during the course of the treatment are changes in the stratum spinosum/stratum granulosum during the first month and then in the superior layers of the epidermis, in the stratum corneum with hyperkeratosis, and focal parakeratosis after the first month [82].

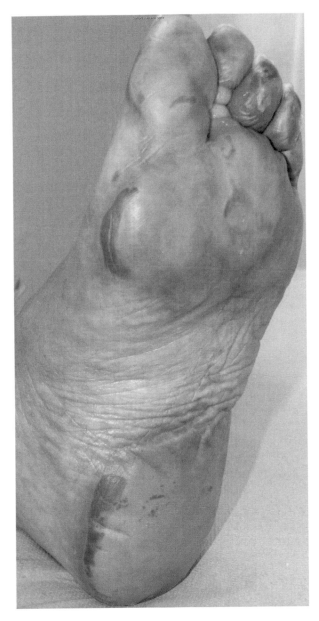

FIGURE 10.5 Grade 3 hand-foot skin reaction of a patient treated with 5-fluorouracil

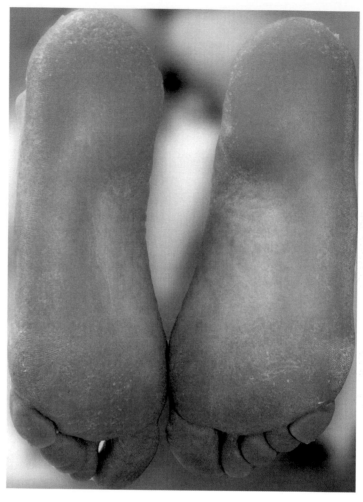

FIGURE 10.6 Grade 1 hand-foot skin reaction in a patient treated with sorafenib

## Management

HFSR is clearly dose dependent and may improve with dose reductions or treatment interruptions. Management has not yet been evaluated by controlled studies and is currently based on prescribers' experience and advice by experts' consensus [83]. Guidance can be split into preventive measures and management strategies.

## Preventive Measures

The patients must be clearly informed that an HFSR might occur; ideally, they should have their hands and feet examined prior to treatment initiation. A podiatric examination and preventive treatment of preexisting hyperkeratotic areas by mechanical or chemical keratolytic measures (topical 10–50 % urea, 2–5 % salicylic acid ointments) seem helpful. Emollients can be used to prevent dryness and cracking. Prescription of orthopedic soles may also be helpful in patients with unbalanced sole pressure areas.

Patients should be advised to wear comfortable and flexible shoes and to avoid rubbing and trauma. As a memory aid, these measures can be referred to as the "3C" approach: control calluses, comfort with cushions, and cover with cream [83].

## Treatment

Treatment is based on symptomatic measures and dose adjustment. Therapeutic measures are proposed according to the three HFSR severity grades NCI-CTCAE classification V4:

- Grade 1: Supportive measures include using moisturizing creams, keratolytic agents such as 40 % urea, and/or creams or ointments containing 1–10 % salicylic acid on the callused areas. Cushioning of the affected regions with gel- or foam-based shock absorber soles and soft shoes is recommended. Treatment is maintained at the same dosage.
- Grade 2: The same symptomatic measures as for grade 1 should be initiated promptly; potent topical corticosteroids (clobetasol) can be prescribed on inflammatory lesions for a few days. Analgesic treatment should be considered, if needed. A dose reduction of 50 % should be considered until the HFSR returns to grade 0 or 1, particularly in the event of a second episode of grade 2 HFSR. If

toxicity resolves to grade 0 or 1, reescalation to the initial dose should be done. Decision whether to reescalate the dose after the second or third occurrence of grade 2 HFSR should be based on clinical judgment and patient preference. If toxicity does not resolve to grade 0 or 1 despite dose reduction, treatment should be interrupted for a minimum of 7 days and until toxicity has resolved to grade 0 or 1. When resuming treatment after dose interruption, treatment should begin at reduced dose. If toxicity is maintained at grade 0 or 1 at reduced dose for a minimum of 7 days, initial dose should be given.

- Grade 3: Symptomatic measures as described for grade 2 HFSR should be prescribed as well as antiseptic treatment of blisters and erosions. Treatment should be interrupted for a minimum of 7 days and until toxicity has resolved to grade 0 or 1. When resuming treatment after dose interruption, treatment should begin at a reduced dose. If toxicity is maintained at grade 0 or 1 at reduced dose for a minimum of 7 days, initial dose should be given again. On the second occurrence of grade 3 HFSR, decision whether to reescalate dose should be based on clinical judgment and patient preference. The same principle applies for the decision whether to discontinue therapy after the third occurrence of grade 3 HFSR.

No systemic therapy has demonstrated any beneficial effect until now.

## Subungual Splinter Hemorrhages

Ranging from 3 to 70 %, depending on the series, subungual splinter hemorrhages occur with the three compounds (sorafenib, sunitinib, pazopanib), but their frequency is often underestimated because of their asymptomatic nature. They appear as painless longitudinal black lines beneath the distal part of the nail plate in the first weeks of therapy. They can be clinically identical to those observed in certain systemic diseases such as rheumatoid arthritis, systemic lupus, or Osler's endocarditis, but they are not associated with distant embolic or thrombotic processes, unlike these conditions. Inhibition of the VEGF receptor coupled with local microtraumas could explain the symptom. They disappear progressively at the end of treatment and do not require any treatment [78, 80, 84].

## Erythematous Rash

Various erythematous rashes are observed with these three compounds – in 13–24 % of cases with sunitinib [85, 86], in 10–60 % with sorafenib [78, 85, 87], and in 6–8 % with pazopanib [72–74]. They usually appear during the first weeks of treatment. They are usually minor, relatively asymptomatic maculopapular eruptions, but can sometimes be more severe and diffuse. They can predominate on the face, as is often the case in the first weeks of sorafenib therapy, where a mild erythematous and desquamative facial rash, resembling seborrheic dermatitis, is frequently observed [78]. Rashes can disappear spontaneously despite continued treatment, but temporary discontinuation of therapy may be necessary in some cases. A case of erythema multiforme has been published [88], and signs of severity such as mucosal involvement, epidermal detachment, and general signs (fever, elevated hepatic enzymes) that can be associated with severe manifestations, toxic epidermal necrolysis, or a DRESS syndrome should always be evaluated

## Hair Modification

Largely underreported in the literature, hair modifications are almost always associated with these drugs. It can be only a minor texture change, with hair usually becoming dryer and curlier. Alopecia occurs in 21–44 % of patients on sorafenib [78, 89]. It occurs slightly less frequently with sunitinib (5–21 %) and pazopanib (8–10 %). [72–74] It is usually moderate and develops gradually after several weeks or months. It can be associated with loss of hair in other hairy regions (trunk, arms, pubis).

It is not unusual to see hair growing back even though patients are still on therapy with sorafenib. New-grown hair is usually curlier than it was before treatment.

Reversible hair depigmentation is seen frequently with sunitinib (7–14 %) [85, 90, 91] and pazopanib (27–44 %) [72, 73]. With sunitinib, which is given 4 weeks on and 2 weeks off, characteristic discoloration can occur, with successive depigmented bands related to periods of treatment and normally pigmented bands associated with periods off treatment [91, 92]. The underlying mechanism of the depigmentation is thought to be a melanogenesis defect resulting from the inhibition of the c-kit pathway; however, this must not be a direct effect of kit inhibition since other kit inhibitors, such as imatinib, dasatinib, or nilotinib, do not induce such systematic hair depigmentation.

## Xerosis

The skin becomes dryer with these treatments [1, 78], and symptomatic emollient treatments are usually efficient.

## Genital Rash

Genital rash with erythematous, desquamative psoriasiform, or lichenoid lesions can be observed in the genital areas of both male and female patients (Fig. 10.7) [61, 93]. Lesions can involve the vulvar or scrotal areas and extend to the inguinal region. It can occasionally result in phimosis. Histological analysis, when performed, revealed a psoriasiform or lichenoid pattern. Such genital rashes have been observed with sorafenib, sunitinib, and pazopanib [62]. Their real incidence is unknown. Careful and systematic questioning is necessary. Treatment with topical steroid can be proposed after ruling out a bacterial or fungal infection. A temporary dosage modification is sometimes necessary, resulting in a rapid improvement of the symptoms.

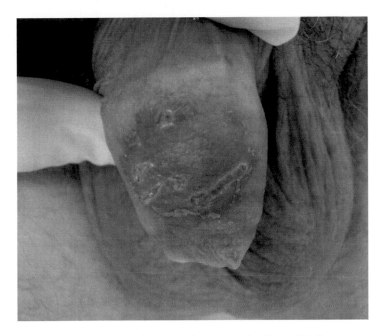

FIGURE 10.7 Genital rash in a patient treated with sunitinib

## Mucositis

Mucositis is characterized by painful inflammation and ulceration of the mucous membranes lining the digestive tracts, whereas stomatitis more specifically refers to inflammation of the mucosae lining the mouth, and cheilitis, to inflammation of the lips. These side effects can give rise to pain and difficulty with speaking or eating. Stomatitis and cheilitis have been reported in 19–35 % of sunitinib-treated patients and 19–26 % of sorafenib-treated patients [71, 78, 85, 94], usually during the first weeks of treatment. They are dose dependent and can require dose modifications [85].

## Adverse Effects Specifically Related to Sunitinib

### Skin Discoloration

A yellow appearance of the skin is seen with sunitinib. It is rapidly reversible and decreases during the 2 weeks off treatment. It is probably due to the bright yellow color of the drug itself [1].

### Facial Edema

A mild to moderate facial edema is seen in 4.5–24 % of patients treated with sunitinib [95]. Hypothyroidism, which is a frequent complication of sunitinib, can exacerbate this edema.

### Xerostomia

Xerostomia is commonly seen with sunitinib and can result in difficulty with speaking and eating as well as in the occurrence of tooth cavities and vulnerability to mouth infection.

## Adverse Effects Related Specifically to Sorafenib

### Eruptive Nevi

In patients treated with sorafenib, several cases of eruptive nevi have been observed on the face, trunk, or limbs, including the palmoplantar areas [89, 96]. Pathologically, the lesions that were biopsied presented as junctional nevi. Because of the pro-senescence effect of BRAF protein in wild-type BRAF cells [97, 98], it can be hypothesized that these nevi eruption could be linked to an "anti-senescence effect" with the appearance and the development of subclinical preexisting nevi.

### Squamous Cell Proliferations: Keratoacanthomas and Squamous Cell Carcinomas

Over the last few years, several cases of skin tumors, keratoa-canthomas (KA) (Fig. 10.8), and squamous cell carcinomas

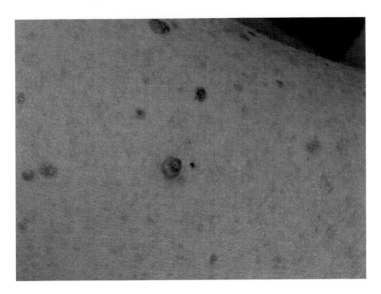

FIGURE 10.8 Keratoacanthoma in a patient treated with sorafenib

(SCC) have been described during the course of sorafenib therapy [99, 100]. These lesions could be multiple and occurred several weeks to months after initiating the treatment with an estimated incidence of less than 10 %. Beside the contexts of uncommon genetic diseases like Ferguson-Smith or Muir-Torre syndromes, KA is a rare lesion preferentially occurring on sun-exposed areas and presenting as a fast-growing, dome-shaped nodule with a central keratotic crust. It does not give rise to metastases and can occasionally spontaneously regress. Pathologically, it is almost undistinguishable from a well-differentiated SCC, with an exoendophytic proliferation and a crateriform zone of well-differentiated squamous epithelium surrounding a central keratotic plug. The existence of KA is still controversial since for some authors this entity should be assimilated to a well-differentiated form of SCC [101–103]. In contrast to KA, SCC is a real malignant lesion that does not regress spontaneously and can give rise to metastases. It is a frequent skin tumor and most of the time related to sun exposure or to the existence of precancerous lesions like actinic keratoses, for example. However, the SCC observed during sorafenib therapy do not appear as the typical and most frequently reported SCC. They all exhibit clinical and pathological aspects close to KA and are usually described pathologically as KA-like SCC with nest of atypical cells invading the dermis as well as a crateriform pattern with bulging borders reminiscent of KA. They are not always located on sun-exposed areas [99]. Until now, no metastatic evolution of any SCC induced by sorafenib has been reported, and they rather appear as low-aggressiveness skin tumors.

Looking at the molecules targeted by sorafenib, it could be deduced that this particular side effect was likely to be due to RAF inhibition. Indeed, no KA or SCC has ever been reported with drugs targeting the molecules inhibited by sorafenib in addition to RAF proteins – that is, PDGFR, FLT3, or VEGFR – like sunitinib (VEGFR, KIT, PDGFR, FLT3) or imatinib (kit, PDGFR), for example. This reasoning proved to be correct since similar tumors are now described with the use of two new drugs, presently in development, that efficiently and specifically target RAF proteins and more particularly the mutant form of BRAF: BRAF$^{V600E}$.

BRAF is a serine/threonine kinase, downstream from the RAS proteins and upstream from MEK and ERK on the MAPK (mitogen-activated protein kinase) signaling pathway [104]. This pathway is constitutively activated in several cancers, including melanomas, favoring cell proliferation and survival. It is activated in more than 65 % of melanomas resulting from the recurrent BRAF$^{V600E}$ mutation in 40–50 % of the cases and NRAS mutation in 15–20 % of the cases [105].

The mechanism explaining the appearance of skin tumors with sorafenib and RAF inhibitors is probably due to a paradoxical RAF-MEK-ERK signaling pathway activation via cells that do not harbor the BRAF mutation, especially if the cells have a mutant RAS protein, as was shown recently in several in vitro models [106–110].

Advice is given that patients' skin should be carefully monitored and that KA and SCC should be removed. These lesions should be completely resected, and simple shaving of the lesions, leading to partial resection only, should not be performed.

In addition to KA and SCC, more or less inflammatory follicular cystic lesions are frequently observed in patients treated with sorafenib: keratosis pilaris [87], microcysts, dystrophic follicular cystic lesions, and perforating folliculitis [78, 87, 99]. Association of these lesions with KA and SCC in the same patients suggests that they could represent various aspects of a wide spectrum of lesions from benign cystic lesions to borderline (KA) and malignant skin tumors (SCC) [99, 109, 110].

# RAF Inhibitors

BRAF is the most frequently mutated protein kinase in human cancer and is the target of several anticancer drugs. The potency and the specificity of BRAF inhibitors available on the market or under clinical development are variable. Sorafenib (Nexavar, Bayer/Onyx) is a pan-RAF inhibitor that also blocks vascular endothelial growth factor receptors (VEGFR)-2, VEGFR-3, platelet-derived growth factor receptor-b (PDGFR-b), fms-like tyrosine kinase 3 (FLT3), and kit. Conversely, vemurafenib (Zelboraf, Plexxikon/Roche) is highly selective and very potent BRAF inhibitor that is effective against tumors harboring BRAF mutations and dependent on the RAF/MEK/ERK pathway, like melanoma with V600E *BRAF* mutation.

## *Skin Neoplasms: Papillomas, Keratoacanthomas, Cutaneous Squamous Cell Carcinomas, and Melanomas*

In spite of their variability in terms of BRAF selectivity and clinical activity, all RAF inhibitors are associated with one and the same intriguing cutaneous side effect, which is the emergence of borderline squamous cell neoplasms: skin papillomas (Fig. 10.9), keratoacanthomas (KA), and squamous cell carcinomas (SCC).

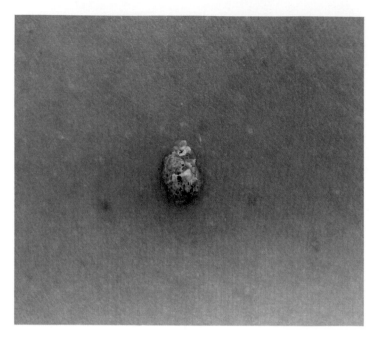

FIGURE 10.9 Skin papilloma in a patient treated with vemurafenib

These paradoxical keratinocyte proliferations arise in less than 10 % of patients treated with sorafenib. They occur much more frequently with vemurafenib, having been described in 15–25 % of the patients [110, 111].

Indeed, vemurafenib frequently induces multiple benign skin tumors resembling human papilloma virus–related papillomas or warts, keratoacanthomas, and cutaneous skin carcinomas during the first weeks or months of treatment. Until now, no metastatic squamous cell carcinoma has been reported, and these skin neoplasms can easily be surgically excised or destroyed.

They are due to a paradoxical activation of the MAPK pathway in keratinocytes associated with BRAF/CRAF heterodimerization and subsequent CRAF activation. Additional somatic events such as a *HRAS* mutation or *EGFR* activation giving rise to MAPK pathway coactivation might be required for full transformation of keratinocytes [109, 112].

Eruptive nevi and thin melanomas have rarely been reported with vemurafenib [113].

They might be related to the same mechanism as keratinocyte proliferation or to an anti-senescence effect of vemurafenib.

The other skin side effects of sorafenib have been reviewed earlier in the antiangiogenic section of this chapter. We will now see the side effects associated with the specific BRAFV600E inhibitor vemurafenib, which is authorized for the treatment of metastatic melanoma after a rapid clinical development reporting a rate of objective response around 50 % and a benefit in terms of overall survival in this population of patients [114–116].

Photosensitivity is frequently observed with vemurafenib in 30–70 % of the patients. It can occur with moderate sun exposure, and patients have to observe strict photoprotection measures: clothes and potent sunscreen with UVA and UVB blockers.

Skin rash, that can present as maculopapular rash or as a keratosis pilaris occur frequently, predominantly on the trunk and the extension parts of the limbs. Rashes are reported in up to 75 % of the patients but rarely impair treatment continuation.

Hair modification and alopecia similar to the ones that are induced by sorafenib are seen.

Hand-foot skin reaction with hyperkeratosis on pressure and rubbing areas, resembling the symptoms observed with VEGFR inhibitors, is associated with vemurafenib, although the symptoms are less severe than those seen with anti-VEGFR and very few patients present with severe inflammatory or bullous lesions (Fig. 10.10). Hyperkeratosis can also be seen on additional skin-rubbing areas like the nipples or the elbows.

Xerosis is reported in 15–20 % of patients and pruritus in 10–30 %.

# mTOR Inhibitors: Everolimus and Temsirolimus

These drugs inhibit the serine/threonine kinase mTOR (mammalian target of rapamycin), inducing downstream dephosphorylation of the mTOR molecular targets and ultimately

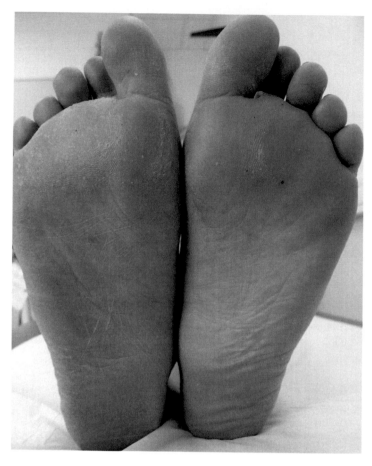

FIGURE 10.10 Grade 2 hand-foot skin reaction in a patient treated with vemurafenib

inhibiting the PI3K/AKT/mTOR signaling pathway. This particular signaling pathway plays a critical role in tumor cell biology, especially in regulating cell growth, survival, and proliferation and apoptosis mechanisms, and is also actively involved in angiogenesis [117–119].

Two compounds are approved in the treatment of advanced or metastatic renal cell cancer: temsirolimus (Torisel, Wyeth,

Madison, NJ, USA) and everolimus (Afinitor, Novartis, New York, NY, USA). These drugs are associated with various side effects, among which mucocutaneous adverse effects are the most frequently represented.

## Rash

Skin rash is reported in 25–61 % of patients on everolimus and 43–76 % of patients on temsirolimus. Usually mild to moderate (0–6 % of grade 3 or 4), it appears during the first weeks of treatment. It rarely requires dose modifications or treatment interruption. The rash is not very well characterized and few series provide details on its clinical presentation. However, the rash is described as papulopustular or acneiform eruptions, in 30–40 % of the patients. There are no associated retention lesions (microcysts, blackheads), which distinguishes this rash from a true acne. A nonspecific neutrophilic dermoepidermal infiltrate has been found pathologically. Therapeutic management is currently, and by analogy, based on that proposed for anti-EGFR inhibitors.

## Stomatitis and Oral Ulcerations

Stomatitis, mucositis, cheilitis, and oral ulcerations resembling aphthous ulcers are very common with both drugs: in up to 40 % of patients with everolimus and 70 % with temsirolimus [117, 120–126]. These side effects are dose dependent and can sometimes entail a dose reduction or treatment interruption, especially in the case of oral ulceration, which is often very painful and can impact patients' food intake.

Xerostomia is reported in 5–11 % of patients treated with everolimus, and a dysguesia has been observed with both compounds [120, 121, 123–125].

Management of these side effects relies on symptomatic measures: topical or systemic analgesics or topical steroids. However, these palliative measures are frequently not effective enough, and dose modification, or temporary treatment discontinuation, is often necessary.

## *Paronychia/Pyogenic Granulomas*

Nail involvement, sometimes described as nail dystrophy or thickening of the nail table, has been reported sporadically with both compounds in 5–46 % of the cases. Paronychia and/or pyogenic granulomas very similar to the lesions observed with EGFR inhibitors are also observed; their incidence is unknown. Management relies on symptomatic measures similar to the ones proposed for anti-EGFR.

Xerosis and pruritus seem common (20 and 30 %, respectively) and are sometimes associated. Pruritus is observed in 40 % of patients treated with temsirolimus with 1 % of grades 3–4.

Edema is also reported in up to 35 % of the patients [95, 122, 127].

# Summary

Systemic cancer, and especially new targeted agents, induces extremely frequent and various skin manifestations that can significantly impact a patient's quality of life and compliance with therapy. Potentially serious adverse events that can require treatment interruption have to be recognized early. Patients must be informed of the risk before the treatments are initiated, and preventive measures can sometimes be advised. Optimal management of these skin side effects requires close interaction between prescribers and dermatologists.

# References

1. Robert C, Soria J-C, Spatz A, Le Cesne A, Malka D, Pautier P, et al. Cutaneous side-effects of kinase inhibitors and blocking antibodies. Lancet Oncol. 2005;6(7):491–500.
2. Agero ALC, Dusza SW, Benvenuto-Andrade C, Busam KJ, Myskowski P, Halpern AC. Dermatologic side effects associated with the epidermal growth factor receptor inhibitors. J Am Acad Dermatol. 2006;55(4):657–70.

3. Osio A, Mateus C, Soria J-C, Massard C, Malka D, Boige V, et al. Cutaneous side-effects in patients on long-term treatment with epidermal growth factor receptor inhibitors. Br J Dermatol. 2009; 161(3):515–21.

4. Laux I, Jain A, Singh S, Agus DB. Epidermal growth factor receptor dimerization status determines skin toxicity to HER-kinase targeted therapies. Br J Cancer. 2006;94(1):85–92.

5. Lacouture ME. Mechanisms of cutaneous toxicities to EGFR inhibitors. Nat Rev Cancer. 2006;6(10):803–12.

6. Surguladze D, Deevi D, Claros N, Corcoran E, Wang S, Plym MJ, et al. Tumor necrosis factor-alpha and interleukin-1 antagonists alleviate inflammatory skin changes associated with epidermal growth factor receptor antibody therapy in mice. Cancer Res. 2009;69(14): 5643–7.

7. Pérez-Soler R. Can rash associated with HER1/EGFR inhibition be used as a marker of treatment outcome? Oncology (Williston Park, NY). 2003;17(11 Suppl 12):23–8.

8. Amador ML, Oppenheimer D, Perea S, Maitra A, Cusatis G, Cusati G, et al. An epidermal growth factor receptor intron 1 polymorphism mediates response to epidermal growth factor receptor inhibitors. Cancer Res. 2004;64(24):9139–43.

9. Lacouture ME. Insights into the pathophysiology and management of dermatologic toxicities to EGFR-targeted therapies in colorectal cancer. Cancer Nurs. 2007;30(4 Suppl 1):S17–26.

10. Janus N, Launay-Vacher V, Robert C, Souquet P-J, Mateus C, Dreno B, et al. Description of erlotinib-related skin effects management in France. Results of the PRECEDE study. Cancer Radiother. 2009;13(2):97–102.

11. Akman A, Yilmaz E, Mutlu H, Ozdogan M. Complete remission of psoriasis following bevacizumab therapy for colon cancer. Clin Exp Dermatol. 2009;34(5):e202–4.

12. Jacot W, Bessis D, Jorda E, Ychou M, Fabbro M, Pujol J-L, et al. Acneiform eruption induced by epidermal growth factor receptor inhibitors in patients with solid tumours. Br J Dermatol. 2004; 151(1):238–41.

13. Scope A, Agero ALC, Dusza SW, Myskowski PL, Lieb JA, Saltz L, et al. Randomized double-blind trial of prophylactic oral minocycline and topical tazarotene for cetuximab-associated acne-like eruption. J Clin Oncol. 2007;25(34):5390–6.

14. Jatoi A, Rowland K, Sloan JA, Gross HM, Fishkin PA, Kahanic SP, et al. Tetracycline to prevent epidermal growth factor receptor inhibitor-induced skin rashes: results of a placebo-controlled trial from the North Central Cancer Treatment Group (N03CB). Cancer. 2008;113(4):847–53.

15. Lacouture ME. The growing importance of skin toxicity in EGFR inhibitor therapy. Oncology (Williston Park, NY). 2009;23(2):194. 196.

412 C. Robert et al.

16. Kerob D, Dupuy A, Reygagne P, Levy A, Morel P, Bernard BA, et al. Facial hypertrichosis induced by Cetuximab, an anti-EGFR monoclonal antibody. Arch Dermatol. 2006;142(12):1656–7.

17. Ellis LM, Hicklin DJ. VEGF-targeted therapy: mechanisms of antitumour activity. Nat Rev Cancer. 2008;8(8):579–91.

18. Breccia M, Carmosino I, Russo E, Morano SG, Latagliata R, Alimena G. Early and tardive skin adverse events in chronic myeloid leukaemia patients treated with imatinib. Eur J Haematol. 2005; 74(2):121–3.

19. Valeyrie L, Bastuji-Garin S, Revuz J, Bachot N, Wechsler J, Berthaud P, et al. Adverse cutaneous reactions to imatinib (STI571) in Philadelphia chromosome-positive leukemias: a prospective study of 54 patients. J Am Acad Dermatol. 2003;48(2):201–6.

20. Basso FG, Boer CC, Corrêa MEP, Torrezan M, Cintra ML, de Magalhães MHCG, et al. Skin and oral lesions associated to imatinib mesylate therapy. Support Care Cancer. 2009;17(4):465–8.

21. Brouard M, Saurat JH. Cutaneous reactions to STI571. N Engl J Med. 2001;345(8):618–9.

22. Kantarjian H, Sawyers C, Hochhaus A, Guilhot F, Schiffer C, Gambacorti-Passerini C, et al. Hematologic and cytogenetic responses to imatinib mesylate in chronic myelogenous leukemia. N Engl J Med. 2002;346(9):645–52.

23. Deininger MWN, O'Brien SG, Ford JM, Druker BJ. Practical management of patients with chronic myeloid leukemia receiving imatinib. J Clin Oncol. 2003;21(8):1637–47.

24. Scheinfeld N. Imatinib mesylate and dermatology part 2: a review of the cutaneous side effects of imatinib mesylate. J Drugs Dermatol. 2006;5(3):228–31.

25. Hensley ML, Ford JM. Imatinib treatment: specific issues related to safety, fertility, and pregnancy. Semin Hematol. 2003;40(2 Suppl 2): 21–5.

26. Hsiao L-T, Chung H-M, Lin J-T, Chiou T-J, Liu J-H, Fan FS, et al. Stevens-Johnson syndrome after treatment with STI571: a case report. Br J Haematol. 2002;117(3):620–2.

27. Severino G, Chillotti C, De Lisa R, Del Zompo M, Ardau R. Adverse reactions during imatinib and lansoprazole treatment in gastrointestinal stromal tumors. Ann Pharmacother. 2005;39(1):162–4.

28. Vidal D, Puig L, Sureda A, Alomar A. Sti571-induced Stevens-Johnson Syndrome. Br J Haematol. 2002;119(1):274–5.

29. Pavithran K, Thomas M. Imatinib induced Stevens-Johnson syndrome: lack of recurrence following re-challenge with a lower dose. Indian J Dermatol Venereol Leprol. 2005;71(4):288–9.

30. Sanchez-Gonzalez B, Pascual-Ramirez JC, Fernandez-Abellan P, Belinchon-Romero I, Rivas C, Vegara-Aguilera G. Severe skin reaction to imatinib in a case of Philadelphia-positive acute lymphoblastic leukemia. Blood. 2003;101(6):2446.

31. Mahapatra M, Mishra P, Kumar R. Imatinib-induced Stevens-Johnson syndrome: recurrence after re-challenge with a lower dose. Ann Hematol. 2007;86(7):537–8.

32. Brouard MC, Prins C, Mach-Pascual S, Saurat JH. Acute generalized exanthematous pustulosis associated with STI571 in a patient with chronic myeloid leukemia. Dermatology (Basel). 2001;203(1):57–9.

33. Schwarz M, Kreuzer K-A, Baskaynak G, Dörken B, le Coutre P. Imatinib-induced acute generalized exanthematous pustulosis (AGEP) in two patients with chronic myeloid leukemia. Eur J Haematol. 2002;69(4):254–6.

34. Le Nouail P, Viseux V, Chaby G, Billet A, Denoeux JP, Lok C. Drug reaction with eosinophilia and systemic symptoms (DRESS) following imatinib therapy. Ann Dermatol Venereol. 2006;133(8–9 Pt 1):686–8.

35. Kantarjian H, Giles F, Wunderle L, Bhalla K, O'Brien S, Wassmann B, et al. Nilotinib in imatinib-resistant CML and Philadelphia chromosome-positive ALL. N Engl J Med. 2006;354(24):2542–51.

36. Kantarjian HM, Giles F, Gattermann N, Bhalla K, Alimena G, Palandri F, et al. Nilotinib (formerly AMN107), a highly selective BCR-ABL tyrosine kinase inhibitor, is effective in patients with Philadelphia chromosome-positive chronic myelogenous leukemia in chronic phase following imatinib resistance and intolerance. Blood. 2007;110(10):3540–6.

37. Woo SM, Huh CH, Park KC, Youn SW. Exacerbation of psoriasis in a chronic myelogenous leukemia patient treated with imatinib. J Dermatol. 2007;34(10):724–6.

38. Brazzelli V, Prestinari F, Roveda E, Barbagallo T, Bellani E, Vassallo C, et al. Pityriasis rosea-like eruption during treatment with imatinib mesylate: description of 3 cases. J Am Acad Dermatol. 2005;53(5 Suppl 1):S240–3.

39. Konstantopoulos K, Papadogianni A, Dimopoulou M, Kourelis C, Meletis J. Pityriasis rosea associated with imatinib (STI571, Gleevec). Dermatology (Basel). 2002;205(2):172–3.

40. Deguchi N, Kawamura T, Shimizu A, Kitamura R, Yanagi M, Shibagaki N, et al. Imatinib mesylate causes palmoplantar hyperkeratosis and nail dystrophy in three patients with chronic myeloid leukemia. Br J Dermatol. 2006;154(6):1216–8.

41. Kuraishi N, Nagai Y, Hasegawa M, Ishikawa O. Lichenoid drug eruption with palmoplantar hyperkeratosis due to imatinib mesylate: a case report and a review of the literature. Acta Derm Venereol. 2010;90(1):73–6.

42. Gómez Fernández C, Sendagorta Cudós E, Casado Verrier B, Feito Rodríguez M, Suárez Aguado J, VidaurrázagaDíazdeArcaya C. Oral lichenoid eruption associated with imatinib treatment. Eur J Dermatol. 2010;20(1):127–8.

43. Kawakami T, Kawanabe T, Soma Y. Cutaneous lichenoid eruption caused by imatinib mesylate in a Japanese patient with chronic myeloid leukaemia. Acta Derm Venereol. 2009;89(3):325–6.

44. Sendagorta E, Herranz P, Feito M, Ramírez P, Feltes R, Floristán U, et al. Lichenoid drug eruption related to imatinib: report of a new case and review of the literature. Clin Exp Dermatol. 2009;34(7): e315–6.

45. Dalmau J, Peramiquel L, Puig L, Fernández-Figueras MT, Roé E, Alomar A. Imatinib-associated lichenoid eruption: acitretin treatment allows maintained antineoplastic effect. Br J Dermatol. 2006;154(6):1213–6.

46. Prabhash K, Doval DC. Lichenoid eruption due to imatinib. Indian J Dermatol Venereol Leprol. 2005;71(4):287–8.

47. Ena P, Chiarolini F, Siddi GM, Cossu A. Oral lichenoid eruption secondary to imatinib (Glivec). J Dermatolog Treat. 2004;15(4):253–5.

48. Arora B, Kumar L, Sharma A, Wadhwa J, Kochupillai V. Pigmentary changes in chronic myeloid leukemia patients treated with imatinib mesylate. Ann Oncol. 2004;15(2):358–9.

49. Tsao AS, Kantarjian H, Cortes J, O'Brien S, Talpaz M. Imatinib mesylate causes hypopigmentation in the skin. Cancer. 2003;98(11):2483–7.

50. Etienne G, Cony-Makhoul P, Mahon F-X. Imatinib mesylate and gray hair. N Engl J Med. 2002;347(6):446.

51. Mcpherson T, Sherman V, Turner R. Imatinib-associated hyperpigmentation, a side effect that should be recognized. J Eur Acad Dermatol Venereol. 2009;23(1):82–3.

52. Dippel E, Haas N, Grabbe J, Schadendorf D, Hamann K, Czarnetzki BM. Expression of the c-kit receptor in hypomelanosis: a comparative study between piebaldism, naevus depigmentosus and vitiligo. Br J Dermatol. 1995;132(2):182–9.

53. Cario-André M, Ardilouze L, Pain C, Gauthier Y, Mahon F-X, Taieb A. Imatinib mesilate inhibits melanogenesis in vitro. Br J Dermatol. 2006;155(2):493–4.

54. Hamm M, Touraud JP, Mannone L, Klisnick J, Ponnelle T, Lambert D. Imatinib-induced purpuric vasculitis. Ann Dermatol Venereol. 2003;130(8–9 Pt 1):765–7.

55. Clark SH, Duvic M, Prieto VG, Prietol VG. Mycosis fungoides-like reaction in a patient treated with Gleevec. J Cutan Pathol. 2003;30(4): 279–81.

56. Rousselot P, Larghero J, Raffoux E, Calvo F, Tulliez M, Giraudier S, et al. Photosensitization in chronic myelogenous leukaemia patients treated with imatinib mesylate. Br J Haematol. 2003;120(6):1091–2.

57. Lacouture ME, Maitland ML, Segaert S, Setser A, Baran R, Fox LP, et al. A proposed EGFR inhibitor dermatologic adverse event-specific grading scale from the MASCC skin toxicity study group. Support Care Cancer. 2010;18(4):509–22.

58. Talpaz M, Shah NP, Kantarjian H, Donato N, Nicoll J, Paquette R, et al. Dasatinib in imatinib-resistant Philadelphia chromosome-positive leukemias. N Engl J Med. 2006;354(24):2531–41.

59. Hochhaus A, Kantarjian HM, Baccarani M, Lipton JH, Apperley JF, Druker BJ, et al. Dasatinib induces notable hematologic and cytogenetic responses in chronic-phase chronic myeloid leukemia after failure of imatinib therapy. Blood. 2007;109(6):2303–9.

60. Robert C. Cutaneous side effects of antiangiogenic agents. Bull Cancer. 2007;94 Spec No:S260–4.

61. Robert C, Mateus C, Spatz A, Wechsler J, Escudier B. Dermatologic symptoms associated with the multikinase inhibitor sorafenib. J Am Acad Dermatol. 2009;60(2):299–305.

62. Abou-Alfa GK, Schwartz L, Ricci S, Amadori D, Santoro A, Figer A, et al. Phase II study of sorafenib in patients with advanced hepatocellular carcinoma. J Clin Oncol. 2006;24(26):4293–300.

63. Blumenschein Jr GR, Gatzemeier U, Fossella F, Stewart DJ, Cupit L, Cihon F, et al. Phase II, multicenter, uncontrolled trial of single-agent sorafenib in patients with relapsed or refractory, advanced non-small-cell lung cancer. J Clin Oncol. 2009;27(26):4274–80.

64. Cheng A-L, Kang Y-K, Chen Z, Tsao C-J, Qin S, Kim JS, et al. Efficacy and safety of sorafenib in patients in the Asia-Pacific region with advanced hepatocellular carcinoma: a phase III randomised, double-blind, placebo-controlled trial. Lancet Oncol. 2009;10(1):25–34.

65. Escudier B, Eisen T, Stadler WM, Szczylik C, Oudard S, Staehler M, et al. Sorafenib for treatment of renal cell carcinoma: Final efficacy and safety results of the phase III treatment approaches in renal cancer global evaluation trial. J Clin Oncol. 2009;27(20):3312–8.

66. Llovet JM, Di Bisceglie AM, Bruix J, Kramer BS, Lencioni R, Zhu AX, et al. Design and endpoints of clinical trials in hepatocellular carcinoma. J Natl Cancer Inst. 2008;100(10):698–711.

67. Ratain MJ, Eisen T, Stadler WM, Flaherty KT, Kaye SB, Rosner GL, et al. Phase II placebo-controlled randomized discontinuation trial of sorafenib in patients with metastatic renal cell carcinoma. J Clin Oncol. 2006;24(16):2505–12.

68. Ryan CW, Goldman BH, Lara Jr PN, Mack PC, Beer TM, Tangen CM, et al. Sorafenib with interferon alfa-2b as first-line treatment of advanced renal carcinoma: a phase II study of the Southwest Oncology Group. J Clin Oncol. 2007;25(22):3296–301.

69. Demetri GD, van Oosterom AT, Garrett CR, Blackstein ME, Shah MH, Verweij J, et al. Efficacy and safety of sunitinib in patients with advanced gastrointestinal stromal tumour after failure of imatinib: a randomised controlled trial. Lancet. 2006;368(9544):1329–38.

70. Gore ME, Szczylik C, Porta C, Bracarda S, Bjarnason GA, Oudard S, et al. Safety and efficacy of sunitinib for metastatic renal-cell carcinoma: an expanded-access trial. Lancet Oncol. 2009;10(8):757–63.

71. Motzer RJ, Hutson TE, Tomczak P, Michaelson MD, Bukowski RM, Rixe O, et al. Sunitinib versus interferon alfa in metastatic renal-cell carcinoma. N Engl J Med. 2007;356(2):115–24.

72. Hurwitz HI, Dowlati A, Saini S, Savage S, Suttle AB, Gibson DM, et al. Phase I trial of pazopanib in patients with advanced cancer. Clin Cancer Res. 2009;15(12):4220–7.

73. Sternberg CN, Davis ID, Mardiak J, Szczylik C, Lee E, Wagstaff J, et al. Pazopanib in locally advanced or metastatic renal cell carcinoma: results of a randomized phase III trial. J Clin Oncol. 2010; 28(6):1061–8.

74. Hutson TE, Davis ID, Machiels J-PH, De Souza PL, Rottey S, Hong B-F, et al. Efficacy and safety of pazopanib in patients with metastatic renal cell carcinoma. J Clin Oncol. 2010;28(3):475–80.

75. Susser WS, Whitaker-Worth DL, Grant-Kels JM. Mucocutaneous reactions to chemotherapy. J Am Acad Dermatol. 1999;40(3):367–98; quiz 399–400.

76. von Moos R, Thuerlimann BJK, Aapro M, Rayson D, Harrold K, Sehouli J, et al. Pegylated liposomal doxorubicin-associated hand-foot syndrome: recommendations of an international panel of experts. Eur J Cancer. 2008;44(6):781–90.

77. Webster-Gandy JD, How C, Harrold K. Palmar-plantar erythrodysesthesia (PPE): a literature review with commentary on experience in a cancer centre. Eur J Oncol Nurs. 2007;11(3):238–46.

78. Autier J, Escudier B, Wechsler J, Spatz A, Robert C. Prospective study of the cutaneous adverse effects of sorafenib, a novel multikinase inhibitor. Arch Dermatol. 2008;144(7):886–92.

79. Lipworth AD, Robert C, Zhu AX. Hand-foot syndrome (hand-foot skin reaction, palmar-plantar erythrodysesthesia): focus on sorafenib and sunitinib. Oncology. 2009;77(5):257–71.

80. Autier J, Mateus C, Wechsler J, Spatz A, Robert C. Cutaneous side effects of sorafenib and sunitinib. Ann Dermatol Venereol. 2008;135(2):148–53; quiz 147, 154.

81. Lacouture ME, Reilly LM, Gerami P, Guitart J. Hand foot skin reaction in cancer patients treated with the multikinase inhibitors sorafenib and sunitinib. Ann Oncol. 2008;19(11):1955–61.

82. Yang C-H, Lin W-C, Chuang C-K, Chang Y-C, Pang S-T, Lin Y-C, et al. Hand-foot skin reaction in patients treated with sorafenib: a clinicopathological study of cutaneous manifestations due to multitargeted kinase inhibitor therapy. Br J Dermatol. 2008;158(3):592–6.

83. Lacouture ME, Wu S, Robert C, Atkins MB, Kong HH, Guitart J, et al. Evolving strategies for the management of hand-foot skin reaction associated with the multitargeted kinase inhibitors sorafenib and sunitinib. Oncologist. 2008;13(9):1001–11.

84. Robert C, Faivre S, Raymond E, Armand J-P, Escudier B. Subungual splinter hemorrhages: a clinical window to inhibition of vascular endothelial growth factor receptors? Ann Intern Med. 2005;143(4): 313–4.

85. Lee WJ, Lee JL, Chang SE, Lee MW, Kang YK, Choi JH, et al. Cutaneous adverse effects in patients treated with the multitar-

geted kinase inhibitors sorafenib and sunitinib. Br J Dermatol. 2009;161(5):1045–51.

86. Motzer RJ, Hutson TE, Tomczak P, Michaelson MD, Bukowski RM, Oudard S, et al. Overall survival and updated results for sunitinib compared with interferon alfa in patients with metastatic renal cell carcinoma. J Clin Oncol. 2009;27(22):3584–90.

87. Kong HH, Turner ML. Array of cutaneous adverse effects associated with sorafenib. J Am Acad Dermatol. 2009;61(2):360–1.

88. MacGregor JL, Silvers DN, Grossman ME, Sherman WH. Sorafenib-induced erythema multiforme. J Am Acad Dermatol. 2007;56(3):5 27–8.

89. Kong HH, Sibaud V, Chanco Turner ML, Fojo T, Hornyak TJ, Chevreau C. Sorafenib-induced eruptive melanocytic lesions. Arch Dermatol. 2008;144(6):820–2.

90. Rosenbaum SE, Wu S, Newman MA, West DP, Kuzel T, Lacouture ME. Dermatological reactions to the multitargeted tyrosine kinase inhibitor sunitinib. Support Care Cancer. 2008;16(6):557–66.

91. Robert C, Spatz A, Faivre S, Armand J-P, Raymond E. Tyrosine kinase inhibition and grey hair. Lancet. 2003;361(9362):1056.

92. Hartmann JT, Kanz L. Sunitinib and periodic hair depigmentation due to temporary c-KIT inhibition. Arch Dermatol. 2008;144(11): 1525–6.

93. Billemont B, Barete S, Rixe O. Scrotal cutaneous side effects of sunitinib. N Engl J Med. 2008;359(9):975–6; discussion 976.

94. Suwattee P, Chow S, Berg BC, Warshaw EM. Sunitinib: a cause of bullous palmoplantar erythrodysesthesia, periungual erythema, and mucositis. Arch Dermatol. 2008;144(1):123–5.

95. Guevremont C, Alasker A, Karakiewicz PI. Management of sorafenib, sunitinib, and temsirolimus toxicity in metastatic renal cell carcinoma. Curr Opin Support Palliat Care. 2009;3(3):170–9.

96. Bennani-Lahlou M, Mateus C, Escudier B, Massard C, Soria J-C, Spatz A, et al. Eruptive nevi associated with sorafenib treatment. Ann Dermatol Venereol. 2008;135(10):672–4.

97. Dhomen N, Reis-Filho JS, da Rocha Dias S, Hayward R, Savage K, Delmas V, et al. Oncogenic Braf induces melanocyte senescence and melanoma in mice. Cancer Cell. 2009;15(4):294–303.

98. Wajapeyee N, Serra RW, Zhu X, Mahalingam M, Green MR. Oncogenic BRAF induces senescence and apoptosis through pathways mediated by the secreted protein IGFBP7. Cell. 2008; 132(3):363–74.

99. Arnault JP, Wechsler J, Escudier B, Spatz A, Tomasic G, Sibaud V, et al. Keratoacanthomas and squamous cell carcinomas in patients receiving sorafenib. J Clin Oncol. 2009;27(23):e59–61.

100. Kwon EJ, Kish LS, Jaworsky C. The histologic spectrum of epithelial neoplasms induced by sorafenib. J Am Acad Dermatol. 2009; 61(3):522–7.

101. Clausen OPF, Aass HCD, Beigi M, Purdie KJ, Proby CM, Brown VL, et al. Are keratoacanthomas variants of squamous cell carcinomas? A comparison of chromosomal aberrations by comparative genomic hybridization. J Invest Dermatol. 2006;126(10):2308–15.
102. Cribier B, Asch P, Grosshans E. Differentiating squamous cell carcinoma from keratoacanthoma using histopathological criteria. Is it possible? A study of 296 cases. Dermatology (Basel). 1999;199(3): 208–12.
103. Hodak E, Jones RE, Ackerman AB. Solitary keratoacanthoma is a squamous-cell carcinoma: three examples with metastases. Am J Dermatopathol. 1993;15(4):332–42; discussion 343–52.
104. Robinson MJ, Cobb MH. Mitogen-activated protein kinase pathways. Curr Opin Cell Biol. 1997;9(2):180–6.
105. Dhomen N, Marais R. BRAF signaling and targeted therapies in melanoma. Hematol Oncol Clin North Am. 2009;23(3):529–45, ix.
106. Heidorn SJ, Milagre C, Whittaker S, Nourry A, Niculescu-Duvas I, Dhomen N, et al. Kinase-dead BRAF and oncogenic RAS cooperate to drive tumor progression through CRAF. Cell. 2010;140(2):209–21.
107. Mateus C, Robert C. New drugs in oncology and skin toxicity. Rev Med Interne. 2009;30(5):401–10.
108. Poulikakos PI, Zhang C, Bollag G, Shokat KM, Rosen N. RAF inhibitors transactivate RAF dimers and ERK signalling in cells with wild-type BRAF. Nature. 2010;464(7287):427–30.
109. Arnault J-P, Mateus C, Escudier B, Tomasic G, Wechsler J, Hollville E, et al. Skin tumors induced by sorafenib; Paradoxical RAS-RAF pathway activation and oncogenic mutations of HRAS, TP53 and TGFBR1. Clin Cancer Res [Internet]. 2012;18(1):263–72. Epub 2011 Nov 17. Available de: http://www.ncbi.nlm.nih.gov/pubmed/22096025. Cité 2011 Dec 18.
110. Robert C, Arnault J-P, Mateus C. RAF inhibition and induction of cutaneous squamous cell carcinoma. Curr Opin Oncol. 2011;23(2): 177–82.
111. Ellard SL, Clemons M, Gelmon KA, Norris B, Kennecke H, Chia S, et al. Randomized phase II study comparing two schedules of everolimus in patients with recurrent/metastatic breast cancer: NCIC Clinical Trials Group IND.163. J Clin Oncol. 2009;27(27):4536–41.
112. Motzer RJ, Escudier B, Oudard S, Hutson TE, Porta C, Bracarda S, et al. Efficacy of everolimus in advanced renal cell carcinoma: a double-blind, randomised, placebo-controlled phase III trial. Lancet. 2008;372(9637):449–56.
113. O'Donnell A, Faivre S, Burris 3rd HA, Rea D, Papadimitrakopoulou V, Shand N, et al. Phase I pharmacokinetic and pharmacodynamic study of the oral mammalian target of rapamycin inhibitor everolimus in patients with advanced solid tumors. J Clin Oncol. 2008;26(10):1588–95.
114. Tabernero J, Rojo F, Calvo E, Burris H, Judson I, Hazell K, et al. Dose- and schedule-dependent inhibition of the mammalian target

of rapamycin pathway with everolimus: a phase I tumor pharmaco-dynamic study in patients with advanced solid tumors. J Clin Oncol. 2008;26(10):1603–10.

115. Punt CJA, Boni J, Bruntsch U, Peters M, Thielert C. Phase I and pharmacokinetic study of CCI-779, a novel cytostatic cell-cycle inhibitor, in combination with 5-fluorouracil and leucovorin in patients with advanced solid tumors. Ann Oncol. 2003;14(6):931–7.

116. Raymond E, Alexandre J, Faivre S, Vera K, Materman E, Boni J, et al. Safety and pharmacokinetics of escalated doses of weekly intravenous infusion of CCI-779, a novel mTOR inhibitor, in patients with cancer. J Clin Oncol. 2004;22(12):2336–47.

117. Flaherty KT, Puzanov I, Kim KB, Ribas A, McArthur GA, Sosman JA, et al. Inhibition of mutated, activated BRAF in metastatic melanoma. N Engl J Med. 2010;363(9):809–19.

118. Su F, Viros A, Milagre C, Trunzer K, Bollag G, Spleiss O, et al. RAS mutations in cutaneous squamous-cell carcinomas in patients treated with BRAF inhibitors. N Engl J Med. 2012;366(3):207–15.

119. Dalle S, Poulalhon N, Thomas L. Vemurafenib in melanoma with BRAF V600E mutation. N Engl J Med. 2011;365(15):1448–9; author reply 1450.

120. Chapman PB, Hauschild A, Robert C, Haanen JB, Ascierto P, Larkin J, et al. Improved survival with vemurafenib in melanoma with BRAF V600E mutation. N Engl J Med. 2011;364(26):2507–16.

121. Sosman JA, Kim KB, Schuchter L, Gonzalez R, Pavlick AC, Weber JS, et al. Survival in BRAF V600-mutant advanced melanoma treated with vemurafenib. N Engl J Med. 2012;366(8):707–14.

122. Bjelogrlić SK, Srdić T, Radulović S. Mammalian target of rapamy-cin is a promising target for novel therapeutic strategy against cancer. J BUON. 2006;11(3):267–76.

123. Sehgal SN. Rapamune (RAPA, rapamycin, sirolimus): mechanism of action immunosuppressive effect results from blockade of signal transduction and inhibition of cell cycle progression. Clin Biochem. 1998;31(5):335–40.

124. Nguyen A, Hoang V, Laquer V, Kelly KM. Angiogenesis in cutaneous disease: part I. J Am Acad Dermatol. 2009;61(6):921–42; quiz 943–4.

125. Amato RJ, Jac J, Giessinger S, Saxena S, Willis JP. A phase 2 study with a daily regimen of the oral mTOR inhibitor RAD001 (everoli-mus) in patients with metastatic clear cell renal cell cancer. Cancer. 2009;115(11):2438–46.

126. Atkins MB, Hidalgo M, Stadler WM, Logan TF, Dutcher JP, Hudes GR, et al. Randomized phase II study of multiple dose levels of CCI-779, a novel mammalian target of rapamycin kinase inhibitor, in patients with advanced refractory renal cell carcinoma. J Clin Oncol. 2004;22(5):909–18.

127. Atkins MB, Yasothan U, Kirkpatrick P. Everolimus. Nat Rev Drug Discov. 2009;8(7):535–6.

# Chapter 11
# Myeloid Malignancies

**Laurent Plawny**

**Abstract**  Myeloid malignancies comprise the various myeloid proliferative stem cell disorders. In this chapter, the side effects of the currently used drugs are given as used in the general hematologic clinic. For the various disorders covered, the side effects of the medications are pleomorphic; therefore, for the tyrosine kinase inhibitors in chronic myeloid leukemia, a tabulated summary is given. Hematopoietic stem cells, autologous as well as allogeneic, are not covered. These treatment modalities are used in very specialized units, and the patient's follow-up during the first few months is also done through these units, which are very familiar with the therapies.

**Keywords**  Myelodysplastic syndromes • Acute myeloid leukemia Polycythemia vera • Essential thrombocythemia • Chronic myeloid leukemia

L. Plawny, M.D.
Department of Hematology, Centre Hospitalier de Luxembourg,
Luxembourg, Luxembourg
e-mail: plawny.laurent@chl.lu

M.A. Dicato (ed.), *Side Effects of Medical Cancer Therapy*,
DOI 10.1007/978-0-85729-787-7_11,
© Springer-Verlag London 2013

421

# Myelodysplastic Syndrome

## *5-Azacytidine*

5-Azacytidine [1–6] is a hypomethylating agent that has been approved in the treatment of myelodysplasia with low-intermediate and high-intermediate International Prognostic Scoring System (IPSS) in the United States. In the European Union, 5-azacytidine has been approved for myelodysplasia with high IPSS only. Some data about its efficacy in chronic myelomonocytic leukemia or in acute myeloid leukemia with low blast count have also been noted.

The side effects of 5-azacytidine are listed below. Hematologic toxicity that results mainly in anemia or thrombocytopenia is observed in most patients. Leukopenia or grade III neutropenia occurs in about one patient out of five and may lead to febrile neutropenia or opportunistic infections. Invasive fungal infections remain an issue in patients receiving 5-azacytidine treatment; therefore, prophylactic antifungal treatment with activity against aspergillus should be discussed in selected patients.

Agranulocytosis or irreversible aplasia are exceptional but are a cause of infectious mortality.

Fever may occur at the time of injection but is mostly related to infection. Nausea and vomiting occur frequently but may be reduced with adequate antiemetic medication.

A recurring problem in patients receiving subcutaneous 5-azacytidine is skin reaction at the infusion site. These reactions can vary from rash to pruritic plaques. Most skin rashes disappear with topical antihistamines or anti-inflammatory creams. The injection technique, however, influences the prevalence of skin lesions. Correct injection that avoids skin contact with the product lowers the occurrence of rash and pruritic plaques by more than a half.

The following are side effects of 5-azacytidine treatment:

Hematologic

- Very frequent (>50 % of patients): anemia, thrombocytopenia
- Frequent (>20 % of patients): leukopenia, neutropenia

- Rare (5–10 % of patients): lymphadenopathies, hematomas
- Very rare (<5 % of patients): agranulocytosis, aplasia, splenomegaly

General

- Very frequent (>50 % of patients): fever
- Frequent (>20 % of patients): fatigue, anorexia, injection site pain
- Occasional (>10 % of patients): epistaxis, febrile neutropenia, weight loss, sweating
- Rare (5–10 % of patients): herpes simplex, hypotension
- Very rare (<5 % of patients): anaphylactic shock, opportunistic infections (blastomycosis, toxoplasmosis), dehydration, systemic inflammatory response

Gastrointestinal

- Very frequent (>50 % of patients): nausea, vomiting
- Frequent (>20 % of patients): diarrhea, constipation, pharyngitis
- Occasional (>10 % of patients): abdominal pain and tenderness
- Rare (5–10 % of patients): stomatitis, oral petechiae, mouth hemorrhage
- Very rare (<5 % of patients): gastrointestinal hemorrhage

Renal

- Rare (5–10 % of patients): dysuria, urinary tract infections
- Very rare (<5 % of patients): renal failure, hematuria

Pulmonary

- Frequent (>20 % of patients): cough, dyspnea
- Occasional (>10 % of patients): chest pain, upper respiratory tract infection, pneumonia, rhinorrhea
- Rare (5–10 % of patients): wheezing, pleural effusion

Cardiac

- Rare (5–10 % of patients): tachycardia

Cutaneous

- Frequent (>20 % of patients): injection site erythema, ecchymosis, petechiae
- Occasional (>10 % of patients): pallor, generalized rash, injection site bruising
- Rare (5–10 % of patients): cellulitis, injection site pruritus, injection site swelling, dry skin, skin nodules

Nervous System

- Frequent (>20 % of patients): headache
- Occasional (>10 % of patients): anxiety, depression, insomnia
- Rare (5–10 % of patients): hypoesthesia
- Very rare (<5 % of patients): confusion, convulsions, intracranial hemorrhage

Metabolic

- Occasional (>10 % of patients): hypokalemia

Locomotor

- Frequent (>20 % of patients): rigors, arthralgia, pain in limb, back pain
- Occasional (>10 % of patients): peripheral edema, myalgia

Teratogenic activity is proven in the animal model. An effective contraceptive method is recommended in patients undergoing 5-azacytidine treatment.

## Decitabine

The use of decitabine [1, 2, 7], an intravenous hypomethylating agent, is currently restricted to the United States. It is indicated in myelodysplasia, with low-intermediate or high-intermediate IPSS.

The most common side effects are hematologic, with anemia, thrombopenia, and neutropenia occurring in more than 50 % of the patients. Febrile neutropenia occurs in about 20 % of patients. Opportunistic infections are rare occurrences. Fungal infections like invasive candidiasis have been described in more than 10 % of patients. The issue of antifungal prophylaxis in patients receiving decitabine treatment remains an open question.

Metabolic side effects are rather common and consist mainly of hypoalbuminemia and hyperglycemia and elevation of liver enzymes. Close monitoring of glucose levels is therefore recommended.

The side effects encountered in patients receiving decitabine treatment are as follows:

Hematologic

- Very frequent (>50 % of patients): neutropenia, thrombocytopenia, anemia
- Occasional (>10 % of patients): lymphadenopathy
- Rare (5–10 % of patients): thrombocythemia
- Very rare (<5 %): bone marrow suppression, splenomegaly

General

- Very frequent (>50 % of patients): pyrexia
- Frequent (>20 % of patients): febrile neutropenia, peripheral edema
- Occasional (>10 % of patients): rigors, pain, lethargy, dehydration, anorexia
- Rare (5–10 % of patients): chest discomfort, catheter site erythema, catheter site pain, injection site swelling

Gastrointestinal

- Frequent (>20 % of patients): nausea, vomiting, constipation, diarrhea
- Occasional (>10 % of patients): abdominal pain, oral mucosal petechiae, stomatitis, dyspepsia, ascites
- Rare (5–10 % of patients): gingival bleedings, hemorrhoids, loose stool, tongue ulceration, dysphagia, lip ulceration, abdominal distension, abdominal pain, gastroesophageal reflux, glossodynia
- Very rare (<5 %): cholecystitis

Renal

- Rare (5–10 % of patients): dysuria, urinary frequency

Pulmonary

- Frequent (>20 % of patients): cough
- Occasional (>10 % of patients): pharyngitis, respiratory crackles, hypoxia
- Rare (5–10 % of patients): postnasal drip

Cardiac

- Rare (5–10 % of patients): pulmonary edema
- Very rare (<5 % of patients): myocardial infarction, atrial fibrillation

Cutaneous

- Frequent (>20 % of patients): ecchymosis, petechiae, pallor
- Occasional (>10 % of patients): rash, skin lesions, pruritus, alopecia
- Rare (5–10 % of patients): urticaria, swelling face

Nervous System

- Frequent (>20 % of patients): headache
- Occasional (>10 % of patients): dizziness, hypoesthesia, insomnia, confusion, anxiety
- Rare (5–10 % of patients): blurred vision

Metabolic

- Frequent (>20 % of patients): hyperglycemia, hypoalbuminemia
- Occasional (>10 % of patients): hyperbilirubinemia, hypomagnesemia, hyponatremia
- Rare (5–10 % of patients): hyperkalemia

Locomotor

- Frequent (>20 % of patients): arthralgia
- Occasional (>10 % of patients): limb pain, back pain
- Rare (5–10 % of patients): chest wall pain, myalgia

Infectious

- Frequent (>20 % of patients): pneumonia
- Occasional (>10 % of patients): cellulitis, candidal infection
- Rare (5–10 % of patients): catheter-related infections, urinary tract infection, sinusitis, bacteremia
- Very rare (<5 % of patients): Mycobacterium avium infection

Effective contraceptive methods are recommended for men and women during and for a minimum of 12 months following therapy.

# Acute Myeloid Leukemia

## *Cytarabine*

Cytarabine [1, 2, 8–10], an intravenous antimetabolite cytidine analogue, has been widely used as monotherapy or in combination with other agents on the induction of treatment for acute myeloid leukemia. It also has proven efficacy in the treatment of lymphomas, especially mantle cell lymphomas, in which cytarabine-containing regimens have allowed longer progression-free survivals and higher remission rates. Cytarabine is also used in some ALL regimens, mainly in the consolidation phase.

The most common adverse effects are hematologic. Hematologic toxicity occurs regularly in patients receiving cytarabine and consists of deep bone marrow depression. Leukopenia typically follows a biphasic curve, with a first nadir at 7–9 days and a second more profound nadir at days 15–24. Frequent bleeds have been described as a result of thrombopenia.

About 10 % of patients may experience cytarabine syndrome, which consists of fever, myalgia, chest pain, maculopapular rash, conjunctivitis, and malaise. Cytarabine syndrome can evolve to severe hypotension and requires corticosteroid treatment. Discontinuation of the treatment must be discussed according to the severity of symptoms.

Nausea and vomiting frequently occur and require prophylaxis with antiemetic treatments. In patients receiving high doses of cytarabine (more than 10 g/week), gastroen-terologic side effects can be more marked and include diarrhea and severe colitis, ranging from neutropenic colitis to gastrointestinal bleeding. Rare cases of pancreatitis have been described with experimental doses of cytarabine.

Febrile neutropenia is a common finding in patients receiving cytarabine-based regimens. If bacterial causes are the most frequent, invasive fungal infections are a frequent occurrence, especially in AML patients. In selected patients, antifungal prophylaxis active against aspergillosis must be considered.

Central nervous system toxicity occurs mostly in elderly patients receiving high-dose regimens. Cerebellar toxicity is the main feature in patients; it results in ataxia and slurred speech. Infrequently, patients can experience confusion or fatal encephalitis. The use of prophylactic pyridoxine treatment has been debated. Conjunctivitis is also a frequent finding in patients. Prophylactic topical corticosteroids may be useful in patients receiving high-dose cytarabine.

The following toxicities have been described with cytarabine:

Hematologic

- Bone marrow depression: anemia, leukopenia, thrombopenia
- Thrombophlebitis (frequent)

General

- Cytarabine syndrome.
- Severe sepsis may occur from leukopenia.
- Rare: allergic reaction, anaphylactic shock.

Gastrointestinal

- Frequent: anorexia, nausea, vomiting, diarrhea, oral and anal mucositis, hepatic dysfunction
- Rare: esophageal ulceration, bowel necrosis, pancreatitis

Renal

- Rare: renal dysfunction, urinary retention

Pulmonary

- Rare: pneumonia, interstitial pneumonitis

Cardiac

- Rare: rapidly progressive pulmonary edema with cardiomegaly, pericarditis

Cutaneous

- Frequent : rash, alopecia (complete alopecia with high doses)
- Rare: freckling, pruritus, urticaria, skin ulceration, hand-foot syndrome, cellulitis at injection site

Nervous System

- Rare: peripheral neuritis, headache, conjunctivitis, CNS toxicity, such as encephalitis and cerebellitis (CNS complications have been described in high-dose and very high-dose cytarabine)

Metabolic

- Frequent: ASAT and ALAT
- Rare: jaundice

Cytarabine may be used intrathecally. The toxicities of intrathecal medication are roughly the same as for intravenous use. Toxicity is, however, self-limiting. Neurologic complications include paraplegia, necrotizing leukoencephalopathy, blindness, and spinal cord necrosis.

Cytarabine displays teratogenic effect in animal models. Women of childbearing age should be advised against conceiving a child during cytarabine therapy. An effective contraceptive method is recommended in both men and women.

## Idarubicin

Idarubicin [1, 2, 11–13], an anthracycline-type topoisomerase II inhibitor, has been recommended in combination with other drugs for the treatment of acute myeloid leukemia.

The main side effects of idarubicin treatment involve hematologic toxicity. Severe myelosuppression is a constant and requires treatment with transfusions and granulocyte colony-stimulating factors. Severe febrile neutropenia may result from idarubicin-containing regimens. Idarubicin should be used with extreme caution in patients displaying cytopenias resulting from prior chemotherapies, as cases of permanent bone marrow suppression have been described.

Alopecia is a frequent complication of idarubicin-based chemotherapies.

Cardiac side effects occur frequently and mostly result from restrictive cardiomyopathy with a decline in left ventricle ejection fraction (LVEF). Decline of LVEF depends on the cumulative dose and the age of the patients. Caution should be applied in patients with preexisting cardiomyopathy or in patients who have been treated with anthracyclines previously.

Extravasation of anthracyclines may lead to extended skin necrosis, which may require surgery. In case of extravasation, intermittent cold packs should be applied and surgical advice should be taken.

Secondary neoplasias have been attributed to anthracyclines. Side effects of idarubicin are as follows:

Hematologic

- Severe myelosuppression

Gastrointestinal

- Frequent: grade I–III nausea, vomiting, mucositis abdominal pain, and diarrhea; grade IV complications are seen in less than 5 % of patients.
- Rare severe enterocolitis with perforation.

Dermatologic

- Frequent: alopecia.
- Occasional: rash, urticaria, and bullous erythrodermous rash of palms and soles. Dermatologic reactions are seen more frequently in patients receiving concurrent antibiotic therapy or with a history of radiotherapy.

Cardiac

- Congestive heart failure, serious arrhythmias, including atrial fibrillation, myocardial infarction

Neurologic

- Very rare (<5 %): peripheral neuropathy, seizures, cerebellar palsy

Pulmonary

- Pneumonitis in less than 5 % of patients

## Daunorubicin

Daunorubicin [1, 2, 11, 12] is an intravenous anthracycline that is used in combination with other drugs for the treatment of acute myeloid leukemia.

Side effects of daunorubicin are roughly the same as for idarubicin. Oral mucositis, bone marrow depression, and decrease in left ventricular function, however, seem less severe than with idarubicin in patients older than 60 years of age.

The maximal cumulative dose of daunorubicin is 550 mg/$m^2$. Some authors propose the dose of 400 mg/$m^2$ in patients who have undergone radiotherapy encompassing the heart.

## Amsacrine

Amsacrine [1, 2, 14] has been approved for the salvage treatment of AML resistant to anthracyclines. In some European countries, amsacrine is used in the consolidation of AML.

Toxicity of amsacrine is essentially hematologic, resulting in constant pancytopenia requiring supportive treatment with red blood cell transfusion and platelet transfusion as well as granulocyte colony-stimulating factor. Amsacrine should not be used if the patient has previous profound chemo-induced pancytopenia.

Gastrointestinal toxicity is frequent and ranges from simple diarrhea to grade IV neutropenic colitis.

Cardiologic side effects consist mostly of arrhythmias, which can be triggered by coexisting hypokalemia. Close monitoring of the electrocardiogram and of serum kalium levels is recommended if using amsacrine.

The side effects of amsacrine are as follows:

Hematologic

- Very frequent: pancytopenia
- Frequent: febrile neutropenia
- Rare: major hemorrhage

Gastrointestinal

- Frequent: grade I–II nausea or vomiting, grade I–IV mucositis

Renal

- Rare: renal dysfunction, anuria, acute renal failure

Hepatic

- Elevation of serum liver tests, hyperbilirubinemia requiring dose adaptation

Neurologic

- Grand mal seizures in heavily pretreated patients with preexisting neurologic conditions

Cardiac

- Frequent: congestive heart failure, cardiac arrest, ventricular tachycardia

Cutaneous

- Reactions at injection site ranging from simple rash to necrosis

Amsacrine has proven teratogenic in mice. Effective methods of contraception are recommended in both men and women.

## Clofarabine (Intravenous)

Clofarabine [1, 2, 15–17], a purine nucleoside analogue, has been approved in the treatment of pediatric ALL. Some studies indicate a benefit in progression-free survival in combination treatment with other drugs in relapsed AML.

Toxicity is mainly hematologic, with febrile neutropenia occurring in about a half of the patients.

Gastrointestinal toxicity is frequent and may lead to severe abdominal pain in 35 % of the patients.

Palmoplantar erythrodysesthesia is a common occurrence and requires topical steroids or topical NSAIDS. Systemic corticosteroids have been discussed as prophylactic treatment.

The side effects of clofarabine are as follows:

Hematologic

- Frequent: bone marrow depression

Cardiologic

- Tachycardia in about a third of the patients
- Pericardial effusion in 35 % of patients

Gastrointestinal

- Frequent: nausea, diarrhea, and vomiting in more than half of the patients. Abdominal pain occurs in 35 % of patients.
- Occasional: sore throat, constipation.

General Disorders

- Fatigue pyrexia and rigors in more than one-third of the patients.
- Mucositis in 17 % of patients.
- Anorexia occurs in 30 % of patients.

Hepatobiliary

- Occasional: jaundice, hepatomegaly

Infectious

- Bacteremia, cellulitis, candidiasis, bacterial, and fungal pneumonia

Neurologic

- Headaches in 44 % of patients
- Rare: somnolence, tremor, depression, anxiety

Respiratory

- Frequent: epistaxis
- Rare: respiratory distress, pleural effusion, cough

Cutaneous

- Frequent: dermatitis, petechiae
- Palmar planter erythrodysesthesia syndrome

## Mylotarg (Intravenous)

Mylotarg [1, 2, 18, 19] is a monoclonal anti-CD33 antibody (gemtuzumab) linked to ozogamycin. It has been used as single-agent treatment of elderly patients with CD33-positive AML. Gemtuzumab ozogamycin has been withdrawn from the market owing to an unfavorable risk-benefit ratio.

Acute infusion-related adverse reactions occur frequently and have led in some cases to grade IV adverse events. Frequent (>30 % of patients) side effects are fever, nausea, chills, vomiting, and headache. About 20–30 % of patients experience dyspnea, hypotension, or hypertension, in some cases with hemodynamic instability. Less frequent acute side effects upon injection may be hyperglycemia and hypoxia. Although no antibodies to gemtuzumab have been detected to date, some severe allergic reaction has been described. Two patients have developed antibodies against ozogamycin.

Hematologic toxicity results in profound neutropenia with a mean time to recovery of 40–43 days. Anemia and thrombopenia are longer lasting. Median time to recovery is 50–56 days.

Hepatotoxicity is an issue in about one-third of patients undergoing treatment with gemtuzumab and ozogamycin and results in grade III–IV elevation of liver enzymes or hyperbilirubinemia. Veno-occlusive disease is a well-known but rare side effect of treatment with gemtuzumab and ozogamycin, occurring in about 1 % of patients. Most cases, however, have been described in the context of allogeneic stem cell transplantation.

The delayed side effects are as follows:

Hematologic

- Very frequent: grade III–IV neutropenia with
- Anemia and thrombopenia
- More than 13 % of patients experienced grade III–IV bleedings

Infectious

- Frequent: septic shock, pneumonia
- Rare: stomatitis, herpes simplex

Hepatotoxicity

- Grade III–IV increase of liver enzymes or hyperbilirubinemia
- Rare: ascites
- Veno-occlusive disease

Gastrointestinal

- Frequent: constipation, anorexia, dyspepsia, nausea stomatitis

Metabolic

- Frequent: hypokalemia
- Occasional: hyperglycemia, hypocalcemia
- Rare: hypomagnesemia, hypophosphatemia

Respiratory

- Frequent (>20 %): cough, dyspnea, epistaxis
- Occasional (20–30 %): pneumonia, pharyngitis

Cutaneous

- Rare: pruritus, rash

# Chronic Myeloproliferative Diseases

The drugs used here are the most common ones for polycythemia vera, essential thrombocythemia, and chronic myeloid
leukemia. For the latter disease, a compilation of the side
effects is given in a tabulated form.

## *Hydrea*

Hydroxyurea [1, 2, 20–22] is an oral inhibitor of nucleoside
reductase and is widely used in melanoma, resistant chronic
myeloid leukemia, recurrent carcinoma of the ovary, and
myeloproliferative diseases (essential thrombocythemia, polycythemia vera).

Bone marrow toxicity is the major side effect of hydroxyurea. Treatment should not be initiated in patients displaying
marked bone marrow depression. Recovery from leukopenia
and thrombopenia is rapid after interruption of treatment.

Cutaneous toxicities are rare but may lead to skin ulcers.
The development of ulcers requires interruption of hydroxyurea
treatment.

In patients treated with hydroxyurea for myeloproliferative syndromes, the rate of secondary leukemias seems slightly increased.

Side effects of hydroxyurea treatment are the following:

Hematologic

- Frequent: neutropenia, thrombopenia, megaloblastic anemia

Cutaneous

- Exacerbation of postirradiation erythema in previously
  irradiated patients.
- Rare: vasculitic toxicities, ulceration, and gangrene are
  seen in patients with myeloproliferative disease with a history
  of interferon.

- Rare: dermatomyositis-like skin changes, maculopapular rash.
- Very rare: alopecia.

### Renal

- Dysuria.
- Impairment of renal tubular function with hyperuricemia and increase of creatinine levels. Renal insufficiency should require dose reduction.

### Gastrointestinal

- Pancreatitis has been described in patients treated with didanosine or stavudine.
- Occasional: stomatitis, nausea, vomiting, diarrhea, constipation.

### Neurologic

- Rare: dizziness, headache, hallucinations, convulsions

### Pulmonary

- Very rare: pulmonary fibrosis

### Carcinogenesis

- Secondary leukemias have been described in patients receiving long-term treatment.

### Laboratory

- Spurious gamma-GT elevations are observed, probably without any clinical consequences.

Multiple fetal malformations have been described in animal models. Men and women considering childbirth should be reassessed for the utility of their treatment, and treatment should be interrupted whenever possible.

## Anagrelide

Anagrelide [1, 2, 22–24] is used in essential thrombocythemia to reduce platelet levels.

Main side effects of anagrelide are cardiologic and consist of supraventricular tachycardia. Anagrelide should be used with caution in patients with preexisting heart disease and prescribed only if the potential benefit outweighs the risks.

Interstitial lung disease (allergic alveolitis, eosinophilic pneumonia, and interstitial pneumonitis), though a very rare occurrence, has been associated with anagrelide. Time of onset is between 1 week and several years after initiation of therapy.

Side effects of anagrelide are the following:

## Hematologic

- Very rare (1–5 %): anemia, leukopenia, and thrombopenia <100,000/uL. Thrombopenia recovers after treatment discontinuation.

### General

- Frequent (20–30 %): asthenia
- Occasional (10–20 %): dizziness, pain, fever
- Rare (5–10 %): malaise
- Very rare (<5 %): flu-like symptoms, chills, photosensitivity, thromboses

### Cardiac

- Frequent (20–30 %): palpitations, edema
- Rare (5–10 %): tachycardia
- Very rare (<5 %): arrhythmia, hypertension, orthostatic hypotension, angina pectoris, heart failure

### Pulmonary

- Interstitial lung diseases

### Locomotor

- Very rare: arthralgia, myalgia, cramps

Cutaneous

- Rare (5–10 %): pruritus
- Very rare (<5 %): alopecia

Gastrointestinal

- Occasional (10–20 %): nausea, abdominal pain, flatulence
- Rare (5–10 %): vomiting
- Very rare (<5 %): GI hemorrhage, melena, aphthous stomatitis, constipation

Special Senses

- Very rare (<5 %): amblyopia, abnormal vision, tinnitus, diplopia, visual field abnormality

Some cases of pregnancies occurring while on anagrelide treatment have been described with no fetal harm. It is, however, recommended that treatment be stopped during pregnancy or if there is a desire to conceive.

## Imatinib, Nilotinib, and Dasatinib [1, 2, 25, 26]

Tyrosine kinase inhibitors are indicated in the treatment of CML. Imatinib and dasatinib have shown efficacy in GIST. Hypereosinophilic syndromes displaying FIP-1L1PDGFR-alpha translocation are also responsive to imatinib.

The spectrum of side effects is comparable between the three molecules. However, the frequency of the respective side effects varies from one molecule to another and may influence treatment decision. Table 11.1 compares the major side effects of imatinib, dasatinib, and nilotinib.

In 2011, a warning was issued by the FDA concerning the risk of pulmonary hypertension in patients receiving dasatinib. Caution is recommended in patients with previous pulmonary hypertension. Close monitoring by cardiac ultrasound is recommended.

TABLE 11.1 Comparative side effects of current tyrosine kinase inhibitors

| Side effects | Frequency Imatinib[a] | | Nilotinib[b] | | Dasatinib | |
|---|---|---|---|---|---|---|
| | All grades | Grade III–IV | All grades | Grade III–IV | All grades | Grade III–IV |
| *Hematologic side effects* (%) | | | | | | |
| Neutropenia | 58–68 | 20 | 38–43 | 10–12 | 65 | 21 |
| Thrombocytopenia | 56–62 | 9–10 | 48 | 10–12 | 70 | 19 |
| Anemia | 47–84 | 5–7 | 38–47 | 3 | 90 | 10 |
| *Nonhematologic side effects* (%) | | | | | | |
| Peripheral edema | 14–36 | 0 | 5 | 0 | 9 | 0 |
| Eyelid edema | 13 | <1 | 2–5 | <1 | 0 | 0 |
| Pleural effusion | 0 | 0 | 0 | 0 | 19 | 1 |
| Periorbital edema | 34 | 0 | 1–2 | 0 | 0 | 0 |
| Diarrhea | 17–60 | 1 | 18–22 | 1 | 17 | <1 |

| | | | | | |
|---|---|---|---|---|---|
| Nausea | 20–31 | 0 | 32–54 | 1 | 8 | 0 |
| Vomiting | 10–14 | 0 | 5–9 | 0 | 5 | 0 |
| Myalgia | 10–12 | 0 | 10 | 0 | 6 | 0 |
| Muscle inflammation | 17 | <1 | NA | NA | 4 | 0 |
| Muscle pain | 14–24 | <1 | 6–7 | 0 | 11 | 0 |
| Rash | 11–17 | 1 | 31–36 | 1–3 | 11% | 0 |
| Headache | 8–10 | 0 | 14–21 | 1 | 12 | 0 |
| Fatigue | 8 | <1 | 9–11 | 0–1 | 10 | 0 |
| Alopecia | 11 | 0 | 22–36 | 0 | 0 | 0 |

*Metabolic side effects* (%)

(continued)

TABLE 11.1  (continued)

| Side effects | Frequency Imatinib[a] | | Nilotinib[b] | | Dasatinib | |
|---|---|---|---|---|---|---|
| | All grades | Grade III–IV | All grades | Grade III–IV | All grades | Grade III–IV |
| Increased bilirubin | 10 | <1 | 53–62 | 4–8 | NA | |
| Increased alkaline phosphatase | 33 | <1 | 21–27 | 0 | | |
| Hypophosphatemia | 45 | 8 | 32–34 | 5 | | |
| Hyperglycemia | 20 | 0 | 41–36 | 4–6 | | |
| Increased lipase | 11 | 3 | 24–29 | 6 | | |
| Increased amylase | 12 | <1 | 15–18 | 1 | | |
| Increased ALT | 20 | 2 | 66–73 | 4–9 | | |
| Increased AST | 23 | 1 | 40–48 | 1–3 | | |
| Increased creatinine | 13 | <1 | 5 | 0 | | |

Adapted from [25, 26]

[a]Ranges for imatinib depend on the study analyzed

[b]Ranges for nilotinib depend on the dosage (300 or 400 mg)

# References

1. Chabner B, Wilson W, Supko J. Pharmacology and toxicity of antineoplastic drugs in Williams. Haematol. 7th edition. 2006, pp. 249–74.
2. Fernandez H. New trends in the standard of care for initial therapy of AML. Haematol. 30th edition. 2010, pp. 56–61.
3. Fenaux P, Gattermann N, Seymour JF, Hellström-Lindberg E, Mufti GJ, Duehrsen U, et al. Prolonged survival with improved tolerability in higher-risk myelodysplastic syndromes: azacitidine compared with low dose ara-C. Br J Haematol. 2010;149(2):244–9. Epub 2010 Feb 5.
4. Santini V, Fenaux P, Mufti GJ, Hellström-Lindberg E, Silverman LR, List A, et al. Management and supportive care measures for adverse events in patients with myelodysplastic syndromes treated with azacitidine. Eur J Haematol. 2010;85(2):130–8. Epub 2010 Apr 12.
5. Almeida AM, Pierdomenico F. Generalized skin reactions in patients with MDS and CMML treated with azacitidine: effective management with concomitant prednisolone. Leuk Res. 2012;36(9):e211–3. Epub 2012 May 22.
6. Fenaux P, Mufti GJ, Hellstrom-Lindberg E, Santini V, Finelli C, Giagounidis A, et al. Efficacy of azacitidine compared with that of conventional care regimens in the treatment of higher-risk myelodysplastic syndromes: a randomised, open-label, phase III study. Lancet Oncol. 2009;10(3):223–32. Epub 2009 Feb 21.
7. Kantarjian HM, Thomas XG, Dmoszynska A, Wierzbowska A, Mazur G, Mayer J, et al. Multicenter, randomized, open-label, phase III trial of decitabine versus patient choice, with physician advice, of either supportive care or low-dose cytarabine for the treatment of older patients with newly diagnosed acute myeloid leukemia. J Clin Oncol. 2012;30(21):2670–7. Epub 2012 Jun 11.
8. Lazarus HM, Herzig RH, Herzig GP, Phillips GL, Roessmann U, Fishman DJ. Central nervous system toxicity of high-dose systemic cytosine arabinoside. Cancer. 1981;48(12):2577–82.
9. Johnson H, Smith TJ, Desforges J. Cytosine-arabinoside-induced colitis and peritonitis: nonoperative management. J Clin Oncol. 1985; 3(5):607–12.
10. Löwenberg B, Pabst T, Vellenga E, van Putten W, Schouten HC, Graux C, et al. Cytarabine dose for acute myeloid leukemia. N Engl J Med. 2011;364(11):1027–36.
11. Mandelli F, Vignetti M, Suciu S, Stasi R, Stasi R, Petti MC, Meloni G, et al. Daunorubicin versus mitoxantrone versus idarubicin as induction and consolidation chemotherapy for adults with acute myeloid leukemia: the EORTC and GIMEMA Groups Study AML-10. J Clin Oncol. 2009;27(32):5397–403. Epub 2009 Oct 13.

12. Moreb JS, Oblon DJ. Outcome of clinical congestive heart failure induced by anthracycline chemotherapy. Cancer. 1992;70:2637.
13. Leoni F, Ciolli S, Nozzoli C, Marrani C, Caporale R, Ferrini PR. Idarubicin in induction treatment of acute myeloid leukemia in the elderly. Haematologica. 1997;82(5 Suppl):13–8.
14. Legha SS, Keating MJ, McCredie KB, Bodey GP, Freireich EJ. Evaluation of AMSA in previously treated patients with acute leukemia: results of therapy in 109 adults. Blood. 1982;60(2):484–90.
15. Faderl S, Wetzler M, Rizzieri D, Schiller G, Jagasia M, Stuart R, et al. Clofarabine plus cytarabine compared with cytarabine alone in older patients with relapsed or refractory acute myelogenous leukemia: results from the CLASSIC I Trial. J Clin Oncol. 2012;30(20):2492–9. Epub 2012 May 14.
16. Claxton D, Erba HP, Faderl S, Arellano M, Lyons RM, Kovacsovics T, et al. Outpatient consolidation treatment with clofarabine in a phase 2 study of older adult patients with previously untreated acute myelogenous leukemia. Leuk Lymphoma. 2012;53(3):435–40. Epub 2011 Oct 24.
17. Kantarjian HM, Erba HP, Claxton D, Arellano M, Lyons RM, Kovascovics T, et al. Phase II study of clofarabine monotherapy in previously untreated older adults with acute myeloid leukemia and unfavorable prognostic factors. J Clin Oncol. 2010;28(4):549–55. Epub 2009 Dec 21.
18. Candoni A, Martinelli G, Toffoletti E, Chiarvesio A, Tiribelli M, Malagola M, et al. Gemtuzumab-ozogamicin in combination with fludarabine, cytarabine, idarubicin (FLAI-GO) as induction therapy in CD33-positive AML patients younger than 65 years. Leuk Res. 2008;32(12):1800–8. Epub 2008 Jul 14.
19. de Lima M, Champlin RE, Thall PF, Wang X, Martin 3rd TG, Cook JD, et al. Phase I/II study of gemtuzumab ozogamicin added to fludarabine, melphalan and allogeneic hematopoietic stem cell transplantation for high-risk CD33 positive myeloid leukemias and myelodysplastic syndrome. Leukemia. 2008;22(2):258–64. Epub 2007 Nov 8.
20. Baz W, Najfeld V, Yotsuya M, Talwar J, Terjanian T, Forte F. Development of myelodysplastic syndrome and acute myeloid leukemia 15 years after hydroxyurea use in a patient with sickle cell anemia. Clin Med Insights Oncol. 2012;6:149–52. Epub 2012 Mar 7.
21. Antonioli E, Guglielmelli P, Pieri L, Finazzi M, Rumi E, Martinelli V, et al. Hydroxyurea-related toxicity in 3,411 patients with Ph'-negative MPN. Am J Hematol. 2012;87(5):552–4. doi:10.1002/ajh.23160. Epub 2012 Apr 4.
22. Kluger N, Naud M, Françès P. Toenails melanonychia induced by hydroxyurea. Presse Med. 2012;41(4):444–5.
23. Gugliotta L, Tieghi A, Tortorella G, Scalzulli PR, Ciancia R, Lunghi M, et al. Low impact of cardiovascular adverse events on anagrelide treatment discontinuation in a cohort of 232 patients with essential thrombocythemia. Leuk Res. 2011;35(12):1557–63. Epub 2011 Jul 20.

24. Birgegård G, Björkholm M, Kutti J, Lärfars G, Löfvenberg E, Markevärn B, et al. Adverse effects and benefits of two years of anagrelide treatment for thrombocythemia in chronic myeloproliferative disorders. Haematologica. 2004;89(5):520–7.
25. Saglio G, Kim DW, Issaragrisil S, le Coutre P, Etienne G, Lobo C, et al. Nilotinib versus imatinib for newly diagnosed chronic myeloid leukemia. N Engl J Med. 2010;362:2251–9.
26. Kantarjian H, Shah NP, Hochhaus A, Cortes J, Shah S, Ayala M, et al. Dasatinib versus imatinib in newly diagnosed chronic-phase chronic myeloid leukemia. N Engl J Med. 2010;362:2260–70.

# Chapter 12
# Lymphoma

**Sigrid Cherrier-De Wilde**

**Abstract**   Lymphomas are subdivided in Hodgkin's disease (HD) and non-Hodgkin's lymphomas (NHL). Essentially the medications used are of two types: monoclonal antibodies and chemotherapy. The side effects of treatment are grouped accordingly. The most commonly used treatment protocol in NHL is a combination of a monoclonal antibody with poly-chemotherapy. Hence, this chapter is subdivided according to these two treatment modalities.

**Keywords**   Hodgkin's disease • Non-Hodgkin's lymphomas Chemotherapy • Monoclonal antibodies

## Introduction

Lymphoma has multiple subtypes. It is variable in its histopathology, symptomatology, area of involvement, and prognosis and treatment. Lymphoma represents about 5 % of cancers and more than 55 % of hematologic cancers.

S. Cherrier-De Wilde, M.D.
Department of Hematology, Centre Hospitalier de Luxembourg,
Luxembourg, Luxembourg
email: cherrier.sigrid@che.lu

M.A. Dicato (ed.), *Side Effects of Medical Cancer Therapy,*     447
DOI 10.1007/978-0-85729-787-7_12,
© Springer-Verlag London 2013

Lymphomas are divided into two groups: the Hodgkin's and the non-Hodgkin's lymphomas. However, sometimes, it is not possible to classify lymphoma in one of those groups; these cases are labeled B-cell lymphoma unclassifiable.

The classical chemotherapy schedule for a non-Hodgkin's lymphoma is the CHOP (cyclophosphamide, hydroxorubicin, Oncovin, and prednisone) regimen and its derivatives (CVP, CHOEP, COMP, etc.), but purine nucleoside-based combinations are also possible.

More intensive schedules include ifosfamide, platins, cytarabine, and melphalan.

Treatment of lymphoma is based on a combination of chemotherapy, radiotherapy, and monoclonal antibodies or a monotherapy with either one of them.

In case of relapse or even for high-grade lymphomas in first remission, an intensification of the treatment can be done by means of high-dose chemotherapy followed by the infusion of stem cells. Mostly these are autologous stem cells, but allografting is a therapeutic option for a relapsing lymphoma.

On the other hand, there is also the treatment of secondary manifestations like pain, hypercalcemia, hyperuricemia, spontaneous tumor lysis, spinal cord compression, seizures, renal insufficiency, anemia, thrombopenia, and so forth. These aspects are covered in other chapters of this book.

Lymphomatous meningitis is treated by high-dose intravenous chemotherapy (cytarabine or methotrexate) and intrathecal chemotherapy (methotrexate, cytarabine, hydrocortisone). More novel treatments include, for example, intrathecal rituximab.

# Monoclonal Antibodies [1–5]

## *Rituximab*

Rituximab is one of the most commonly used intravenous drugs in the treatment of CD20-positive lymphomas.

The possibility of severe or even fatal infusion reaction necessitates the use of adequate premedication (antipyretics, antihistamine, and glucocorticoid). Resuscitation equipment should be available, and close monitoring is indispensable, especially in patients with a preexisting cardiac condition.

The initial infusion rate (250 mg/h) has to be increased every 30 min to a maximum of 400 mg/h. If a severe reaction happens, stop immediately. In case of a less severe reaction, the diffusion rate is to be decreased.

Tumor lysis syndrome occurs frequently when there is a large tumor burden and necessitates adequate hydration, rasburicase, or allopurinol.

Because of suppression of the B-lymphocytes with increased sensitivity to infections, prophylaxis against pneumocystis and herpes may be necessary.

The most frequent side effects are fever, hypertension, peripheral edema, pain, rash, pruritus, nausea, diarrhea, cytopenia, arthralgia, cough, and weakness.

Less frequent adverse events include hypotension, anxiety, dizziness, hyperglycemia, progressive multifocal leukoencephalopathy (JC virus), bowel obstruction and perforation, ventricular tachycardia, viral reactivation, and mucocutaneous reactions.

Drug interactions with anticoagulants or antiplatelet agents, immunosuppressants, vaccines, and so forth need to be considered.

In order to prevent pregnancy, effective contraceptive methods, as discussed in another chapter in this book, are recommended during and for a minimum of 12 months following therapy.

## Ibritumomab (Zevalin)

Ibritumomab is an intravenous radioimmunotherapy for CD20-positive lymphomas in relapsed or refractory setting or as a part of intensification.

The necessary premedication is similar to that for rituximab, and serious fatal infusion reactions may occur (see section "Rituximab").

No administration should be considered if the platelets are below 100,000 cells/mm$^3$ or in case of 25 % bone marrow involvement because of the risk of prolonged cytopenia.

The most frequent side effects are fatigue, chills, fever, pain, headache, nausea and vomiting, diarrhea, abdominal pain, nasopharyngitis, cough or dyspnea, infection, and hematologic toxicity.

Less frequent adverse reactions occur as peripheral edema, hypertension or hypotension, flushing, pruritus, rash, myalgia or arthralgia, melena, myelodysplastic syndromes, bronchospasm, and apnea.

There is a risk of formation of human antimouse antibodies (HAMA).

Severe mucocutaneous reactions or extravasation and radiation necrosis are possible.

Delayed radiation injury in the region of lymphoma can occur.

One should pay attention to drug interactions with anticoagulants or antiplatelet agents, immunosuppressants, and vaccines.

The B-cell recovery starts only at 3 months and reaches normal range in 9 months.

## Alemtuzumab

Alemtuzumab is an intravenous or subcutaneous drug with the following action: antibody-dependent lysis by binding the CD52 of B-cell chronic lymphocytic leukemia (CLL), T-cell lymphoma, and T-cell prolymphocytic leukemia.

In the beginning, dose escalation is required. Because of a possible infusion reaction, it is necessary to initiate effective antiallergic and antipyretic treatment before administration. There is a high infection rate if no prophylactic treatment is administered.

In case of subcutaneous injection, a local site reaction can be observed.

The most frequent side effects are hypotension, peripheral edema, hypertension, dysrhythmias, fever, fatigue, headache, dizziness, rash, urticaria and dizziness, nausea and vomiting, anorexia, rigors, myalgias, and skeletal pain.

Less frequent side effect reactions include chest pain, purpura, dyspepsia, positive Coombs' test without hemolysis, autoimmune thrombocytopenia, and hemolytic anemia.

A serious and fatal cytopenia can occur, and transfusion with irradiated blood product is recommended because of the potential for graft-versus-host disease (GVHD) during lymphopenia.

## Ofatumumab

Ofatumumab is a new intravenous drug for relapses of CD20-positive lymphomas and leukemias after treatment with rituximab.

The possible adverse effects are flu-like signs, fatigue, nausea, diarrhea, infections, cough, temperature, mouth sores, anal itching, and difficulty speaking.

## Tositumomab

Tositumomab is an intravenous radioimmunotherapeutic drug acting on depletion of CD20-positive cells by apoptosis, complement-dependent cytotoxicity, and antibody-dependent cellular cytotoxicity.

As for rituximab administration, premedication is necessary to avoid infusion-related toxicity.

The administration of thyroid-protective agents is recommended 24 h before administration of the dosimetric dose.

The most frequent adverse events are fever, pain, chills, headache, rash, hypothyroidism, nausea, anorexia, myelosuppression, myalgia, cough, dyspnea, and infections.

Less frequent side reactions can occur as hypotension, peripheral edema, dizziness, pruritus, arthralgia, rhinitis, and secondary malignancies.

Tositumomab should not be used in patients with impaired bone marrow reserve or marrow involvement over 25 %.

## Temsirolimus

Temsirolimus is a new intravenous drug in the treatment of mantle cell lymphoma.

Premedication with an H1 antagonist is indispensable. In case of a hypersensitivity reaction, the infusion rate should be slowed.

Drug interactions and concomitant administration of CYP3A4 inhibitors or inducers as well as anticoagulants and sunitinib should be avoided. The patient should also avoid drinking grapefruit juice.

This drug is contraindicated in moderate to severe hepatic dysfunction.

The dose must be adapted for hematologic toxicity. The dose may need to be adapted to the complete blood count.

The most frequent adverse reactions are edema, chest pain, fever, headache, insomnia, rash, hyperglycemia, hypercholesterolemia, hypophosphatemia, hypokalemia, mucositis, nausea and anorexia, diarrhea, dyspnea, and infections.

Less frequent side effects are hypertension, venous thromboembolism, depression, acne, bowel perforation, hyperbilirubinemia, myalgia, interstitial lung disease, and seizure.

To prevent pregnancy, effective contraceptive methods for men and women during and for a minimum of 3 months following therapy are recommended for all the aforementioned drugs.

# Chemotherapy [2, 6]

## Fludarabine

Fludarabine [7–9] is a widely used oral and intravenous treatment in cases of CLL, acute leukemia, follicular lymphoma, Waldenström's macroglobulinemia, and stem cell transplant.

An adjustment to renal creatinine clearance must be made.

A major problem can be hematotoxicity, with even very long cytopenias (2 months to 1 year), and common autoimmune effects such as hemolysis, ITP, Evans syndrome, and acquired hemophilia. These side effects may recur if the patient is given the drug again.

Because of the frequent opportunistic infections, prophylactic anti-infectives should be considered.

The most frequent adverse reactions are edema, fever, fatigue, rash, nausea, diarrhea, neuromuscular weakness, visual disturbance, paresthesia, cough, and pneumonia. Less frequent side effects include headache, neurotoxicity (coma, confusion, seizure, PML), arrhythmia, thromboembolic event, alopecia, hyperglycemia, stomatitis, dysuria, hearing loss, hematuria, allergic pneumonitis, flu-like syndrome, and cortical blindness.

Fludarabine should not be used in combination with pentostatin because of the risk of severe or fatal pulmonary toxicity.

If transfusion is necessary, only irradiated blood products should be used because of the possibility of transfusion-related GVHD.

The combination with alcohol can induce gastrointestinal irritation.

Drug interactions with trastuzumab, clozapine, immunosuppressants, and vaccines can occur.

In order to prevent pregnancy, effective contraceptive methods are recommended for men and women during and for a minimum of 6 months following therapy.

## Chlorambucil

Chlorambucil is an old oral chemotherapeutic given to treat CLL, non-Hodgkin's lymphoma, Hodgkin's lymphoma, and Waldenström's macroglobulinemia.

Frequent adverse events are drug fever, skin reaction (discontinue promptly), edema, syndrome of inappropriate antidiuretic hormone (SIADH) secretion, hematologic toxicity, hepatotoxicity, neuropathy, interstitial pneumonia, secondary malignancies, and seizures (especially if there is a history of seizure, nephrotic syndrome, or head trauma).

A dosage reduction is needed in case of hepatic impairment.

The absorption is reduced with food.

Drug interactions with trastuzumab, clozapine, immunosuppressants, and vaccines can occur.

It can affect human fertility and probably has mutagenic and teratogenic effects, which are covered elsewhere in this book.

## Bleomycin

Bleomycin is a drug administered intravenously, intramuscularly, subcutaneously, and intrapleurally for a wide range of indications, such as Hodgkin's lymphoma, testicular cancer, ovarian germ cell cancer, malignant pleural effusion, and squamous cell carcinoma.

The best known toxicity is pulmonary, and this risk increases with cumulative lifetime dose (>400 mg). It is diagnosed as an interstitial pneumonitis and pulmonary fibrosis, and the response to corticoids is variable. It is more frequent in the elderly, smokers, and patients with prior radiation therapy or who are undergoing oxygen therapy. Filgrastim may enhance the adverse effects and pulmonary toxicity.

There is a risk for an anaphylactoid reaction. It is controversial whether an initial test dose should be given because of false-negative results. The onset may be immediate or delayed for several hours.

The dose must be adjusted in cases of renal impairment.

The most frequent adverse reactions are phlebitis, pain at tumor site, hyperpigmentation, alopecia, mucositis, anorexia, and acute febrile reactions.

Rare side effects include angioedema, chest pain, cerebrovascular accident (CVA), hepatotoxicity, Raynaud's phenomenon, and thrombotic microangiopathy.

Women should avoid becoming pregnant during treatment.

## Carmustine (BCNU)

Carmustine is an intravenous medication for Hodgkin's lymphoma, multiple myeloma, brain tumors, non-Hodgkin's lymphoma, glioblastoma, stem cell transplant, and mycosis fungoides.

This product is an irritant at the injection site and should be prepared in glass or polyolefin containers. The infusion must go slowly for 2 h to avoid flushing, hypotension, and agitation.

The most frequent adverse events are arrhythmia, ataxia, headache, hyperpigmentation, vomiting, nausea, hematologic toxicity, hepatic toxicity, conjunctival suffusion, renal failure, interstitial pneumonitis, and pulmonary fibrosis (with delayed onset).

Melphalan favors the adverse effects and sensitizes patients to carmustine lung toxicity.

Attention needs to be paid to drug interactions with trastuzumab, clozapine, immunosuppressants, and vaccines.

Women should avoid becoming pregnant while on treatment.

## Dacarbazine

Dacarbazine is an intravenous chemotherapeutic drug for Hodgkin's lymphoma, metastatic melanoma, and sarcoma.

In case of extravasation, immediately apply cold packs and protect the site of extravasation from daylight.

The most frequent adverse reactions are alopecia, nausea and vomiting, anorexia, myelosuppression, flu-like syndrome, hepatic necrosis, anaphylactic reactions, and renal and liver impairment.

One should pay attention to drug interactions with trastuzumab, clozapine, immunosuppressants, and vaccines; patients should avoid ethanol and St. John's wort.

Because of its known carcinogenic and teratogenic effects, dacarbazine should be used in pregnancy only if the benefit outweighs the potential risk to the fetus.

## Bendamustine

Bendamustine [4, 5, 10, 11] is an old but newly available intravenous drug for CLL, non-Hodgkin's lymphoma, mantle cell lymphoma, and multiple myeloma.

Its use is not recommended if moderate or severe hepatic insufficiency is present or if clearance is under 40 mL/min.

Hypersensitivity reactions during infusion are possible (chills, pruritus, rash, fever, anaphylactic reactions).

The most frequent adverse events are peripheral edema, fatigue, fever, headache, chills, rash, nausea and vomiting, diarrhea, stomatitis, abdominal pain, myelosuppression, weakness, cough, and dyspnea.

Rare side effects can be tachycardia, anxiety, pain, chest pain, hypotension, xerostomia, increase in transaminases, infusion site pain, infection, and toxic skin reactions.

One should pay attention to drug interactions with clozapine and inducers or inhibitors of CYP1A2.

In case of possible pregnancy, effective contraceptive methods during and for a minimum of 3 months following therapy are recommended.

# References

1. Smith MR. Antibodies and hematologic malignancies. Cancer J. 2008;14(3):184–90.
2. Armitage JO. How I treat patients with diffuse large B-cell lymphoma. Blood. 2007;110(1):29–36.
3. Cheson BD, Leonard JP. Monoclonal antibody therapy for B-cell non-Hodgkin's lymphoma. N Engl J Med. 2008;359:613–26.
4. Friedberg JW, Vose JM, Kelly JL, Young F, Bernstein SH, Peterson D, et al. The combination of bendamustine, bortezomib, and rituximab for patients with relapsed/refractory indolent and mantle cell non-Hodgkin lymphoma. Blood. 2011;117:2807–12. doi:10.1182/blood-2010-11-314708.
5. Rummel MJ, Niederle N, Maschmeyer G, Banat AG, von Gruenhagen U, Losem C, et al. Bendamustine plus rituximab (B-R) versus CHOP plus rituximab (CHOP-R) as first-line treatment in patients with indolent and mantle cell lymphomas (MCL): updated results from the StiL NHL1 study. J Clin Oncol. 2012;30(suppl; abstr 3).
6. Savage KJ, Skinnider B, Al-Mansour M, Sehn LH, Gascoyne RD, Connors JM. Treating limited-stage nodular lymphocyte predominant Hodgkin lymphoma similarly to classical Hodgkin lymphoma with ABVD may improve outcome. Blood. 2011;118:4585–90. doi:10.1182/blood-2011-07-365932.
7. Zinzani PL. Clinical experience with fludarabine in indolent non-Hodgkin's lymphoma. Hematol J. 2004;5 Suppl 1:S38–49.

8. Economopoulos T, Psyrri A, Fountzilas G, Tsatalas C, Anagnostopoulos A, Papageorgiou S, et al. Phase II study of low-grade non-Hodgkin lymphomas with fludarabine and mitoxantrone followed by rituximab consolidation: promising results in marginal zone lymphoma. Leuk Lymphoma. 2008;49(1):68–74.

9. Johnson SA. Use of fludarabine in the treatment of mantle cell lymphoma, Waldenström's macroglobulinemia and other uncommon B- and T-cell lymphoid malignancies. Hematol J. 2004;5 Suppl 1:S50–61.

10. Weidmann E, Kim SZ, Rost A, Schuppert H, Seipelt G, Hoelzer D, Mitrou PS. Bendamustine is effective in relapsed or refractory aggressive non-Hodgkin's lymphoma. Ann Oncol. 2012;13(8):1285–9.

11. Ohmachi K, Ando K, Ogura M, Uchida T, Itoh K, Kubota N, et al.; Japanese Bendamustine Lymphoma Study Group. Multicenter phase II study of bendamustine for relapsed or refractory indolent B-cell non-Hodgkin lymphoma and mantle cell lymphoma. Cancer Sci. 2010;101(9):2059–64.

# Chapter 13
## Multiple Myeloma

**Mario A. Dicato**

**Abstract** The treatment and prognosis of multiple myeloma have completely changed over the past decade with the advent of the new nonchemotherapeutic agents thalidomide, lenalidomide, and bortezomib. Their side effects are completely different from those seen with standard treatment. Some are common, like peripheral neuropathy for thalidomide and bortezomib, blood count changes for lenalidomide and bortezomib, or venous thromboembolic events for thalidomide and lenalidomide. These different toxicity profiles allow combinations and sequences of administration, thus avoiding cumulative toxicities.

**Keywords** Myeloma • Plasma cell dyscrasias • Side effects Thalidomide • Lenalidomide • Bortezomib

## Introduction

With the availability over the past decade of three new drugs—thalidomide, lenalidomide, and bortezomib—multiple myeloma is one of the few instances in neoplastic diseases

M.A. Dicato, M.D.
Department of Hematology-Oncology, Centre Hospitalier
de Luxembourg, Luxembourg, Luxembourg
e-mail: dicato.mario@chl.lu, mdicato@gmail.com

M.A. Dicato (ed.), *Side Effects of Medical Cancer Therapy,*  459
DOI 10.1007/978-0-85729-787-7_13,
© Springer-Verlag London 2013

where a poor prognostic malignancy has been changed into a more chronic disease with a substantial improvement in quality of life and survival.

Before the availability of these agents, the side effects of chemotherapy were, and still are, those of bone marrow depression, which occurs with standard- and high-dose chemotherapy, with and without autologous stem cell transplantation. Chemotherapy's side effects of anemia, neutropenia, and thrombocytopenia, as well as mucositis, hair loss, and so forth, are similar to those that occur in other oncological situations, namely, hypo-oxygenation, infections, and bleeding, and they are described elsewhere in this book.

These new nonstandard chemotherapeutic drugs have a different toxicity profile that will be covered in this chapter. Various nonspecific side effects, such as constipation and fatigue, are treated symptomatically.

## Thalidomide

Thalidomide, which was used some 40–50 years ago to treat emesis in pregnancy and as a light sedative, was taken off the market because of its major teratogenic effect of phokomelia due to its antiangiogenic properties. By the end of the 1990s, thalidomide became available for multiple myeloma. Very rapidly, this drug was used fairly frequently at various dosages as a primary treatment, as maintenance, and in combination with other treatments, such as chemotherapy, and also with lenalidomide, corticosteroids, and bortezomib. Several side effects are characteristic, but we will discuss peripheral neuropathy, which is a major side effect of this drug. The second major side effect is the risk of venous thromboembolic events. This complication is the same as for lenalidomide, as discussed below.

*Peripheral neuropathy* (PN) is one of the major side effects of this drug. The neuropathy is mostly sensorial with dysesthesias and less frequently of the motor type. Often patients with myeloma already have some neuropathic symptoms owing to the disease itself, other medical problems like diabetes or alcohol consumption, or to previous peripheral nerve-damaging treatments like vincristine, which was part of the standard VAD therapy (vincristine, Adriamycin, and dexamethasone). The precise mechanism of thalidomide-induced PN is not established. A dose-dependent neuropathy occurs frequently, and often this side effect becomes irreversible and may have a major negative impact on quality of life. EMG testing is not really useful, and early clinical diagnosis is of prime importance. One should ask the patient about early signs like dysesthesia, pain, and so forth in order to modify the dose, lengthen the interval of administration, or to stop the medication. Side effects may be alleviated by standard pain medication or gabapentin, pregabalin, and so on [1]. Vitamin B preparations have not been a major contribution to therapy.

## Lenalidomide

Lenalidomide is of the same group as thalidomide, but it has a different toxicity profile. The bone marrow toxicity of thalidomide is very minor or nonexistent, but lenalidomide may present major hematologic toxicity.

*Neutropenia* is common with lenalidomide when given as single agent, as, for instance, in maintenance therapy. However, the incidence of neutropenia is notably increased when lenalidomide is used in combination with chemotherapeutic agents [1]. Febrile neutropenia, on the other hand, is notably less frequent. Neutropenia may be such that treatment will have to be adapted, the more so when used in association with chemotherapeutic agents.

*Secondary cancers* like myelodysplastic syndromes (MDS) and acute myeloid leukemia (AML) have been reported in about 6 % of patients, with an expected 2 % in the placebo group [2, 3]. The interpretation of this observation is difficult, however. Of note, the same malignancies, MDS and AML, are also increased in untreated monoclonal gammopathies of unknown significance [2, 3]. For thalidomide, no increased risk has been reported [4].

*Venous thromboembolic events* (VTE) are reported with both thalidomide and lenalidomide. The incidence is markedly increased if patients are treated in combination with a corticosteroid, mostly dexamethasone, erythropoietin, and/or a chemotherapeutic agent. In these situations, the standard prophylaxis set forth in all guidelines for VTE in cancer patients is recommended [5]. In addition to these recommendations, it is notable that prophylaxis with aspirin is useful and can be an option [6]. Skin rashes are seen occasionally with lenalidomide. Symptomatic treatment is advisable. Often dexamethasone can be added as antimyeloma therapy, and skin rashes may be controlled.

Lenalidomide does not have peripheral neuropathy as a side effect and can be an alternative to thalidomide or bortezomib [7]. Renal failure can be induced or worsened by lenalidomide. A rare renal complication is *acute interstitial nephritis*. A renal biopsy is necessary to diagnose this complication because in myeloma, renal failure can present due to other causes. Often myeloma patients are on bisphosphonates, including zoledronic acid; these nephrotoxic agents are covered in another chapter in this book. With these agents, accompanying lesions are tubular necrosis and not interstitial nephritis. In lenalidomide-induced interstitial nephritis, some authors presume the cause is immune mediated [8].

# Bortezomib

This proteasome inhibitor, first in class, has also been a major advance in treatment of myeloma. Side effects include also peripheral neuropathy. Usually PN is less severe than the one seen with thalidomide, and if the medication is stopped when not far advanced, this side effect is mostly reversible.

As with thalidomide, questioning the patient and paying attention to early clinical signs of dysesthesia can be helpful.

One major side effect is *thrombocytopenia*. This is not due to bone marrow toxicity, as seen with chemotherapeutic agents, but is a transient effect on platelet release by megakaryocytes. It is advisable to stop or decrease the dosage when platelet levels are below 50,000 mm$^3$; however, platelet transfusions are rarely necessary.

*Herpes zoster-varicella* virus reactivation can occur with bortezomib and increase the incidence of debilitating postherpetic neuralgia, especially when bortezomib is used in combination with high-dose dexamethasone. Acyclovir has to be considered as a prophylactic measure [9].

*Renal insufficiency* is a frequent complication of myeloma. The incidence is about 20–40 % at presentation and can be 50 % or more in the course of the disease. Renal failure can be induced or worsened with nonsteroidal anti-inflammatory drugs or bisphosphonates. Bortezomib has been shown to rapidly improve kidney function and may sometimes prevent or even reverse dialysis [10]. If for some reason bortezomib is not indicated, thalidomide or lenalidomide can be an option [11].

# Summary

Overall, in myeloma, the new agents, thalidomide, lenalidomide, and bortezomib, though they have a different profile of side effects, are much easier to administer, and their side effects are less severe, resulting in a remarkably improved quality of life for the patient.

# References

1. Mateos MV. Management of treatment related adverse events in patients with multiple myeloma. Cancer Treat Rev. 2010;36 Suppl 2:S24–32. http://www.ncbi.nlm.nih.gov/pubmed/20472185.
2. Attal M, Lauwers VC, Marit G, Caillot D, Facon T, Hulin C, et al. Maintenance treatment with lenalidomide after transplantation for myeloma: final analysis of the IMF 2005–02. Blood (ASH annual meeting abstracts) 2010;116:Abstract 310.
3. McCarthy PL, Owzar K, Anderson KC, Hofmeister CC, Hurd DD, Hassoun H, et al. Phase III Intergroup study of lenalidomide versus placebo maintenance therapy following single autologous hematopoietic stem cell transplantation for multiple myeloma: CALGB 100104 abstract. Blood (ASH annual meeting abstracts). 2010;116:Abstract 37.

4. Stewart AK, Trudel S, Bahlis N, et al. A randomized phase III trial of thalidomide and prednisone as maintenance therapy following autologous stem cell transplantation in patients with multiple myeloma: the NCIC CTG My.10 trial (abstract). Blood. 2010;116(21). Abstract 39.

5. Mandala M, Falanga A, Roila F. Management of venous thromboembolism in cancer patients. ESMO Clinical Practice Guidelines. Ann Oncol. 2011;22 Suppl 6:85–92.

6. Palumbo A, Rajkumar SV, Dimopoulos MA, Richardson PG, San Miguel J, Barlogie B, et al. Prevention of thalidomide and lenalidomide associated thrombosis in myeloma. Leukemia. 2008;22:414–23.

7. Delforge M, Bladé J, Dimopoulos MA, Facon T, Kropff M, Ludwig H, et al. Treatment- related peripheral neuropathy in multiple myeloma. The challenge continues. Lancet Oncol. 2010;11:1086–95.

8. Lipson EJ, Huff CA, Holanda DG, McDevitt MA, Fine DM. Lenalidomide-induced acute interstitial nephritis. Oncologist. 2010;15:961–4.

9. Vickrey E, Allen S, Singhal S. Acyclovir to prevent reactivation of varicella-zoster virus (herpes zoster) in multiple myeloma patients receiving bortezomib therapy. Cancer. 2009;115:229–32.

10. Ludwig H, Adam Z, Hajek R, Greil R, Tóthová E, Keil F, et al. Light chain induced acute renal failure can be reversed by bortezomib-doxorubicin-dexamethasone in multiple myeloma: results of a phase II study. J Clin Oncol. 2010;28:4635–41.

11. Dimopoulos M, Alegre A, Stadtmauer EA, Goldschmidt H, Zonder JA, de Castro CM, et al. The efficacy and safety of lenalidomide plus dexamethasone in relapsed and/or refractory multiple myeloma patients with impaired renal function. Cancer. 2010;116:3807–14.

# Chapter 14
# Preservation of Fertility in the Cancer Patient

**Duhem Caroline and Fernand Ries**

**Abstract** Preservation of fertility is a key determinant of long-term quality of life of adolescents and young adults treated for curable forms of cancer. The risk of developing primary or secondary infertility after completion of their treatment is variable and difficult to predict. Moreover, evaluation of the extent and reversibility of gonadotoxicity of cancer therapies is currently imperfect, especially in young women.

The most established method of preserving fertility is sperm banking in men and embryo cryopreservation in young women who have a partner. However, many alternative, though still experimental, options are in development that can already be proposed to young patients in well-defined conditions.

Despite the progress and refinement of fertility preservation techniques and the increase in educational resources, an information gap between patients and healthcare teams still persists. As the new field of oncofertility goes forward, concerted efforts must be made to improve communication of information to patients by integrating these features in pretreatment discussion and in definition of therapeutic strategies.

D. Caroline, M.D. (✉) • F. Ries, M.D.
Department of Hematology-Oncology,
Centre Hospitalier de Luxembourg, Luxembourg, Luxembourg

M.A. Dicato (ed.), *Side Effects of Medical Cancer Therapy,*
DOI 10.1007/978-0-85729-787-7_14,
© Springer-Verlag London 2013

**Keywords**    Fertility preservation • Quality of life • Information
Communication • Reproductive medicine • Methods of medically
assisted procreation

# Introduction

As the curability of most cancer subtypes in children and young
adults has improved, preservation of an optimal quality of life
has become a major issue and requires from oncologists an
increasing acknowledgment and prevention of long-term adverse
effects of their treatments. Among these, the loss of reproductive
potential of cancer survivors has major repercussions on their
quality of life [1–4]. It is often reported by young women treated
for breast cancer as one of the most devastating experiences,
even more stressful than the diagnosis of cancer itself [5].

Approximately 5–6 % of cancer patients are younger than
40 years, and a large proportion of them have not completed
their parenthood. About 50 % of current oncologic treatments may have severe repercussions on their reproductive
potential. Fertility items and potential fertility preservation
(FP) modalities are challenging in young patients but much
less complex in men than in women.

# Fertility Preservation in Men

## *Risk Factors for Infertility*

Cancer itself can be correlated with azoospermia in conditions like Hodgkin's disease and testicular cancer. Moreover,
several surgical procedures (like pelvic surgery for testicular
or prostate cancer) can cause severe damage, interfering with
ejaculation. However, the primary threat for fertility in men
is compromised sperm production, quality and mobility, and
DNA damage secondary to chemotherapy and/or radiotherapy exposure (Table 14.1).

If permanent infertility can result from quantitative and
qualitative damage to spermatogenesis stem cells, more

TABLE 14.1 Risk of azoospermia according to treatment regimen

*Major (prolonged or definitive azoospermia)*:

Total body irradiation

Testicular irradiation at a dose ≥ 2.5 Gy

High-dose alkylating agents ± radiotherapy for transplant conditioning

Cyclophosphamide >7.5 $g/m^2$ (cumulative dose)

Cranial brain radiation (≥40 Gy)

*Intermediate (prolonged azoospermia)*:

Uncommon at standard dose (BEP regimen for 2–4 cycles)

Cumulative cisplatin dose < 400 $mg/m^2$ or carboplatin < 2 $g/m^2$

*Low risk (temporary azoospermia)*: nonalkylating chemotherapy (ABVD)

*Unknown*: irinotecan, oxaliplatin, bevacizumab, cetuximab, erlotinib, etc.

frequently, temporary impairment of spermatogenesis occurs with most cytotoxic agents, up to 2 years after completion of therapy, with a nadir in sperm count during the first 6 months. As in women, the extent of damage to gametogenesis depends on the age of the patient and on the type, the cumulative dose, and the schedule of chemotherapy.

Radiotherapy, even at low dose, is toxic for developing sperm tissue; the delivery of high-dose pelvic irradiation (as required for prostate and rectal cancer or testicular seminoma) can induce permanent damage to testicular function and also possibly some level of erectile dysfunction.

## Options to Preserve Fertility in Men

### Sperm Banking

The best option for FP in males is cryopreservation of semen before treatment. Collection of three or four samples after an approximately 48-h period of abstinence between sampling (a total of more than 5 days) is ideal. Long-term follow-up studies of cryopreservation (up to 28 years) suggest a very prolonged conservability of sperm capacity for fertilization [6]. The significance of notifying the patient of potential risk (even if minimal) of iatrogenic infertility as early as possible remains critical. It is strongly advisable to complete sperm banking before starting therapy to avoid increased genetic damage in sperm collected after the start of therapy.

Limitations to this intervention include the inability to masturbate and/or ejaculate as a result of age, discomfort, or level of illness. In these rare situations, some alternative, though more invasive, procedures can be offered, such as electroejaculation under general anesthesia or microsurgical epididymal sperm aspiration.

## Alternative Options

Cryopreservation of spermatogonial stem cells and testicular tissue is an outpatient procedure that can be considered for prepubescent boys or when sperm banking is impossible for any other reason. As for ovarian cortex cryopreservation in females, this method is still experimental (with no live births reported to date) and carries a theorical risk of contamination of testicular tissue by cancer cells.

There is currently no substantial evidence supporting the use of hormonal suppression by LH-RH (luteinizing hormone-releasing hormone) analogues together with chemotherapy in men for the purpose of FP.

The use of gonadal shielding during radiotherapy to reduce the dose of radiation delivered to the testis can be offered when feasible (eventually in combination with sperm banking).

# Fertility Preservation in Women

The issue of FP is much more complex in young women than in men because simple, rapid, and validated procedures like sperm banking are not available. Moreover, reliable methods to predict and evaluate the gonadal toxicity of treatments in females are still lacking.

## Risk Factors and Evaluation of Gonadal Repercussions of Treatment

If the diagnosis of cancer itself does not seem to affect female fertility, most anticancer treatments may induce a variety of reproductive disorders, including immediate, definitive infertility, premature menopause, and compromized ability to carry a pregnancy due to uterine damage. The evaluation of risk of gonadotoxicity is hampered by several factors. First, long-term follow-up studies of reproductive function in female survivors are lacking, precluding the distinction between acute and permanent ovarian failure. Moreover, the assessment of secondary ovarian failure relies mostly on clinical parameters like the rate of prolonged chemotherapy-induced amenorrhea (CIA) rather than on objective indicators of ovarian reserve such as ultrasonic parameters (antral follicle counts or AFCs) or serum hormonal levels [7]. Some recent papers report on the value of anti-Müllerian hormone (AMH) assessment as a reliable predictor of primary follicle reserve before, during, and after chemotherapy, preferable in that setting to any other conventional dosage (estradiol, follicle-stimulating hormone [FSH], and inhibin B) [8].

The risk of secondary ovarian failure depends greatly on the age of the treated patient, on her pretreatment fertility status, and on the type and dose of chemotherapy (high dose of alkylating agents being the more toxic). Definitive infertility can also result from abdominal and/or pelvic radiotherapy (according to doses and fields of irradiation) and obviously from most forms of nonconservative gynecologic surgery.

If the effects of cytotoxic regimens depend partly on the baseline ovarian reserve, they become particularly pronounced by the time the patients reach 40 years of age. As young women have a large primordial follicle pool, they are less likely to lose all their reserves immediately after chemotherapy, but even those women who resume regular menses after treatment will eventually experience premature ovarian failure as a consequence of a significant loss of primary follicles.

TABLE 14.2 Risk of prolonged CIA in women

| Degree of risk | Treatment protocol |
|---|---|
| High (>80 % CIA) | Whole abdominal or pelvic irradiation ($\geq 6$ Gy in adults) |
| | Total body irradiation |
| | Cyclophosphamide $\geq 5$ g/m$^2$ in women >40 |
| | Any high cumulative dose of alkylating agent |
| | Cranial radiation $\geq 40$ Gy |
| Intermediate (30–70 % CIA) | CMF, CEF, or CAF ×6 in women aged 30–39 (breast cancer) |
| | AC in women >40 (breast cancer) |
| | BEACOPP in women <40 (Hodgkin's disease) |
| Low risk (<20 % CIA) | AC in women aged 30–39 (breast cancer) |
| | CMF, CEF, or CAF in women <30 |
| | Nonalkylating chemotherapy (ABVD) |
| Unknown | Taxanes |
| | Oxaliplatin |
| | Irinotecan |
| | Targeted therapies (bevacizumab, cetuximab, trastuzumab, erlotinib, imatinib, etc.) |

Taken together, all these variables make any accurate prediction or evaluation of the incidence and reversibility of iatrogenic infertility difficult at an individual level. Table 14.2 reports grossly on the rate of prolonged CIA during and after treatment, which is the only available (but quite imperfect) surrogate measure of impact on female fertility. However, these data are even lacking for many modern treatments already used in the routine.

TABLE 14.3 Techniques of FP in young women

| Options | Benefits | Concerns |
| --- | --- | --- |
| 1. IVF and embryo cryopreservation | Well-established technique | Requires a male partner |
| | Clinical availability | Ovarian stimulation |
| | | Delay |
| 2. Oocyte cryopreservation | No male partner required | Efficacy unknown |
| | | Ovarian stimulation |
| | | Delay |
| 3. Cryopreservation of ovarian tissue | No male partner required | Pregnancy rate unknown |
| | No ovarian stimulation | Potential malignant tissue grafting |
| | No delay | Laparoscopy |
| 4. Ovarian suppression by LH-RH analogues | No male partner required | Unproven efficacy |
| | Noninvasive technique | Safety concerns |
| | No delay | |

## Options to Preserve Fertility in Women

Currently, the choices for FP in female patients undergoing chemotherapy are limited; most are still investigational, and highly variable success rates are reported. The potential benefits and drawbacks of the four main FP methods in young women are summarized in Table 14.3.

### In Vitro Fertilization

In vitro fertilization (IVF) and embryo banking are the most successful and the only validated forms of FP with excellent chances of future pregnancy, with a success rate per embryo transfer of 15–45 % . The main downside of IVF in cancer patients is that a single cycle can take up to 6 weeks from the first day of the menstrual cycle to complete; this includes a sequence of hormonal injections during 10–12 days to stimulate egg development and oocyte retrieval after a close monitoring of growth. In practice, it entails a delay in onset of cancer treatment that sometimes exceeds 2 months (e.g., if more than one cycle of IVF is needed). However, this can be significantly shortened by early referral of potential candidates to reproductive specialists. For this reason, some authors suggest a global implication and awareness of multidisciplinary teams caring for young patients (like breast units) and a real shift in responsibilities. In the case of young breast cancer patients, a rapid referral of potential young candidates for FP techniques from surgeons and even from radiologists (instead of medical oncologists) to specialists in reproductive medicine could shorten this delay by 2–6 weeks. Another emerging approach that attempts to reduce the delays required by IVF is an emergency ovarian stimulation at a random cycle date without waiting for the spontaneous cycle to start [9].

A second barrier to adopt IVF as a routine procedure of FP in breast cancer patients is the concern about estradiol peak (sometimes 30 times above baselines values) secondary to ovarian stimulation. Several alternative regimens of ovarian stimulation can be proposed in that setting. Patients can undergo ovulation induction with the aromatase inhibitor letrozole, either as a sole agent or as an adjunct to standard stimulation protocols, to avoid an extreme rise in estradiol levels [10]. Up to now, preliminary data suggest comparable outcomes (recurrence of breast cancer and survival rate) in young women stimulated with this IVF regimen and a control group of unstimulated patients [11].

## Oocyte Banking

For many years, the fragility of mature oocytes compared to fertilized embryos has hampered the relative success of this procedure, mainly due to viability concerns after thawing.

This method is still experimental, but rapid advances are currently being made in freezing-thawing protocols (like vitrification methods) that should make it a more viable alternative in the future.

Oocyte banking can be an option for single women who are not interested in using donor sperm, but, similarly to IVF, it requires an ovarian hyperstimulation followed by oocyte retrieval and entails a delay in treatment ranging from 2 to 6 weeks.

## Cryopreservation of Ovarian Tissue

Surgical excision of ovarian cortex tissue and freezing of dissected slices have emerged as an innovative, promising, though still experimental, option for female FP. The theoretical advantages include the rapidity of this laparoscopic procedure, which can provide a large number of follicles and oocytes at any time during the menstrual cycle and without any previous ovarian stimulation in young women but also in prepubertal young girls (the only option in this population). The ovarian tissue can be used for orthotopic transplantation, with a possibility to restore both endocrine function and egg production for spontaneous pregnancy but also for in vitro growth and maturation of oocytes as emerging options in the future [12].

However, though highly publicized in the media since the first publication in 2004, the success rate of this attractive procedure is unknown; to date, fewer than 20 pregnancies have been reported after orthotopic transplantation of thawed ovarian tissue [13].

Moreover, despite screening for tumor cells before freezing and again before reimplantation with appropriate histologic, immunologic, and molecular biology techniques, the risk of viable malignant cell contamination and restoration persists. This risk could be higher in leukemia patients than in patients with Hodgkin's lymphoma or breast cancer [14, 15].

Very active research tracks are ongoing in this domain, aimed at optimizing the efficacy and safety of the procedure. Examples include avoidance of ischemic injury (transplantation of whole cryopreserved ovary), isolated follicles transplant, in vitro follicular culture, pharmacological protection of oocytes, and new freezing-thawing techniques.

## Ovarian Suppression by LH-RH Analogues

During the last two decades, animal studies and small observational series have suggested that LH-RH agonists, given together with chemotherapy, might offer protection against premature ovarian failure; however, no consistent explanation nor biologic plausibility can be hypothesized, FSH receptors being exclusively expressed on follicles during advanced stages of development. Speculative mechanisms of action include the reduction of blood flow to the ovaries.

Monthly LH-RH injections (triptorelin or goserelin) have to begin at least 2 weeks prior to the first cycle of chemotherapy; this time is required to obtain hormonal suppression after an initial stimulatory "flare." During this period of ovarian overactivity, the ovary would be placed at particular risk from the toxic effect of chemotherapy.

Recently, the results of three randomized controlled trials and one meta-analysis have been published, investigating the preventive effect of LH-RH analogues given together with chemotherapy, on ovarian failure, mostly in young women treated for breast cancer or lymphoma [16–18]. In general, these studies have not provided consistent, reproducible evidence of the protective effect on ovarian function, especially when reliable indicators of ovarian reserve (like AMH levels or AFC at ultrasound) were evaluated [19]; at best, available data suggest a certain degree of prevention on incidence and duration of CIA.

In breast cancer, this approach raises theorical safety concerns, both as interfering with the efficacy of systemic treatments and as a consequence of the initial flare effect (potential stimulatory effect and delay of at least 2 weeks in treatment onset).

In reality, the greatest danger in administering LH-RH analogues for the purpose of FP outside clinical trials is that it may divert patients from more relevant options.

## Other Options of FP in Females

Adapted surgical and/or radiotherapy procedures can be offered in selected cases of pelvic or abdominal tumors:

- Ovarian transposition (or oophoropexy): this intervention can be done laparoscopically and allows the moving of ovaries as far as possible from the radiation fields, though scatter radiation and alteration of ovarian blood supply can be reasons behind ovarian failure.
- Gonadal shielding during radiation therapy.
- Conservative gynecologic surgery, like trachelectomy in early cervical cancer or limited surgical staging for border-line or early ovarian cancer. These surgical approaches can be considered in very selected cases and after careful mul-tidisciplinary discussion.

Donor embryos, donor eggs, gestational surrogacy, and adoption are other potential options subject to national bio-ethics. Nevertheless, some evidence suggests that cancer sur-vivors prefer biologic offspring over adoption and third-party reproduction opportunities and are rather interested in pro-tecting their own reproductive capacity [2].

# Attitude Toward FP in Cancer Patients

When questioned specifically on this issue, most young cancer patients manifest a huge interest in FP questions, as they pres-ent, when feasible, a positive perspective for the future; however, these issues are still suboptimally approached by oncologists in daily practice, despite international guideline recommendations like the 2006 guidelines of the American Society of Clinical Oncology (Table 14.4) [20]. Retrospective series report a consis-tent proportion of 30–60 % of oncologists appropriately tackling these issues before treatment, even in male patients despite the wide and rapid accessibility to sperm banking [1–3, 21, 22].

The most apparent barriers to communicate in that field are as follows:

TABLE 14.4 Summary of FP procedures: an algorithm

Evaluation of risk of gonadotoxicity

Discussion with the patient

↓

Interest and feasibility of FP techniques

↙                                              ↘

*Validated techniques*                         *Experimental techniques*

↙        ↘

| Males | Females | Cryopreservation of ovarian/testicular tissue |
|---|---|---|
| Sperm banking | IVF and cryopreservation of embryos | Cryopreservation of oocytes |
| | Gonadal shielding | Ovarian suppression by LH-RH analogues |
| | Oophoropexy | |

Adapted from [20]

- Lack of physicians' knowledge about real risks of infertility from their treatments, about FP techniques, and about inherent risks (mainly delay and stimulation of hormone-responsive tumors)
- Lack of appropriate collaboration with a team of fertility specialists
- Lack of time to discuss this issue and wrong appreciation of patient's interest for FP procedures according to her/his parenting or marital status
- Anticipation of patient's wish to begin the treatment rapidly and to give priority to optimal chances of cure

The topic of FP may be understated when it is presented by oncologists along with a myriad of other potential, sometimes severe, adverse effects; additional educational material (booklets, website, etc.) may be required to help facilitate conversation and decision making [23].

Moreover, pretreatment fertility and FP counseling delivered not exclusively by an oncologist but also by a fertility specialist significantly improve long-term quality of life in reproductive-age women with cancer [24]; this issue has been evaluated by validated quality-of-life scales (like the Decision Regret Score), but most potential candidates, sometimes under pressure from their families or their physicians, believe they have no time to pursue such consultation.

In parallel to technical and practical issues, two major issues must be pointed out by oncologists early enough in the complex discussion about FP:

- It is mostly recommended to female patients to wait 2–5 years after cancer treatment completion before trying to achieve spontaneous or medically assisted pregnancy. Recent data seem very reassuring about the outcome of breast cancer survivors who became pregnant after their treatment. There is even an observed lower risk of death compared with that of breast cancer patients who did not become pregnant, though selection bias partly could contribute to this decreased risk ("healthy mother effect") [25].
- There is currently no evidence that a history of cancer, cancer treatment, or fertility intervention increase the rate of congenital abnormalities or of cancer in the progeny compared to general population; the risk of miscarriage and of preterm delivery can be a concern, but it is limited to a small fraction of women who had radiation to their pelvic area or some fertility-sparing surgery.

Finally, as the FP decisions are made in the context of a life-changing and potentially life-threatening diagnosis, the broader application of FP techniques to young cancer patients will undoubtedly raise new difficult ethical and legal problems in the future (like ownership of embryos after death of one partner, preimplantation genetic diagnosis in conjunction with IVF, reimplantation of embryos in oligometastatic setting). It could require an adaptation of bioethical legislation to this specific population. These problems are beyond the scope of this chapter.

# Summary

Young patients confronted with a diagnosis of cancer have unmet needs for information about the potential risks of infertility and available options of FP. Although choices (at least for young women) are still limited, advances in both gamete and gonadal tissue cryopreservation as well as assisted reproductive technologies are quickly developing. Oncofertility has emerged as a new hybrid specialty, requiring from all oncologists minimal basic knowledge, communication skills, and effective collaboration with fertility specialists, as emergency decisions and measures have to be taken before any cytotoxic treatment. Basic information delivered by oncology teams to their young patients can be relayed by educational material, but, more importantly, the potential candidates must be rapidly referred to reproductive medicine specialists for optimal individualized management.

On the other hand, young patients must be made aware of the limitations of the currently available FP techniques in order to establish reasonable expectations; sperm banking and embryo cryopreservation are actually considered the only standard procedures. Other new options, while promising, are still experimental and must be proposed as such. Patients must be informed of persisting uncertainties in up-to-date knowledge about potential repercussions of modern therapies on their fertility, success rate of different procedures, and possible additional risks from available options. However, a multidisciplinary approach that integrates both realism and medical progress should facilitate a meaningful discussion that assists young patients in making the parenthood decisions that are right for them.

# References

1. Knopman JM, Papadopoulos EB, Grifo JA, Fino ME, Noyes N. Surviving childhood and reproductive-age malignancy: effects on fertility and future parenthood. Lancet Oncol. 2010;11(5):490–8.
2. Levine J, Canada A, Stern CJ. Fertility preservation in adolescents and young adults with cancer. J Clin Oncol. 2010;28(32):4831–41.
3. Sonmezer M, Oktay K. Fertility preservation in young women undergoing breast cancer therapy. Oncologist. 2006;11(5):422–34.
4. Jeruss JS, Woodruff TK. Preservation of fertility in patients with cancer. N Engl J Med. 2009;360(9):902–11.
5. Peate M, Meiser B, Friedlander M, Zorbas H, Rovelli S, Sansom-Daly U, et al. It's now or never: fertility-related knowledge, decision-making preferences, and treatment intentions in young women with breast cancer – an Australian fertility decision aid collaborative group study. J Clin Oncol. 2011;29(13):1670–7.
6. Feldschuh J, Brassel J, Durso N, Levine A. Successful sperm storage for 28 years. Fertil Steril. 2005;84(4):1017.
7. Sukumvanich P, Case LD, Van Zee K, Singletary SE, Paskett ED, Petrek JA, et al. Incidence and time course of bleeding after long-term amenorrhea after breast cancer treatment: a prospective study. Cancer. 2010;116(13):3102–11.
8. Reh A, Oktem O, Oktay K. Impact of breast cancer chemotherapy on ovarian reserve: a prospective observational analysis by menstrual history and ovarian reserve markers. Fertil Steril. 2008;90(5):1635–9.
9. Sönmezer M, Türkçüoğlu I, Coşkun U, Oktay K. Random start controlled ovarian hyperstimulation for emergency fertility preservation in letrozole cycles. Fertil Steril. 2011;95(6):2125.e9–11.
10. Oktay K, Buyuk E, Libertella N, Akar M, Rosenwaks Z. Fertility preservation in breast cancer patients: a prospective controlled comparison of ovarian stimulation with tamoxifen and letrozole for embryo cryopreservation. J Clin Oncol. 2005;23(19):4347–53.
11. Azim AA, Costantini-Ferrando M, Oktay K. Safety of fertility preservation by ovarian stimulation with letrozole and gonadotropins in patients with breast cancer: a prospective controlled study. J Clin Oncol. 2008;26(16):2630–5.
12. Sonmezer M, Oktay K. Orthotopic and heterotopic ovarian tissue transplantation. Best Pract Res Clin Obstet Gynaecol. 2010;24(1):113–26.
13. Donnez J, Dolmans MM, Demylle D, Jadoul P, Pirard C, Squifflet J, et al. Livebirth after orthotopic transplantation of cryopreserved ovarian tissue. Lancet. 2004;364(9443):1405–10. Erratum in: Lancet. 2004;364(9450):2020.

14. Dolmans MM, Marinescu C, Saussoy P, Van Langendonckt A, Amorim C, Donnez J. Reimplantation of cryopreserved ovarian tissue from patients with acute lymphoblastic leukemia is potentially unsafe. Blood. 2010;116(16):2908–14.

15. Rosendahl M, Timmermans Wielenga V, Nedergaard L, Kristensen SG, Ernst E, et al. Cryopreservation of ovarian tissue for fertility preservation: no evidence of malignant cell contamination in ovarian tissue from patients with breast cancer. Fertil Steril. 2011;95(6): 2158–61.

16. Gerber B, von Minckwitz G, Stehle H, Reimer T, Felberbaum R, Maass N, et al. Effect of luteinizing hormone-releasing hormone agonist on ovarian function after modern adjuvant breast cancer chemotherapy: the GBG 37 ZORO study. J Clin Oncol. 2011;29(17): 2334–41.

17. Del Mastro L, Boni L, Michelotti A, Gamucci T, Olmeo N, Gori S, et al. Effect of the gonadotropin-releasing hormone analogue triptorelin on the occurrence of chemotherapy-induced early menopause in premenopausal women with breast cancer: a randomized trial. JAMA. 2011;306(3):269–76.

18. Bedaiwy MA, Abou-Setta AM, Desai N, Hurd W, Starks D, El-Nashar SA, et al. Gonadotropin-releasing hormone analog cotreatment for preservation of ovarian function during gonadotoxic chemotherapy: a systematic review and meta-analysis. Fertil Steril. 2011;95(3):906–14. e1–4.

19. Behringer K, Wildt L, Mueller H, Mattle V, Ganitis P, van den Hoonaard B, et al. No protection of the ovarian follicle pool with the use of GnRH-analogues or oral contraceptives in young women treated with escalated BEACOPP for advanced-stage Hodgkin lymphoma. Final results of a phase II trial from the German Hodgkin Study Group. Ann Oncol. 2010;21(10):2052–60.

20. Lee SJ, Schover LR, Partridge AH, Patrizio P, Hamish Wallace W, Hagerty K, et al. American Society of Clinical Oncology recommendations on fertility preservation in cancer patients. J Clin Oncol. 2006;24(18):2917–31.

21. Quinn GP, Vadaparampil ST, Lee JH, Jacobsen PB, Bepler G, Lancaster J, et al. Physician referral for fertility preservation in oncology patients: a national study of practice behaviors. J Clin Oncol. 2009;27(35):5952–7.

22. Schover LR, Brey K, Lichtin A, Lipshultz LI, Jeha S. Oncologists' attitudes and practices regarding banking sperm before cancer treatment. J Clin Oncol. 2002;20(7):1890–7.

23. Quinn GP, Vadaparampil ST, Malo T, Reinecke J, Bower B, Albrecht T, et al. Oncologists' use of patient educational materials about cancer and fertility preservation. Psychooncology. 2011. doi:10.1002/pon.2022.

24. Letourneau JM, Ebbel EE, Katz PP, Katz A, Ai WZ, Chien AJ, et al. Pretreatment fertility counseling and fertility preservation improve quality of life in reproductive age women with cancer. Cancer. 2011. doi:10.1002/cncr.26459.
25. Azim Jr HA, Santoro L, Pavlidis N, Gelber S, Kroman N, Azim H, et al. Safety of pregnancy following breast cancer diagnosis: a meta-analysis of 14 studies. Eur J Cancer. 2011;47(1):74–83.

# Chapter 15
# Cardiotoxicity

**Irene Braña, Esther Zamora, and Josep Tabernero**

**Abstract**   Although outcomes in cancer patients have dramatically improved with the development of novel cancer chemotherapies and combination treatment, these developments are nonetheless associated with emerging concerns over drug-induced cardiotoxicity. Moreover, recent incorporation of targeted therapies into therapeutic regimens has widened the cardiotoxic spectrum. Knowledge of these side effects and the main risk factors associated with cardiotoxicity in cancer patients is essential for adequate monitoring and early treatment of such events in these patients. This concern is reflected in drug development with an emphasis on improved characterization of potential cardiotoxicity of new compounds during the early phases of development and designing safer drugs. This chapter summarizes the major cardiotoxic effects and pathophysiology of a large number of antineoplastic treatments currently in use. Current recommendations for early treatment and future development are also described.

I. Braña, M.D. (✉) • E. Zamora, M.D. • J. Tabernero, M.D.
Medical Oncology Department, Vall d'Hebron University Hospital,
Barcelona, Spain
email: ibrana@vhebron.net

M.A. Dicato (ed.), *Side Effects of Medical Cancer Therapy*,
DOI 10.1007/978-0-85729-787-7_15,
© Springer-Verlag London 2013

483

**Keywords**    Cardiotoxicity • Side effect • Left ventricular dysfunction
Heart failure • Angina • Arrhythmia • QTc interval

# Introduction

Oncologists are becoming increasingly concerned about the presence of cardiotoxicity associated with many antineoplastic agents currently used to effectively treat patients, particularly in light of the observation that such chronic adverse events may worsen the long-term outcomes of survivors [1–4]. It is especially important given that the general population is aging and that cancer and cardiovascular diseases are common in this elderly population. In addition, novel mechanisms of cardiotoxicity associated with classic cytotoxics and new targeted therapies have been described. There is thus a need for cooperation between cardiologists and oncologists to improve prevention and management of cancer-associated cardiovascular events. Various authors have recently proposed the need for a novel discipline that has been referred to as cardio-oncology or onco-cardiology [5].

Cardiotoxicity is defined by the National Cancer Institute (NCI) as "toxicity that affects the heart" [5], which not only includes direct effects on the heart but also hemodynamic flow alterations or thrombotic events associated with cancer treatment. The most common complications related to anticancer treatment include dilated cardiomyopathy due to myocardial necrosis, rhythm disturbances, and angina or myocardial infarction secondary to vasoocclusion or vasospasm. Several drugs act via a combination of the underlying mechanisms that result in these conditions, but typically one is predominant in the clinical landscape for each drug [5–7].

The incidence of both cancer and heart disease increase with age. Additionally, the presence of an underlying heart condition increases the risk of cardiotoxicity of any kind [8], leaving the elderly population more prone to developing cardiotoxicity.

TABLE 15.1 Drug-induced ventricular dysfunction classification

|  | Type I | Type II |
|---|---|---|
| Reversibility | No | Yes |
| Cumulative dose-related | Yes | No |
| Ultrastructural changes | Vacuoles, sarcomere disruption, necrosis | Not relevant |
| Drugs | Doxorubicin | Trastuzumab |
|  | Mitoxantrone | Sunitinib |
|  | Cyclophosphamide | Lapatinib |
|  |  | Imatinib |
|  |  | Bortezomib |

# Cardiomyopathy: Left Ventricular Dysfunction

Anthracycline-related cardiomyopathy is the paradigm of chemotherapy-induced cardiotoxicity, but in recent years, other agents have also been shown to induce cardiomyopathy, such as trastuzumab and the tyrosine kinase inhibitors sunitinib, lapatinib, and imatinib.

A classification of cardiomyopathy developed in association with an anticancer treatment has been proposed, based on its reversibility and observed pathological features (Table 15.1) [9], Type I agents, such anthracyclines, mitoxantrone, or cyclophosphamide, induce irreversible myocardial damage, which correlates with the cumulative dose. On the other hand, type II agents, such as trastuzumab or tyrosine kinase inhibitors, induce potentially reversible cardiomyopathy without ultrastructural myocyte damage. Based on the transient nature of this cardiotoxicity, the anticancer agent may be resumed after recovery from toxicity, assuming an acceptable risk.

## Anthracyclines

Anthracyclines, the cornerstone treatment of breast cancer, sarcoma, and hematological malignancies, can potentially induce cardiotoxicity as either an early event after administration or as a chronic side effect [6–8, 10].

Acute/subacute cardiovascular complications include those occurring within the first 2 weeks after dosing. They consist of electrocardiographic abnormalities, supraventricular or ventricular arrhythmias [11], or a pericarditis-myocarditis syndrome [12]. Chronic cardiotoxicity is manifested as clinical heart failure or subclinical decline in myocardial function. For some patients, this toxicity constitutes an early event (within the first year) after chemotherapy completion, while others experience it as a delayed effect manifesting more than 1 year after treatment completion [13].

The main mechanism associated with anthracycline-related cardiotoxicity is oxidative stress, which generates free radicals that induce cellular membrane damage due to lipid peroxidation [5]. Other proposed mechanisms include mitochondrial DNA mutations, calcium imbalance, direct DNA damage, and deregulation of cardiac transcription factors. Endomyocardial biopsies show several specific features under electron microscopy such as vacuole formation, disarray of the contractile elements, and myocyte necrosis [14–16]. Furthermore, these findings have been shown to correlate with cumulative dose, which is considered by some to be the main risk factor associated with anthracycline-induced cardiomyopathy [10]. For instance, cumulative doxorubicin doses of 400–450 mg/m$^2$ result in a 5 % likelihood of congestive heart failure [17]. An additional risk factor identified is the rate of infusion, with lower infusion rates appearing to be less harmful [17, 18].

Various studies have observed anthracycline toxicity at lower cumulative doses than expected in specific susceptible patient populations, based on the following risk factors: planned cumulative doxorubicin dose >300 mg/m$^2$ [8, 19], prior cardiac irradiation [20], previous heart disease [21], hypertension [21], coronary artery disease [21], and age greater than 65 years [17]. Patients can be stratified according to these risk factors in low-risk (no risk factors), moderate-risk (one to two risk factors), and high-risk (more than two risk factors) categories [8]. Evaluation of these risk factors, adequate correction of reversible risk factors prior to anthracycline treatment, and subsequent close monitoring of high-risk patients are paramount.

One approach to reducing anthracycline cardiotoxicity involves the development of new compounds and formulations. Epirubicin and liposomal formulations are good examples. Epirubicin is a semisynthetic epimer of doxorubicin that induces less cardiotoxicity than doxorubicin at equivalent myelosuppressive doses, allowing administration of approximately one-third more equivalent treatment cycles [22–25]. Liposomal formulations confer substantial cardioprotection, as they induce changes in the drug distribution pattern, achieving lower concentrations in the heart and higher concentrations in the tumor. Thus, pegylated liposomal doxorubicin allows administration of twice as many cycles compared to the native compound [26, 27]. Moreover, high distribution to peripheral tissues has widened its oncological spectrum, leading to approval for use in ovarian cancer, multiple myeloma, and AIDS-related Kaposi's sarcoma, in addition to breast cancer. Pegylated liposomal doxorubicin is thus a possible chemotherapeutic alternative in patients requiring anthracycline treatment when a cardiac-sparing agent is sought.

## Mitoxantrone

Structurally related to anthracyclines, mitoxantrone induces similar ultrastructural changes in myocytes. Its potential to induce cardiotoxicity is linked to its cumulative dose or of any other type I agents [28].

## Cyclophosphamide

This alkylating agent produces myocardial hemorrhagic necrosis, especially with high-dose regimens. Distinct from anthracyclines and mitoxantrone, cyclophosphamide-induced cardiotoxicity is less dependent on the cumulative dose and more closely related to the dose administered in an individual cycle [29, 30].

## Trastuzumab

This humanized monoclonal antibody against HER2 tyrosine kinase receptor is effective in patients with HER2-positive breast cancers (20–25 % of all breast cancers). Trastuzumab induces left ventricular dysfunction, which mimics the stunning or hibernation phenomenon described in myocardial ischemia [9]. Extensive data supporting the underlying mechanism for this toxicity have been published; HER2 is also expressed in the heart, and preclinical studies suggest that perturbation of downstream pathways affects cardiomyocyte survival and adaptation to stress. According to trastuzumab adjuvant trials [31–33], associated cardiotoxicity is not dependent on cumulative dose, is reversible, and does not result in endomyocardial ultrastructural changes [9].

A number of risk factors have been associated with higher incidence of trastuzumab-induced cardiotoxicity: age greater than 50 years, borderline left ventricular ejection fraction (LVEF) prior to trastuzumab treatment, history of cardiovascular disease, cardiovascular risk factors (diabetes, dyslipidemia, or body mass index greater than 30), the sequence in which chemotherapy is administered, and prior anthracycline treatment (cumulative dose greater than 300 mg/m$^2$) [6, 34–38]. In a metastatic setting, the incidence of LVEF decrease or asymptomatic heart failure with single-agent trastuzumab was 7 %, increasing to 13 % when administered concurrently with paclitaxel and to 27 % when administered sequentially with anthracyclines [38]. The synergistic toxicity seen with trastuzumab and anthracyclines, which was also observed in adjuvant trials, may be related to two aspects of the regimen. Firstly, anthracyclines induce loss of cardiomyocytes, and thus, by the time trastuzumab is administered, several remodeling processes are underway. This favors anti-HER2 treatment-induced toxicity [39]. Secondly, HER2 appears to be required for cell repair in the heart. Trastuzumab administration might inhibit downstream pathways, leading ultimately to increased damage and myocyte death [36, 40, 41].

It is important to note that a higher incidence of heart failure was observed in trials in which trastuzumab was administered concurrently with, or shortly after, anthracycline treatment [38]. Results of the Breast Cancer International Research Group study (BCIRG-006) are of particular interest. This study assessed the efficacy and safety of trastuzumab combined with a non-anthracycline regimen (paclitaxel, cyclophosphamide, and trastuzumab) compared to sequential administration of trastuzumab in an anthracycline-containing group (four cycles of doxorubicin and cyclophosphamide, followed by four cycles of docetaxel and trastuzumab) and in comparison to an anthracycline-containing regimen without trastuzumab [32]. In this trial, the risk of developing New York Heart Association (NYHA) class III or IV heart failure was significantly lower in the non-anthracycline arm (0.38 %) versus the anthracycline-containing arm (1.96 %).

## Lapatinib

Lapatinib is an oral dual inhibitor of the epidermal growth factor receptor and of HER2. Pooled data from 44 studies suggest that 1.6 % of patients treated with lapatinib developed clinical failure or experienced an absolute LVEF decrease of $\geq 20$ % [42]. In most cases cardiac events were reversible. The mechanism of toxicity is related to impaired myocyte response following injury secondary to inhibition of HER2 downstream pathways [36, 40, 41]. The reasons why the rates of cardiotoxicity induced by trastuzumab and lapatinib, both targeting HER2, are so different remain controversial.

## Sunitinib

Sunitinib is an oral inhibitor of vascular endothelial growth factor receptors (VEGFRs) 1–3, platelet-derived growth factor receptors (PDGFRs)-(alpha)$\alpha$ and (beta)$\beta$, KIT, fms-related tyrosine kinase 3 (FLT3), colony-stimulating factor 1 receptor (CSFIR), and rearranged during transfection (RET). Chu et al. retrospectively analyzed the cardiotoxicity of this agent in 75 patients with gastrointestinal stromal tumors enrolled in phase I and II trials using sunitinib. The incidence of LVEF decrease >10 % was 28 %, while the incidence of heart failure was 8 % [43]. LVEF significantly improved after sunitinib discontinuation, and no cumulative dose relationship was observed.

It is thought that the underlying mechanism is a so-called "off-target" effect mediated by ribosomal S6 kinase inhibition, which causes ATP depletion and activates the intrinsic apoptotic pathway [36]. In contrast to trastuzumab-induced cardiomyopathy, some changes in myocardial biopsies, such as alterations in mitochondria, have been observed [43]. An additional potential mechanism is that sunitinib induces hypertension, but also impairs heart adaptation to pressure overload through VEGFR inhibition, as is the case for other antiangiogenic treatments [36]. It is still unknown whether angiotensin-converting enzyme inhibitors or beta-blockers, now commonly used to treat sunitinib-induced hypertension, have a role in preventing sunitinib-induced left ventricular dysfunction [8].

## Imatinib

This is a small molecule tyrosine kinase inhibitor of ABL, ABL-related gene (ARG), PDGFRs-(alpha)$\alpha$ and (beta)$\beta$, and KIT. Peripheral edema has been described along with a 0.6 % incidence of heart failure, usually in older patients with prior cardiovascular disease [44]. This toxicity is considered to be secondary to endoplasmic reticulum stress response activation, and it is mediated by PKR-like ER kinase (PERK) [45].

## Bortezomib

This proteasome inhibitor is associated with a 5 % incidence of heart failure [46]. It is believed that proteasome inhibition causes endoplasmic reticulum stress, leading ultimately to myocyte dysfunction [6, 47].

# Coronary Artery Disease

Systemic anticancer treatments have been shown to induce coronary events, mainly via two different mechanisms: coronary artery vasospasm and arterial thrombotic events. 5-Fluorouracil is the most commonly used drug associated with the first mechanism, while antiangiogenic drugs are the archetype of the second. Additionally, other antineoplastic agents commonly linked to cardiac ischemia include purine analogues, topoisomerase inhibitors such as etoposide, and antitumor antibiotics.

## Fluoropyrimidines

Treatment with 5-fluorouracil and capecitabine may lead to cardiac ischemia, myocardial infarction, and malignant ventricular arrhythmia through coronary vasospasm. The incidence of 5-fluorouracil-induced angina varies widely between studies, from as little as 1 % to up to 68 % [6, 48–51], with a mean onset of 72 h after treatment initiation [52]. The incidence of capecitabine-induced toxicity ranges from 3 to 9 % [6, 49], and its onset is typically in the range of 3 h to 4 days after treatment initiation. In a study of over 600 patients treated with 5-fluorouracil, 4 % developed clinical symptoms, electrographic changes, or both [6, 53]. In most cases, patients had a prior coronary condition. Treatment with nitrates and calcium-channel blockers has successfully prevented new episodes of ischemia in these patients [51]. 5-fluouroracil-induced toxicity appears to be dose- and rate-dependent, with continuous infusion and high doses ($>800$ mg/m$^2$) associated with higher rates of toxicity [52].

## Antiangiogenic Therapies

One of the proposed mechanisms for antiangiogenic drug-induced arterial thrombosis is mediated by inhibition of the vascular endothelial growth factor (VEGF), which may impair endothelial cell regeneration after incidental trauma, leading to subendothelial collagen exposure followed by activation of tissue factors that ultimately induce arterial thrombosis. Interference with platelet aggregation has also been described as playing a role. A third mechanism associated with sorafenib-induced ischemia has been proposed, with RAF inhibition activating two proapoptotic kinases involved in oxidant stress-induced injury in cardiomyocytes, making them more prone to ischemic damage [54].

The incidence of angina and myocardial infarction with bevacizumab, a monoclonal antibody against VEGF, varies in the literature from 0.6 to 1.5 % [55, 56]. This toxicity has not been shown to be dose-dependent, and the median time to a coronary event is 3 months. Proposed risk factors include age over 65 years and previous history of arterial thrombotic event [55].

Regarding antiangiogenic multi-targeted kinase inhibitors, in an observational study of 86 patients with metastatic renal cell carcinoma treated with sunitinib or sorafenib, 33.8 % experienced a cardiovascular event, most of which were related to myocardial damage of varying degrees. Approximately half of the cases (16.2 % of the total population) were asymptomatic and had cardiac enzyme elevations or electrocardiogram (ECG) changes. The remaining cases (17.6 % of the total population) experienced mild to life-threatening clinical symptoms. Seven patients (9.4 %) required intermediate or intensive care admission. As is discussed later, a high proportion of the patients in this study had at least one coronary artery disease risk factor [57].

# Cardiac Arrythmias

Cancer patients are prone to arrhythmic events, secondary to systemic treatment as well as to other conditions and concomitant medications [58–60]. Fortunately, most arrhythmogenic events are not clinically significant rhythm alterations; in some cases, however, life-threatening arrhythmias can occur. Their early identification and treatment as well as correction of the associated risk factors are essential [59, 60].

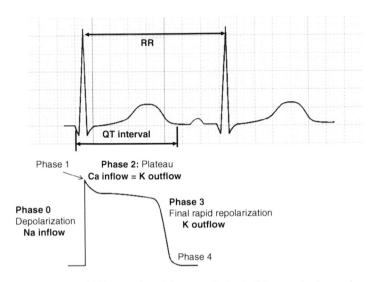

FIGURE 15.1 QT interval and its correlation with ventricular action potential. QT interval is measured from the beginning of the QRS complex to the end of the T wave; RR is the interval from the onset of one QRS complex to the onset of the next QRS complex. The lower part of the figure shows the correlation between QT interval and ventricular action potential: phase 0 or depolarization is mainly caused by sodium influx into the cells; while in phase 2 or plateau there is equilibrium between calcium influx and potassium efflux. Phase 3 or rapid final repolarization is caused by a potassium efflux

## QT Interval and Prolonged QTc Interval-Associated Arrhythmias

### QTc Interval Prolongation: Definition and Physiopathology

The QT interval is measured from the beginning of the QRS complex to the end of the T wave [61, 62] (Fig. 15.1) and represents ventricular activation and recovery (depolarization and repolarization) on an ECG. Depolarization is a result of sodium and calcium influx into the cardiomyocyte. Conversely, when potassium efflux exceeds sodium and calcium influx,

TABLE 15.2  QTc interval correction formulas

| References | Formula |
| --- | --- |
| Fridericia [66, 67] | $QT_F = QT / RR^{1/3}$ |
| Bazett [66, 68, 69] | $QTc = QT / RR^{1/2}$ |
| Framingham (Sagie) [70] | $QT_{LC} = QT + 0.154(1 - RR)$ |

*Abbreviation*: *RR* interval from the onset of one QRS complex to the onset of the next QRS complex

repolarization occurs [61]. Any drug affecting these channels, especially hERG potassium channels involved in potassium efflux during repolarization [63], can potentially cause changes in the QT interval [64, 65]. Additionally, electrolytic disturbances may also interfere in the normal process of depolarization and repolarization [58, 59].

The QT interval is prolonged with slower heart rates and shortened with faster rates. To avoid the variability associated with heart rate, several formulas have been developed that mathematically correct the QT interval, known as the QTc interval (Table 15.2) [7, 58, 59, 61, 71]. This is the most common measurement used to evaluate the arrhythmogenic potential of a drug secondary to repolarization interference. There is currently no agreement regarding which is the most appropriate method. Automatic measurements usually provide QTc intervals adjusted according to the Bazett formula. This formula is known to overestimate QTc interval at high heart rates, while the Fridericia formula seems to be more accurate in this setting [72, 73].

An international consensus regarding what can be considered as normal versus prolonged QTc intervals is also currently lacking. Generally, QTc intervals ≤430 for males and ≤450 ms for females are considered normal, while QTc intervals >450 ms in men and >470 ms in women are considered prolonged [58, 59]. These different values reflect the physiological variation of the QTc interval between genders [74]. Based on experience in patients with congenital long-QT

TABLE 15.3 Drugs inducing QTc interval prolongation

| Drug class | Known drugs |
|---|---|
| Serotonin agonists/ antagonists | Cisapride, ketanserin, zimeldine |
| Antibiotics | Clarithromycin, erythromycin, gatifloxacin, sparfloxacin, pentamidine |
| Antifungal | Ketoconazole, miconazole, itraconazole |
| Antipsychotics | Phenothiazine, droperidol, haloperidol, pimozide, ziprasidone, olanzapine, risperidone |
| Antidepressants | Amitriptyline, clomipramine, desipramine, imipramine, sertraline, venlafaxine |
| Vasodilators | Bepridil, perhexiline |
| Antiarrhythmic drugs | IA: Procainamide, quinidine, amaline, disopyramide |
| | IC: Flecainide, propafenone |
| | III: Amiodarone, sotalol, dofetilide, ibutilide |
| Other | Methadone |

syndrome, it is considered that the risk of ventricular arrhythmias, particularly Torsade des Pointes, is increased when the QTc interval exceeds 500 ms [73]; however, there is no threshold below which the QTc interval prolongation is considered free of proarrhythmic risk [58].

While several anticancer agents that induce QTc interval prolongation have been identified, a review of the literature shows other conditions with the potential to cause prolongation are commonly associated with cancer patients. This includes concomitant medications (Table 15.3), other comorbidities, and electrolytic disturbances (Table 15.4) [59,71,73,75]. Identification and correction of any reversible risk factors present in a patient are paramount to limiting additional toxicity when prescribing drugs with the potential to prolong the QTc interval.

TABLE 15.4 Drug-induced QTc interval prolongation risk factors

| Parameter | Risk factor |
|---|---|
| Gender | Female |
| Related to drug administration | High drug concentration |
| | Rapid rate of intravenous infusion with a QT-prolonging drug |
| Electrolyte disturbances | Hypocalcemia |
| | Hypokalemia |
| | Hypomagnesemia |
| Previous cardiovascular disease | Myocardial ischemia |
| | Cardiac hypertrophy |
| | Congestive heart failure |
| | Bradycardia |
| | Atrioventricular block |
| | Myocarditis |
| Baseline ECG alteration | Subclinical long-QT syndrome |
| | Baseline QT prolongation |
| Endocrine disorders | Hyperaldosteronism |
| | Hypothyroidism |
| | Hyperparathyroidism |
| Neurologic disorders | Stroke |
| | Subarachnoid hemorrhage |
| | Intracranial trauma |
| Other diseases | Diabetes |
| | Cirrhosis |

After the post-marketing withdrawal of several chemically unrelated drugs in the early 1990s due to their arrhythmogenic risk secondary to QTc interval prolongation [76], evaluation of drug-induced QTc interval changes became a clinical issue for both anticancer agents and other medications. The International Conference Harmonization Guideline for the clinical evaluation of QT interval prolongation and proarrhythmic potential for non-antiarrhythmic drugs (ICH E14) was published in 2005 [66]. This guideline requires every new drug to undergo clinical assessment for its repolarization effects before entering phase II trials. Nonetheless, such guidelines have limitations when evaluating anticancer agents because in most cases, studies cannot be performed in healthy volunteers; thus, studies including placebo are likely to be unethical [58, 73, 77].

Furthermore, the risk-benefit balance must be taken into account when evaluating anticancer drugs. Thus, while drugs such as terfenadine were removed from the market for inducing a mean QTc interval prolongation of 6 ms, approval has been maintained for others with similar or longer intervals. Examples include the antiemetic granisetron, which induces a 5 ms mean QTc interval prolongation [73], and drugs such as nilotinib or romidepsin, approved on the basis of their efficacy, despite inducing mean QTc interval prolongations of 10 ms [78] and 14 ms [79], respectively.

## Anticancer Agents Associated with QTc Interval Prolongation

Both classic chemotherapeutic agents and targeted therapies have been shown to induce QTc interval prolongation [80]. These are summarized in the following sections and in Table 15.5.

### Chemotherapeutic Agents

Anthracyclines have been associated with prolonged QTc intervals and an increased arrhythmogenic risk [83, 105, 106]. Even years after having received chemotherapy, women receiving anthracycline pretreatment for breast cancer have been observed to have longer baseline QTc and significant differences in QTc interval prolongation after isoflurane anesthesia [107].

TABLE 15.5 Anticancer agent-induced QTc interval prolongation

| Drug | Effect measured[a] | Percentage of patients/ interval duration | Reference |
|---|---|---|---|
| *Chemotherapeutic agents* | | | |
| Arsenic trioxide | QTc interval prolongation (any grade) | 38.4 % | Barbey et al. [81] |
| | QTc interval prolongation ≥500 ms | 26.5 % | Barbey et al. [81] |
| | Ventricular tachycardia | 4 of 14 patients | Ohnishi et al. [82] |
| Anthracyclines | QTc prolongation after first dose | 11.5 % | Pudil et al. [83] |
| | QTc prolongation 6 months after chemo | 34.6 % | Pudil et al. [83] |
| *Histone deacetylase inhibitors* | | | |
| Romidepsin | Mean QTc prolongation | 14 ms | Piekarz et al. [79] |
| | QTc prolongation 480 ms (grade 2) | 10 % | Bates et al. [73] |

| | | | |
|---|---|---|---|
| Vorinostat | QTc prolongation grade 2 | 1–3 % | Munster et al. [84] |
| | QTc prolongation grade 3 | 0.8–4 % | |
| | QTc prolongation >60 ms enlargement from baseline | 2 % | |
| Panobinostat | | | |
| IV, daily × 7 days every 3 weeks | DLT due to QTc interval prolongation >500 ms | 4 of 6 patients | Giles et al. [85] |
| | Grade 2 QTc interval prolongation | 1 of 2 patients | |
| IV, day 1, 3, and 5 every 3 weeks | QTc interval prolongation >500 ms | 1 of 44 patients | Sharma et al. [86] |
| Dose 20 mg | QTc interval prolongation 480–500 ms | 2 of 44 patients | Zhang et al. [87] |

TABLE 15.5 (continued)

| Drug | Effect measured[a] | Percentage of patients/interval duration | Reference |
|---|---|---|---|
| LAQ824 | Mean QTc prolongation | 14 ms | De Bono et al. [88] |
| Plitidepsin | Mean QT prolongation | 2.51 ms | Soto-Matos et al. [89] |
| *Multi-targeted tyrosine kinase inhibitors* | | | |
| Vandetanib | | | |
| Single agent | | | Tamura et al. [90] |
| Single-agent dose 100 mg | QTc interval prolongation (any grade) | 23 % | |
| Single-agent dose 200 mg | QTc interval prolongation (any grade) | 50 % | |
| | Grade 3 | 5 % | |
| Single-agent dose 300 mg | QTc interval prolongation (any grade) | 47 % | |
| | Grade 3 | 5 % | |

| | | | |
|---|---|---|---|
| | Combination with docetaxel NSCLC | | | Heymach et al. [91] |
| | Control arm (docetaxel) | Median QTc interval prolongation after 6 weeks of treatment | 2 ms | |
| | Vandetanib 100 mg + docetaxel | Median QTc interval prolongation after 6 weeks treatment | 14 ms | |
| | | QTc interval prolongation grade 3 or more | 5 % | |
| | Vandetanib 300 mg + docetaxel | Median QTc interval prolongation after 6 week of treatment | 26 ms | |
| | | QTc interval prolongation grade 3 or more | 11 % | |
| | Sunitinib | Torsade de pointes | <0.1 % | Food and Drug Administration [92] |

(continued)

TABLE 15.5 (continued)

| Drug | Effect measured[a] | Percentage of patients/interval duration | Reference |
|---|---|---|---|
| Nilotinib | QTc interval prolongation >30 ms | 33–40.8 % | Hazarika et al. [93] |
| | QTc interval prolongation >60 ms | 1.9–2.5 % | |
| Dasatinib | Mean QTc interval changes | 7.0–13.4 ms | Food and Drug Administration [94] |
| | QTc interval prolongation <30 ms | 54 % | Johnson et al. [95] |
| | QTc interval prolongation 30–60 ms | 36 % | |
| | QTc interval prolongation >60 ms | 11 % | |
| | QTc interval prolongation 450–500 ms | 21 % | |
| | QTc interval prolongation >500 ms | 1 % | |
| *Other agents* | | | |
| Lonafarnib | QTc interval prolongation grade 3 | 1 out 15 patients | Hanrahan et al. [96] |

| | | | |
|---|---|---|---|
| Combretastatin A4 phosphate | QTc interval prolongation grades 1–2 | 5 % | Dowlati et al. [97] |
| Enzastaurin | | | |
| Single agent | | | |
| 800 mg daily | QTc interval prolongation grade 3 | 1 out of 9 | Kreisl et al. [98] |
| 250 mg twice daily | QTc interval prolongation grade 3 | 1 out of 5 | |
| Multiple doses | QTc interval prolongation grades 1–2 | 23 % | |
| 350 mg twice daily | QTc interval prolongation grade 2 | 1 out of 7 | Rademaker-Lakhai et al. [99] |
| 500–525 mg daily | QTc interval prolongation grade 2 | | Kreisl et al. [100] |
| 500 mg daily | QTc interval prolongation >50 ms | 5 % | Oh et al. [101] |

(continued)

TABLE 15.5  (continued)

| Drug | Effect measured[a] | Percentage of patients/interval duration | Reference |
|------|-------------------|------------------------------------------|-----------|
| Multiple doses (healthy volunteers) | QTc interval prolongation >450 ms | 1 out of 25 | Welch et al. [102] |
|  | QTc interval prolongation >30 ms | 5 out of 25 |  |
| Combination with capecitabine |  |  |  |
| Enzastaurin 350 mg | QTc interval prolongation >500 ms | 1 out of 7 | Camidge et al. [103] |
| Multiple doses | QTc interval prolongation grades 1–2 | 23 % |  |
| Goserelin-bicalutamide | QTc interval prolongation 30–60 ms | 46 % | Garnick [104] |
|  | QTc interval prolongation >60 ms | 8 % |  |
| Leuprolide-bicalutamide | QTc interval prolongation 30–60 ms | 26 % | Garnick [104] |
|  | QTc interval prolongation >60 ms | 6 % |  |

*Abbreviation: DLT* dose-limiting toxicity
[a]Graded according to NCI-CTCAE, version 3

The chemotherapeutic agent most closely associated with QTc interval prolongation is probably arsenic trioxide. Its potential to induce QTc interval prolongation was first described in an acute promyelocytic leukemia study in which 16 of the 40 enrolled patients experienced QTc interval prolongation >500 ms, accompanied in one case by a single, asymptomatic, brief, self-limited episode of Torsade de Pointes [108]. Pooled analysis of 99 patients enrolled in phase I and II trials with arsenic trioxide showed that 38 patients experienced QT interval prolongation, 26 of whom experienced QT interval prolongation >500 ms. Arsenic trioxide-induced QTc interval prolongation is reversible before the following cycle, dose-dependent, and also more likely to occur in females, in patients with hypokalemia, or those with an underlying heart disease [81].

Other chemotherapeutic agents associated with QTc interval prolongation are amsacrine [80], 5-fluorouracil, generally in the context of a coronary event [109, 110], and cyclophosphamide [111]. The magnitude of QTc interval prolongation associated with cyclophosphamide appears to correlate with further risk of heart failure.

### Histone Deacetylase Inhibitors

Histone deacetylase (HDAC) inhibitors are a group of compounds that modulate histone acetylation, which ultimately induces epigenetic changes in transcription. Several chemically unrelated HDAC inhibitors induce QTc interval prolongation. The first HDAC inhibitor that showed arrhythmogenic potential was romidepsin, also known as depsipeptide. A phase II study of romidepsin in metastatic neuroendocrine tumors was prematurely terminated because two patients experienced ventricular tachycardia and a sudden death was described in a third patient [112]. Pooled analysis of NCI-sponsored clinical trials including more than 500 patients showed a 10 % incidence of QTc interval >480 ms [73]. Moreover, mean QTc interval prolongation in the cardiac substudy of a phase II trial of romidepsin in T-cell lymphoma was 14 ms [79]. Romidepsin, now approved for T-cell lymphoma, merits further development that takes into account QTc data; Food and Drug Administration (FDA) approval includes several recommendations regarding QTc interval monitoring and management of its potential prolongation [113].

Vorinostat, a phenylbutyrate-derived HDAC, led to a QTc interval >470 ms in 1 of 74 patients enrolled in a phase II study in refractory T-cell lymphoma [114]. The incidence of grade 2 QTc interval prolongation according to CTCAE v3.0 was 1–3 %, and that of grade 3 was 0.8–4 % [84]. A dedicated phase I cardiac study in advanced solid tumors showed that a single overdose of vorinostat did not significantly increase QTc interval [84]. FDA approval includes a specific recommendation for electrolyte monitoring prior to vorinostat administration to diminish the risk of QTc interval prolongation and arrhythmia [115].

Another chemically unrelated molecule, panobinostat, showed dose- and schedule-related QTc interval prolongation, with a much higher incidence of grade 3 QTc interval prolongation observed following daily intravenous administration compared to the intermittent schedule [85–87].

## Multi-targeted Kinase Inhibitors

Several approved multi-targeted kinase inhibitors have the potential to induce QTc interval prolongation [59], all of which have been shown preclinically to interact with HERG $K^+$ channels. In the phase III randomized trial of vandetanib in medullary thyroid cancer [116], vandetanib induced a QTc interval prolongation of any grade in approximately 14 % of patients, but only 8 % had grade 3 QTc interval prolongations (i.e., which could potentially be serious) [117]. FDA approval of this drug incorporates specific guidelines for QTc interval and electrolyte monitoring and dose adjustment in the event of QTc interval prolongation [117].

FDA approval of sunitinib described a <0.1 % incidence of Torsade de Pointes risk in patients exposed to this drug [92]. For this reason, caution is recommended when administering it to any patients with electrolyte disturbances, previous history of QT interval prolongation, or other preexisting cardiac conditions.

Nilotinib and dasatinib, both ABL inhibitors, have been associated with heart failure and QTc prolongation (see Table 15.5), with specific guidelines for the management of this toxicity in the FDA approval [78, 94].

Other Agents

Other agents such as vascular disruptors (lonafarnib [96] and combretastatin A4 phosphate [97]), protein kinase C inhibitors (enzastaurin) [98–102], or Hdm-2 inhibitors (serdemetan) [118] were shown to induce QTc interval prolongation in phase I clinical trials. Even hormonotherapy has been described as inducing QTc interval prolongation (see Table 15.5) [104, 119].

## Other Chemotherapy-Induced Arrhythmias

Arrhythmias other than those associated with QTc interval prolongation have also been described. Post-chemotherapy arrhythmias are one of the most common reasons for cardiology consultations in cancer centers [120]. A variety of types have been reported, mainly sinus bradycardia, atrioventricular block, atrial fibrillation, or ventricular tachycardia; however, others have been described [60, 120].

The chemotherapeutic agent most commonly associated with rhythm disturbances is paclitaxel. The most frequent events are asymptomatic sinus bradycardia (29 %) and first-degree atrioventricular block (25 %) [121]. Fortunately, more severe conduction abnormalities are rare [122]; among 3,400 patients in an NCI database, only four experienced second- or third-degree heart block [121]. The physiopathology of these rhythm disturbances is as yet unclear; it is unknown whether it is a direct toxicity of paclitaxel on the Purkinje system, secondary to histamine release induced by the Cremophor EL vehicle, or both [121]. Paclitaxel itself might have some proarrhythmogenic potential. In the phase III randomized trial of nab-paclitaxel versus paclitaxel in metastatic breast cancer patients, bradycardia is described as an important, although infrequent (<1 %), side effect of nab-paclitaxel, which does not require the Cremophor EL vehicle [123]. Other anticancer agents have been associated with rhythm disturbance, including 5-fluorouracil, cisplatin, gemcitabine, IL-2, anthracyclines, and melphalan (Table 15.6) [11].

TABLE 15.6  Patients with chemotherapy-induced arrhythmia

| Drug | Bradycardia | Atrial fibrillation | Ventricular tachycardia | Reference |
|---|---|---|---|---|
| Paclitaxel | 29 % bradycardia | 0.18 % | 0.26 % | Rowinsky and Donehower [121] |
| | 25 % first-degree atrioventricular block | | | Guglin et al. [120] |
| | <0.1 % second- to third-degree atrioventricular block | | | |
| Fluorouracil | 2.8 % | 4.2–6.5 % | 1.1 % | Talapatra et al. [124] |
| | | | | De Forni et al. [48] |
| | | | | Guglin et al. [120] |
| Cisplatin | Case reports | Case reports | x-x | Hashimi et al. [125] |
| | | | | Canobbio et al. [126] |
| | | | | Altundag et al. [127] |
| | | | | Guglin et al. [120] |

| Drug | | | | Notes | References |
|---|---|---|---|---|---|
| Gemcitabine | 2.3 % | 8.1 % | 1.6 % | | Lin et al. [128]; Gridelli et al. [129]; Santini et al. [130]; Sauer-Heilborn et al. [131]; Zwitter et al. [132] |
| Anthracyclines | 3.4 % | 2.2–10 % | 6 % | | Kilickap et al. [133]; Guglin et al. [120]; Kilickap et al. [134]; Steinberg et al. [11] |
| IL-2 | 1.08 % | 4.3–13.3 % | 0.2–1.1 % | Associated to polychemotherapy | Lee et al. [135]; Margolin et al. [136]; Guglin et al. [120] |
| Melphalan | 5 % | 6.6–11.8 % | 0.7–1.5 % | In combination with bortezomib | Lonial et al. [137]; Moreau et al. [138]; Phillips et al. [139]; Mileshkin et al. [140]; Palumbo et al. [141] |

# Hypertension

Hypertension is one of the most common toxicities associated with VEGF pathway inhibitors for both monoclonal antibodies (such as bevacizumab) or multi-targeted tyrosine kinase inhibitors such as sunitinib, sorafenib, axitinib, cediranib, and telatinib, among others. Several mechanisms of action have been identified. First, inhibition of the VEGF pathway decreases nitric oxide levels, which leads to vasoconstriction. This might be responsible for the rapid increase in blood pressure after initiation of anti-VEGF therapy [142]. Additionally, sustained VEGF pathway inhibition induces endothelial cell apoptosis, which ultimately causes a reduction in the number of capillaries and increases overall vascular resistance. This second mechanism has been observed in patients treated with bevacizumab [143], sunitinib [144], and telatinib [145] and appears to be reversible within 2 weeks of treatment discontinuation [146, 147].

Incidence of drug-induced hypertension ranges from 15 to 25 % with sunitinib [148, 149], 20 % with sorafenib [150], and up to 35 % with bevacizumab, all of which are dose-dependent [151, 152]. Serious complications have been reported, such as intracranial hemorrhage and hypertensive urgency. Prior uncontrolled hypertension is a relevant risk factor for developing these complications; therefore, blood pressure normalization prior to antiangiogenic treatment initiation is essential.

# Venous Thromboembolic Disease

## Chemotherapy and Other Drugs

A number of agents are associated with an increased incidence of venous thromboembolic events, including cisplatin [153], vorinostat [114, 154], thalidomide [155, 156], and erlotinib [157]. Proposed mechanisms include alterations in platelet aggregation as well as direct effects on the endothelium [8].

The role of prophylactic administration of aspirin or low-molecular-weight heparin in this setting is uncertain and may benefit some high-risk patients [158].

## Hormonotherapy

Tamoxifen, an estrogen receptor antagonist, has shown an increased incidence of thromboembolic events [159] and should be used cautiously in women with previous thromboembolic events. This higher risk has not been observed in the same patient population when treated with aromatase inhibitors, although a higher incidence of adverse cardiac events has been described [160]. Some data suggest a cardioprotective role for tamoxifen, supporting these differences.

## Radiation-Induced Heart Disease

Although it is not a systemic therapy, radiation therapy is included in the current review because it has been shown to increase toxicities secondary to systemic therapy. External radiation therapy to the mediastinum can induce toxicity in the pericardium, coronary arteries, heart valves, and myocardium [161, 162]. A number of factors have been associated with cardiotoxicity risk – namely, radiation dose [4], the heart volume exposed, radiation delivery technique, and patient's age at the time of exposure, with patients under the age of 20 years apparently more susceptible to DNA damage [162, 163]. Two large studies of survivors of childhood cancer show an increased risk of cardiotoxicity after radiation therapy, with hazard ratios between 2 and 25, depending on the radiation doses [4, 164]. The underlying mechanism is microvascular destruction and apoptosis due to direct cellular injury, which produces fibrosis in the years subsequent to therapy. Incidence of cardiac damage from radiation has been reducing with improvements in radiation techniques.

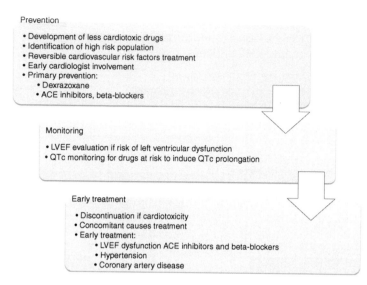

FIGURE 15.2 Proposed algorithm for cardiotoxicity prevention, monitoring, and management

# Cardiotoxicity Prevention and Management

As described in Fig. 15.2, several approaches are available to limit the occurrence of cardiotoxicity and to treat it optimally in the event that it does occur [5, 7, 165, 166].

## Prevention

### Drug Development

Prevention of cardiotoxicity has been integrated into the early phases of drug development. Extensive efforts have been invested in the design of less cardiotoxic drugs. One of the first examples was the alternative formulations of anthracyclines; epirubicin is a semisynthetic epimer of doxorubicin with an improved cardiotoxic profile, while liposomal anthracycline formulations diminish the distribution of the drug into the heart [27]. More recent examples are nab-paclitaxel, in which paclitaxel is associated with albumin in an attempt to improve its activity and reduce its toxicity [123], and plitidepsin, a romidepsin analog that has reduced QTc interval prolongation in the early phases of clinical development [89].

Regarding tyrosine kinase inhibitors, some of the cardiotoxic effects are thought to be a result of off-target effects of the drug, resulting from the inhibition of another kinase not involved in the drug's anticancer activity [167]. In some cases, drug reformulation to decrease its affinity for this off-target kinase could improve its cardiotoxic profile. The successfully redesigned formulation of imatinib for GIST is a good example of this approach [168].

In addition to the guidelines described in this chapter for the evaluation of QTc interval during clinical development [66], specific guidelines have been issued for preclinical evaluation of the arrhythmogenic risk of non-antiarrhythmic drugs [169], which also applies to anticancer agents.

## Identification of High-Risk Populations

Cardiovascular risk factors are often underestimated in cancer patients. Some studies show that a high proportion of patients have at least one cardiovascular risk factor. Based on observational data published by Schmidinger et al., 48.8 % of patients had hypertension, 26 % had hypercholesterolemia, 22 % had type II diabetes, and 12.8 % were hypertriglyceridemic [57].

As has been described throughout this chapter, adequate control of these reversible risk factors and electrolyte disturbances are essential to diminish and control cardiotoxicity [59]. Early involvement of cardiologists in the clinical management should be encouraged in patients with a preexisting heart condition or those taking drugs that can significantly prolong the QTc interval [59].

## Primary Prevention

Two randomized studies have evaluated preventive strategies for chemotherapy-related cardiomyopathy. Cardinale et al. studied enalapril, an angiotensin-converting enzyme inhibitor, versus placebo in a patient population with increased troponin I levels soon after the start of chemotherapy [170]. Results showed a significantly reduced incidence of left ventricular dysfunction at 12 months with enalapril compared to placebo ($p<0.001$). In a smaller study by Kalay et al., 25 patients treated with anthracyclines were randomly assigned to beta-blocker treatment (carvedilol) or placebo. A lower incidence of anthracycline-induced myocardiopathy at 6 months was observed in the carvedilol group compared with placebo. These studies suggest that optimizing hemodynamic and neurohumoral status before left ventricular dysfunction onset could be beneficial and these two agents might be the preferred treatment for hypertension in this setting [171].

Dexrazoxane is an iron chelator similar to ethylenediaminetetraacetic acid. Although dexrazoxane has been shown to reduce heart failure incidence in children and adults treated with anthracyclines [172], concerns have been raised regarding a possible increased risk of secondary malignancies and a potential decrease in antitumor efficacy. In light of this, the FDA has limited its use to cumulative doxorubicin doses exceeding 300 mg/m$^2$ [173].

## Monitoring

### Left Ventricular Ejection Fraction Evaluation

Cardiac assessment prior, during, and after anthracycline treatment is a subject of controversy because many guidelines and algorithms have been published but none have been validated. Cardiac monitoring should include the patient's medical history, with a physical examination focusing on signs and symptoms of heart failure and assessing LVEF by echocardiography or radionuclide angiography. For patients without increased risk of cardiotoxicity, an estimation of LVEF after the patient has completed four to five chemotherapy cycles (200–300 mg/m$^2$ of doxorubicin or equivalent) is recommended to identify patients with an asymptomatic decrease in systolic function and then to reconsider further therapies. Patients at higher risk should be monitored more frequently [8].

In general, a 15 % decrease within the normal range or a 10 % decrease to a value below the lower limit of normal

LVEF is considered a significant decline of left ventricular function. These events should trigger additional evaluations, and a less cardiotoxic regimen should be considered.

Studies of optimal monitoring intervals to maximize sensitivity and specificity for detection of anthracycline-related cardiomyopathy are unclear, and further investigation will be extremely valuable.

In addition to imaging techniques, a number of serum cardiac markers are under evaluation. Serum troponin I levels are thought to reflect myocyte death and correlate with cumulative doxorubicin dose and congestive heart failure. For example, elevation of troponin I levels 72 h and 1 month after chemotherapy administration predict a late decline in LVEF and cardiac events. Similar results with troponin T have been documented [174, 175]. Elevated B-type natriuretic peptide (BNP) levels after anthracycline administration may also correlate with left ventricular dysfunction and clinical heart failure, but no standard cutoff has been established owing to interindividual variability [176–178]. Additional research is needed before the incorporation of these markers into routine practice.

## QTc Interval Assessment

As previously noted, specific guidelines for drugs undergoing clinical development have been issued, ensuring evaluation of QTc interval changes related to drug administration. In addition, a number of approved drugs known to induce QTc interval prolongation, such as romidepsin, vandetanib, or nilotinib, have specific recommendations for cardiac monitoring during administration in the FDA label [78, 113, 117].

## Early Treatment

Any anticancer drug should be immediately discontinued in the event of a cardiovascular event such as a significant decrease in LVEF or the occurrence of a QTc prolongation

>500 ms. Reversible associated factors should be ruled out prior to further treatment and corrected, if present.

Little information regarding cardiac dysfunction once treatment is established is available. An observational study showed an improvement in LVEF in patients with LVEF ≤ 45 % if treatment with enalapril and carvedilol was established during the 6 months after completion of anthracycline treatment [179]. A number of studies have evaluated the effect of enalapril in childhood cancer survivors with asymptomatic cardiac dysfunction. Although temporary improvement of LVEF has been observed, it is unclear whether this would impact the global outcome in the future [180, 181].

No specific guidelines have been issued for chemotherapy-induced heart failure treatment, but it is widely believed that evidence-based guidelines for the general population would also be useful for cancer patients, despite not having been specifically validated in this setting. In individual cases with reasonable prognosis and good quality of life, an implanted cardioverter-defibrillator [182] and cardiac resynchronization therapy may be used to improve left ventricular dysfunction. Data regarding the potential use of stem cell therapy for anthracycline-induced cardiomyopathy treatment are yet to be published.

# Summary

Cancer patients have an increased risk of developing heart disease as a result of chemotherapy, targeted therapies, and radiation therapy. Individuals at a high risk of developing such toxicity need to be identified prior to treatment initiation to minimize this risk through cardioprotective measures or modifications to the proposed treatment regimen. Cardiovascular monitoring is essential, both during and after antineoplastic treatment, for early detection and effective management of cardiotoxicity.

An interdisciplinary approach between oncologists and cardiologists is needed to ensure optimal patient outcomes. A new discipline termed cardio-oncology or onco-cardiology is currently being developed.

# References

1. Oeffinger KC, Mertens AC, Sklar CA, Kawashima T, Hudson MM, Meadows AT, et al. Chronic health conditions in adult survivors of childhood cancer. N Engl J Med. 2006;355(15):1572–82.
2. Armstrong GT, Liu Q, Yasui Y, Neglia JP, Leisenring W, Robison LL, et al. Late mortality among 5-year survivors of childhood cancer: a summary from the Childhood Cancer Survivor Study. J Clin Oncol. 2009;27(14):2328–38.
3. Armenian SH, Bhatia S. Cardiovascular disease after hematopoietic cell transplantation – lessons learned. Haematologica. 2008;93(8): 1132–6.
4. Tukenova M, Guibout C, Oberlin O, Doyon F, Mousannif A, Haddy N, et al. Role of cancer treatment in long-term overall and cardiovascular mortality after childhood cancer. J Clin Oncol. 2010;28(8): 1308–15.
5. Albini A, Pennesi G, Donatelli F, Cammarota R, De Flora S, Noonan DM. Cardiotoxicity of anticancer drugs: the need for cardio-oncology and cardio-oncological prevention. J Natl Cancer Inst. 2010;102(1):14–25.
6. Yeh ET, Bickford CL. Cardiovascular complications of cancer therapy: incidence, pathogenesis, diagnosis, and management. J Am Coll Cardiol. 2009;53(24):2231–47.
7. Brana I, Tabernero J. Cardiotoxicity. Ann Oncol. 2010;21 suppl 7:vii173–9.
8. Ewer MS, Ewer SM. Cardiotoxicity of anticancer treatments: what the cardiologist needs to know. Nat Rev Cardiol. 2010;7(10):564–75.
9. Ewer MS, Lippman SM. Type II chemotherapy-related cardiac dysfunction: time to recognize a new entity. J Clin Oncol. 2005;23(13):2900–2.
10. Jones RL, Swanton C, Ewer MS. Anthracycline cardiotoxicity. Expert Opin Drug Saf. 2006;5(6):791–809.
11. Steinberg JS, Cohen AJ, Wasserman AG, Cohen P, Ross AM. Acute arrhythmogenicity of doxorubicin administration. Cancer. 1987;60(6):1213–8.
12. Harrison DT, Sanders LA. Pericarditis in a case of early daunorubicin cardiomyopathy. Ann Intern Med. 1976;85(3):339–41.
13. Lipshultz SE, Lipsitz SR, Sallan SE, Dalton VM, Mone SM, Gelber RD, et al. Chronic progressive cardiac dysfunction years after doxorubicin therapy for childhood acute lymphoblastic leukemia. J Clin Oncol. 2005;23(12):2629–36.
14. Billingham ME, Bristow MR, Glatstein E, Mason JW, Masek MA, Daniels JR. Adriamycin cardiotoxicity: endomyocardial biopsy evidence of enhancement by irradiation. Am J Surg Pathol. 1977;1(1): 17–23. Epub 1977 Mar 1.
15. Billingham ME, Mason JW, Bristow MR, Daniels JR. Anthracycline cardiomyopathy monitored by morphologic changes. Cancer Treat Rep. 1978;62(6):865–72. Epub 1978 June 1.

16. Mackay B, Ewer MS, Carrasco CH, Benjamin RS. Assessment of anthracycline cardiomyopathy by endomyocardial biopsy. Ultrastruct Pathol. 1994;18(1–2):203–11. Epub 1994 Jan 1.
17. Swain SM, Whaley FS, Ewer MS. Congestive heart failure in patients treated with doxorubicin: a retrospective analysis of three trials. Cancer. 2003;97(11):2869–79.
18. van Dalen Elvira C, van der Pal Helena JH, Caron Huib N, Kremer Leontien CM. Different dosage schedules for reducing cardiotoxicity in cancer patients receiving anthracycline chemotherapy. Cochrane Database Syst Rev. 2009;(4):CD005008. Available from: http://www.mrw.interscience.wiley.com/cochrane/clsysrev/articles/CD005008/frame.html.
19. Von Hoff DD, Layard MW, Basa P. Risk factors for doxorubicin-induced congestive heart failure. Ann Intern Med. 1979;91(5):710–7.
20. Steinherz LJ, Steinherz PG, Tan CTC, Heller G, Murphy ML. Cardiac toxicity 4 to 20 years after completing anthracycline therapy. J Am Med Assoc. 1991;266(12):1672–7.
21. Hershman DL, McBride RB, Eisenberger A, Wei YT, Grann VR, Jacobson JS. Doxorubicin, cardiac risk factors, and cardiac toxicity in elderly patients with diffuse B-cell non-Hodgkin's lymphoma. J Clin Oncol. 2008;26(19):3159–65.
22. Bonneterre J, Roché H, Kerbrat P, Fumoleau P, Goudier MJ, Fargeot P, et al. Long-term cardiac follow-up in relapse-free patients after six courses of fluorouracil, epirubicin, and cyclophosphamide, with either 50 or 100 mg of epirubicin, as adjuvant therapy for node-positive breast cancer: French Adjuvant Study Group. J Clin Oncol. 2004;22(15):3070–9.
23. Jain KK, Casper ES, Geller NL. A prospective randomized comparison of epirubicin and doxorubicin in patients with advanced breast cancer. J Clin Oncol. 1985;3(6):818–26.
24. Ryberg M, Nielsen D, Cortese G, Nielsen G, Skovsgaard T, Andersen PK. New insight into epirubicin cardiac toxicity: competing risks analysis of 1097 breast cancer patients. J Natl Cancer Inst. 2008;100(15):1058–67.
25. Bedano PM, Brames MJ, Williams SD, Juliar BE, Einhorn LH. Phase II study of cisplatin plus epirubicin salvage chemotherapy in refractory germ cell tumors. J Clin Oncol. 2006;24(34):5403–7.
26. Valero V, Buzdar AU, Theriault RL, Azarnia N, Fonseca GA, Willey J, et al. Phase II trial of liposome-encapsulated doxorubicin, cyclophosphamide, and fluorouracil as first-line therapy in patients with metastatic breast cancer. J Clin Oncol. 1999;17(5):1425–34.
27. van Dalen Elvira C, Michiels Erna MC, Caron Huib N, Kremer Leontien CM. Different anthracycline derivates for reducing cardiotoxicity in cancer patients. Cochrane Database Syst Rev. 2010;(5):CD005006. Available from: http://www.mrw.interscience.wiley.com/cochrane/clsysrev/articles/CD005006/frame.html.

28. Posner LE, Dukart G, Goldberg J. Mitoxantrone: an overview of safety and toxicity. Invest New Drugs. 1985;3(2):123–32.
29. Dow E, Schulman H, Agura E. Cyclophosphamide cardiac injury mimicking acute myocardial infarction. Bone Marrow Transplant. 1993;12(2):169–72.
30. Katayama M, Imai Y, Hashimoto H, Kurata M, Nagai K, Tamita K, et al. Fulminant fatal cardiotoxicity following cyclophosphamide therapy. J Cardiol. 2009;54(2):330–4.
31. Piccart-Gebhart MJ, Procter M, Leyland-Jones B, Goldhirsch A, Untch M, Smith I, et al. Trastuzumab after adjuvant chemotherapy in HER2-positive breast cancer. N Engl J Med. 2005;353(16):1659–72.
32. Slamon D, Eiermann W, Robert N, Pienkowski T, Martin M, Press M, et al. Adjuvant trastuzumab in HER2-positive breast cancer. N Engl J Med. 2011;365(14):1273–83.
33. Costa RB, Kurra G, Greenberg L, Geyer CE. Efficacy and cardiac safety of adjuvant trastuzumab-based chemotherapy regimens for HER2-positive early breast cancer. Ann Oncol. 2010;21(11):2153–60.
34. Seidman A, Hudis C, Pierri MK, Shak S, Paton V, Ashby M, et al. Cardiac dysfunction in the trastuzumab clinical trials experience. J Clin Oncol. 2002;20(5):1215–21.
35. Tan-Chiu E, Yothers G, Romond E, Geyer CE, Ewer M, Keefe D, et al. Assessment of cardiac dysfunction in a randomized trial comparing doxorubicin and cyclophosphamide followed by paclitaxel, with or without trastuzumab as adjuvant therapy in node-positive, human epidermal growth factor receptor 2Â–overexpressing breast cancer: NSABP B-31. J Clin Oncol. 2005;23(31):7811–9.
36. Force T, Krause DS, Van Etten RA. Molecular mechanisms of cardiotoxicity of tyrosine kinase inhibition. Nat Rev Cancer. 2007;7(5):332–44.
37. Serrano C, Cortés J, De Mattos-Arruda L, Bellet M, Gómez P, Saura C, et al. Trastuzumab-related cardiotoxicity in the elderly: a role for cardiovascular risk factors. Ann Oncol. 2012 Apr; 23(4):897–902. Epub 2011 Aug 9.
38. Slamon DJ, Leyland-Jones B, Shak S, Fuchs H, Paton V, Bajamonde A, et al. Use of chemotherapy plus a monoclonal antibody against HER2 for metastatic breast cancer that overexpresses HER2. N Engl J Med. 2001;344(11):783–92. Epub 2001 Mar 15.
39. Mann DL. Mechanisms and models in heart failure: a combinatorial approach. Circulation. 1999;100(9):999–1008.
40. de Korte MA, de Vries EGE, Lub-de Hooge MN, Jager PL, Gietema JA, van der Graaf WTA, et al. 111Indium-Trastuzumab visualises myocardial human epidermal growth factor receptor 2 expression shortly after anthracycline treatment but not during heart failure: a clue to uncover the mechanisms of trastuzumab-related cardiotoxicity. Eur J Cancer. 2007;43(14):2046–51.
41. Grazette LP, Boecker W, Matsui T, Semigran M, Force TL, Hajjar RJ, et al. Inhibition of ErbB2 causes mitochondrial dysfunction in

cardiomyocytes: implications for herceptin-induced cardiomyopathy. J Am Coll Cardiol. 2004;44(11):2231–8.

42. Perez EA, Koehler M, Byrne J, Preston AJ, Rappold E, Ewer MS. Cardiac safety of lapatinib: pooled analysis of 3689 patients enrolled in clinical trials. Mayo Clin Proc. 2008;83(6):679–86.

43. Chu TF, Rupnick MA, Kerkela R, Dallabrida SM, Zurakowski D, Nguyen L, et al. Cardiotoxicity associated with tyrosine kinase inhibitor sunitinib. Lancet. 2007;370(9604):2011–9.

44. Atallah E, Durand JB, Kantarjian H, Cortes J. Congestive heart failure is a rare event in patients receiving imatinib therapy. Blood. 2007;110(4):1233–7.

45. Kerkela R, Grazette L, Yacobi R, Iliescu C, Patten R, Beahm C, et al. Cardiotoxicity of the cancer therapeutic agent imatinib mesylate. Nat Med. 2006;12(8):908–16.

46. Food & Drug Administration US. VELCADE ® prescribing information. 2011. Available from: http://www.accessdata.fda.gov/drug-satfda_docs/label/2011/021602s029s030lbl.pdf. Cited 14 Nov 2011.

47. Fu HY, Minamino T, Tsukamoto O, Sawada T, Asai M, Kato H, et al. Overexpression of endoplasmic reticulum-resident chaperone attenuates cardiomyocyte death induced by proteasome inhibition. Cardiovasc Res. 2008;79(4):600–10.

48. De Forni M, Malet-Martino MC, Jaillais P, Shubinski RE, Bachaud JM, Lemaire L, et al. Cardiotoxicity of high-dose continuous infusion fluorouracil: a prospective clinical study. J Clin Oncol. 1992;10(11): 1795–801.

49. Van Cutsem E, Hoff PM, Blum JL, Abt M, Osterwalder B. Incidence of cardiotoxicity with the oral fluoropyrimidine capecitabine is typical of that reported with 5-fluorouracil [2]. Ann Oncol. 2002;13(3):484–5.

50. Rezkalla S, Kloner RA, Ensley J, Al-Sarraf M, Revels S, Olivenstein A, et al. Continuous ambulatory ECG monitoring during fluorouracil therapy: a prospective study. J Clin Oncol. 1989;7(4):509–14.

51. Kosmas C, Kallistratos MS, Kopterides P, Syrios J, Skopelitis H, Mylonakis N, et al. Cardiotoxicity of fluoropyrimidines in different schedules of administration: a prospective study. J Cancer Res Clin Oncol. 2008;134(1):75–82.

52. Saif MW, Shah MM, Shah AR. Fluoropyrimidine-associated cardiotoxicity: revisited. Expert Opin Drug Saf. 2009;8(2):191–202.

53. Jones RL, Ewer MS. Cardiac and cardiovascular toxicity of nonanthracycline anticancer drugs. Expert Rev Anticancer Ther. 2006;6(9): 1249–69.

54. Kilickap S, Abali H, Celik I. Bevacizumab, bleeding, thrombosis, and warfarin. J Clin Oncol. 2003;21(18):3542.

55. Scappaticci FA, Skillings JR, Holden SN, Gerber HP, Miller K, Kabbinavar F, et al. Arterial thromboembolic events in patients with metastatic carcinoma treated with chemotherapy and bevacizumab. J Natl Cancer Inst. 2007;99(16):1232–9.

56. Sugrue M, Yi J, Purdie D, Dong W, Grothey A, Kozloff M. Serious arterial thromboembolic events (sATE) in patients (pts) with metastatic colorectal cancer (mCRC) treated with bevacizumab (BV): Results from the BRiTE registry. Proc Am Soc Clin Oncol. 2007;25:4136.

57. Schmidinger M, Zielinski CC, Vogl UM, Bojic A, Bojic M, Schukro C, et al. Cardiac toxicity of sunitinib and sorafenib in patients with metastatic renal cell carcinoma. J Clin Oncol. 2008;26(32):5204–12.

58. Strevel EL, Ing DJ, Siu LL. Molecularly targeted oncology therapeutics and prolongation of the qt interval. J Clin Oncol. 2007;25(22): 3362–71.

59. Ederhy S, Cohen A, Dufaitre G, Izzedine H, Massard C, Meuleman C, et al. QT interval prolongation among patients treated with angiogenesis inhibitors. Target Oncol. 2009;4(2):89–97.

60. Morgan C, Tillett T, Braybrooke J, Ajithkumar T. Management of uncommon chemotherapy-induced emergencies. Lancet Oncol. 2011;12(8):806–14.

61. Al-Khatib SM, Allen LaPointe NM, Kramer JM, Califf RM. What clinicians should know about the qt interval. J Am Med Assoc. 2003;289(16):2120–7.

62. Viskin S, Rosovski U, Sands AJ, Chen E, Kistler PM, Kalman JM, et al. Inaccurate electrocardiographic interpretation of long QT: the majority of physicians cannot recognize a long QT when they see one. Heart Rhythm. 2005;2(6):569–74.

63. Curran ME, Splawski I, Timothy KW, Vincent GM, Green ED, Keating MT. A molecular basis for cardiac arrhythmia: HERG mutations cause long QT syndrome. Cell. 1995;80(5):795–803.

64. Mitcheson JS, Chen J, Lin M, Culberson C, Sanguinetti MC. A structural basis for drug-induced long QT syndrome. Proc Natl Acad Sci USA. 2000;97(22):12329–33.

65. Raschi E, Vasina V, Poluzzi E, De Ponti F. The hERG K + channel: target and antitarget strategies in drug development. Pharmacol Res. 2008;57(3):181–95.

66. International Conference on Harmonisation of Technical Requirements for Registration of Pharmaceuticals for Human Use. ICH Harmonised Tripartite Guideline: the clinical evaluation of QT/ QTc interval prolongation and proarrhythmic potential for non-antiarrhythmic drugs E14. 2005. Available from: http://www.ich.org/ fileadmin/Public_Web_Site/ICH_Products/Guidelines/Efficacy/E14/ Step4/E14_Guideline.pdf. Cited 17 Nov 2011.

67. Fridericia LS. Die Systolendauer im Elektrokardiogramm bei normalen Menschen und bei Herzkranken. Acta Med Scand. 1920;53(1):489–506.

68. Bazett HC. An analysis of the time-relations of electrocardiograms. Heart. 1920;7:353–70.

69. Bazett HC. An analysis of the time-relations of electrocardiograms. Ann Noninvasive Electrocardiol. 1997;2(2):177–94.

70. Sagie A, Larson MG, Goldberg RJ, Bengtson JR, Levy D. An improved method for adjusting the QT interval for heart rate (the Framingham Heart Study). Am J Cardiol. 1992;70(7):797–801.
71. Varterasian M, Fingert H, Agin M, Meyer M, Cooney M, Radivoyevitch T, et al. Consideration of QT/QTc interval data in a phase I study in patients with advanced cancer (multiple letters) [1]. Clin Cancer Res. 2004;10(17):5967–9.
72. Davey P. How to correct the QT interval for the effects of heart rate in clinical studies. J Pharmacol Toxicol Methods. 2002;48(1):3–9.
73. Bates SE, Rosing DR, Fojo T, Piekarz RL. Challenges of evaluating the cardiac effects of anticancer agents. Clin Cancer Res. 2006;12(13):3871–4.
74. Yarnoz MJ, Curtis AB. More reasons why men and women are not the same (gender differences in electrophysiology and arrhythmias). Am J Cardiol. 2008;101(9):1291–6.
75. Zeltser D, Justo D, Halkin A, Prokhorov V, Heller K, Viskin S. Torsade de pointes due to noncardiac drugs: most patients have easily identifiable risk factors. Medicine. 2003;82(4):282–90.
76. Lasser KE, Allen PD, Woolhandler SJ, Himmelstein DU, Wolfe SM, Bor DH. Timing of new black box warnings and withdrawals for prescription medications. J Am Med Assoc. 2002;287(17):2215–20.
77. Sarapa N, Britto MR. Challenges of characterizing proarrhythmic risk due to QTc prolongaton induced by nonadjuvant anticancer agents. Expert Opin Drug Saf. 2008;7(3):305–18.
78. Food and Drug Administration US. TASIGNA® Label information. 2011. Available from: http://www.accessdata.fda.gov/drugsatfda_docs/label/2011/022068s007lbl.pdf. Cited 14 Nov 2011.
79. Piekarz RL, Frye AR, Wright JJ, Steinberg SM, Liewehr DJ, Rosing DR, et al. Cardiac studies in patients treated with depsipeptide, FK228, in a phase II trial for T-cell lymphoma. Clin Cancer Res. 2006;12(12):3762–73.
80. Becker TK, Yeung SCJ. Drug-induced QT interval prolongation in cancer patients. Oncol Rev. 2010;4(4):223–32.
81. Barbey JT, Pezzullo JC, Soignet SL. Effect of arsenic trioxide on QT interval in patients with advanced malignancies. J Clin Oncol. 2003;21(19):3609–15.
82. Ohnishi K, Yoshida H, Shigeno K, Nakamura S, Fujisawa S, Naito K, et al. Arsenic trioxide therapy for relapsed or refractory Japanese patients with acute promyelocytic leukemia: need for careful electrocardiogram monitoring. Leukemia. 2002;16(4):617–22.
83. Pudil R, Horacek J, Vojacek J, Jakl M. Anthracycline therapy induces very early increase in QT dispersion and QTc prolongation. Circulation. 2010;122(2):e385.
84. Munster PN, Rubin EH, Van Belle S, Friedman E, Patterson JK, Van Dyck K, et al. A single supratherapeutic dose of vorinostat does not prolong the QTc interval in patients with advanced cancer. Clin Cancer Res. 2009;15(22):7077–84.

85. Giles F, Fischer T, Cortes J, Garcia-Manero G, Beck J, Ravandi F, et al. A phase I study of intravenous LBH589, a novel cinnamic hydroxamic acid analogue histone deacetylase inhibitor, in patients with refractory hematologic malignancies. Clin Cancer Res. 2006;12(15):4628–35.
86. Sharma S, Vogelzang N, Beck J, Patnaik A, Mita M, Dugan M. Phase I pharmacokinetic and pharmacodynamic study of once-weekly iv panobinostat (LBH589). ECCO Poster presented. 2007. p. 23–7.
87. Zhang L, Lebwohl D, Masson E, Laird G, Cooper MR, Prince HM. Clinically relevant QTc prolongation is not associated with current dose schedules of LBH589 (panobinostat) [1]. J Clin Oncol. 2008; 26(2):332–3.
88. De Bono JS, Kristeleit R, Tolcher A, Fong P, Pacey S, Karavasilis V, et al. Phase I pharmacokinetic and pharmacodynamic study of LAQ824, a hydroxamate histone deacetylase inhibitor with a heat shock protein-90 inhibitory profile, in patients with advanced solid tumors. Clin Cancer Res. 2008;14(20):6663–73.
89. Soto-Matos A, Szyldergemajn S, Extremera S, Miguel-Lillo B, Alfaro V, Coronado C, et al. Plitidepsin has a safe cardiac profile: a comprehensive analysis. Mar Drugs. 2011;9(6):1007–23.
90. Tamura T, Minami H, Yamada Y, Yamamoto N, Shimoyama T, Murakami H, et al. A phase I dose-escalation study of ZD6474 in Japanese patients with solid, malignant tumors. J Thorac Oncol. 2006;1(9):1002–9.
91. Heymach JV, Johnson BE, Prager D, Csada E, Roubec J, Pešek M, et al. Randomized, placebo-controlled phase II study of vandetanib plus docetaxel in previously treated non-small-cell lung cancer. J Clin Oncol. 2007;25(27):4270–7.
92. Food and Drug Administration US. SUTENT®. Prescription information. 2011. Available from: http.//www.accessdata.fda.gov/drug-satfda_docs/label/2011/021938s13s17s18lbl.pdf. Cited 14 Nov 2011.
93. Hazarika M, Jiang X, Liu Q, Lee SL, Ramchandani R, Garnett C, et al. Tasigna for chronic and accelerated phase philadelphia chromosome-positive chronic myelogenous leukemia resistant to or intolerant of imatinib. Clin Cancer Res. 2008;14(17):5325–31.
94. Food and Drug Administration US. SPRYCEL® Prescribing information. 2011. Available from: http://www.accessdata.fda.gov/drug-satfda_docs/label/2011/021986s009s010lbl.pdf. Cited 14 Nov 2011.
95. Johnson FM, Agrawal S, Burris H, Rosen L, Dhillon N, Hong D, et al. Phase 1 pharmacokinetic and drug-interaction study of dasatinib in patients with advanced solid tumors. Cancer. 2010;116(6):1582–91.
96. Hanrahan EO, Kies MS, Glisson BS, Khuri FR, Feng L, Tran HT, et al. A phase II study of Lonafarnib (SCH66336) in patients with chemorefractory, advanced squamous cell carcinoma of the head and neck. Am J Clin Oncol. 2009;32(3):274–9. Epub 2009 May 13.
97. Dowlati A, Robertson K, Cooney M, Petros WP, Stratford M, Jesberger J, et al. A phase I pharmacokinetic and translational

study of the novel vascular targeting agent combretastatin A-4 phosphate on a single-dose intravenous schedule in patients with advanced cancer. Cancer Res. 2002;62(12):3408–16.

98. Kreisl TN, Kim L, Moore K, Duic P, Kotliarova S, Walling J, et al. A phase I trial of enzastaurin in patients with recurrent gliomas. Clin Cancer Res. 2009;15(10):3617–23.

99. Rademaker-Lakhai JM, Beerepoot LV, Mehra N, Radema SA, Van Maanen R, Vermaat JS, et al. Phase I pharmacokinetic and pharmacodynamic studyof the oral protein kinase C b-inhibitor enzastaurin in combination with gemcitabine and cisplatinin patients with advanced cancer. Clin Cancer Res. 2007;13(15):4474–81.

100. Kreisl TN, Kotliarova S, Butman JA, Albert PS, Kim L, Musib L, et al. A phase I/II trial of enzastaurin in patients with recurrent high-grade gliomas. Neuro Oncol. 2010;12(2):181–9. Epub 2010 Feb 13.

101. Oh Y, Herbst RS, Burris H, Cleverly A, Musib L, Lahn M, et al. Enzastaurin, an oral serine/threonine kinase inhibitor, as second- or third-line therapy of non-small-cell lung cancer. J Clin Oncol. 2008;26(7):1135–41.

102. Welch PA, Sinha VP, Cleverly AL, Darstein C, Flanagan SD, Musib LC. Safety, tolerability, QTc evaluation, and pharmacokinetics of single and multiple doses of enzastaurin HCl (LY317615), a Protein kinase C-b inhibitor, in healthy subjects. J Clin Pharmacol. 2007;47(9):1138–51.

103. Camidge DR, Gail Eckhardt S, Gore L, O'Bryant CL, Leong S, Basche M, et al. A phase I safety, tolerability, and pharmacokinetic study of enzastaurin combined with capecitabine in patients with advanced solid tumors. Anticancer Drugs. 2008;19(1):77–84. Epub 2007 Nov 29.

104. Garnick MB, Pratt CM, Campion M, Shipley J. The effect of hormonal therapy for prostate cancer on the electrocardiographic QT interval: phase 3 results following treatment with leuprolide and goserelin, alone or with bicalutamide, and the GnRH antagonist abarelix. ASCO meeting abstracts. 2004;22(14 suppl):4578.

105. Nousiainen T, Vanninen E, Rantala A, Jantunen E, Hartikainen J. QT dispersion and late potentials during doxorubicin therapy for non-Hodgkin's lymphoma. J Intern Med. 1999;245(4):359–64. Epub 1999 June 5.

106. Kuittinen T, Jantunen E, Vanninen E, Mussalo H, Nousiainen T, Hartikainen J. Late potentials and QT dispersion after high-dose chemotherapy in patients with non-Hodgkin lymphoma. Clin Physiol Funct Imaging. 2010;30(3):175–80. Epub 2010 Feb 6.

107. Owczuk R, Wujtewicz MA, Sawicka W, Wujtewicz M, Swierblewski M. Is prolongation of the QTc interval during isoflurane anaesthesia more prominent in women pretreated with anthracyclines for breast cancer? Br J Anaesth. 2004;92(5):658–61. Epub 2004 Apr 6.

108. Soignet SL, Frankel SR, Douer D, Tallman MS, Kantarjian H, Calleja E, et al. United States multicenter study of arsenic trioxide in

relapsed acute promyelocytic leukemia. J Clin Oncol. 2001;19(18): 3852–60.

109. Stewart T, Pavlakis N, Ward M. Cardiotoxicity with 5-fluorouracil and capecitabine: more than just vasospastic angina. Intern Med J. 2010;40(4):303–7. Epub 2010 June 10.

110. Wacker A, Lersch C, Scherpinski U, Reindl L, Seyfarth M. High incidence of angina pectoris in patients treated with 5-fluorouracil. A planned surveillance study with 102 patients. Oncology. 2003;65(2):108–12. Epub 2003 Aug 22.

111. Nakamae H, Tsumura K, Hino M, Hayashi T, Tatsumi N. QT dispersion as a predictor of acute heart failure after high-dose cyclophosphamide. Lancet. 2000;355(9206):805–6.

112. Shah MH, Binkley P, Chan K, Xiao J, Arbogast D, Collamore M, et al. Cardiotoxicity of histone deacetylase inhibitor depsipeptide in patients with metastatic neuroendocrine tumors. Clin Cancer Res. 2006;12(13):3997–4003.

113. Food and Drug Administration US. ISTODAX® Prescribing information. 2011. Available from: http://www.accessdata.fda.gov/drugsatfda_docs/label/2011/022393s006lbl.pdf. Cited 14 Nov 2011.

114. Olsen EA, Kim YH, Kuzel TM, Pacheco TR, Foss FM, Parker S, et al. Phase IIB multicenter trial of vorinostat in patients with persistent, progressive, or treatment refractory cutaneous t-cell lymphoma. J Clin Oncol. 2007;25(21):3109–15.

115. Food and Drug Administration US. ZOLINZA® Prescribing information. 2011. Available from: http://www.accessdata.fda.gov/drugsatfda_docs/label/2011/021991s002lbl.pdf. Cited 14 Nov 2011.

116. Wells S, Robinson B, Gagel R, Dralle H, Fagin J, Santoro M, et al., editors. Vandetanib (VAN) in locally advanced or metastatic medullary thyroid cancer (MTC): a randomized, double-blind phase III trial (ZETA). ASCO annual meeting, Chicago, 2010. Abstract 5503.

117. Food and Drug Administration US. CAPRELSA® (vandetanib) Tablets. Prescription information. 2011. Available from: http://www.accessdata.fda.gov/drugsatfda_docs/label/2011/022405s001lbl.pdf. Cited 14 Nov 2011.

118. Tabernero J, Dirix L., Schöfski P, Cervantes A, Lopez-Martin JA, Capdevila J, et al. A phase I first-in-human pharmacokinetic and pharmacodynamic study of serdemetan in patients with advanced solid tumors. Clin Cancer Res. 2011;17(19):6313–21.

119. Slovacek L, Ansorgova V, Macingova Z, Haman L, Petera J. Tamoxifen-induced QT interval prolongation. J Clin Pharm Ther. 2008;33(4):453–5.

120. Guglin M, Aljayeh M, Saiyad S, Ali R, Curtis AB. Introducing a new entity: chemotherapy-induced arrhythmia. Europace. 2009;11(12): 1579–86.

121. Rowinsky EK, Donehower RC. Drug therapy: paclitaxel (taxol). N Engl J Med. 1995;332(15):1004–14.

122. Rowinsky EK, McGuire WP, Guarnieri T, Fisherman JS, Christian MC, Donehower RC. Cardiac disturbances during the administration of taxol. J Clin Oncol. 1991;9(9):1704–12.
123. Food and Drug Administration US. ABRAXANE® for Injectable Suspension (paclitaxel protein-bound particles for injectable suspension) labeling revision. 2009. Available from: http://www.accessdata.fda.gov/drugsatfda_docs/label/2009/021660s022lbl.pdf. Cited 14 Nov 2011.
124. Talapatra K, Rajesh I, Rajesh B, Selvamani B, Subhashini J. Transient asymptomatic bradycardia in patients on infusional 5-fluorouracil. J Cancer Res Ther. 2007;3(3):169–71.
125. Hashimi LA, Khalyl MF, Salem PA. Supraventricular tachycardia. A probable complication of platinum treatment. Oncology. 1984;41(3):174–5.
126. Canobbio L, Fassio T, Gasparini G. Cardiac arrhythmia: possible complication from treatment with cisplatin. Tumori. 1986;72(2):201–4.
127. Altundağ O, Çelik I, Kars A. Recurrent asymptomatic bradycardia episodes after cisplatin infusion. Ann Pharmacother. 2001;35(5): 641–2.
128. Lin LL, Picus J, Drebin JA, Linehan DC, Solis J, Strasberg SM, et al. A phase II study of alternating cycles of split course radiation therapy and gemcitabine chemotherapy for inoperable pancreatic or biliary tract carcinoma. Am J Clin Oncol. 2005;28(3):234–41.
129. Gridelli C, Cigolari S, Gallo C, Manzione L, Ianniello GP, Frontini L, et al. Activity and toxicity of gemcitabine and gemcitabine + vinorelbine in advanced non-small-cell lung cancer elderly patients: phase II data from the Multicenter Italian Lung Cancer in the Elderly Study (MILES) randomized trial. Lung Cancer. 2001;31(2–3):277–84.
130. Santini D, Tonini G, Abbate A, Di Cosimo S, Gravante G, Vincenzi B, et al. Gemcitabine-induced atrial fibrillation: a hitherto unreported manifestation of drug toxicity. Ann Oncol. 2000;11(4):479–81.
131. Sauer-Heilborn A, Kath R, Schneider CP, Höffken K. Severe non-haematological toxicity after treatment with gemcitabine. J Cancer Res Clin Oncol. 1999;125(11):637–40.
132. Zwitter M, Kovac V, Smrdel U, Kocijancic I, Segedin B, Vrankar M. Phase I-II trial of low-dose gemcitabine in prolonged infusion and cisplatin for advanced non-small cell lung cancer. Anticancer Drugs. 2005;16(10):1129–34.
133. Kilickap S, Akgul E, Aksoy S, Aytemir K, Barista I. Doxorubicin-induced second degree and complete atrioventricular block. Europace. 2005;7(3):227–30.
134. Kilickap S, Barista I, Akgul E, Aytemir K, Aksoy S, Tekuzman G. Early and late arrhythmogenic effects of doxorubicin. South Med J. 2007;100(3):262–5.
135. Lee RE, Lotze MT, Skibber JM, Tucker E, Bonow RO, Ognibene FP, et al. Cardiorespiratory effects of immunotherapy with interleukin-2. J Clin Oncol. 1989;7(1):7–20.

136. Margolin KA, Raynor AA, Hawkins MJ, Atkins MB, Dutcher JP, Fisher RI, et al. Interleukin-2 and lymphokine-activated killer cell therapy of solid tumors: analysis of toxicity and management guidelines. J Clin Oncol. 1989;7(4):486–98.

137. Lonial S, Kaufman J, Tighiouart M, Nooka A, Langston AA, Heffner LT, et al. A Phase I/II trial combining high-dose melphalan and autologous transplant with bortezomib for multiple myeloma: a dose- and schedule-finding study. Clin Cancer Res. 2010; 16(20):5079–86.

138. Moreau P, Milpied N, Mahé B, Juge-Morineau N, Rapp MJ, Bataille R, et al. Melphalan 220 mg/m2 followed by peripheral blood stem cell transplantation in 27 patients with advanced multiple myeloma. Bone Marrow Transplant. 1999;23(10):1003–6.

139. Phillips GL, Meisenberg B, Reece DE, Adams VR, Badros A, Brunner J, et al. Amifostine and autologous hematopoietic stem cell support of escalating-dose melphalan: a phase I study. Biol Blood Marrow Transplant. 2004;10(7):473–83.

140. Mileshkin LR, Seymour JF, Wolf MM, Gates P, Januszewicz EH, Joyce P, et al. Cardiovascular toxicity is increased, but manageable, during high-dose chemotherapy and autologous peripheral blood stem cell transplantation for patients aged 60 years and older. Leuk Lymphoma. 2005;46(11):1575–9.

141. Palumbo A, Bringhen S, Caravita T, Merla E, Capparella V, Callea V, et al. Oral melphalan and prednisone chemotherapy plus thalidomide compared with melphalan and prednisone alone in elderly patients with multiple myeloma: randomised controlled trial. Lancet. 2006;367(9513):825–31.

142. Maitland ML, Kasza KE, Karrison T, Moshier K, Sit L, Black HR, et al. Ambulatory monitoring detects sorafenib-induced blood pressure elevations on the first day of treatment. Clin Cancer Res. 2009;15(19):6250–7.

143. Morere JF, Des Guetz G, Mourad J, Lévy BI, Breau J. Mechanism of bevacizumab-induced arterial hypertension: Relation with skin capillary rarefaction in patients treated for metastatic colorectal cancer. 2007 ASCO annual meeting. 2007:Abst 3557.

144. de Boer MP, van der Veldt AAM, Lankheet NA, Wijnstok NJ, van den Eertwegh AJM, Boven E, et al. Sunitinib-induced reduction in skin microvascular density is a reversible phenomenon. Ann Oncol. 2010;21(9):1923–4.

145. Steeghs N, Gelderblom H, Roodt JO, Christensen O, Rajagopalan P, Hovens M, et al. Hypertension and rarefaction during treatment with telatinib, a small molecule angiogenesis inhibitor. Clin Cancer Res. 2008;14(11):3470–6.

146. Steeghs N, Rabelink TJ, op't Roodt J, Batman E, Cluitmans FHM, Weijl NI, et al. Reversibility of capillary density after discontinuation of bevacizumab treatment. Ann Oncol. 2010;21(5):1100–5.

147. van der Veldt AAM, de Boer MP, Boven E, Eringa EC, van den Eertwegh AJM, van Hinsbergh VW, et al. Reduction in skin microvascular density and changes in vessel morphology in patients treated with sunitinib. Anticancer Drugs. 2010;21(4):439–46. doi:10.1097/CAD.0b013e3283359c79.

148. Demetri GD vOA, Blackstein M, Garrett C, Shah M, Heinrich M, McArthur G, Judson I, Baum CM, Casali PG. Phase 3, multicenter, randomized, double-blind, placebo-controlled trial of SU11248 in patients following failure of imatinib for metastatic GIST. ASCO annual meeting 2005. Abstract 4000.

149. Motzer RJ, Rini BI, Bukowski RM, Curti BD, George DJ, Hudes GR, et al. Sunitinib in patients with metastatic renal cell carcinoma. J Am Med Assoc. 2006;295(21):2516–24.

150. Kane RC, Farrell AT, Saber H, Tang S, Williams G, Jee JM, et al. Sorafenib for the treatment of advanced renal cell carcinoma. Clin Cancer Res. 2006;12(24):7271–8.

151. Kabbinavar F, Hurwitz HI, Fehrenbacher L, Meropol NJ, Novotny WF, Lieberman G, et al. Phase II, randomized trial comparing bevacizumab plus fluorouracil (FU)/leucovorin (LV) with FU/LV alone in patients with metastatic colorectal cancer. J Clin Oncol. 2003; 21(1):60–5.

152. Hurwitz H, Fehrenbacher L, Novotny W, Cartwright T, Hainsworth J, Heim W, et al. Bevacizumab plus irinotecan, fluorouracil, and leucovorin for metastatic colorectal cancer. N Engl J Med. 2004;350(23): 2335–42.

153. Czaykowski PM, Moore MJ, Tannock IF. High risk of vascular events in patients with urothelial transitional cell carcinoma treated with cisplatin based chemotherapy. J Urol. 1998;160(6, Part 1): 2021–4.

154. Duvic M, Talpur R, Ni X, Zhang C, Hazarika P, Kelly C, et al. Phase 2 trial of oral vorinostat (suberoylanilide hydroxamic acid, SAHA) for refractory cutaneous T-cell lymphoma (CTCL). Blood. 2007;109(1):31–9.

155. Rajkumar SV. Thalidomide therapy and deep venous thrombosis in multiple myeloma. Mayo Clin Proc. 2005;80(12):1549–51.

156. Rodeghiero F, Elice F. Thalidomide and thrombosis. Pathophysiol Haemost Thromb. 2003;33 Suppl 1:15–8.

157. Food and Drug Administration US. TARCEVA® Prescribing information. 2010. Available from: http://www.accessdata.fda.gov/drugsatfda_docs/label/2010/021743s14s16lbl.pdf. Cited 14 Nov 2011.

158. Palumbo A, Rajkumar SV, Dimopoulos MA, Richardson PG, San Miguel J, Barlogie B, et al. Prevention of thalidomide- and lenalidomide-associated thrombosis in myeloma. Leukemia. 2008;22(2):414–23.

159. Deitcher SR, Gomes MPV. The risk of venous thromboembolic disease associated with adjuvant hormone therapy for breast carcinoma: a systematic review. Cancer. 2004;101(3):439–49.

160. Thürlimann B, Keshaviah A, Coates AS, Mouridsen H, Mauriac L, Forbes JF, et al. A comparison of letrozole and tamoxifen in post-menopausal women with early breast cancer. N Engl J Med. 2005;353(26):2747–57.

161. Adams MJ, Lipsitz SR, Colan SD, Tarbell NJ, Treves ST, Diller L, et al. Cardiovascular status in long-term survivors of Hodgkin's disease treated with chest radiotherapy. J Clin Oncol. 2004;22(15):3139–48.

162. Hancock SL, Tucker MA, Hoppe RT. Factors affecting late mortality from heart disease after treatment of Hodgkin's disease. J Am Med Assoc. 1993;270(16):1949–55.

163. Mulrooney DA, Yeazel MW, Kawashima T, Mertens AC, Mitby P, Stovall M, et al. Cardiac outcomes in a cohort of adult survivors of childhood and adolescent cancer: Retrospective analysis of the childhood cancer survivor study cohort. BMJ. 2010;340(7736):34.

164. Mulrooney DA, Yeazel MW, Kawashima T, Mertens AC, Mitby P, Stovall M, et al. Cardiac outcomes in a cohort of adult survivors of childhood and adolescent cancer: retrospective analysis of the Childhood Cancer Survivor Study cohort. BMJ (Clin Res Ed). 2009;339: b4606.

165. Bovelli D, Plataniotis G, Roila F. Cardiotoxicity of chemotherapeutic agents and radiotherapy-related heart disease: ESMO clinical practice guidelines. Ann Oncol. 2010;21 Suppl 5:v277–82.

166. Eschenhagen T, Force T, Ewer MS, de Keulenaer GW, Suter TM, Anker SD, et al. Cardiovascular side effects of cancer therapies: a position statement from the Heart Failure Association of the European Society of Cardiology. Eur J Heart Fail. 2011; 13(1):1–10.

167. Cheng H, Force T. Why do kinase inhibitors cause cardiotoxicity and what can be done about it? Prog Cardiovasc Dis. 2010; 53(2):114–20.

168. Fernandez A, Sanguino A, Peng Z, Ozturk E, Chen J, Crespo A, et al. An anticancer C-Kit kinase inhibitor is reengineered to make it more active and less cardiotoxic. J Clin Invest. 2007;117(12):4044–54.

169. International Conference on Harmonisation of Technical Requirements for Registration of Pharmaceuticals for Human Use. ICH Harmonised Tripartite Guideline: the non-clinical evaluation of the potential for delayed ventricular repolarization (QT interval prolongation) by human pharmaceuticals. S7B. 2005. Available from: http://www.ich.org/fileadmin/Public_Web_Site/ICH_Products/ Guidelines/Safety/S7B/Step4/S7B_Guideline.pdf. Cited 14 Nov 2011.

170. Cardinale D, Colombo A, Sandri MT, Lamantia G, Colombo N, Civelli M, et al. Prevention of high-dose chemotherapy-induced cardiotoxicity in high-risk patients by angiotensin-converting enzyme inhibition. Circulation. 2006;114(23):2474–81.

171. Kalay N, Basar E, Ozdogru I, Er O, Cetinkaya Y, Dogan A, et al. Protective effects of carvedilol against anthracycline-induced cardiomyopathy. J Am Coll Cardiol. 2006;48(11):2258–62.

172. van Dalen EC, Caron HN, Dickinson HO, Kremer LC. Cardioprotective interventions for cancer patients receiving anthracyclines. Cochrane Database Syst Rev. 2005;(1):CD003917.
173. Food and Drug Administration US. ZINECARD® Approved Labeling. 2005. Available from: http://www.accessdata.fda.gov/drugsatfda_docs/label/2005/020212s008lbl.pdf. Cited 14 Nov 2011.
174. Cardinale D, Sandri MT, Colombo A, Colombo N, Boeri M, Lamantia G, et al. Prognostic value of troponin I in cardiac risk stratification of cancer patients undergoing high-dose chemotherapy. Circulation. 2004;109(22):2749–54.
175. Auner HW, Tinchon C, Linkesch W, Tiran A, Quehenberger F, Link H, et al. Prolonged monitoring of troponin T for the detection of anthracycline cardiotoxicity in adults with hematological malignancies. Ann Hematol. 2003;82(4):218–22.
176. Sandri MT, Salvatici M, Cardinale D, Zorzino L, Passerini R, Lentati P, et al. N-terminal pro-B-type natriuretic peptide after high-dose chemotherapy: a marker predictive of cardiac dysfunction? Clin Chem. 2005;51(8):1405–10.
177. Nousiainen T, Vanninen E, Jantunen E, Puustinen J, Remes J, Rantala A, et al. Natriuretic peptides during the development of doxorubicin-induced left ventricular diastolic dysfunction. J Intern Med. 2002;251(3):228–34.
178. Suzuki T, Hayashi D, Yamazaki T, Mizuno T, Kanda Y, Komuro I, et al. Elevated B-type natriuretic peptide levels after anthracycline administration. Am Heart J. 1998;136(2):362–3.
179. Cardinale D, Colombo A, Lamantia G, Colombo N, Civelli M, De Giacomi G, et al. Anthracycline-induced cardiomyopathy. Clinical relevance and response to pharmacologic therapy. J Am Coll Cardiol. 2010;55(3):213–20.
180. Sieswerda E, van Dalen Elvira C, Postma A, Cheuk Daniel KL, Caron Huib N, Kremer Leontien CM. Medical interventions for treating anthracycline-induced symptomatic and asymptomatic cardiotoxicity during and after treatment for childhood cancer. Cochrane Database Syst Rev [Internet]. 2011;(9). Available from: http://www.mrw.interscience.wiley.com/cochrane/clsysrev/articles/CD008011/frame.html.
181. Lipshultz SE, Lipsitz SR, Sallan SE, Simbre 2nd VC, Shaikh SL, Mone SM, et al. Long-term enalapril therapy for left ventricular dysfunction in doxorubicin-treated survivors of childhood cancer. J Clin Oncol. 2002;20(23):4517–22.
182. Rudzinski T, Ciesielczyk M, Religa W, Bednarkiewicz Z, Krzeminska-Pakula M. Doxorubicin-induced ventricular arrhythmia treated by implantation of an automatic cardioverter-defibrillator. Europace. 2007;9(5):278–80.

# Chapter 16
## Toxicity of Bone-Targeted Agents in Malignancy

**Caroline Wilson, Fiona G. Taylor, and Robert E. Coleman**

**Abstract**   The bisphosphonates have been in clinical use for three decades. During this time, the adverse event profile and favorable risk-benefit ratio have become clearly defined, and strategies have been identified for minimizing the impact of these side effects on patients. More recently, denosumab has been incorporated into clinical practice and so far demonstrated mild and treatable side effects, although long-term data are lacking.

In this chapter, we review the side effects of the four bisphosphonates licensed for use in malignancy, including clodronate, ibandronate, pamidronate, and zoledronic acid, as well as the new targeted agent denosumab.

**Keywords**   Bisphosphonates • Zoledronic acid • Denosumab Toxicity • Acute phase reactions • Renal impairment Osteonecrosis of the jaw

C. Wilson, MBChB, MRCP, M.Sc.
Academic Unit of Clinical Oncology, Weston Park Hospital, Sheffield University , Sheffield, South Yorkshire, UK

F.G. Taylor, B.Sc., MB ChB, MRCP
Medical Oncology, Weston Park Hospital , Sheffield, South Yorkshire, UK

R.E. Coleman, M.S., B.S., M.D., FRCP (✉)
Academic Unit of Clinical Oncology, Weston Park Hospital, Sheffield, South Yorkshire, UK
email: r.e.coleman@sheffield.ac.uk

M.A. Dicato (ed.), *Side Effects of Medical Cancer Therapy,*
DOI 10.1007/978-0-85729-787-7_16,
© Springer-Verlag London 2013

531

# Introduction

Bone metastases are a common feature of many tumor types, including those arising in the breast, prostate, kidney, lung, and multiple myeloma. Metastasis to bone can lead to skeletal-related events (SREs), including hypercalcemia of malignancy, spinal cord compression, pathologic fracture, and surgery to bone, thus adversely affecting the quality of life of patients with advanced malignancy [1].

Therapies targeting bone metastasis have been a focus of research and development over the past three decades. These include the bone matrix homing bisphosphonates that are taken up during osteoclast bone resorption and the more recently developed RANK ligand inhibitor, denosumab, which prevents the activation of osteoclasts. Inhibition of osteoclast activity strengthens bone, thus largely preventing the devastating complications associated with bone metastasis.

# Bisphosphonates

## *Clinical Indications and Pharmacology*

Bisphosphonates are effective in the treatment of established metastatic bone disease and the prevention of SREs, including hypercalcemia of malignancy, spinal cord compression, pathologic fracture, and surgery to bone. Four bisphosphonates are currently approved for use in malignancy-associated metastatic bone disease in Europe and America and include oral clodronate, oral or intravenous ibandronic acid, intravenous pamidronate, and zoledronic acid (Fig. 16.1) [2].

Bisphosphonates have also been used in the adjuvant setting to prevent bone loss associated with anticancer therapy. The bisphosphonates used in this setting also include alendronate, etidronate, and risedronate. None of the bisphosphonates have been FDA labeled for this use but remain approved for the treatment of osteoporosis in high-risk populations, and as such their use has been extrapolated to

| | Clodronate | Ibandronate | Pamidronate | Zoledronate |
|---|---|---|---|---|
| Dose (mg) | 1600-3200 | 6 50 | 90 | 4 |
| Route of administration | Oral | IV Oral | IV | IV |
| Frequency of administration | Twice daily | 3-4 weeks Daily | 3-4 weeks | 3-4 weeks |
| Chemical structure | | | | |
| Launced indications | Bone metastasis Hypercalcemia of malignancy | Bone metastasis Hypercalcemia of malignancy | Bone metastasis Bone cancer Hypercalcemia of malignancy | Bone metastasis Bone cancer Hypercalcemia of malignancy |
| Relative potency* | 1 | 100 | 1000 | >10,000 |
| Pivotal trials [references] | [28,42,43,97-105] | [43,44,45,106-109] | [110-116] | [33,58,61,117-119] |

FIGURE 16.1 Summary of approved bisphosphonates for use in malignancy. *, dose response for the inhibition of 1,25-(OH)2 vitamin D3-induced hypercalcemia in thyroparathyroidectomized rats

patients at high risk of bone loss during anticancer therapy. The evidence supporting the use of bisphosphonates for prevention of metastasis is currently insufficient for this to be recommended as part of standard practice; it remains an ongoing area of research.

Bisphosphonates are stable synthetic analogues of pyrophosphate with a P-C-P backbone and an $R_1$ side chain that acts as a "bone hook," resulting in avid binding to the bone surface. There are two main classes of bisphosphonates: aminobisphosphonates, which contain an $R_2$ covalently bonded nitrogen atom (i.e., zoledronic acid, pamidronate, and ibandronic acid), and non-nitrogen-containing compounds such as clodronate. The mechanisms of action of these two classes are different; nitrogen-containing bisphosphonates inhibit farnesyl diphosphate synthase in the mevalonate pathway, leading to a reduction in signaling GTPases [34], while non-nitrogen-containing bisphosphonates are metabolized to hydrolysis-resistant ATP analogues [35].

Bisphosphonates are taken up by osteoclasts during bone resorption and result in osteoclast apoptosis and, thus, reduced bone turnover. Their bioavailability is determined by the route of administration, with poor absorption (0.5–3 %) when given by mouth. Following intravenous administration, the half-life in serum is less than 1 h, with approximately 30–60 % of the infused dose rapidly binding to the bone surface, and the remainder excreted by the kidney. The half-life in bone is, however, substantially longer and measurable in years, with evidence of ongoing biological activity after a single infusion of 4 mg for more than 3 years [36].

## Animal Toxicology and Teratogenicity

### Animal Studies

Bisphosphonates are excreted in a nonmetabolized form in the kidneys of mammals. Preclinical studies in rats demonstrated that the renal toxicity is not only linked to renal excretion rates but also varies according to the particular bisphosphonate. A comparison of ibandronic acid, 10–20 mg/kg; zoledronic acid, 3–10 mg/kg; and intraperitoneal clodronate injection, 200 mg/kg twice daily demonstrated tubular degeneration and single cell necrosis of proximal convoluted tubules on the fourth day of dosing, with zoledronic acid showing the strongest dose-effect relationship [37]. These data were further supported in a rat model using clinically relevant doses of zoledronic acid (1 or 3 mg/kg) and ibandronic acid (1 mg/kg). The rats were treated on a single infusion protocol or an intermittent intravenous dosing protocol every 3 weeks. Ibandronic acid induced similar proximal tubular damage in both dosing protocols; however, zoledronic acid demonstrated increased renal toxicity at the intermittent dosing versus the single dose. Thus, the cumulative use of zoledronic acid appears to increase toxicity in rats, but ibandronic acid may have a safer profile when used repeatedly [38]. The longer renal half-life of zoledronic acid (150–200 days) compared to ibandronic acid (24 days) may explain the differences in cumulative toxicity since zoledronic acid will take longer to excrete [39].

Bisphosphonates have been associated with various adverse reproductive toxicities in animal studies, including dystocia, teeth abnormalities, visceral anomalies, and failure of embryo implantation. As such, they are contraindicated during pregnancy. However, human case studies have reported safe use of pamidronate [40] and ibandronic acid [41]. In a review of 51 case studies of bisphosphonate use during pregnancy reported from 1950 to 2008, no skeletal or congenital abnormalities were reported [42]. Furthermore, the outcome of 21 pregnancies exposed to bisphosphonates in the first trimester compared to matched control subjects did not demonstrate any adverse events in the pregnancy, suggesting bisphosphonates may not pose a significant teratogenic risk in humans [43]. The balance of risks to the pregnancy, with consideration of the potential teratogenic risk in humans, must always be weighed against the benefits of bisphosphonate treatment.

Postpartum, there is evidence, in vivo, of passage of bisphosphonates into milk; thus, it is recommended that use during breast-feeding should be avoided. A clinical case report of intravenous monthly pamidronate use during breast-feeding did not demonstrate pamidronate in breast milk collected for 48 h after the first infusion, suggesting pamidronate may be safe during lactation in humans [44].

## Systemic Effects

### Acute Phase Response

The acute phase response is a systemic inflammatory reaction characterized by flu-like symptoms, including fever, arthralgia, myalgia, exhaustion, and leucocytosis. These reactions have most commonly been described with the intravenous bisphosphonates, zoledronic acid, ibandronic acid, and pamidronate. They occur more commonly after the first infusion, and symptoms dissipate with subsequent infusions. Treatment involves paracetamol and nonsteroidal anti-inflammatory agents. All components of the acute phase response have a peak onset within 1 day, with a median duration of 3 days. Severity is mild to moderate in 90 % of cases [45] and self-limiting in nature.

The cause of the acute phase reaction is thought to be due to an increase in gamma/delta ($\gamma/\Delta$) T lymphocytes and release of tumor necrosis factor alpha and interleukin-6 following use of an aminobisphosphonate [46, 47]. The incidence of the acute phase response appears to be similar between intravenous bisphosphonates. In breast cancer and myeloma patients treated with zoledronic acid or pamidronate, the frequency of fever was 38 % versus 31 %, respectively [48]. When zoledronic acid (4 mg every 4 weeks) was compared to oral ibandronic acid (50 mg daily) in a phase 3 trial of breast cancer patients, fever expectedly occurred more frequently in the zoledronic acid group (16.8 % zoledronic acid vs. 0 % oral ibandronic acid) [49]. However, intravenous ibandronic acid (6 mg day 1 followed by oral 50 mg daily) demonstrated an acute phase reaction incidence, on days 1–3, of 13 % [50], indicating that the incidence of the acute phase reaction may be more dependent on the route of administration than the specific type of aminobisphosphonate. The incidence of acute phase reactions may be less common in immunocompromised cancer patients than in healthy subjects or patients with malignancy who do not have metastasis [51].

## Metabolic

Prolonged use of bisphosphonates can be associated with alterations in calcium, magnesium, phosphate, and vitamin D metabolism. Hypocalcemia is the most commonly reported metabolic side effect of bisphosphonates. In studies of bisphosphonates, without supplementation with calcium and vitamin D, the incidence of hypocalcemia compared to placebo was greater with zoledronic acid (39 % vs. 7 %) [52], but only slightly higher than placebo with ibandronic acid, pamidronate, and clodronate [53]. Concomitant use of oral calcium and vitamin D supplements is recommended as routine with zoledronic acid and advised for ibandronic acid or pamidronate if dietary intake or sunlight exposure is felt to be insufficient, both of which are common in cancer patients [54].

The severity of hypocalcemia is usually mild and often subclinical. However, there are recognized exacerbating factors such as concurrent use of aminoglycosides, which can lower calcium and magnesium; preexisting vitamin D deficiency; hypomagnesemia; and hypoparathyroidism [53]. In an exploratory study comparing changes in bone biochemistry in metastatic breast cancer patients on prolonged bisphosphonate therapy compared to healthy controls matched for age, gender, and renal function, bisphosphonate use was associated with elevated PTH (5.7 vs. 4.8 pmol/L, $p = 0.043$) when serum calcium was at the lower range. Sixty-two percent of patients demonstrated a suboptimal level of vitamin D, and 18 % were deficient in 25-hydroxy vitamin D, despite supplementation with 400 IU of vitamin D daily [55].

Hypomagnesemia, hypokalemia, and hypophosphatemia have all been described with zoledronic acid but are less common than hypocalcemia [56].

## Renal Toxicity

Rat models indicated that proximal tubular necrosis was the predominant mechanism of renal injury associated with several

TABLE 16.1 Recommended dosing and schedule of bisphosphonates according to creatinine clearance

| Bisphosphonate | Baseline creatinine clearance (mL/min) | Recommended dose in malignant bone disease (infusion time) |
|---|---|---|
| Clodronate | >30 | 1,600 mg daily |
| | 10–30 | 800 mg daily |
| | <10 | Not recommended |
| Ibandronate | >50 | 6 mg q3–4 weeks (15 min) |
| | ≥30 | 4 mg q3–4 weeks (1 h) |
| | <30 | 2 mg q3–4 weeks (1 h) |
| Pamidronate | ≥30 | 90 mg q3–4 weeks (1.5–4 h dependent on creatinine) |
| | <30 | Not recommended |
| Zoledronate | >60 | 4 mg q3–4 weeks |
| | 50–60 | 3.5 mg q3–4 weeks |
| | 40–49 | 3.3 mg q3–4 weeks |
| | 30–39 | 3 mg q3–4 weeks |
| | <30 | Not recommended |

bisphosphonates. However, in clinical studies, different bisphosphonates demonstrate distinctive patterns of renal damage. Zoledronic acid-induced renal toxicity is characterized by acute tubular necrosis and apoptosis [57]. Pamidronate, however, may induce a collapsing focal segmental glomerulosclerosis [58].

Toxicity is dependent on dose, scheduling, and, for intravenous preparations, the infusion rates (Table 16.1). Oral bisphosphonates have not been demonstrated to cause clinically relevant renal impairment in human studies. Clodronate had a similar rate of renal impairment to that of placebo in breast cancer [3, 4]. Renal adverse events with ibandronic acid (6 mg via a 1- to 2-h infusion 3–4 times weekly) in metastatic breast cancer appear to be similar in frequency to placebo-treated patients (4.5 % ibandronic acid vs. 4 % placebo). Pamidronate, at doses higher than 90 mg, may cause renal impairment [59, 60], and this may occasionally occur at standard doses [61].

Early dose-finding studies with zoledronic acid use in metastatic bone disease suggested that an 8 or 4-mg dose infused over 5 min was efficacious, and this dose was taken forward into phase III trials. However, a dose- and schedule-dependent effect on renal function was seen that resulted in the abandonment of the 8-mg dose and lengthening of infusion time to 15 min. With the 4-mg dose and longer infusion time, the phase III randomized trials of zoledronic acid in prostate, breast, myeloma, and lung cancer patients demonstrated the incidence of renal impairment to be approximately 10–15 % (as defined by an increase in serum creatinine of $\geq 0.5$ mg/dL [if baseline < 1.4 mg/dL] or 1.0 mg/dL [if baseline $\geq 1.4$ mg/dL] and an increase in glomerular filtration rate [GFR] $\geq 25$ % from baseline). This incidence was not dissimilar to that observed in advanced cancer patients receiving placebo [28, 62]. Clinically significant renal deterioration with zoledronic acid is uncommon and is exacerbated by previous exposure to bisphosphonates, underlying malignancy, increased age, dehydration, cumulative doses, and concurrent use of nephrotoxic drugs (i.e., nonsteroidal anti-inflammatories and cisplatin) [63].

Limited comparison studies of bisphosphonates have been performed in an attempt to identify the safest renal profile. A retrospective comparison of risk of renal impairment with ibandronic acid versus zoledronic acid in 333 breast, myeloma, prostate, and non-small-cell lung cancer patients found the renal impairment incidence rates (number of events per patient per year of treatment with bisphosphonate) to be significantly higher with zoledronic acid for all tumor sites (0.56 vs. 0.21, $p < 0.0001$ when assessed by serum creatinine and 1.92 vs. 1.01, $p < 0.0001$ when assessed using GFR for zoledronic acid and ibandronic acid, respectively). Even after adjustment of patient characteristics between both groups, the hazard ratio (HR) for a decline in renal function with zoledronic acid compared to ibandronic acid persisted (HR serum creatinine 1.99, $p = 0.08$, HR GFR 1.94, $p = 0.02$) [64]. Similar results were demonstrated in myeloma patients, while the risk of renal impairment with ibandronic acid increased if patients had received prior zoledronic acid [65]. Comparison of pamidronate, 90 mg over 2 h every 3–4 weeks, with zoledronic acid, 4 mg over 15 min at similar intervals, in breast and myeloma patients demonstrated no significant difference in renal safety profiles between the two drugs over a period of up to 2 years [66].

In general, provided bisphosphonates are used at the recommended dose and schedule, renal toxicity is unlikely, and serious complications are rare, with an incidence of <0.5 % [67] (see Table 16.1). The ability to reliably discern which bisphosphonate represents a "safer" option, with lower renal toxicity, would need prospective analysis in appropriately powered comparative trials [51].

## Gastrointestinal Toxicity

The most common side effect of oral bisphosphonates is gastrointestinal toxicity, notably to the esophagus or the colon. Recommendations for administration stipulate that oral bisphosphonates should be taken with water, on an empty stomach to prevent food interaction, and the patient remain upright for at least 30 min post ingestion.

Placebo-controlled trials of clodronate reported rates of gastrointestinal disorders at 3–10 % [68] due mainly to increased diarrhea during the initial treatment phase rather than upper gastrointestinal (GI) side effects [69]. Further studies reported clodronate-associated diarrhea at 19.9 % versus 10 % placebo, with only mild upper GI toxicity, including nausea and difficulty swallowing tablets [5].

Ibandronic acid placebo trials have reported an overall upper GI toxicity rate of 10 %, with upper GI symptoms reported as abdominal pain (2.1 %), dyspepsia (7 %), nausea

(3.5 %), and esophagitis (2.1 %), all of which were twice as likely to occur on ibandronic acid compared to placebo; however, diarrhea occurred at similar frequency to placebo [6, 15]. Coleman et al. reported on four oral dosing regimens of ibandronic acid at 5, 10, 20, and 50 mg compared to placebo and found the frequency of GI adverse events occurring in the first month to be 30 % with placebo and 33, 39, 41, and 50 % at the four increasing dose levels [16].

Gastrointestinal toxicity may result in poor compliance with oral bisphosphonates, and studies in malignancy have suggested that up to one-third of patients will not continue or comply with treatment [70]. Thus, intravenous preparations may be preferable if oral preparations become intolerable.

Two recent papers have reported conflicting findings in relation to the risk of esophageal cancer with the use of oral bisphosphonates. Both studies examined the UK General Practice database over similar time periods, with one study reporting no association with esophageal or gastric cancer [71] and the other an increased risk of esophageal malignancy with oral bisphosphonate use for longer than 5 years when compared to no bisphosphonate use (relative risk [RR] 2.24, CI 1.47–3.4) [72]. Green et al. conclude that with an incidence of esophageal cancer in patients aged 60–79 of 1 per 1,000 population over 5 years, this would increase to 2 per 1000 population over 5 years of treatment with oral bisphosphonates, thus still remaining at very low risk [72].

A consistent reduction in risk of colon cancer has been demonstrated in studies of oral bisphosphonate use. A case control study of more than 900 postmenopausal females diagnosed with colorectal cancer demonstrated that bisphosphonate use for at least a year prior to diagnosis was associated with a significantly reduced relative risk, even when other confounders were taken into account such as diet, body mass index, and use of low-dose aspirin (RR, 0.41; 95 % CI 0.25–0.67) [73]. These data are supported by the lack of association of oral bisphosphonates with colorectal cancer in the study by Green et al. [72].

## Osteonecrosis of the Jaw

Osteonecrosis of the jaw (ONJ) was first reported in 2003 in association with pamidronate and zoledronic acid use [74, 75]. Painful bone exposure in the mandible and maxilla was described, commonly occurring after tooth extraction and exacerbated by dental/gingival or jawbone disease, cancer diagnosis, increased age, smoking, diabetes, concurrent chemotherapy or steroids, and potency and duration of bisphosphonate use. The lesions were nonhealing and resistant to antibiotic therapy or debridement. ONJ is a clinical diagnosis and defined as an area of exposed bone in the maxillofacial region that does not heal within 8 weeks after identification in a patient who has not had radiation therapy to the craniofacial region [76].

The causes of ONJ in malignancy are likely to be multifactorial, and although proposed mechanisms include suppressed angiogenesis from aminobisphosphonates and oversuppression of bone turnover, the evidence for either of these processes being causative is weak. Immune dysfunction during anticancer therapy can also provide an opportunity for infection and inflammation in the oral cavity, which may exacerbate the potential detrimental effect of bisphosphonates on the jawbone [77].

Because of global market share, most ONJ cases have been associated with the use of pamidronate and/or zoledronic acid. There have been isolated cases with intravenous ibandronic acid, but reports are few, and the incidence associated with this agent is not known [78]. ONJ is rare with oral bisphosphonates, and the prevalence is reported as less than 0.1 % in patients receiving chronic oral bisphosphonate administration for a range of nonmalignant medical conditions, but whether this reflects the prevalence in malignancy is not known [79]. The incidence with monthly intravenous bisphosphonates has been reported from retrospective trials as approximately 5 % in patients with metastatic bone disease; however, prospective randomized trials of zoledronic acid versus denosumab indicate the incidence is probably lower, at approximately 1.5–3 % over 2–3 years of use [80, 81]. The incidence is less when administration is less frequent as used to prevent cancer treatment-induced bone loss. Data from a large prospective randomized trial of zoledronic acid in early breast cancer with a median follow-up of approximately 5 years reported an ONJ incidence of 1.1 % (CI 0.6–1.7) [29]. Despite the potential risk for developing ONJ during treatment with an intravenous bisphosphonate, the benefits of bisphosphonates in metastatic malignancy far outweigh this small risk.

Treatment of ONJ is difficult despite local debridement, antibiotics, and oxygen therapy. Thus, the management focus should be on prevention by increasing awareness among oncologists, dentists, and maxillofacial surgeons. Good dental hygiene and avoidance of dental procedures during therapy significantly reduce the risk of ONJ with zoledronic acid [82, 83].

## Cardiovascular

Atrial fibrillation (AF) is the only cardiovascular side effect potentially associated with bisphosphonates. Untreated, it can increase risk of stroke, thromboembolism, and cardiac failure. Atrial fibrillation has been described in association with the use of pamidronate and zoledronic acid. The first data describing AF as a side effect came from trials in osteoporosis. In an osteoporosis clinical trial of annual zoledronic acid versus placebo in around 3,800 postmenopausal women, there was an increased incidence of serious adverse events due to AF with zoledronic acid (1.3 % vs. 0.6 %, $p < 0.001$). The majority of these cases occurred more than 30 days after a zoledronic acid infusion when serum levels would be undetectable; thus, the mechanism for any relationship was obscure. The increase in AF did not translate to an increase in stroke or thrombosis in the patients [30].

A systematic review and meta-analysis of placebo-controlled trials of bisphosphonates used in osteoporosis, including over 26,000 patients, demonstrated a significant increased risk of AF serious adverse events with bisphosphonate exposure (odds ratio 1.47; CI 1.01–2.14, $p = 0.04$). However, a further meta-analysis of serious and nonserious AF events from the same trials failed to demonstrate a significant association, and there was no increase in risk of stroke or cardiovascular mortality [84]. Three further observational studies involving over 120,000 patients treated with bisphosphonates compared to untreated controls have failed to demonstrate an increased risk of AF [85–87]. Two analyses of large prospective databases of over 47,000 patients registered as part of cardiac intervention follow-up showed no link between AF and bisphosphonate administration and no increase in the long-term incidence of myocardial infarction [88]. Any possible association would therefore appear to be very weak and probably not clinically relevant.

The extrapolation of these data to oncology patients is difficult, but none of the studies to date have demonstrated an increased risk of AF [89, 90]. A recent large adjuvant breast cancer trial of zoledronic acid did not demonstrate any excess cardiac toxicity in those receiving zoledronic acid compared to standard therapy (0.8 % vs. 0.6 %, respectively) [29].

## Eye

Eye complications are rare, with an incidence of about 0.05 % [53], but have been reported with pamidronate [91, 92], zoledronic acid [93–95], clodronate [96], and, in postmarketing experience, with ibandronic acid. The possible complications include cataract, ocular inflammation, conjunctivitis, uveitis, scleritis, episcleritis, and cranial nerve palsies due to extraocular muscle edema [97].

The onset of ocular inflammation appears to start soon after administration of a bisphosphonate, and the mechanism of action has been proposed to be related to the acute phase response with infiltration of inflammatory cytokines, including interleukin 1 and 6, into the extraocular muscles [98].

Management involves referral to a specialist of ophthalmology care. Conjunctivitis is usually self-limiting and often decreases in severity with ongoing bisphosphonate therapy.

Several ocular side effects can occur in conjunction and usually resolve over several weeks with termination of therapy [92]. Severe cases of global ocular inflammation, scleritis, or uveitis may need hospitalization and intravenous high-dose steroids [98]. Rechallenge with the causative bisphosphonate is not recommended [53].

## Central Nervous System

Case reports of seizures associated with zoledronic acid have been published, although in all cases there was an underlying neurologic disorder in elderly patients treated for osteoporosis [99]. Many of the reported neurologic side effects during bisphosphonate use in malignancy, including headache, dizziness, and lethargy, are likely to relate to the acute phase response discussed earlier.

## *Conclusion*

The use of bisphosphonates in malignancy has been supported by clear evidence from clinical trials of a reduction in SREs from bone metastases arising from numerous tumor sites, including breast, prostate, myeloma, lung, and other solid tumors. Bisphosphonates have also demonstrated efficacy in reducing bone loss associated with adjuvant therapy and may have a role in the prevention of metastasis [51].

The benefits and risks of bisphosphonate use in both the palliative and adjuvant settings must be carefully considered to ensure that the former offset the latter. Although there can be occasional serious toxicities with bisphosphonates (Table 16.2), the majority of these can be avoided with increased awareness of potential side effects, appropriate monitoring, and strict adherence to recommended administration guidelines and dosage.

Although renal impairment and ONJ are two potentially serious side effects, they only occasionally lead to a need for discontinuation of the bisphosphonate. Alteration of the infusion

TABLE 16.2  Summary of side effects of bisphosphonates and denosumab

| Frequency | Oral bisphosphonates | Intravenous bisphosphonates | Denosumab |
|---|---|---|---|
| Common | Asymptomatic hypocalcemia | Symptomatic hypocalcemia | Urinary tract infection |
| ≥1/100 | ↑AST/ALT (within normal range) | Hypophosphatemia | Upper respiratory tract infection |
| <1/10 | Diarrhea | Hypomagnasemia | Sciatica |
| | Abdominal pain | Parathyroid disorder | Cataracts |
| | Nausea/dyspepsia | ↑GGT | Constipation |
| | Vomiting | ↑Creatinine | Rash |
| | Constipation | Diarrhea | Pain in extremities |
| | Headache | Abdominal pain | |
| | Musculoskeletal pain | Nausea/dyspepsia | |
| | | Vomiting | |
| | | Constipation | |

| | | | |
|---|---|---|---|
| Uncommon | Iritis | Pharnygitis | Osteonecrosis of the jaw[a] |
| | | Influerza-like illness | |
| | | Headache | |
| | | Bone/joint pain | |
| | | Cataract/conjunctivitis | |
| | | Bundle branch block | |
| | | Osteonecrosis of the jaw[a] | |
| ≥1/1,000 | Gastritis | Uveitis | Diverticulitis |
| <1/100 | Esophagitis | Gastritis | Cellulitis |
| | Dysphagia | Gastroenteritis | Ear infection |
| | Duodenitis | Mouth ulceration | Eczema |
| | Esophageal ulcer | Dysphagia | |
| | | Cholelithiasis | |
| | | Myalgia | |
| | | Anemia/blood dyscrasia | |

(continued)

TABLE 16.2  (continued)

| Frequency | Oral bisphosphonates | Intravenous bisphosphonates | Denosumab |
|---|---|---|---|
| | | Migraine/neuralgia | |
| | | Deafness | |
| | | Myocardial ischemia | |
| | | Atrial fibrillation | |
| | | Pulmonary edema | |
| | | Rash/pruritus | |
| | | Hair loss | |
| | | Urine retention/ARF | |
| Rare | Symptomatic hypocalcemia | Ocular inflammation | Hypocalcemia (<1.88 mmol/L) |
| ≥1/10,000 | ↑PTH | Focal segmental glomerulosclerosis | |
| <1/1,000 | ↑Alk phos | Nephrotic syndrome | |
| | ↑AST/ALT (>2× normal range) | | |
| | Mild skin hypersensitivity (i.e., pruritus, urticaria) | | |
| | Bronchospasm | | |

Glossitis

Esophageal stricture

Osteonecrosis of the jaw

Very rare

<1/10,000

Anaphylaxis

Bronchospasm

Osteonecrosis of the jaw

Infection

Leukopenia

Scleritis

Episcleritis

Xanthopsia

Hyperkalemia

Hypernatremia

(continued)

TABLE 16.2 (continued)

| Frequency | Oral bisphosphonates | Intravenous bisphosphonates | Denosumab |
|---|---|---|---|
| Frequency unknown | Uveitis | | |
| | Severe bone, joint, and/or muscle pain | | |
| | Severe hypersensitivity reaction, including angioedema, bullous reaction, Stevens-Johnson, toxic epidermal necrolysis, anaphylaxis | | |
| | Hair loss | | |
| | Impaired renal function | | |

Adapted from [100–104]

[a]Estimated rates for osteonecrosis of the jaw relate to annual risk

time and/or dose with appropriate dental hygiene and management should ensure these are mild, self-limiting side effects. To put the risk benefit into context, the reduction in skeletal complications with zoledronic acid exceeds the risk of ONJ by a factor of >10 [105]. Bisphosphonates have established themselves as an integral part of the treatment of cancer-related bone disease, have a favorable safety profile, and contribute to an enhanced quality of life for cancer patients.

# Denosumab

## Clinical Indication and Pharmacology

Denosumab is a fully human IgG2 monoclonal antibody given by subcutaneous injection that targets receptor activator of nuclear factor-kB ligand (RANKL). RANKL controls the differentiation and activation of osteoclasts [106] by binding to RANK receptors on osteoclasts [107] and its precursors [108]. RANKL-mediated bone resorption is increased in osteoporosis and malignant bone disease due to breast and prostate cancer [109]. Denosumab inhibits RANKL receptor interaction, and this leads to diminished osteoclast activity and survival. As a consequence, bone resorption is reduced, and bone mineral density (BMD) is enhanced. This effect has been observed in trabecular as well as cortical bones of patients [110]. In addition, there is evidence that RANKL may be involved in facilitating the development of metastasis to bone from breast cancer [111]. Denosumab is administered as a subcutaneous injection.

Denosumab has been approved by both the Food and Drug Administration in the United States and the European Medicines Evaluation Agency. It is currently licensed as Prolia (Amgen, Thousand Oaks, CA, USA), 60 mg every 6 months to improve bone mass and reduce fracture in osteoporotic postmenopausal females [112]. In the cancer setting, denosumab is approved to reduce treatment-induced bone loss and fracture in nonmetastatic prostate cancer patients having hormone ablation therapy [113] as well as adjuvant breast cancer patients on aromatase inhibitors [110]. More recently, denosumab, 120 mg every 4 weeks (Xgeva, Amgen, Thousand Oaks, CA, USA), has been shown to be more effective than zoledronic acid for prevention of skeletal morbidity in patients with bone metastases from breast cancer, prostate cancer, and other solid tumors [80, 81, 114]. Trials are currently under way to establish the role of denosumab in preventing cancer recurrence in the adjuvant setting in high-risk breast cancer patients undergoing chemotherapy (NCT01077154) as well as the benefit of treatment in bisphosphonate refractory hypercalcemia (NCT0896454).

In the first single-dose phase I study, carried out in postmenopausal women, denosumab caused marked dose-dependent reduction in bone turnover markers compared to placebo. Effects upon the markers – namely, urine N-telopeptide corrected for creatinine (uNTX/Cr) as well as serum N-telopeptide – were observed 12 h post dose and were sustained for up to 6 months, demonstrating a rapid response and a long plasma half-life. UNTX/Cr levels eventually returned to normal, indicating that suppression of osteoclast activity was reversible. Pharmacokinetics of denosumab was found to be nonlinear. No significant safety issues were identified, and, importantly, no reductions were noted in lymphocyte counts to substantiate concerns regarding increased infection risk [115].

Denosumab is administered at a dose of 60 mg subcutaneously every 6 months in postmenopausal patients to treat osteoporosis or to cancer patients receiving aromatase inhibitors or androgen-deprivation therapy. In patients with metastatic bone disease, a higher dose and frequency of administration, 120 mg subcutaneously every 3–4 weeks, are recommended.

In contrast to intravenous bisphosphonates, there are no requirements to reduce the dose of denosumab in patients with renal impairment. The safety of denosumab has not been studied in patients with hepatic impairment, but, as monoclonal antibodies are thought to be eliminated by being broken down to peptides and amino acids by an "immunoglobulin clearance" pathway within the reticuloendothelial system and not excreted by the liver, specific dosing recommendations do not appear to be required. Importantly, significant levels of neutralizing antibodies against denosumab have not been demonstrated in clinical trials [80, 81, 110]. There is no experience in drug overdose. The highest dose used in a phase II trial – 180 mg every 4 weeks over 21 weeks – was well tolerated by breast cancer patients with bone metastases, although hypocalcemia was more common at this dose than the approved 120-mg dose [116].

## Animal Toxicology and Teratogenicity

RANK/RANKL "knockout" mice demonstrated reduced lymph node formation and partial inhibition of early T- and B-lymphocyte development as well as reduced bone growth and lack of tooth eruption [117, 118]. Denosumab is not recommended for use in the pediatric population. The safety and efficacy in children remain to be established, and the effect on developing bone may be detrimental. Inhibition of mammary gland formation has been observed in vitro [119]. For this reason, denosumab should not be administered if there are plans to breast-feed, as postpartum lactation potentially may be impaired. In addition, it is unknown whether denosumab is excreted in breast milk. No data exist for humans on the effect of denosumab on fertility or the developing fetus; therefore, its usage is not recommended during pregnancy or in subjects intending to conceive.

## Systemic Side Effects

### Metabolic

Hypocalcemia is the most common metabolic side effect. However, in clinical trials where patients also received calcium and vitamin D supplements, clinical manifestations were rarely observed, even with prolonged monthly treatment [81, 110, 114]. In 3,933 postmenopausal patients treated with denosumab, 60 mg every 6 months over 3 years, plus calcium and vitamin D supplements, there were no reported cases of hypocalcemia (adjusted calcium <2 mmol/L) [112]. In trials of patients with bony metastases from solid tumors treated with denosumab, 120 mg every 3–4 weeks, the overall incidences of hypocalcemia were 10.8 and 13 % with grade 3 or 4 hypocalcemia (<1.75 mmol/L) in 2.3 % [81] and 5 %, respectively [114]. Most events were asymptomatic, occurred once, and only infrequently required intravenous replacement. None were fatal. In one study, 5.7 and 2.7 % of patients required intravenous calcium during treatment with denosumab on zoledronic acid, respectively [81].

There is an increased risk of hypocalcemia in patients with a history indicative of abnormal calcium metabolism such as previous hypoparathyroidism, thyroid surgery, or severe renal impairment. Furthermore, patients with a creatinine clearance of <30 mL/min or a patient on renal dialysis is at higher risk and must have calcium levels monitored closely. Denosumab is contraindicated in patients with hypocalcemia, but, once corrected, treatment may be initiated or resumed. The manufacturer recommends that all patients should be well supplemented with calcium and vitamin D.

Phosphate levels can also be seen to transiently drop as bone turnover is reduced [115], although none of the large clinical trials have reported this specifically as an adverse metabolic effect.

## Musculoskeletal

Musculoskeletal events were rarely reported in patients treated with 60 mg of denosumab every 6 months, except in adjuvant breast cancer patients taking aromatase inhibitors. In this study, arthralgia (24 %), pain in the extremities (14.7 %), and back pain (14 %) were documented. However, most cases were attributed to the aromatase inhibitor, and few cases in each symptom group were attributed to the study drug by the investigator. Furthermore, no significant difference in incidence or severity was found compared to placebo [110]. In fact, back pain and arthralgia were significantly more common in patients with bone metastases from breast cancer treated with zoledronic acid compared to high-dose denosumab in one study [80].

## Osteonecrosis of the Jaw

Osteonecrosis of the jaw has been defined earlier in this chapter. It is very rare in patients treated with denosumab, 60 mg every 6 months. As with bisphosphonates, the frequency of ONJ appears to be related to the dose, frequency, and duration of action. The incidence in advanced cancer patients treated with denosumab, 120 mg every 4 weeks, remains low and similar to that associated with use of zoledronic acid. In 2,046 patients with bone metastases from breast cancer, the incidence of ONJ was 2.0 % with denosumab compared to 1.4 % with zoledronic acid ($P = 0.39$) [80]. In a trial of 1904 patients with bone metastases from prostate cancer, the incidence of ONJ was 2.0 % with denosumab compared to 1.0 % with zoledronic acid ($P = 0.09$) [114]. A similar incidence was also seen in patients with bone metastases from other solid organs (excluding breast and prostate) or myeloma. Here, the incidence of ONJ was 1.3 % with denosumab compared to 1.1 % with zoledronic acid ($P = 1.0$) [81]. Risk factors for ONJ in these three studies included poor dental hygiene, concurrent chemotherapy, comorbidities, dental extraction, and previous treatment with bisphosphonates [76]. Most cases could be managed with oral rinses and antibiotics, but occasionally surgical debridement or bone resection was necessary. Approximately 40 % of the cases resolved. As with the use of bisphosphonates, regular dental examinations, patient education, and avoidance of invasive dental procedures while on treatment are vital.

## Skin

Dermatologic side effects such as rash, eczema, and injection site reaction have been reported rarely. Only for eczema has a significant difference been found compared to placebo in the incidence rates (3 % denosumab vs. 1.7 % placebo [$p < 0.001$]) [112]. However, an excess frequency of eczema has not been reported in other trials.

## Gastrointestinal

Constipation in patients with bone metastases from solid tumors has been reported in the three bone metastases trials with incidences of 17.3, 24, and 25 %. However, constipation was more commonly noted in patients on zoledronic acid in each trial. At lower doses of denosumab, constipation has not been reported as an adverse effect.

## Ophthalmic

In prostate cancer patients receiving androgen-deprivation therapy and denosumab, 60 mg every 6 months, rates of cataracts were 4.7 % compared to 1.2 % for placebo [113]. Although none of these cases were considered related to denosumab, a prospective evaluation is under way to assess the risk prospectively for cataracts associated with deno-sumab use (NCT00925600).

## Infections and Immune Function

In patients having low-dose denosumab as part of the FREEDOM trial, the rate of serious adverse infection was 4.1 % compared to placebo 3.4 % ($P = 0.14$). There was an increased incidence of cellulitis with denosumab, but overall rates remained very low (0.3 % denosumab vs. <0.1 % pla-cebo [$P = 0.002$]). In the bone metastasis trials, infections were more common owing to the underlying malignancy and concomitant treatments, but no significant excess was seen with denosumab. Initial concerns of an increased risk of infection with denosumab have not been supported by the many large randomized trials.

In terms of new primary cancers, cancer recurrence, or disease progression, no significant differences between denosumab and either placebo or zoledronic acid across different patient groups and trials have been reported.

## Late Effects

The effects of long-term bone suppression with denosumab are yet to be established. Iliac crest biopsies from postmenopausal females treated with denosumab, 60 mg every 6 months for 2 years, showed normal bone architecture and no evidence of bone mineralization defects, woven bone, or marrow fibrosis [120]. Concerns still exist regarding increased risk of atypical fractures and delayed fracture healing. Although no large trial has reported any significant findings regarding this issue, follow-up data are currently limited.

## *Conclusions*

Overall, denosumab is very well tolerated. There is a higher incidence of hypocalcemia with denosumab compared to zoledronic acid. The incidence of ONJ is similar to that seen with intravenous zoledronic acid. Hypocalcemia is manageable with adequate calcium and vitamin D supplementation. Denosumab is safe in patients with renal impairment, and no dose modification is required. The long-term effects of bone suppression are unknown, and this is of particular relevance in the adjuvant setting. Ease of administration, low toxicity profile, and continued use in patients with worsening renal function make denosumab an attractive therapeutic agent.

# References

1. Coleman RE. Skeletal complications of malignancy. Cancer. 1997;80(8 Suppl):1588–94 [Review].
2. Coleman RE. Bisphosphonates in breast cancer. Ann Oncol. 2005;16(5):687–95.
3. Kristensen B, Ejlertsen B, Groenvold M, Hein S, Loft H, Mouridsen HT. Oral clodronate in breast cancer patients with bone metastases: a randomized study. J Intern Med. 1999;246(1):67–74.
4. Tubiana-Hulin M, Beuzeboc P, Mauriac L, Barbet N, Frenay M, Monnier A, et al. Double-blinded controlled study comparing clodronate versus placebo in patients with breast cancer bone metastases. Bull Cancer. 2001;88(7):701–7.
5. Powles T, Paterson S, Kanis JA, McCloskey E, Ashley S, Tidy A, et al. Randomized, placebo-controlled trial of clodronate in patients with primary operable breast cancer. J Clin Oncol. 2002; 20(15):3219–24.
6. Body JJ, Diel IJ, Lichinitzer M, Lazarev A, Pecherstorfer M, Bell R, et al. Oral ibandronate reduces the risk of skeletal complications in breast cancer patients with metastatic bone disease: results from two randomised, placebo-controlled phase III studies. Br J Cancer. 2004;90(6):1133–7.
7. Elomaa I, Kylmala T, Tammela T, Viitanen J, Ottelin J, Ruutu M, et al. Effect of oral clodronate on bone pain. A controlled study in patients with metastic prostatic cancer. Int Urol Nephrol. 1992;24(2):159–66.
8. McCloskey EV, MacLennan IC, Drayson MT, Chapman C, Dunn J, Kanis JA. A randomized trial of the effect of clodronate on skeletal morbidity in multiple myeloma. MRC Working Party on Leukaemia in Adults. Br J Haematol. 1998;100(2):317–25.
9. Lahtinen R, Laakso M, Palva I, Virkkunen P, Elomaa I. Randomised, placebo-controlled multicentre trial of clodronate in multiple myeloma. Finnish Leukaemia Group. Lancet. 1992;340(8827): 1049–52.
10. Paterson AH, Powles TJ, Kanis JA, McCloskey E, Hanson J, Ashley S. Double-blind controlled trial of oral clodronate in patients with bone metastases from breast cancer. J Clin Oncol. 1993;11(1): 59–65.
11. Diel IJ, Solomayer EF, Costa SD, Gollan C, Goerner R, Wallwiener D, et al. Reduction in new metastases in breast cancer with adjuvant clodronate treatment. N Engl J Med. 1998;339(6):357–63.
12. Saarto T, Vehmanen L, Virkkunen P, Blomqvist C. Ten-year follow-up of a randomized controlled trial of adjuvant clodronate treatment in node-positive breast cancer patients. Acta Oncol. 2004;43(7):650–6.
13. Dearnaley DP, Sydes MR, Mason MD, Stott M, Powell CS, Robinson AC, et al. A double-blind, placebo-controlled, randomized trial of

oral sodium clodronate for metastatic prostate cancer (MRC PR05 Trial). J Natl Cancer Inst. 2003;95(17):1300–11.

14. Mason MD, Sydes MR, Glaholm J, Langley RE, Huddart RA, Sokal M, et al. Oral sodium clodronate for nonmetastatic prostate cancer–results of a randomized double-blind placebo-controlled trial: Medical Research Council PR04 (ISRCTN61384873). J Natl Cancer Inst. 2007;99(10):765–76.

15. Tripathy D, Lichinitzer M, Lazarev A, MacLachlan SA, Apffelstaedt J, Budde M, et al. Oral ibandronate for the treatment of metastatic bone disease in breast cancer: efficacy and safety results from a randomized, double-blind, placebo-controlled trial. Ann Oncol. 2004;15(5):743–50.

16. Coleman RE, Purohit OP, Black C, Vinholes JJ, Schlosser K, Huss H, et al. Double-blind, randomised, placebo-controlled, dose-finding study of oral ibandronate in patients with metastatic bone disease. Ann Oncol. 1999;10(3):311–6.

17. Diel IJ, Body JJ, Lichinitser MR, Kreuser ED, Dornoff W, Gorbunova VA, et al. Improved quality of life after long-term treatment with the bisphosphonate ibandronate in patients with metastatic bone disease due to breast cancer. Eur J Cancer. 2004;40(11):1704–12.

18. Mancini I, Dumon JC, Body JJ. Efficacy and safety of ibandronate in the treatment of opioid-resistant bone pain associated with metastatic bone disease: a pilot study. J Clin Oncol. 2004;22(17):3587–92.

19. Heras P, Kritikos K, Hatzopoulos A, Georgopoulou AP. Efficacy of ibandronate for the treatment of skeletal events in patients with metastatic breast cancer. Eur J Cancer Care. 2009;18(6):653–6.

20. Clemons M, Dranitsaris G, Ooi W, Cole DE. A Phase II trial evaluating the palliative benefit of second-line oral ibandronate in breast cancer patients with either a skeletal related event (SRE) or progressive bone metastases (BM) despite standard bisphosphonate (BP) therapy. Breast Cancer Res Treat. 2008;108(1):79–85.

21. Conte PF, Giannessi PG, Latreille J, Mauriac L, Koliren L, Calabresi F, et al. Delayed progression of bone metastases with pamidronate therapy in breast cancer patients: a randomized, multicenter phase III trial. Ann Oncol. 1994;5 Suppl 7:S41–4.

22. Glover D, Lipton A, Keller A, Miller AA, Browning S, Fram RJ, et al. Intravenous pamidronate disodium treatment of bone metastases in patients with breast cancer. A dose-seeking study. Cancer. 1994;74(11):2949–55.

23. Berenson JR, Lichtenstein A, Porter L, Dimopoulos MA, Bordoni R, George S, et al. Efficacy of pamidronate in reducing skeletal events in patients with advanced multiple myeloma. Myeloma Aredia Study Group. N Engl J Med. 1996;334(8):488–93.

24. Hortobagyi GN, Theriault RL, Porter L, Blayney D, Lipton A, Sinoff C, et al. Efficacy of pamidronate in reducing skeletal complications in patients with breast cancer and lytic bone metastases. Protocol 19

Aredia Breast Cancer Study Group. N Engl J Med. 1996; 335(24):1785–91.

25. Hultborn R, Gundersen S, Ryden S, Holmberg E, Carstensen J, Wallgren UB, et al. Efficacy of pamidronate in breast cancer with bone metastases: a randomized, double-blind placebo-controlled multicenter study. Anticancer Res. 1999;19(4C):3383–92.

26. Theriault RL, Lipton A, Hortobagyi GN, Leff R, Gluck S, Stewart JF, et al. Pamidronate reduces skeletal morbidity in women with advanced breast cancer and lytic bone lesions: a randomized, placebo-controlled trial. Protocol 18 Aredia Breast Cancer Study Group. J Clin Oncol. 1999;17(3):846–54.

27. Small EJ, Smith MR, Seaman JJ, Petrone S, Kowalski MO. Combined analysis of two multicenter, randomized, placebo-controlled studies of pamidronate disodium for the palliation of bone pain in men with metastatic prostate cancer. J Clin Oncol. 2003;21(23):4277–84.

28. Saad F, Gleason DM, Murray R, Tchekmedyian S, Venner P, Lacombe L, et al. A randomized, placebo-controlled trial of zoledronic acid in patients with hormone-refractory metastatic prostate carcinoma. J Natl Cancer Inst. 2002;94(19):1458–68.

29. Coleman RE, Marshall H, Cameron D, Dodwell D, Burkinshaw R, Keane M, et al. Breast-cancer adjuvant therapy with zoledronic acid. N Engl J Med. 2011;365(15):1396–405.

30. Black DM, Delmas PD, Eastell R, Reid IR, Boonen S, Cauley JA, et al. Once-yearly zoledronic acid for treatment of postmenopausal osteoporosis. N Engl J Med. 2007;356(18):1809–22.

31. Gnant M, Mlineritsch B, Luschin-Ebengreuth G, Kainberger F, Kassmann H, Piswanger-Solkner JC, et al. Adjuvant endocrine therapy plus zoledronic acid in premenopausal women with early-stage breast cancer: 5-year follow-up of the ABCSG-12 bone-mineral density substudy. Lancet Oncol. 2008;9(9):840–9.

32. Rosen LS, Gordon D, Tchekmedyian S, Yanagihara R, Hirsh V, Krzakowski M, et al. Zoledronic acid versus placebo in the treatment of skeletal metastases in patients with lung cancer and other solid tumors: a phase III, double-blind, randomized trial – the Zoledronic Acid Lung Cancer and Other Solid Tumors Study Group. J Clin Oncol. 2003;21(16):3150–7.

33. Major PP, Cook RJ, Chen BL, Zheng M. Survival-adjusted multiple-event analysis for the evaluation of treatment effects of zoledronic Acid in patients with bone metastases from solid tumors. Support Cancer Ther. 2005;2(4):234–40.

34. Luckman SP, Hughes DE, Coxon FP, Graham R, Russell G, Rogers MJ. Nitrogen-containing bisphosphonates inhibit the mevalonate pathway and prevent post-translational prenylation of GTP-binding proteins, including Ras. J Bone Miner Res. 1998;13(4):581–9.

35. Rogers MJ, Gordon S, Benford HL, Coxon FP, Luckman SP, Monkkonen J, et al. Cellular and molecular mechanisms of action of bisphosphonates. Cancer. 2000;88(12 Suppl):2961–78.

36. Brown JE, Ellis SP, Lester JE, Gutcher S, Khanna T, Purohit OP, et al. Prolonged efficacy of a single dose of the bisphosphonate zoledronic acid. Clin Cancer Res. 2007;13(18 Pt 1):5406–10.
37. Pfister T, Atzpodien E, Bohrmann B, Bauss F. Acute renal effects of intravenous bisphosphonates in the rat. Basic Clin Pharmacol Toxicol. 2005;97(6):374–81.
38. Pfister T, Atzpodien E, Bauss F. The renal effects of minimally nephrotoxic doses of ibandronate and zoledronate following single and intermittent intravenous administration in rats. Toxicology. 2003;191(2–3):159–67.
39. Body JJ, Pfister T, Bauss F. Preclinical perspectives on bisphosphonate renal safety. Oncologist. 2005;10 Suppl 1:3–7.
40. Mastaglia SR, Watman NP, Oliveri B. Intravenous bisphosphonate treatment and pregnancy: its effects on mother and infant bone health. Osteoporos Int. 2010;21(11):1959–62.
41. Hellmeyer L, Kuhnert M, Ziller V, Schmidt S, Hadji P. The use of i.v. bisphosphonate in pregnancy-associated osteoporosis – case study. Exp Clin Endocrinol Diabetes. 2007;115(2):139–42.
42. Djokanovic N, Klieger-Grossmann C, Koren G. Does treatment with bisphosphonates endanger the human pregnancy? J Obstet Gynaecol Can. 2008;30(12):1146–8.
43. Levy S, Fayez I, Taguchi N, Han JY, Aiello J, Matsui D, et al. Pregnancy outcome following in utero exposure to bisphosphonates. Bone. 2009;44(3):428–30.
44. Siminoski K, Fitzgerald AA, Flesch G, Gross MS. Intravenous pamidronate for treatment of reflex sympathetic dystrophy during breast feeding. J Bone Miner Res. 2000;15(10):2052–5.
45. Reid IR, Gamble GD, Mesenbrink P, Lakatos P, Black DM. Characterization of and risk factors for the acute-phase response after zoledronic acid. J Clin Endocrinol Metab. 2010;95(9):4380–7.
46. Dicuonzo G, Vincenzi B, Santini D, Avvisati G, Rocci L, Battistoni F, et al. Fever after zoledronic acid administration is due to increase in TNF-alpha and IL-6. J Interferon Cytokine Res. 2003;23(11):649–54.
47. Sauty A, Pecherstorfer M, Zimmer-Roth I, Fioroni P, Juillerat L, Markert M, et al. Interleukin-6 and tumor necrosis factor alpha levels after bisphosphonates treatment in vitro and in patients with malignancy. Bone. 1996;18(2):133–9.
48. Rosen LS, Gordon D, Kaminski M, Howell A, Belch A, Mackey J, et al. Long-term efficacy and safety of zoledronic acid compared with pamidronate disodium in the treatment of skeletal complications in patients with advanced multiple myeloma or breast carcinoma: a randomized, double-blind, multicenter, comparative trial. Cancer. 2003;98(8):1735–44.
49. Body JJ, Lichinitser M, Tjulandin S, Garnero P, Bergstrom B. Oral ibandronate is as active as intravenous zoledronic acid for reducing bone turnover markers in women with breast cancer and bone metastases. Ann Oncol. 2007;18(7):1165–71.

50. Bergstrom B, Lichinitser M, Body JJ. Intravenous and oral iban-dronate have better safety and tolerability profiles than zoledronic acid: evidence from comparative phase II/III trials. Bone. 2006;38 suppl 1:S68.
51. Coleman RE. Risks and benefits of bisphosphonates. Br J Cancer. 2008;98(11):1736–40.
52. Kohno N, Aogi K, Minami H, Nakamura S, Asaga T, Iino Y, et al. Zoledronic acid significantly reduces skeletal complications compared with placebo in Japanese women with bone metastases from breast cancer: a randomized, placebo-controlled trial. J Clin Oncol. 2005;23(15):3314–21.
53. Tanvetyanon T, Stiff PJ. Management of the adverse effects associated with intravenous bisphosphonates. Ann Oncol. 2006;17(6): 897–907.
54. Pearce SH, Cheetham TD. Diagnosis and management of vitamin D deficiency. BMJ. 2010;340:b5664.
55. Simmons C, Amir E, Dranitsaris G, Clemons M, Wong B, Veith R, et al. Altered calcium metabolism in patients on long-term bisphosphonate therapy for metastatic breast cancer. Anticancer Res. 2009;29(7):2707–11.
56. Chennuru S, Koduri J, Baumann MA. Risk factors for symptomatic hypocalcemia complicating treatment with zoledronic acid. Intern Med J. 2008;38(8):635–7.
57. Markowitz GS, Fine PL, Stack JI, Kunis CL, Radhakrishnan J, Palecki W, et al. Toxic acute tubular necrosis following treatment with zoledronate (Zometa). Kidney Int. 2003;64(1):281–9.
58. Markowitz GS, Appel GB, Fine PL, Fenves AZ, Loon NR, Jagannath S, et al. Collapsing focal segmental glomerulosclerosis following treatment with high-dose pamidronate. J Am Soc Nephrol. 2001;12(6): 1164–72.
59. Desikan R, Veksler Y, Raza S, Stokes B, Sabir T, Li ZJ, et al. Nephrotic proteinuria associated with high-dose pamidronate in multiple myeloma. Br J Haematol. 2002;119(2):496–9.
60. Banerjee D, Asif A, Striker L, Preston RA, Bourgoignie JJ, Roth D. Short-term, high-dose pamidronate-induced acute tubular necrosis: the postulated mechanisms of bisphosphonate nephrotoxicity. Am J Kidney Dis. 2003;41(5):E18.
61. Kunin M, Kopolovic J, Avigdor A, Holtzman EJ. Collapsing glomerulopathy induced by long-term treatment with standard-dose pamidronate in a myeloma patient. Nephrol Dial Transplant. 2004;19(3): 723–6.
62. Rosen LS, Gordon D, Tchekmedyian NS, Yanagihara R, Hirsh V, Krzakowski M, et al. Long-term efficacy and safety of zoledronic acid in the treatment of skeletal metastases in patients with nonsmall cell lung carcinoma and other solid tumors: a randomized, phase III, double-blind, placebo-controlled trial. Cancer. 2004;100(12):2613–21.

63. McDermott RS, Kloth DD, Wang H, Hudes GR, Langer CJ. Impact of zoledronic acid on renal function in patients with cancer: clinical significance and development of a predictive model. J Support Oncol. 2006;4(10):524–9.

64. Diel IJ, Weide R, Koppler H, Antras L, Smith M, Green J, et al. Risk of renal impairment after treatment with ibandronate versus zoledronic acid: a retrospective medical records review. Support Care Cancer. 2009;17(6):719–25.

65. Weide R, Koppler H, Antras L, Smith M, Chang MP, Green J, et al. Renal toxicity in patients with multiple myeloma receiving zoledronic acid vs. ibandronate: a retrospective medical records review. J Cancer Res Ther. 2010;6(1):31–5.

66. Rosen LS, Gordon D, Kaminski M, Howell A, Belch A, Mackey J, et al. Zoledronic acid versus pamidronate in the treatment of skeletal metastases in patients with breast cancer or osteolytic lesions of multiple myeloma: a phase III, double-blind, comparative trial. Cancer J. 2001;7(5):377–87.

67. Guarneri V, Donati S, Nicolini M, Giovannelli S, D'Amico R, Conte PF. Renal safety and efficacy of i.v. bisphosphonates in patients with skeletal metastases treated for up to 10 years. Oncologist. 2005;10(10):842–8.

68. Diel IJ, Bergner R, Grotz KA. Adverse effects of bisphosphonates: current issues. J Support Oncol. 2007;5(10):475–82.

69. Atula S, Powles T, Paterson A, McCloskey E, Nevalainen J, Kanis J. Extended safety profile of oral clodronate after long-term use in primary breast cancer patients. Drug Saf. 2003;26(9):661–71.

70. Conte P, Guarneri V. Safety of intravenous and oral bisphosphonates and compliance with dosing regimens. Oncologist. 2004;9 Suppl 4:28–37.

71. Cardwell CR, Abnet CC, Cantwell MM, Murray LJ. Exposure to oral bisphosphonates and risk of esophageal cancer. JAMA. 2010;304(6):657–63.

72. Green J, Czanner G, Reeves G, Watson J, Wise L, Beral V. Oral bisphosphonates and risk of cancer of oesophagus, stomach, and colorectum: case–control analysis within a UK primary care cohort. BMJ. 2010;341:c4444.

73. Rennert G, Pinchev M, Rennert HS, Gruber SB. Use of bisphosphonates and reduced risk of colorectal cancer. J Clin Oncol. 2011;29(9):1146–50.

74. Marx RE. Pamidronate (Aredia) and zoledronate (Zometa) induced avascular necrosis of the jaws: a growing epidemic. J Oral Maxillofac Surg. 2003;61(9):1115–7.

75. Migliorati CA. Bisphosphonates and oral cavity avascular bone necrosis. J Clin Oncol. 2003;21(22):4253–4.

76. Khosla S, Burr D, Cauley J, Dempster DW, Ebeling PR, Felsenberg D, et al. Bisphosphonate-associated osteonecrosis of the jaw: report

of a task force of the American Society for Bone and Mineral Research. J Bone Miner Res. 2007;22(10):1479–91.
77. Yamashita J, McCauley LK, Van Poznak C. Updates on osteonecrosis of the jaw. Curr Opin Support Palliat Care. 2010;4(3):200–6.
78. Migliorati CA, Armonis BN, Nicolatou-Galitis O. Oral osteonecrosis associated with the use of ibandronate: report of a case and clinical implications. Oral Surg Oral Med Oral Pathol Oral Radiol Endod. 2008;106(1):e18–21.
79. Lo JC, O'Ryan FS, Gordon NP, Yang J, Hui RL, Martin D, et al. Prevalence of osteonecrosis of the jaw in patients with oral bisphosphonate exposure. J Oral Maxillofac Surg. 2010;68(2):243–53.
80. Stopeck AT, Lipton A, Body JJ, Steger GG, Tonkin K, de Boer RH, et al. Denosumab compared with zoledronic acid for the treatment of bone metastases in patients with advanced breast cancer: a randomized, double-blind study. J Clin Oncol. 2010;28(35):5132–9.
81. Henry DH, Costa L, Goldwasser F, Hirsh V, Hungria V, Prausova J, et al. Randomized, double-blind study of denosumab versus zoledronic acid in the treatment of bone metastases in patients with advanced cancer (excluding breast and prostate cancer) or multiple myeloma. J Clin Oncol. 2011;29(9):1125–32.
82. Dimopoulos MA, Kastritis E, Bamia C, Melakopoulos I, Gika D, Roussou M, et al. Reduction of osteonecrosis of the jaw (ONJ) after implementation of preventive measures in patients with multiple myeloma treated with zoledronic acid. Ann Oncol. 2009;20(1):117–20.
83. Ripamonti CI, Maniezzo M, Campa T, Fagnoni E, Brunelli C, Saibene G, et al. Decreased occurrence of osteonecrosis of the jaw after implementation of dental preventive measures in solid tumour patients with bone metastases treated with bisphosphonates. The experience of the National Cancer Institute of Milan. Ann Oncol. 2009;20(1):137–45.
84. Loke YK, Jeevanantham V, Singh S. Bisphosphonates and atrial fibrillation: systematic review and meta-analysis. Drug Saf. 2009; 32(3):219–28.
85. Vestergaard P, Schwartz K, Pinholt EM, Rejnmark L, Mosekilde L. Risk of atrial fibrillation associated with use of bisphosphonates and other drugs against osteoporosis: a cohort study. Calcif Tissue Int. 2010;86(5):335–42.
86. Grosso A, Douglas I, Hingorani A, MacAllister R, Smeeth L. Oral bisphosphonates and risk of atrial fibrillation and flutter in women: a self-controlled case-series safety analysis. PLoS One. 2009;4(3): e4720.
87. Huang WF, Tsai YW, Wen YW, Hsiao FY, Kuo KN, Tsai CR. Osteoporosis treatment and atrial fibrillation: alendronate versus raloxifene. Menopause. 2010;17(1):57–63.
88. Bunch TJ, Anderson JL, May HT, Muhlestein JB, Horne BD, Crandall BG, et al. Relation of bisphosphonate therapies and risk of developing atrial fibrillation. Am J Cardiol. 2009;103(6):824–8.

89. Bisphosphonates and atrial fibrillation: clinical trial data suggest possible link. Prescrire Int. 2011;20(115):96–7.

90. Howard PA, Barnes BJ, Vacek JL, Chen W, Lai SM. Impact of bisphosphonates on the risk of atrial fibrillation. Am J Cardiovasc Drugs. 2010;10(6):359–67.

91. Macarol V, Fraunfelder FT. Pamidronate disodium and possible ocular adverse drug reactions. Am J Ophthalmol. 1994;118(2): 220–4.

92. Fraunfelder FW. Ocular side effects associated with bisphosphonates. Drugs Today (Barc). 2003;39(11):829–35.

93. Benderson D, Karakunnel J, Kathuria S, Badros A. Scleritis complicating zoledronic acid infusion. Clin Lymphoma Myeloma. 2006;7(2):145–7.

94. ElSaghir NS, Otrock ZK, Bleik JH. Unilateral anterior uveitis complicating zoledronic acid therapy in breast cancer. BMC Cancer. 2005;5:156.

95. Colucci A, Modorati G, Miserocchi E, Di Matteo F, Rama P. Anterior uveitis complicating zoledronic acid infusion. Ocul Immunol Inflamm. 2009;17(4):267–8.

96. Fietta P, Manganelli P, Lodigiani L. Clodronate induced uveitis. Ann Rheum Dis. 2003;62(4):378.

97. Fraunfelder FW, Fraunfelder FT. Bisphosphonates and ocular inflammation. N Engl J Med. 2003;348(12):1187–8.

98. Sharma NS, Ooi JL, Masselos K, Hooper MJ, Francis IC. Zoledronic acid infusion and orbital inflammatory disease. N Engl J Med. 2008;359(13):1410–1.

99. Tsourdi E, Rachner TD, Gruber M, Hamann C, Ziemssen T, Hofbauer LC. Seizures associated with zoledronic acid for osteoporosis. J Clin Endocrinol Metab. 2011;96(7):1955–9.

100. Electronic Medicines Compendium. Summary of product characteristics for denosumab. Datapharm Communications Ltd.; 2010. www.emc.medicines.org.uk.

101. Electronic Medicines Compendium. Summary of product characteristics for zometa 4 mg/100 ml solution. Datapharm Communications Ltd.; 2011. www.emc.medicines.org.uk

102. Electronic Medicines Compendium. Summary of product characteristics for sodium clodronate. Datapharm Communications Ltd.; 2011. www.emc.medicines.org.uk.

103. Electronic Medicines Compendium. Summary of product characteristics for pamidronate disodium. Datapharm Communications Ltd.; 2009. www.emc.medicines.org.uk.

104. Electronic Medicines Compendium. Summary of product characteristics for ibandronic acid. Datapharm Communications Ltd.; 2011. www.emc.medicines.org.uk.

105. Coleman R, Burkinshaw R, Winter M, Neville-Webbe H, Lester J, Woodward E, et al. Zoledronic acid. Expert Opin Drug Saf. 2011;10(1):133–45.

106. Lacey DL, Timms E, Tan HL, Kelley MJ, Dunstan CR, Burgess T, et al. Osteoprotegerin ligand is a cytokine that regulates osteoclast differentiation and activation. Cell. 1998;93(2):165–76.

107. Burgess TL, Qian Y, Kaufman S, Ring BD, Van G, Capparelli C, et al. The ligand for osteoprotegerin (OPGL) directly activates mature osteoclasts. J Cell Biol. 1999;145(3):527–38.

108. Nakagawa N, Kinosaki M, Yamaguchi K, Shima N, Yasuda H, Yano K, et al. RANK is the essential signalling receptor for osteoclast differentiation factor in osteoclastogenesis. Biochem Biophys Res Commun. 1998;253(2):395–400.

109. Kearns AE, Khosla S, Kostenuik PJ. Receptor activator of nuclear factor kB ligand and osteoprotegerin regulation of bone remodeling in health and disease. Endocr Rev. 2008;29(2):155–92.

110. Ellis GK, Bone HG, Chlebowski R, Paul D, Spadafora S, Smith J, et al. Randomised trial of denosumab in patients receiving adjuvant aromatase inhibitors for nonmetastatic breast cancer. J Clin Oncol. 2008;26(30):4875–82.

111. Jones DH, Nakashima T, Sanchez OH, Kozieradzki I, Komarova SV, Sarosi I, Morony S, et al. Regulation of cancer cell migration and bone metastasis by RANKL. Nature. 2006;440(7084):692–6.

112. Cummings SR, San Martin J, McClung MR, Siris ES, Eastell R, Reid IR, et al. Denosumab for prevention of fractures in postmenopausal women with osteoporosis. N Engl J Med. 2009;361(8): 756–65.

113. Smith MR, Egerdie B, Hernández Toriz N, Feldman R, Tammela TL, Saad F, et al. Denosumab in men receiving androgen-deprivation therapy for prostate cancer. N Engl J Med. 2009;361(8):745–55.

114. Fizazi K, Carducci M, Smith M, Damião R, Brown J, Karsh L, et al. Denosumab versus zoledronic acid for treatment for bone metastases in men with castration-resistant prostate cancer: a randomised, double-blind study. Lancet. 2011;377:813–22.

115. Bekker PJ, Holloway DL, Rasmussen AS, Murphy R, Martin SW, Leese PT, et al. A single-dose placebo-controlled study of amg 162, a fully human monoclonal antibody to RANKL, in postmenopausal women. J Bone Miner Res. 2004;19(7):2274–82.

116. Lipton A, Steger GG, Figueroa J, Alvarado C, Solal-Celigny P, Body JJ, et al. Extended efficacy and safety of denosumab in breast cancer patients with bone metastases not receiving prior bisphosphonate therapy. Clin Cancer Res. 2008;14:6690–6.

117. Dougall WC, Glaccum M, Charrier K, Rohrbach K, Brasel K, De Smedt T, et al. RANK is essential for osteoclast and lymph node development. Genes Dev. 1999;13(18):2412–24.

118. Kong YY, Yoshida H, Sarosi I, Tan HL, Timms E, Capparelli C, et al. OPGL is a key regulator of osteoclastogenesis, lymphocyte development and lymph-node organogenesis. Nature. 1999;397(6717): 315–23.

119. Fata JE, Kong YY, Li J, Sasaki T, Irie-Sasaki J, Moorehead RA, et al. The osteoclast differentiation factor osteoprotegerin-ligand is essential for mammary gland development. Cell. 2000;103(1): 41–50.
120. Reid IR, Miller PD, Brown JP, Kendler DL, Fahrleitner-Pammer A, Valter I, et al. Effects of denosumab on bone histomorphometry: the FREEDOM and STAND studies. J Bone Miner Res. 2010; 25(10):2256–65.

# Chapter 17
## State of the Art
## of Antiemetic Therapy

**Sonia Fatigoni and Fausto Roila**

**Abstract** Despite relevant progress achieved in the last 20 years for the prevention of chemotherapy-induced emesis, nausea and vomiting continue to be among the most distressing adverse events induced by chemotherapy. Emesis is a complex phenomenon, and the precise mechanism by which chemotherapy induces nausea and vomiting is not well known. Many neurotransmitters are involved, and several antiemetic drugs are available. The complete control of vomiting could be achieved in about 70–90 % of patients with the better combination of antiemetic drugs.

Recently, international guidelines to prevent chemotherapy-induced nausea and vomiting have been updated, and it is very important to know these recommendations and to use them in our clinical practice correctly. However, several aspects of antiemetic therapy will be clarified in the coming years: the improvement of nausea control, the best prophylaxis of delayed emesis induced by multiple days of cisplatin, the prevention of nausea and vomiting induced by high-dose chemotherapy, the control of emesis induced by chemoradiation therapy, and the emesis in children.

S. Fatigoni, M.D. (✉) • F. Roila, M.D.
Department of Oncology, Santa Maria Hospital,
Terni, Italy
e-mail: fatisoni@libero.it

M.A. Dicato (ed.), *Side Effects of Medical Cancer Therapy*,
DOI 10.1007/978-0-85729-787-7_17,
© Springer-Verlag London 2013

**Keywords** Antiemetics • Chemotherapy • Nausea •
Vomiting • Side effect • Chemoreceptor trigger zone (CTZ)

# Introduction

Significant progress has been achieved in the last years for
the prevention of chemotherapy-induced nausea and vomiting. Nevertheless, vomiting and especially nausea continue to
be the most important chemotherapy-induced side effects,
with significant consequences for patients' quality of life and
patients' adherence to chemotherapy.

For these reasons, it is very important in clinical practice to
know the different risks of emesis induced by different chemotherapeutic agents, the antiemetic drugs available, and the
international antiemetic guidelines.

In the 1990s several professional organizations published
recommendations for antiemetic treatment in patients submitted to chemotherapy and radiotherapy. In the following
years these recommendations have been updated, and the
last update was published in 2010 [1], after the third Consensus
Conference on Antiemetics, organized in Perugia, Italy, on
June 20–21, 2009 by the European Society of Medical
Oncology (ESMO) and the Multinational Association of
Supportive Care in Cancer (MASCC). The majority of suggestions (Table 17.1) refer only to intravenous agents, because
no randomized trial has been carried out in patients receiving
oral antineoplastic agents. Recently, the American Society of
Clinical Oncology (ASCO) guidelines have been updated,
and these recommendations are similar to the European
guidelines [2]. The National Comprehensive Cancer Network
(NCCN) antiemetic guidelines have been updated as well,
but it is important to remember that these recommendations,
as opposed to the ESMO-MASCC and ASCO recommendations, are opinion-based rather than evidence-based [3].

TABLE 17.1 ESMO and MASCC guidelines for the prevention of chemotherapy-induced emesis

| Emetogenic potential | Chemotherapy | Recommendations |
|---|---|---|
| High (>90 %) | Cisplatin (see Table 17.2) | Day 1: 5-HT3 antagonist + dex + (fos) aprepitant |
| | | Days 2–3: dex + aprepitant |
| | | Day 4: dex |
| Moderate (30–90 %) | AC | Day 1: 5-HT3 antagonist + dex + (fos) aprepitant[a] |
| | | Days 2–3: aprepitant |
| | Non-AC (see Table 17.2) | Day 1: palo + dex |
| | | Days 2–3: no routine prophylaxis |
| Low (10–30 %) | See Table 17.2 | Day 1: dex or 5-HT3 antagonist or dopamine-receptor antagonist |
| | | Days 2–3: no routine prophylaxis |
| Minimal (<10 %) | See Table 17.2 | Day 1: no routine prophylaxis |
| | | Days 2–3: no routine prophylaxis |

*Abbreviations*: *Dex* dexamethasone, *AC* anthracycline and cyclophosphamide combination, *palo* palonosetron
[a]If an NK1 receptor antagonist is not available for AC chemotherapy, palonosetron should be the preferred 5-HT3 receptor antagonist

## Definition and Classification

Nausea is the perception that emesis may occur; it can be judged only by the patient. The incidence of nausea correlates with the incidence of vomiting, but nausea generally occurs more frequently than vomiting. Vomiting is forcing the stomach contents up through the esophagus and out of the mouth; it may occur with or without nausea. Chemotherapy-induced nausea and vomiting should be classified as acute, delayed, and anticipatory arbitrarily, based on the time of onset: acute nausea and vomiting occur within the first 24 h after chemotherapy; delayed nausea and vomiting occur 24 h after chemotherapy; anticipatory nausea and vomiting occur before chemotherapy, usually in patients with acute and/or delayed nausea and vomiting experiences, in the previous courses of chemotherapy. When the patient comes back to receive the following cycle of chemotherapy, emesis could be induced by the smells, sights, and sounds of the treatment room.

Several factors may influence the incidence and severity of chemotherapy-induced emesis.

Some are patient-related: gender, age (females and young patients more frequently have nausea and vomiting), history of alcohol intake, history of emesis during pregnancy or due to motion sickness, and anxiety. Other factors are therapy-related: chemotherapy type and dose, infusion rate, and route of administration. However, the most important factor is the presence or absence of acute nausea and vomiting and emesis in previous courses of chemotherapy.

The emetogenic potential of antineoplastic agents should be classified as high (>90 % incidence), moderate (30–90 %), low (10–30 %), and minimal (<10 %). However, every classification is arbitrary, because many characteristics of emetogenic potential (frequency, intensity, duration, latency) are not so well known for many chemotherapeutic agents, especially oral antineoplastic agents (Table 17.2).

# Pathogenesis of Chemotherapy-Induced Emesis

Emesis is a complex side effect, and the precise mechanisms by which chemotherapy induces nausea and vomiting are not well known. There are probably two principal pathways,

TABLE 17.2 Emetogenic potential of intravenous and oral antineoplastic agents

| Emetogenic potential | Intravenous agents | Oral agents |
|---|---|---|
| High (>90 %) | Cisplatin | Hexamethylmelamine |
| | Mechlorethamine | Procarbazine |
| | Streptozotocin | |
| | Ciclofosfamide $\geq 1{,}500$ mg/m$^2$ | |
| | Carmustine | |
| | Dacarbazine | |

(continued)

TABLE. 17.2 (continued)

| Emetogenic potential | Intravenous agents | Oral agents |
|---|---|---|
| Moderate (30–90 %) | Oxaliplatin | Cyclophosphamide |
| | Cytarabine > 1 g/m$^2$ | Temozolomide |
| | Carboplatin | Vinorelbine |
| | Ifosfamide | Imatinib |
| | Cyclophosphamide < 1,500 mg/m$^2$ | |
| | Doxorubicin | |
| | Daunorubicin | |
| | Epirubicin | |
| | Idarubicin | |
| | Irinotecan | |
| | Azacitidine | |
| | Bendamustine | |
| | Clofarabine | |
| | Alentuzumab | |

| Low (10–30 %) | Paclitaxel | Capecitabine |
| --- | --- | --- |
| | Docetaxel | Tegafur uracil |
| | Mitoxantrone | Fludarabine |
| | Doxorubicin HCl liposome injection | Etoposide |
| | Ixabepilone | Sunitinib |
| | Topotecan | Everolimus |
| | Etoposide | Lapatinib |
| | Pemetrexed | Lenalidomide |
| | Methotrexate | Thalidomide |
| | Mitomycin | |
| | Gemcitabine | |
| | Cytarabine $\leq 1{,}000$ mg/m$^2$ | |
| | 5-Fluorouracil | |
| | Temsirolimus | |
| | Bortezomib | |
| | Cetuximab | |
| | Trastuzumab | |
| | Panitumumab | |
| | Catumaxumab | |

(continued)

TABLE. 17. 2 (continued)

| Emetogenic potential | Intravenous agents | Oral agents |
|---|---|---|
| Minimal (<10 %) | Bleomycin | Chlorambucil |
| | Busulfan | Hydroxyurea |
| | 2-Chlorodeoxyadenosine | L-Phenylalanine mustard |
| | Fludarabine | 6-Thioguanine |
| | Vinblastine | Methotrexate |
| | Vincristine | Gefitinib |
| | Vinorelbine | Erlotinib |
| | Bevacizumab | Sorafenib |

central and peripheral [4], and some mechanisms of activation are described in the following sections.

## Central Pathway

The principal mechanism is the activation of the chemoreceptor trigger zone (CTZ), located in the area postrema in the brain. The CTZ works through the release of various neurotransmitters, including substance P, dopamine, serotonin, histamine, norepinephrine, apomorphine, neurotensin, angiotensin II, gastrin, and vasopressin. These neurotransmitters activate the vomiting center, located in the brain, near the CTZ. The CTZ can receive and transmit information from/to the other central and peripheral sites.

The nucleus of tractus solitarius, an area of the medulla oblongata, also plays an important role, because it probably contains the highest concentration of serotonin type 3 (5-HT3) and neurokinin 1 (NK1) receptors in the brain.

Moreover, there may be a cortical mechanism, with direct or indirect (psychogenic) cerebral activation; for example, patients with previous experience of nausea and vomiting are more likely to have emesis.

## Peripheral Pathway

It is activated primarily by the damage of gastrointestinal mucosa with release of neurotransmitters or by the direct activation of peripheral neurotransmitter receptors. Serotonin plays a central role: it is released by enterochromaffin cells, and it activates the serotonin type 3 (5-HT3) receptors along the vagus nerve in the gastrointestinal tract.

Many chemotherapeutic agents can induce taste and smell alterations, which may lead to nausea and vomiting.

The vestibular system also may be involved in chemotherapy-induced emesis, and patients with a history of motion sickness are more likely to have chemotherapy-induced emesis.

# Antiemetic Drugs

Several antiemetic drugs are available, and the optimal combination can achieve vomiting control in about 80–90 % of patients, with minimal side effects. The most important agents are reported as follows [5, 6]:

1. Corticosteroids (Dexamethasone, Methylprednisolone). Their antiemetic mechanism is still unclear; they probably work without the blockage of specific neurotransmitters. Their adverse events as antiemetic drugs may be limited to insomnia, euphoria, facial flush, increased appetite, and anal pruritus when administered rapidly. They can decompensate diabetes or reactivate gastrin/duodenal ulcers, but these side effects are unlikely in short-term use, and their use is contraindicated only in cases of diabetic ketoacidosis and active peptic ulcers.

2. 5-HT3 Receptor Antagonists (Granisetron, Ondansetron, Palonosetron, Tropisetron). They block the serotonin type 3 receptors, both central and peripheral (in the small bowel). Palonosetron, the newest of these agents, has a potent and selective 5-HT3 antagonist action with a plasma-elimination half-life of about 40 h, longer than that of ondansetron (4–6 h), granisetron (5–8 h), tropisetron (7 h), and dolasetron (7 h). Constipation and headaches are drug-class adverse effects and appear in about 10 % of patients. All the 5-HT3-receptor antagonists have similar tolerability.

3. NK1 Receptor Antagonists (Aprepitant, Fosaprepitant). The NK1 antagonists are the most recent antiemetic agents, introduced about 10 years ago. This receptor is usually bound by substance P. The substance P, an 11-amino acid neuropeptide located primarily within the gastrointestinal tract and the central nervous system, can induce emesis when injected into the ferret, by binding the NK1 receptor. The NK1 antagonists are able to antagonize this effect of substance P and also the emetic stimulus induced by morphine, chemotherapy, radiation, and anesthesia. They usually are well tolerated.

4. NK1 receptor antagonists present several drug-drug inter-actions, because they are metabolized by the cytochrome P-450 isoenzyme 3A4 (CYP3A4), the major metabolic pathway for drugs in humans [7]. NK1 antagonists may decrease, for example, the plasmatic level of oral contra-ceptives and tolbutamide; they may increase the plasmatic level of benzodiazepines and corticosteroids, which require a dose reduction of around 50 %; they can influence the plasmatic level of warfarin. They can also influence the metabolism of some chemotherapeutic agents (docetaxel, vinorelbine), but generally dose adjustments are not required. Therefore, it is very important to verify the drug-drug interactions during antiemetic treatment.

5. Dopamine Antagonists (Metoclopramide, Domperidone, Prochlorperazine, Aloperidol). They have antiemetic activ-ity by the blockage of dopamine receptors. Metoclopramide may induce extrapyramidal adverse effects, especially in young women when used at high dosage.

6. Benzodiazepines (Lorazepam, Alprazolam). They are use-ful as combination therapy, for their sedative, anxiolytic, and amnesic effects. They may induce somnolence.

# Nausea and Vomiting Induced by Highly Emetogenic Chemotherapy

## Prevention of Acute Emesis

Before the introduction of aprepitant, a combination of a 5-HT3 receptor antagonist plus dexamethasone was indi-cated for the prevention of acute nausea and vomiting in cisplatin-treated patients.

Aprepitant showed antiemetic activity in several phase II double-blind studies and in two phase III trials with an identi-cal design. The two phase III studies, published in 2003 [8, 9], compared ondansetron, 32 mg, plus dexamethasone, 20 mg on day 1, followed by dexamethasone, 8 mg twice a day on days 2–4, with the combination of ondansetron, 32 mg; dexamethasone,

12 mg; and aprepitant, 125 mg on day 1, followed by dexamethasone, 8 mg daily on days 2–4, and aprepitant, 80 mg on days 2 and 3. In the first study 530 patients were enrolled and in the second, 569 patients.

The dexamethasone dose was reduced in the aprepitant arm because aprepitant increases dexamethasone plasma concentrations with an approximately twofold increase in the plasmatic level; because different dexamethasone doses could change the efficacy of the antiemetic regimen, a 40–50 % reduction of the oral dexamethasone dose was made in the aprepitant arm.

The primary endpoint was complete response (no emesis, no use of rescue antiemetics) over the 5-day study period. In both studies complete response was significantly superior with aprepitant (73 % vs. 52 %, 63 % vs. 43 %). The complete response on day 1 was also significantly superior with aprepitant (89 % vs. 78 %, 83 % vs. 68 %). Complete response from nausea was significantly superior with aprepitant only in the second study. In both the studies side effects were mild, with no difference between the two arms.

Another study used a similar design [10], but with prolonged ondansetron in the control arm on days 2–4, with the dose of 8 mg orally twice a day. The aprepitant arm was superior in this case also.

Concerning the type of 5-HT3 antagonist, at the present all the 5-HT3 antagonists available are to be considered with similar efficacy and tolerability in this setting of patients [11]. The single lowest tested fully effective dose, intravenous or oral, should be used before chemotherapy.

Based on these results, a combination of a 5-HT3 antagonist, dexamethasone, and aprepitant should be recommended to prevent acute nausea and vomiting induced by highly emetogenic chemotherapy.

Recently, fosaprepitant, a new NK1 receptor antagonist, has been approved. When administered intravenously, fosaprepitant is converted within 30 min into aprepitant. A phase III, randomized study [12] compared the standard combination of dexamethasone, ondansetron, and aprepitant (125 mg orally, day 1; 80 mg orally, days 2–3) with dexamethasone, ondansetron, and fosaprepitant (150 mg intravenously, day 1). The study, in which 2,322 patients were enrolled, showed the noninferiority of the fosaprepitant arm.

## Prevention of Delayed Emesis

The main risk factor for delayed nausea and vomiting is the presence of acute nausea and vomiting, so the incidence of delayed emesis is high in those patients who experienced acute emesis. Therefore, the guidelines recommend that all patients submitted to cisplatin-based chemotherapy receive the adequate prophylaxis for acute and delayed emesis.

Before the introduction of NK1 receptor antagonists, the recommended therapy was with dexamethasone (8 mg twice a day on days 23, and 4 mg twice a day on days 4–5) and oral metoclopramide (0.5 mg/kg four times a day on days 2–5) or a 5-HT3 receptor antagonist.

In the two previously mentioned phase III trials, complete response on days 2–5 was significantly superior with aprepitant plus dexamethasone than with dexamethasone alone (75 % vs. 56 % and 68 % vs. 47 %, respectively).

Therefore, the combination of aprepitant and dexamethasone should be recommended in patients submitted to cisplatin-based chemotherapy and receiving a combination of aprepitant, 5-HT3 receptor antagonist, and dexamethasone for the prevention of acute emesis. The recommended doses are aprepitant, 80 mg orally on days 2–3, and dexamethasone, 8 mg orally on days 2–4.

Unfortunately, in both studies, patients received two different combinations of drugs for acute emesis prevention, and the difference in acute emesis protection may influence the incidence of delayed emesis between the two arms.

Moreover, the combination of aprepitant and dexamethasone has been compared with dexamethasone alone and not with the standard delayed emesis prophylaxis, such as the combination of dexamethasone and metoclopramide.

In conclusion, the real impact of aprepitant in the prevention of delayed emesis is not well known: aprepitant is more efficacious than placebo, and, combined with dexamethasone, it is more efficacious than dexamethasone alone; the efficacy with respect to the combination of dexamethasone and metoclopramide or 5-HT3 antagonists remains to be evaluated. An ongoing randomized, double-blind trial of Italian Group for Antiemetic Research (IGAR) is evaluating this aspect: the patients submitted for the first time to cisplatin-based chemotherapy receive a combination of aprepitant, dexamethasone, and palonosetron on day 1; they are randomized to receive aprepitant on days 2–3 and dexamethasone on days 2–4 or dexamethasone and metoclopramide on days 2–4.

Moreover, the better aprepitant schedule is not perfectly clarified: pilot studies showed no differences between 1 day versus 3 days of aprepitant therapy, and further trials are necessary to validate the use of single-day aprepitant.

# Nausea and Vomiting Induced by Moderately Emetogenic Chemotherapy

## Prevention of Acute Emesis

For the prevention of acute emesis induced by moderately emetogenic chemotherapy, not including a combination of anthracycline and cyclophosphamide, a combination of dexamethasone and palonosetron should be used.

This suggestion is based on three studies evaluating the efficacy of palonosetron in this situation.

In the first two trials, two different doses of palonosetron (0.25 and 0.75 mg intravenously) were compared with dolasetron, 100 mg intravenously [13], and ondansetron, 32 mg intravenously [14], in patients chemotherapy-naïve or pretreated, receiving moderately emetogenic chemotherapy. Palonosetron was superior in both trials. Unfortunately, in these trials the 5-HT3 receptor antagonist was not combined with dexamethasone, as recommended by guidelines.

Moreover, in both studies only 5 % of patients received dexamethasone combined with 5-HT3 antagonist in the acute phase and no one in the delayed phase, and this may be a confounding factor.

In the third trial [15] palonosetron, 0.75 mg intravenously, was compared with granisetron, both combined with dexamethasone, 16 mg, in patients receiving high emetogenic cisplatin-based or anthracycline-cyclophosphamide-based chemotherapy. The acute emesis control was similar in both arms, while palonosetron showed superior efficacy for delayed emesis control. In this study, patients with a different emetogenic risk were randomized, and dexamethasone was used at different doses with respect to those recommended by guidelines. In conclusion, the real efficacy of palonosetron, when combined with dexamethasone, as recommended by guidelines, has not been definitely clarified.

The combination of anthracycline and cyclophosphamide represents a particular situation, with high risk of nausea and vomiting, especially in young women.

A double-blind study [16], randomizing 866 patients receiving anthracycline and cyclophosphamide, evaluated the efficacy of aprepitant combined with a 5-HT3 antagonist and dexamethasone. The patients received on day 1 aprepitant, 125 mg orally, plus dexamethasone, 12 mg intravenously, plus ondansetron, 8 mg before and 8 mg after chemotherapy, or dexamethasone, 20 mg intravenously, plus ondansetron, 8 mg before and 8 mg after chemotherapy. On days 2–3, the patients received aprepitant, 80 mg orally, once a day or ondansetron, 8 mg, twice a day.

The complete response over the 5-day study period was significantly superior with aprepitant (51 % vs. 42 %); the complete response was also significantly superior with aprepitant on day 1 (76 % vs. 69 %) and on days 2–5 (55 % vs. 49 %). Complete response from nausea was not significantly different. In both the studies side effects were mild, with no difference between the two arms.

Therefore, to prevent acute nausea and vomiting in women receiving a combination of anthracycline and cyclophosphamide, a three-drug regimen, including a single dose of 5-HT3 antagonist, dexamethasone, and aprepitant given before chemotherapy, is recommended. If aprepitant is not available for anthracycline-cyclophosphamide-based chemotherapy, palonosetron should be used in combination with dexamethasone, based on the results of the study reported above.

## Prevention of Delayed Emesis

The guidelines recommend the prophylaxis of delayed emesis induced by moderately emetogenic chemotherapy.

The incidence of delayed emesis depends on the incidence of acute emesis: in fact, it is low (12 % delayed vomiting and 14 % delayed nausea) if the patients did not have acute emesis; instead, it is high (55 % delayed vomiting and 75 % delayed nausea) if the patients had acute emesis. The patients submitted to moderately emetogenic chemotherapy, without the combination of anthracycline and cyclophosphamide, receiving palonosetron plus dexamethasone for the prevention of acute emesis, should receive dexamethasone orally on days after chemotherapy.

This recommendation has been based especially on a large trial of the IGAR that demonstrated oral dexamethasone superior with respect to placebo with 10 % difference in complete response [17]. The recommended dose is 4 mg orally twice a day on days 2–4.

For the women submitted to the combination of anthracycline and cyclophosphamide, receiving aprepitant plus 5-HT3 antagonist plus dexamethasone for the prevention of acute emesis, aprepitant is recommended to prevent delayed emesis. The dose of aprepitant is 80 mg orally once a day on days 2–3.

Unfortunately, in the previously evaluated study [16], the patients received a different antiemetic combination on day 1, and the different acute emesis protection may influence the incidence of delayed emesis in the two arms.

Moreover, aprepitant was compared with ondansetron to prevent delayed emesis and not with the standard therapy, represented by dexamethasone. So it is unknown if dexamethasone is as effective as aprepitant or if the combination of dexamethasone and aprepitant could be more effective than aprepitant alone to prevent delayed emesis. An ongoing randomized, double-blind trial of IGAR is evaluating this aspect: the patients submitted for the first time to anthracycline-cyclophosphamide chemotherapy receive a combination of aprepitant, dexamethasone, and palonosetron on day 1; they are randomized to receive aprepitant on days 2–3 or dexamethasone on days 2–4.

Recently, two randomized phase III, noninferiority trials evaluated the possibility of reducing the duration of dexamethasone therapy in delayed emesis, using palonosetron as 5-HT3 antagonist, to minimize the possible side effects related to corticosteroids.

In the first study [18], 300 female chemotherapy-naive patients with breast cancer were enrolled. The patients were submitted to anthracycline-cyclophosphamide chemotherapy, and they received a combination of palonosetron, 0.25 mg intravenously, and dexamethasone, 8 mg, on day 1; then, they were randomized to receive placebo or dexamethasone, 4 mg orally twice a day on days 2–3.

During the overall period of study of 5 days, the complete response was similar in both arms: 53.6 % versus 53.7 %, respectively; similar noninferiority results were achieved in the acute phase (69.5 % vs. 68.5 %) and in the delayed phase (62.3 % vs. 65.8 %).

In the second study [19], 322 patients receiving moderately emetogenic chemotherapy for the first time were enrolled. The chemotherapy included anthracycline-cyclophosphamide combination, oxaliplatin, carboplatin, or irinotecan-based therapy. The patients received palonosetron, 0.25 mg intravenously, and dexamethasone, 8 mg intravenously, on day 1; then, they were randomized to receive no additional therapy or dexamethasone, 8 mg orally, on days 2–3.

During the overall period of study of 5 days, the complete response was similar in both arms: 67.5 % versus 71.1 %, respectively; similar noninferiority results were also achieved in the acute phase (88.6 % vs. 84.3 %) and in the delayed phase (68.7 % vs. 77.7 %). Therefore, both the studies seem

S. Fatigoni and F. Roila

to demonstrate a lack of efficacy against delayed emesis of dexamethasone when used in patients receiving palonosetron. On the other hand, the studies are noninferiority studies with a sample size calculated considering equivalent of the drug if the complete response was inferior to 15 %. We think that further larger studies should be conducted to clarify the problem.

# Nausea and Vomiting Induced by Low or Minimally Emetogenic Chemotherapy

Only a few trials have been carried out in patients submitted to low and minimal emetogenic chemotherapy, so there is very little evidence. Moreover, the number of agents with low and minimal emetogenic risk was increased with the addition of several target therapies, and there is the possibility of an over- or undertreatment by antiemetics.

Nevertheless, the guidelines recommend that the patients submitted to chemotherapy with low emetogenic risk should receive a single antiemetic agent, such as dexamethasone, or a 5-HT3 antagonist or a dopamine-receptor antagonist to prevent acute emesis.

The patients submitted to chemotherapy with minimal emetogenic risk should not routinely receive antiemetic prophylaxis before chemotherapy, if they do not have a history of nausea and vomiting.

No antiemetic prophylaxis should be administered for the prevention of delayed emesis induced by chemotherapy with low and minimal emetogenic risk.

# Chemotherapy-Induced Anticipatory Nausea and Vomiting

Anticipatory emesis occurs before chemotherapy, usually in patients who experienced nausea and vomiting in previous chemotherapy courses. Several other factors may be associated with anticipatory nausea and vomiting: the number of

TABLE 17.3 ESMO and MASCC guidelines for prevention of radiotherapy-induced emesis

| Emetogenic potential | Radiotherapy | Recommendations |
|---|---|---|
| High (>90 %) | Total body irradiation; total nodal irradiation | Dex + 5-HT3 antagonist |
| Moderate (60–90 %) | Upper abdomen, half body or upper body irradiation | 5-HT3 antagonist + optional dex |
| Low (30–60 %) | Cranium, craniospinal, head and neck, lower thorax region, pelvis | 5-HT3 antagonist (prophylaxis or rescue) |
| Minimal (<30 %) | Extremities, breast | Dopamine-receptor antagonist or 5-HT3 antagonist (rescue) |

*Abbreviation*: *Dex* dexamethasone

chemotherapy cycles, age, sex, and anxiety. In fact, young patients, females, with a history of anxiety have a higher incidence of anticipatory emesis.

The guidelines recommend the best control of acute and delayed emesis as the best way to prevent anticipatory nausea and vomiting. Antiemetic agents usually given in the prevention of acute and delayed nausea and vomiting are often ineffective in treating anticipatory emesis. Behavioral techniques could be effective in reducing anticipatory symptoms, including progressive relaxation technique, desensitization, and hypnosis. Benzodiazepines may help to reduce the incidence of anticipatory emesis, but their efficacy decreases during the treatment.

# Radiotherapy-Induced Nausea and Vomiting

Radiotherapy also is often associated with nausea and vomiting. Incidence and severity of radiotherapy-induced emesis depend on several factors, similar to chemotherapy-induced emesis. Some factors are patient-related (age, gender, state of health, previous history of emesis), and others are treatment-related (irradiated site, single and total dose, fractionation, irradiate volume, radiotherapy techniques). Concurrent or recent chemotherapy is also an important factor. Overall cumulative incidence of emesis is estimated to be around 50–80 % of patients undergoing radiotherapy.

This may be a major problem, considering that fractionated radiotherapy involves a period of 6–8 weeks and prolonged nausea and vomiting may significantly decrease patients' quality of life.

Only a few randomized studies, and often with a small number of patients, evaluated the problem of radiotherapy-induced emesis, so only a little evidence is available. It is very important to investigate the role of individual risk factors, the incidence of delayed nausea and vomiting, the potential role of NK1 receptor antagonists, and the optimal duration of antiemetic prophylaxis [20].

Nevertheless, the guidelines proposed new recommendations, considering four levels of risk (high, moderate, low, and minimal), based on the irradiation area as the most important risk factor (Table 17.3). In the case of chemoradiotherapy, the antiemetic regimen is determined by the chemotherapy antiemetic recommendations of the corresponding risk level, unless the radiotherapy-related risk is higher.

# Special Topics

## Nausea and Vomiting Induced by Multiple-Day Cisplatin Therapy

Only a few studies evaluated antiemetic therapies in these patients. About 55–83 % of complete protection from vomiting has been achieved with a combination of dexamethasone and 5-HT3 antagonist administered all days of chemotherapy.

The guidelines recommend a combination of dexamethasone and 5-HT3 antagonist to prevent acute emesis and dexamethasone to prevent delayed emesis, but the optimal dose of dexamethasone and 5-HT3 antagonist is unknown, as well as the optimal duration of antiemetic therapy [21].

Patients have more severe nausea and vomiting on days 4 and 5, both in studies evaluating dexamethasone, 20 mg, on each day of cisplatin therapy or only on days 1 and 2, and it is unclear if this could reflect delayed emesis from days 1 and 2. The use of dexamethasone for 5 consecutive days, followed by three additional doses on days 6–8 (for delayed emesis prevention), may be an overtreatment, especially if repeated every 3 weeks for three or four courses, with side effects such as insomnia, agitation, weight gain, epigastric discomfort, and risk of femur osteonecrosis.

The possible role of NK1 antagonists is still undefined, because no large randomized clinical trial compared the addiction of NK1 antagonists to dexamethasone and 5-HT3 antagonist in this type of patient.

Recently, a small, double-blind, crossover study, presented at the 2011 ASCO meeting, was carried out in 68 patients with germ cell cancer, submitted to 5-day cisplatin chemotherapy [22]. The patients were randomized to receive aprepitant, 125 mg on day 3 and 80 mg on days 4–7, plus dexamethasone, 4 mg orally twice a day on days 6–8, or placebo plus dexamethasone, 8 mg twice a day on days 6–7 and 4 mg twice a day on day 8. A 5-HT3 receptor antagonist on days 1–5 plus dexamethasone, 20 mg on days 1 and 2, were utilized in both arms. A complete response was achieved in 47 % of patients in aprepitant arm versus 19 % in the placebo arm.

Further larger studies are necessary to confirm these interesting results and to clarify the better combination of antiemetic drugs in these patients.

## Nausea and Vomiting in Children

This aspect of chemotherapeutic treatment for children is often underevaluated. It has been estimated that about 70 %

of children receiving chemotherapy experienced nausea and vomiting. Published studies present many problems, such as a low number of patients and nonoptimal design, so it is impossible to give a specific recommendation for many aspects of antiemetic therapy. Moreover, it is inappropriate to assume that the adult therapy can be directly applied to children, because efficacy and side effects of antiemetics may be different.

Nevertheless, the guidelines [23] recommend a combination of a 5-HT3 receptor plus dexamethasone to prevent acute nausea and vomiting in children receiving high or moderate emetogenic chemotherapy. The optimal dose and schedule are not well known, such as the optimal therapy for delayed emesis or for anticipatory emesis and the possible role of NK1 antagonists.

## High-Dose Chemotherapy

In this case there are very few data on the effective use of antiemetics for patients treated with high-dose chemotherapy with stem cell support. The combination of a 5-HT3 receptor antagonist with dexamethasone represents the current standard of care, but complete protection is reached in a minority of patients. One of the major problems is that in these patients nausea and vomiting depend on several factors, including prophylactic antibiotics, narcotic analgesics, the administration of several highly emetogenic antineoplastic agents over consecutive days, and the use of total body irradiation [21]. All these factors make the research more difficult; nevertheless, randomized trials evaluating new antiemetic drugs are necessary to optimize the prophylaxis.

## Summary

Major improvements have been achieved in the last 20 years in chemotherapy-induced emesis, especially in the control of vomiting. However, chemotherapy-induced nausea is still hard to control, and it is one of the most important challenges in the following years. Future trials should be oriented to develop new antinausea drugs and to incorporate new agents into current antiemetic regimens.

Despite the increasing use of new antineoplastic agents (e.g., monoclonal antibodies or tyrosine kinase inhibitors) with minimal emetogenic potential and despite several antiemetic agents being available, nausea and vomiting are still disabling side effects. Therefore, the diffusion and the right utilization of the guidelines is a major objective.

Future improvement in antiemetic therapy will require well-designed clinical trials to define several unresolved questions: the best prophylaxis of delayed emesis induced by multiple days of cisplatin, control of nausea and vomiting induced by high-dose chemotherapy, chemoradiation therapy-induced emesis, and emesis in children.

# References

1. Roila F, Herrstedt J, Aapro M, Gralla RJ, Einhorn LH, Ballatori E, et al. Guideline update for MASCC and ESMO in the prevention of chemotherapy- and radiotherapy-induced nausea and vomiting: results of the Perugia multinational Consensus Conference. Ann Oncol. 2010;21 Suppl 5:228–39.
2. Basch E, Prestrud AA, Hesketh PJ, Kris MG, Feyer PC, Somerfield MR, et al. Antiemetics: American Society of Clinical Oncology clinical practice guideline update. J Clin Oncol. 2011;29:4189–98.
3. Ettinger DS, Armstrong DK, Barbour S, Berger MJ, Bierman PJ, Bradbury B, et al. Antiemesis. J Natl Compr Canc Netw 2009;7:572–95.www.nccn.org
4. Frame DG. Best practice management of CINV in oncology patients: physiology and treatment of CINV. J Support Oncol. 2010;8 Suppl 1:5–9.
5. Herrstedt J, Dombernowsky P. Anti-emetic therapy in cancer chemotherapy: current status. Basic Clin Pharmacol Toxicol. 2007;101:143–50.
6. Herrstedt J, Matti AS, John F. Corticosteroids, dopamine antagonists and other drugs. Support Care Cancer. 1998;6:204–14.
7. Aapro MS, Walko CM. Aprepitant: drug-drug interactions in perspective. Ann Oncol. 2010;21:2316–23.

8. Poli-Bigelli S, Rodrigues-Pereira J, Carides AD, Julie MG, Eldridge K, Hipple A, et al. Addition of the neurokinin 1 receptor antagonist aprepitant to standard antiemetic therapy improves control of chemotherapy-induced nausea and vomiting. Cancer. 2003;97:3090–8.

9. Hesketh PJ, Grunberg SM, Gralla RJ, Warr DG, Roila F, de Wit R, et al. The oral neurokinin-1 antagonist aprepitant for the prevention of chemotherapy-induced nausea and vomiting: a multinational, randomized, double-blind, placebo-controlled trial in patients receiving high-dose cisplatin – the Aprepitant Protocol 052 Study Group. J Clin Oncol. 2003;21(22):4112–9.

10. Schmoll HJ, Aapro MS, Poli-Bigelli S, Kim HK, Park K, Jordan K, et al. Comparison of an aprepitant regimen with multiple-day ondansetron regimen, both with dexamethasone, for antiemetic efficacy in high dose cisplatin treatment. Ann Oncol. 2006;17: 1000–6.

11. Kris MG, Tonato M, Bria E, Ballatori E, Espersen B, Herrstedt J, et al. Consensus recommendations for the prevention of vomiting and nausea following high-emetic-risk chemotherapy. Support Care Cancer. 2011;19 Suppl 1:25–32.

12. Grunberg SM, Chua D, Maru A, Dinis J, DeVandry S, Boice JA, et al. Single-dose fosaprepitant for the prevention chemotherapy-induced nausea and vomiting associated with cisplatin therapy: randomized, double-blind study protocol-EASE. J Clin Oncol. 2011;29: 1495–501.

13. Eisenberg P, Figueroa-Vadillo J, Zamora R, Charu V, Hajdenberg J, Cartmell A, et al. Improved prevention of moderately emetogenic chemotherapy-induced nausea and vomiting with palonosetron, a pharmacologically novel 5-HT3 receptor antagonist. Results of a phase III, single-dose trial versus dolasetron. Cancer. 2003;98: 2473–82.

14. Gralla R, Lichinitser M, Van der Vegt S, Sleeboom H, Mezger J, Peschel C, et al. Palonosetron improves prevention of chemotherapy-induced nausea and vomiting following moderately emetogenic chemotherapy: results of a double-blind randomized phase III trial comparing single doses of palonosetron with ondansetron. Ann Oncol. 2003;14:1570–7.

15. Saito M, Aogi K, Sekine I, Yoshizawa H, Yanagita Y, Sakai H, et al. Palonosetron plus dexamethasone versus granisetron plus dexamethasone for prevention of nausea and vomiting during chemotherapy: a double-blind, double-dummy, randomised, comparative phase III trial. Lancet Oncol. 2009;10:115–24.

16. Warr DG, Hesketh PJ, Gralla RJ, Muss HB, Herrstedt J, Eisenberg PD, et al. Efficacy and tolerability of aprepitant for the prevention of chemotherapy-induced nausea and vomiting in patients with breast cancer after moderately emetogenic chemotherapy. J Clin Oncol. 2005;23:2822–30.

17. The Italian Group for Antiemetic Research. Dexamethasone alone or in combination with ondansetron for the prevention of delayed nausea and vomiting induced by chemotherapy. N Engl J Med. 2000;342:1554–9.
18. Aapro M, Fabi A, Nolè F, Medici M, Steger G, Bachmann C, et al. Double-blind, randomized, controlled study of the efficacy and tolerability of palonosetron plus dexamethasone for 1 day with or without dexamethasone on days 2 and 3 in the prevention of nausea and vomiting induced by moderately emetogenic chemotherapy. Ann Oncol. 2010;21(5):1083–8.
19. Celio L, Frustaci S, Denaro A, Buonadonna A, Ardizzoia A, Piazza E, et al. Palonosetron in combination with 1-day versus 3-day dexamethasone for prevention of nausea and vomiting following moderately emetogenic chemotherapy: a randomized, metacentre, phase III trial. Support Care Cancer. 2011;19:1217–25.
20. Feyer PC, Maranzano E, Molassiotis A, Roila F, Clark-Snow RA, Jordan K, et al. Radiotherapy-induced nausea and vomiting (RINV): MASCC/ESMO guideline for antiemetics in radiotherapy: update 2009. Support Care Cancer. 2011;19 suppl 1:5–14.
21. Einhorn LH, Grunber SM, Rapoport B, Rittenberg C, Feyer P. Antiemetic therapy for multiple-day chemotherapy and additional topics consisting of rescue antiemetics and high-dose chemotherapy with stem cell transplant: review and consensus statement. Support Care Cancer. 2011;19 suppl 1:1–4.
22. Brames MJ, Picus J, Yu M, Johnston E, Bottema B, Williams C, et al. Phase III, double-blind, placebo-controlled, crossover study evaluating a 5-HT3 antagonist plus dexamethasone with or without aprepitant in patients with germ cell tumour receiving 5-days cisplatin combination chemotherapy: A Hoosier Oncology Group (HOG) study. J Clin Oncol. 2011;29(suppl; abstr 9013):553s.
23. Jordan K, Roila F, Molassiotis A, Maranzano E, Clark-Snow RA, Feyer P, MASCC/ESMO. Antiemetics in children receiving chemotherapy. MASCC/ESMO guideline update 2009. Support Care Cancer. 2011;19 suppl 1:37–42.

# Chapter 18
## Side Effects of Nociceptive Cancer Pain Treatments in Adults

**Ivan Krakowski and Aline Henry**

**Abstract**   Pain is unfortunately a frequent symptom of cancer, especially in the advanced stages of disease. Its treatment must be integrated into a comprehensive supportive care approach, which itself must be conducted in parallel with specific therapeutic cancer agents, if indicated, and then integrated into the process of palliative care in the advanced phase.

Several classes of pain killers are available:

- Nociceptive pain medications uses non-opioid analgesics, weak opioids, and strong opioids, described in the three levels of the WHO ladder.
- "Pure" neuropathic pain is treated by different drug classes, at least in the front line, such as antidepressants, antiepileptics, and some anesthetics such as ketamine. The analgesics in the WHO ladder, including opioids, are generally less effective for this indication, but they, as well as nondrug treatments, will be tried in case of refractory pain.

For the two types of pain, analgesics are often used in combination with co-analgesics (anxiolytics, corticosteroids, anti-osteoclast, antispasmodic, etc.).

I. Krakowski, M.D. (✉) • A. Henry, M.D.
Supportive Care Department, Centre Alexis Vautrin, 6 Avenue de Bourgogne - CS 30519 - 54519, Vandœuvre Les Nancy Cedex, France
e-mail: i.krakowski@nancy.unicancer.fr

M.A. Dicato (ed.), *Side Effects of Medical Cancer Therapy,*     595
DOI 10.1007/978-0-85729-787-7_18,
© Springer-Verlag London 2013

It is obviously important to know the main side effects of these different drug classes, in order to prevent them, to inform patients of their possible occurrence, and thereby to promote better compliance. The problem of compliance is indeed particularly acute in the area of pain therapy because patients want to use pain as an indicator of a possible disease progression or of an expected response to specific treatments of cancer, and they fear the side effects of analgesics in general and opioids in particular. The main side effects of analgesics are discussed in this chapter.

**Keywords**   Cancer • Pain • Side effect • Pain killer • Analgesic

# Introduction

Pain is unfortunately a frequent symptom of cancer, especially in the advanced stages of disease. Its treatment must be integrated into a comprehensive supportive care approach, which itself must be conducted in parallel with specific cancer therapy, if indicated, and then integrated into the process of palliative care in the advanced phase.

At diagnosis and in the early stages of cancer, 30–45 % of patients have moderate to severe pain [1, 2]. This percentage increases on average to 75 % in advanced stages. Concerning the intensity of pain, 40–50 % of patients have moderate or high pain, and 25–30 % describe very strong pain [3]. Finally, a number of cured patients (it is difficult to estimate the number) present with sequellar pain from cancer and/or treatments used [4, 5].

We traditionally distinguish two main mechanisms of cancer pain, knowing that these two mechanisms are often entangled with advanced disease:

- Nociceptive pain, which represents 70 % of the pain [6]
- Neuropathic pain, corresponding to 30–40 % of cancer pain [6]

Several classes of drugs are available:

- The treatment of nociceptive pain uses non-opioid analgesics, weak opioids, and strong opioids, which are described in the three levels of the WHO ladder (Fig. 18.1).

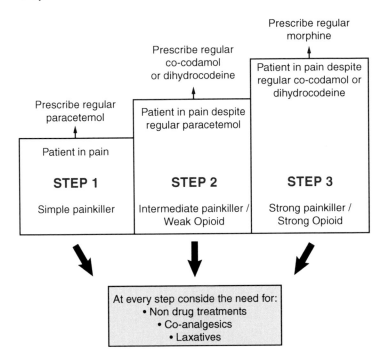

FIGURE. 18.1 The treatment of nociceptive pain uses non-opioid analgesics, weak opioids, and strong opioids, which are described in the three levels of the WHO ladder (Adapted by permission from MacMillan Publishers Ltd. on behalf of Cancer Research UK: British Journal of Cancer, Krakowski et al. [65], Copyright 2003)

- "Pure" neuropathic pain is treated by different drug classes, at least in the front line, such as antidepressants, antiepileptics, and some anesthetics, such as ketamine. The analgesics in the WHO ladder, including opioids, are generally less effective in this indication, but they, as well as nondrug treatments, will be tried in case of refractory pain.

In the two types of pain, analgesics are often used in combination with co-analgesics (anxiolytics, corticosteroids, antiosteoclast, antispasmodic, etc.).

It is obviously important to know the main side effects of these different drug classes, in order to prevent them, to inform patients of their possible occurrence, and thereby to promote better compliance. The problem of compliance is indeed particularly important in pain therapy because patients often use pain as an indicator of disease progression and as a response to specific treatment for cancer, and they fear the side effects of analgesics in general and opioids in particular.

# Side Effects of Non-opioid Analgesics (WHO Level I)

The non-opioid analgesics are used in the treatment of pain of mild intensity (see Fig. 18.1). The main drugs used are paracetamol, anti-inflammatory drugs (NSAIDs at low doses; at high dosages, they are primarily anti-inflammatory), and nefopam.

## *Paracetamol*

Paracetamol is recommended as first choice in mild to moderate pain at a dose of 1,000 mg every 4–6 h [7]. Paracetamol can be toxic to the liver when overdosed, justifying precaution for use in cases of liver failure. Liver cell necrosis does occur rarely and with high doses: 8–10 g in a single dose, according to most authors [8]. This product does not alter bleeding time and does not cause thrombocytopenia or leukopenia; it causes neutropenia only in exceptional cases [9]. Finally, in very exceptional circumstances, cases of asthma have been described [10]. It does not alter the renal excretion of water and salts, which facilitates its prescription in patients receiving chemotherapy and renal insufficiency. Liver cell necrosis can occur in three situations: overdose, intoxication in adults with doses beyond 6 g and/or a single dose, and in case of acute alcohol intoxication [7].

Rare cases of hypersensitivity reactions such as anaphylactic shock, angioedema, rash, hives, and skin rash have been reported. These patients should not be treated with this medication and related drugs [8].

Overall, this drug is generally very well tolerated at standard doses [11] and when given up to 6 g/day, if necessary, taking into account the benefit/risk ratio. It is appropriate to take particular care in all patients who have hepatic impairment and/or are taking other hepatotoxic drugs.

## *NSAIDs*

The anti-inflammatory drugs include all drugs inhibiting prostaglandin synthesis. These prostaglandins have a purely local, but almost ubiquitous, distribution, acting in many physiological and pathological processes [7].

Prostaglandins are synthesized from arachidonic acid through cyclooxygenase (COX) isoenzymes:

- The COX1 catalyzes the formation of prostaglandins involved in the cytoprotection of gastric mucosa and preservation of renal function and the production of thromboxane A2 (vasoconstrictive prostaglandins and pro-aggregating) by platelets.
- The COX2, essentially an inducible isoenzyme, leads to the release of prostaglandins having a pathological role (fever, pain, inflammation, cell proliferation) but also a beneficial role in various processes (wound healing, kidney function, ovulation). It governs the synthesis of prostacyclin (vasodilator prostaglandins and anti-aggregating) by endothelial cells.

The decreased synthesis of prostaglandins by NSAIDs is following the more or less selective inhibition of COX isoenzymes. This common mechanism of action of NSAIDs confers their properties and side effects.

COX2 inhibitors (also called coxibs) have not been studied in the context of cancer pain and have no market approval in cancer [4].

Adverse reactions are common to all NSAIDs and can be classified into several groups [12].

## Gastrointestinal Side Effects

Several different side effects must be distinguished:

- The functional symptoms (dyspepsia, gastric pain, nausea): frequent and rapidly upon discontinuation of product. They are not systematically correlated with the presence of mucosal esophageal or gastroduodenal lesion.
- Peptic ulcers discovered at endoscopy: They are more common with NSAIDs than with coxibs but asymptomatic in half the cases. Small bowel ulcers have been described.
- The symptomatic ulcer, simple or complicated (gastrointestinal bleeding, perforation), of occasionally rapid onset, which occurs in 2–4 % per patient year with traditional NSAIDs.

The main predisposing circumstances are a high dosage of NSAIDs, old age, an active or former ulcer, concomitant anti-coagulant, a corticosteroid, or other NSAIDs, including aspirin. This risk is about two times lower with coxibs, but this advantage is lost when the patient is given antithrombotic aspirin.

The treatment of gastrointestinal adverse events is by a proton pump inhibitor [4].

The occurrence of gastrointestinal symptoms while the patient is taking NSAIDs should alert one to reconsider the usefulness of NSAID treatment and/or prescription of a proton pump inhibitor and/or the appropriateness of gastroscopy.

Finally, prevention of these injuries must be a priority and can be achieved by a rational prescription of NSAIDs and especially respect for these simple rules:

- Limit the duration of prescriptions.
- Do not associate with other NSAIDs.
- Challenge dangerous associations (antiplatelet agents, anticoagulants).
- Observe the effect, especially in the elderly.

## Mucocutaneous Reactions

Mucocutaneous reactions consist of pruritus, various eruptions, stomatitis, rhinitis, bronchospasm, and, to a much lesser extent, angioedema or anaphylactic shock. They are the expression of an allergy to the molecule or idiosyncratic state, including the Widal triad (asthma, nasal polyposis, and aspirin intolerance) and other NSAIDs.

## Renal Complications

The most common renal complications are early, dose dependent, and consecutive to the inhibition of renal COX:

- Sodium and water retention resulting in lower limb edema, increased blood pressure, or congestive heart failure.
- Acute renal failure, oliguria early on, reversible upon discontinuation of the NSAID. Its occurrence is favored by prior renal hypoperfusion (nephropathy, dehydration, diuretics, etc.) and taking inhibitors of angiotensin converting enzyme or angiotensin II antagonists.
- The concomitant prescription of NSAIDs and other nephrotoxic drugs, including cisplatin, whose elimination is over several weeks, is not to be prescribed owing to risk of renal failure [13].

## Vascular Complications

All NSAIDs seem likely to favor thrombotic events (myocardial infarction, stroke) through an increase in systolic blood pressure. In combination with anticoagulants, they increase the risk of bleeding.

The blood cytopenias are rare, as well as hepatitis with a clinical expression [13]. Erythema multiforme (Lyell and Stevens-Johnson) is exceptional.

NSAIDs can sometimes cause neurosensory disorders (headache, dizziness, tinnitus, etc.).

## Drug Interactions with NSAIDs Are Numerous

Some associations can be a risky choice and, if indicated, should be discussed with the treatment team – for example, the NSAIDs and low-molecular-weight heparin in a bedridden patient suffering from prolonged difficult-to-control bone pain.

Besides the well-known interaction with cisplatin cited above, one must keep in mind the following interactions:

- Anticoagulants and antiplatelet agents: Concomitant use of NSAIDs increases the risk of bleeding, either because of competition for their protein binding or by interference on hemostasis.
- Methotrexate (MTX) [14]: Concomitant use of NSAIDs leads within hours to days to an increase in the overall toxicity of MTX (association formally not to be recommended).
- Lithium: In principle, one must admit that all NSAIDs, except salicylate, reduce the renal clearance of lithium with a risk of overdose.
- Digoxin: Increased plasma levels owing to decreased renal clearance.
- Antihypertensives and diuretics: The antihypertensive effect of diuretics, beta-blockers, inhibitors of angiotensin converting enzyme, and calcium antagonists can be reduced when taking NSAIDs.
- NSAIDs association: The association of two NSAIDs has no pharmacological advantage.
- Special case: Clinical experience shows that some patients with bone pain and who are taking corticosteroids for another indication may have their pain alleviated by the addition of NSAIDs. However, this association cannot be recommended owing to the lack of studies, and prevention of gastrointestinal side effects is recommended.

Finally, NSAIDs, despite their powerful action, especially in inflammatory pain, are second-line analgesics for cancer pain because of their numerous side effects and risks of drug interactions. Their long-term prescription, that is, over several months or years, can only be considered for uncontrollable chronic pain failing paracetamol, steroids, or opioids alone or in combination. They can be very useful in acute situations or during initial breakthrough pain, for example, for bone pain, when looking for a safer alternative. Whatever the class of NSAID, the dosage, the potential side effects, precautions for use, and contraindications are the same.

For any NSAID prescription, it is appropriate to limit the duration of prescription, to not associate two NSAIDs, to avoid dangerous interactions, and to respect the precautions for poly-medicated patients, the elderly, and patients with renal failure.

## Nefopam

Nefopam has an unclear mechanism of action. It has no opi-oid property and no anti-inflammatory activity. It is not anti-pyretic. It inhibits the reuptake of norepinephrine, serotonin, and dopamine [15]. It has anticholinergic effects independent of analgesia. Adverse events [16] reported very frequently are drowsiness, nausea and vomiting, and hyperhidrosis.

Frequently, cases of dizziness, tachycardia, palpitation, dry mouth, and urinary retention have been described.

Rarely, undesirable effects of excitability, irritability, hal-lucinations, drug dependence, seizures, malaise, and hyper-sensitivity reactions have been reported.

It should be used with caution in patients with a history of myocardial ischemia and seizures [17]. Its use with tricyclic antidepressants decreases the seizure threshold.

# Side Effects of Weak Opioids (WHO Level II)

Opioids are used in the treatment of pain of moderate inten-sity. They are represented by codeine, dihydrocodeine, codeine association/paracetamol, tramadol, and tramadol/paracetamol.

## Tramadol and Tramadol-Acetaminophen Association

The main side effects attributable to tramadol are nausea and vomiting, drowsiness, headache, euphoria, sweating, dry mouth, and constipation [4, 18].

Nausea is generally dose dependent, and dose reduction during the first days of treatment improves the tolerance. Constipation, euphoria, and respiratory depression are less severe than with level III analgesics [19].

Because of the mechanism of action (preferential mu-opioid receptor agonist activity and central monoaminergic effect by inhibition of neuronal reuptake of serotonin and norepinephrine), tramadol should not be associated with MAO inhibitors. Precaution for use must be taken when prescribed with anti-depressants. Indeed, their association can cause a serotonin syndrome, characterized by three groups of symptoms: neuro-muscular hyperactivity (tremor, myoclonus, hyperreflexia, pyramidal rigidity), autonomic hyperactivity (hyperthermia, diaphoresis, tachycardia, tachypnea, mydriasis, diarrhea), and altered mental status (agitation, excitement, confusion) [20]. The drugs most frequently responsible for the serotonin syn-drome are paroxetine, sertraline, citalopram, fluoxetine, and venlafaxine [21, 22]. Precautions are also taken in case of sei-zure risk, although the effect of tramadol remains controver-sial. Particular attention should be paid in patients with a history of head trauma, stroke, or excessive consumption of alcohol [20].

## Codeine, Codeine-Paracetamol Combination, and Dihydrocodeine

Codeine and dihydrocodeine generally share the adverse effects of opioids (see below), although they are less intense [23]. They are metabolized by the liver. One must therefore be careful when using them in cases of liver failure.

# Side Effects of Strong Opioids (WHO Level III)

Strong opioids are prescribed in the treatment of pain of moderate to major intensity.

TABLE 18.1  Classification of strong opioids (WHO level 3)

| Strong opioid agonists | Strong opioid partial agonists or agonist-antagonists | Strong opioid antagonists |
|---|---|---|
| Morphine | Buprenorphine | Naloxone |
| Oxycodone | Nalbuphine | |
| Fentanyl | Pentazocine | |
| Hydromorphone | | |
| Methadone | | |
| Meperidine or Pethidine | | |
| Sufentanil | | |

They are classified into several groups, summarized in Table 18.1.

• Strong opioid agonists
• Strong opioid partial agonists or agonist-antagonists
• Strong opioid antagonists

Opioids generally all share the same side effects. The main effects reported in the literature are reported in Table 18.2 [24].

## Nausea and Vomiting

Nausea and vomiting are observed in 15–30 % of patients receiving oral morphine as treatment for chronic cancer pain [24].

No study shows an advantage to a specific antiemetic drug. The most frequently used are metoclopramide, haloperidol, phenothiazines, scopolamine patch, and corticosteroids. The use of antagonists of serotonin 5-HT3 (setrons) has not been specifically evaluated in nausea and vomiting induced by opioids in cancer [4].

TABLE 18.2  Common opioid-induced adverse effects

| | |
|---|---|
| Gastrointestinal | Nausea |
| | Vomiting |
| | Constipation |
| Autonomic | Xerostomia |
| | Urinary retention |
| | Postural hypotension |
| Central nervous system | Drowsiness |
| | Cognitive impairment |
| | Hallucinations |
| | Delirium |
| | Respiratory depression |
| | Myoclonus |
| | Seizure disorders |
| | Hyperalgesia |
| Cutaneous | Itching |
| | Sweating |

Reprinted with permission. © 2001 American Society of Clinical Oncology. All rights reserved. Cherny et al. [24]

Uncontrollable nausea and vomiting must induce, if possible, a drug rotation [25–30] or a different route of administration [31, 32]. The subcutaneous route may be less emetogenic [31, 32].

## Constipation

Constipation is almost constant and must be systematically prevented with the introduction of opioid therapy [4].

Preventive treatment, whose fundamentals remain empirical, combines lifestyle changes and laxatives.

## Dietary Measures

Dietary measures include the following:

- Maintain physical activity whenever possible.
- Increase fluid intake, especially because a dry mouth can occur with morphine.
- Dietary intake balanced with consumption of raw or cooked vegetables, fresh or cooked fruit, dried fruit and nuts (prunes, peanuts, hazelnuts, walnuts, etc.), and preserved fruit. Overconsumption of dietary fiber to fight against constipation related to morphine is not a proven preventive measure. Limitation of foods that slow food transit (rice, chocolate) is empirically recommended.
- Comfortable conditions for a bowel movement (private place, nearness of a commode).

## Laxatives

No one laxative has demonstrated its superiority over another [24]. The effectiveness of laxatives is variable from one patient to another. The use of rectal laxatives may be necessary in case of failure of oral laxatives. Protocols are empirical. It is the experience and clinical supervision that will guide the clinician, depending on patient comfort and the choice of products to use.

Rectal laxatives are usually given because of the poor efficacy of oral laxatives. Digital rectal examination helps with the prescription of the following [33, 34]:

- Hard stools: softening laxatives (paraffin, fiber, mucilage, lactulose, polyethylene glycol, etc.)
- Soft stools: laxatives increasing intrarectal pressure (anthracenes, neostigmine, etc.)
- Rectal ampulla empty: discuss a radiograph of the abdomen without preparation, increase the oral laxative treatment (type preparation for colonoscopy), reconsider the oral morphine treatment, and no rectal laxative

The methylnaltrexone and oxycodone-naloxone combination have demonstrated efficacy [35–37].

Three recent studies have revealed a trend toward reduction of constipation in patients receiving transdermal fentanyl compared to those treated with oral morphine [38, 39, 48].

## Sleepiness

Drowsiness is present, according to studies, in 20–60 % of patients [24]. It occurs mainly during the adjustment phase of therapy and disappears within a few days. Its reappearance or persistence should suggest a metabolic disorder (renal failure, hypercalcemia, etc.), possibly a potentiation by other sedatives. The benefit of amphetamines and psychostimulants is limited. Some studies indicate that methylphenidate may reduce drowsiness [40–45]. Methylphenidate is not approved in all countries for this indication. Rotation to oral or subcutaneous administration would cause less drowsiness [32]. The severity and prevalence of drowsiness may decrease by changing opioids [26, 28, 29, 46, 47].

## Neuropsychiatric Disorders

These disorders can be cognitive (disturbance of consciousness, orientation, memory, attention), behavioral (anxiety, agitation), disorders of perception (hallucinations, dream-like phenomena), and mood disorders (depression, euphoria, exaltation). They are often multifactorial in origin, and an organic cause should always be eliminated.

Reduction of 20–30 % of the dose, when possible, can improve these side effects. If this is insufficient, neuroleptics or antidepressants can be used [4, 24].

## Myoclonus

These are involuntary muscle movements that are generally dose dependent. Reducing the dosage may allow their control.

Drugs such as diazepam, baclofen, midazolam, clonazepam, and valproic acid appear to be able to reduce this side effect [24].

## Pruritus

Pruritus is found in 2–10 % of cases [24]. The hypothesis of a link between pruritus, release of serotonin, and histamine-induced morphine has been raised [4]. Antihistamines are recommended to treat pruritus [24], and one study [48] mentioned a favorable effect of paroxetine. The use of a setron can be discussed as well as naloxone [4]. Note that fentanyl and hydromorphone would release less histamine than other molecules [24], so changing the molecule could be of interest.

## Respiratory Effects

Morphine is a histamine liberator. It thickens the bronchopulmonary secretions and inhibits the cough reflex. Morphine has a respiratory depressant effect, but the pain is a natural agonist of this effect. Therefore, a patient regularly evaluated, suffering from cancer pain and treated with regular escalating doses, has a small risk of respiratory depression [4].

The use of opioids is not indicated in the patient with asthmatic or restrictive respiratory insufficiency. It is advisable to estimate the advantage of the opioid treatment and to be particularly watchful in the therapeutic escalation during an obstructive respiratory failure. A correction of obstruction (mucolytic agents, physiotherapy, etc.), as much as possible, must be implemented. The treatment of respiratory depression involves the prescription of the opioid antagonist naloxone, which is fully effective and rapid. Its dosage should be adjusted considering its half-life (duration of action of intravenous naloxone is 30 min, and 2–3 h for subcutaneous naloxone [4]) and also that of the opioid used.

## Other Effects

Dysuria, urinary retention, and sweating have a poorly defined incidence rate. Reducing dosages would improve these symptoms.

For urinary problems, which are associated with an increase in tone of the detrusor muscle and sphincter, a bladder catheter and neostigmine can easily solve the problem [4].

For sweating, NSAIDs and corticosteroids may be tried, even if they do not have market approval for this indication [4].

Tolerance or habituation reflects the need to increase doses of a product to maintain a given effect. Tolerance to the analgesic effect of opioids is low. Most often, the need to increase doses is related to an increase in clinical pain by infra-clinical evolution. However, there is a tolerance benefit to some side effects: drowsiness, respiratory depression, nausea and vomiting, etc.

Chronic use of morphine, like other products, causes physiological changes in connection with its action on specific receptors. Physical dependence is one of those changes. It can lead in the extreme to a syndrome of opioid withdrawal when opioids are stopped abruptly or if an opioid antagonist is prescribed. This phenomenon should not be confused with addiction. The withdrawal syndrome is characterized by anxiety, irritability, chills, piloerection, flushing, sweating, lacrimation, rhinorrhea, yawning, nausea and vomiting, abdominal cramps, diarrhea, joint pain, and mydriasis.

Addiction and physical dependence are problems in patients treated with opioids for cancer pain. Physical dependence requires continuity of the prescription and avoidance of co-prescription of agonist–antagonist opioid receptors [4]. Psychological dependence is, in turn, exceptional [4].

Psychological dependence or addiction is the development of addictive-like behavior, with craving and obsessive attention to obtain the product. Addiction is rare in cancer patients treated with opioids for pain [4, 49].

Some hyperalgesia with morphine may be encountered. These phenomena are currently poorly explained, even though there are interesting hypotheses based on animal experiments [50]. The decrease in dosage or change of opioid sometimes allows a decrease or disappearance of symptoms.

# Side Effects of Other Drugs for the Treatment of Nociceptive Pain

## Ketamine

Ketamine is a general anesthetic, not a barbiturate, that is fast acting and has been known for over 40 years. It provides a so-called dissociative anesthesia – that is, loss of consciousness, catalepsy, amnesia, sedation, and analgesia without hypnotic effect. Used since the 1990s at subanesthetic doses for its analgesic activity [51–53], ketamine is commonly used as an intravenous continuous low dose associated with opioid therapy. Its mechanism of action involves various receptors, but especially its effect is a noncompetitive antagonist of N-methyl-D-aspartate (NMDA) [52]. Indeed, it is established that the intractable pain, often with a neuropathic component, involves NMDA receptors, located in the central nervous system. Because of repeated stimulation of C fibers and poorly relieved pain, these receptors lead to central sensitization, an increase and an amplification of pain perception. The patient will have an exaggerated pain response during stimulation of C fiber [54, 55].

Adverse effects of ketamine are mainly psychotomimetic [56]. With a subanesthetic dose, patients can express hallucinations or a sense of unreality, sedation, confusion, and salivary or bronchial hypersecretion. These adverse effects can be prevented by adequate prophylaxis based on benzodiazepines, haloperidol, and an anticholinergic and by gradually increasing the dose and the gradual decline of other analgesics [51, 52, 55].

## Entonox

Entonox (equimolar mixture of oxygen and nitrous oxide) is presented as a colorless, odorless gas inhaled by mask. The major effects observed with nitrous oxide are a euphoric and anxiolytic effect, an analgesic surface. The use of nitrous oxide at a concentration of 50 % does not fit into the context of anesthesia because this concentration is insufficient to induce general anesthesia. With Entonox, the patient remains alert, there is no respiratory depression or hemodynamic alteration, and laryngeal reflexes are preserved [57].

Side effects are minor and disappear quickly as the administration of gas is stopped [58]. The following effects may occur during treatment and disappear within minutes after cessation of inhalation of the mixture:

- Euphoria, dreams
- Paresthesia
- Sedation
- Dizziness
- Nausea and vomiting
- Changes in sensory perceptions
- Anxiety, agitation

In patients taking drugs that depress the central nervous system, primarily opioids and benzodiazepines, the risk of drowsiness, desaturation, vomiting, and hypotension is increased. Assessment and monitoring by a physician familiar with the use of gas are required.

Neurologic disorders like myeloneuropathies may occur late in patients chronically exposed to high doses. Neurologic toxicity was observed in a case of prolonged inhalation in a context of addiction. After prolonged or repeated exposure, megaloblastic anemia with leukopenia has been reported. It takes more than 6 h of continuous inhalation and over 9 h of intermittent administration to cause bone marrow megaloblastosis without blood changes or clinical signs, and it is reversible upon discontinuation of treatment [59].

Entonox should not be administered in the following situations:

- Patients requiring ventilation with pure oxygen
- Increased intracranial pressure

- Altered consciousness preventing patient cooperation
- Pneumothorax, emphysema
- Abdominal bloating

## *Ziconotide*

Ziconotide is an N-type voltage-dependent calcium channel blocker (NACC) used intrathecally. It is recommended in the treatment of severe chronic pain in patients who require intrathecal analgesia [60]. The main side effects attributed to ziconotide are neuropsychological disorders (dizziness, nystagmus, confusion, gait disturbance, memory impairment, blurred vision, headache, drowsiness) and gastrointestinal disorders such as nausea and vomiting, and asthenia. These side effects are mild to moderate and often disappear over time [60, 61].

These major problems are described in three major studies, summarized in Table 18.3 [62–64].

## Summary

Analgesic drugs represent a major focus of supportive therapy. They are applied to fight against some symptoms related to cancer or its treatment; in this chapter, their efficacy against pain was discussed. Treatment of these symptoms must be done with maximum efficiency but also with the least possible side effects in order to avoid a situation in which the remedy is worse than the disease. This implies that professionals are familiar with supportive and palliative as well as specific cancer therapy. To achieve this goal, continuous education in this area must be encouraged. It is recalled here that the handling of opioids, a key factor in cancer pain therapy, follows some simple rules applied to the entire class of drugs. These drugs are extremely safe. In case of overdose, the availability of a good antidote is always effective. Few in our pharmacopeia have such an advantage.

TABLE 18.3 Overview of randomized placebo-controlled clinical studies with ziconotide

| | Staats [62] | Wallace et al. [63] | Rauck [64] |
|---|---|---|---|
| Titration schedule | Fast[a] | Fast[a] | Slow[b] |
| Treatment duration (days) | 10–11 | 6–11 | 21 |
| Population | Patients with pain (VASPI score ≥50 mm) associated with cancer or AIDS | Patients with severe chronic pain (VASPI score ≥50 mm) of nonmalignant cause | Patients with severe chronic pain (VASPI score ≥50 mm) of any cause |
| Number of patients given Z/P | 71/40 | 169/86 | 112/108 |
| Pain reported | | | |
| Neuropathic (Z/P) | NR | 75.7 %/76.7 % | 75.9 %/71.3 % |
| Non-neuropathic (Z/P) | NR | 13.0 %/12.8 % | 35.7 %/32.4 % |
| Mean baseline VASPI score for Z/P group (mm) | 74/78 | 80/77 | 81/81 |
| Mean decrease in VASPI scores after Z/P | 51.4 %/18.1 % (p < 0.001) | 31.2 %/6.0 % (p < 0.001) | 14.7 %/7.2 % (p = 0.036) |

Adverse events

| | | | |
|---|---|---|---|
| Nervous system[c] | Dizziness (50.0 %)[d], nystagmus (45.8 %), somnolence (23.6 %)[d], confusion (20.8 %)[d], abnormal gait (12.5 %)[d] | Dizziness (53.5 %)[d] nystagmus (40.0 %)[d] abnormal gait (27.1 %)[d], somnolence (12.4 %), confusion (11.8 %), amblyopia (10.6 %)[d] | Dizziness (47.3 %)[d], somnolence (22.3 %), confusion (17.9 %)[d], ataxia (16.1 %)[d], abnormal gait (15.2 %)[d], memory impairment (11.6 %)[d] |
| Digestive system[c] | Nausea (29.2 %)[d], vomiting (18.1 %)[d], constipation (12.5 %) | Nausea (48.8 %)[d], constipation (18.2 %), vomiting (14.1 %)[d] | Nausea (41.1 %), diarrhea (18.8 %), vomiting (15.2 %) |
| Other systems[c] | Fever (25.0 %)[d], postural hypotension (23.6 %)[d] urinary retention (18.1 %)[d], headache (15.3 %) | Pain (16.5 %)[d] headache (16.5 %), urinary retention (15.3 %)[d], postural hypotension (11.8 %) | Asthenia (22.3 %), headache (15.2 %), pain (10.7 %) |

Adapted from Schmidtko et al. [61], Copyright 2010. With permission from Elsevier

*Abbreviations*: *A* ziconotide, *P* placebo, *NR* not reported

[a]Fast titration: Initial dosage 9.6 (mu) µg/day, a dose increase 7–14 times per week, maximum dosage per protocol 57.6 µg/day, time to maximum dose 5–6 days

[b]Slow titration: Initial dosage 2.4 µg/day, a dose increase 2–3 times per week, maximum dosage per protocol 21.6 µg/day, time to maximum dose 21 days

[c]Adverse events reported in >10 % of patients treated with ziconotide

[d]Occurred with significantly greater frequency with ziconotide than with placebo ($p < 0.05$)

# References

1. Dault RL, Cleeland CS. The prevalence and severity of pain in cancer. Cancer. 1982;50:1913–8.
2. Van den Beuken-van Everdingen MHJ, de Rijke JM, Kessels AG, Schouten HC, van Kleef M, Patijn J. Prevalence of pain in patients with cancer: a systematic review of the past 40 years. Ann Oncol. 2007;18: 1437–49.
3. Bonica JJ, editor. The management of pain. 2nd ed. Philadelphia: Lea & Febiger; 1990.
4. Krakowski I, Theobald S, Balp L, Bonnefoi MP, Chvetzoff G, Collard O, et al. Standards, options, et recommandations: traitements antalgiques médicamenteux des douleurs cancéreuses par excès de nociception chez l'adulte, mise à jours 2002. Paris: Fédération Nationale des Centres de Lutte Contre le Cancer; 2002. http://www.fnclcc.fr.
5. Van den Beuken-van Everdingen MHJ, de Rijke JM, Kessels AG, Schouten HC, van Kleef M, Patijn J. High prevalence of pain in patients with cancer in a large population-based study in The Netherlands. Pain. 2007;132:312–20.
6. Garcia B. Prise en charge de la douleur en cancérologie digestive. Post'U 2011;169–72.
7. Graham GG, Scott KF, Day RO. Tolerability of paracetamol. Drug Saf. 2005;28(3):227–40.
8. Le Dictionnaire Vidal. Paris: Edition du Vidal; 2011.
9. Bougie D, Aster R. Immune thrombocytopenia resulting from sensitivity to metabolites of naproxen and acetaminophen. Blood. 2001;97(12):3846–50.
10. Nuttall SL, Williams J, Kendall MJ. Does paracetamol cause asthma? J Clin Pharm Ther. 2003;28(4):251–7.
11. Graham GG, Scott KF, Day RO. Tolérance du paracétamol. Drugs. 2003;63(2):43–6.
12. Prescriptions et surveillance des antiinflammatoires stéroïdiens et non stéroïdiens. Support de cours. Université Médicale Virtuelle Francophone 2008–2009. http://sist.education.gov.mg/UMVFmiroir/campus-cours-c/rhumato25/site/html/cours.pdf
13. Sunshine A, Olson NZ. Non-narcotic analgesics. In: Wall PD, Melzack R, editors. Textbook of pain. 2nd ed. New York: Churchill Livingstone; 1989. p. 670–85.
14. Frenia ML, Long KS. Methotrexate and nonsteroidal antiinflammatory drug interactions. Ann Pharmacother. 1992;26:234–7.
15. Heel RC, Brogden RN, Pakes GE, Speight TM, Avery GS. Nefopam: review of its pharmacological properties and therapeutic efficacy. Drugs. 1980;19:249–67.
16. Durrieu G, Olivier P, Bagheri H, Montastruc JL. Overview of adverse reactions to nefopam: an analysis of the French Pharmacovigilance database. Fundam Clin Pharmacol. 2007;21(5):555–8.

17. Pillans PI, Woods DJ. Adverse reactions associated with nefopam. N Z Med J. 1995;108(1008):382–4.
18. Leppert W. Tramadol as an analgesic for mild to moderate cancer pain: review. Pharmacol Rep. 2009;61:978–92.
19. Dayer P, Desmeules J, Collart L. Pharmacology of tramadol. Drugs. 1997;53 Suppl 2:18–24.
20. Coulombe A, Thiffault R. Le syndrome sérotoninergique secondaire à l'association du tramadol et des inhibiteurs sélectifs du recaptage de la sérotonine. Pharmactuel. 2008;41(1). Janvier-Février. p. 30–35.
21. Gillman PK. A review of serotonin toxicity data: implications for the mechanisms of antidepressant drug action. Biol Psychiatry. 2006;59:1046–51.
22. Boyer EW, Shannon M. The serotonin syndrome. N Engl J Med. 2005;352:1112–20 [see comment].
23. Leppert W. Pain management in patients with cancer: focus on opioid analgesics. Curr Pain Headache Rep. 2011;15:271–9.
24. Cherny N, Ripamonti C, Pereira J, Davis C, Fallon M, McQuay H, et al. Strategies to manage the adverse effects of oral morphine: an evidence-based report. J Clin Oncol. 2001;19(9):2542–54.
25. Cherny NJ, Chang V, Frager G, Ingham JM, Tiseo PJ, Popp B, et al. Opioid pharmacotherapy in the management of cancer pain: a survey of strategies used by pain physicians for the selection of analgesic drugs and routes of administration. Cancer. 1995;76:1283–93.
26. De Stoutz ND, Bruera E, Suarez-Almazor M. Opioid rotation for toxicity reduction in terminal cancer patients. J Pain Symptom Manage. 1995;10:378–84.
27. Maddocks I, Somogyi A, Abbott F, Hayball P, Parker D. Attenuation of morphine-induced delirium in palliative care by substitution with infusion of oxycodone. J Pain Symptom Manage. 1996;12:182–9.
28. Vigano A, Fan D, Bruera E. Individualized use of methadone and opioid rotation in the comprehensive management of cancer pain associated with poor prognostic indicators. Pain. 1996;67:115–9.
29. Ashby MA, Martin P, Jackson KA. Opioid substitution to reduce adverse effects in cancer pain management. Med J Aust. 1999;170:68 71.
30. Donner B, Zenz M, Tryba M, Strumpf M. Direct conversion from oral morphine to transdermal fentanyl: a multicenter study in patients with cancer pain. Pain. 1996;64:527–34.
31. McDonald P, Graham P, Clayton M, Buhagiar A, Stuart-Harris R. Regular subcutaneous bolus morphine via an indwelling cannula for pain from advanced cancer. Palliat Med. 1991;5:323–9.
32. Drexel H, Dzien A, Spiegel RW, Lang AH, Breier C, Abbrederis K, et al. Treatment of severe cancer pain by low-dose continuous subcutaneous morphine. Pain. 1989;36:169–76.
33. Derby S, Portenoy RK. Assessment and management of opioid-induced constipation. In: Portenoy RK, Bruera E, editors. Topics in palliative care. New York: Oxford University Press; 1997. p. 95–112.

34. Sykes NP. The relationship between opioid use and laxative use in terminally ill cancer patients. Palliat Med. 1998;12:375–82.
35. Sykes NP. An investigation of the ability of oral naloxone to correct opioid-related constipation in patients with advanced cancer. Palliat Med. 1996;10:135–44.
36. Sykes NP. Oral naloxone in opioid-associated constipation. Lancet. 1991;337:1475.
37. Culpepper-Morgan JA, Inturrisi CE, Portenoy RK, Foley K, Houde RW, Marsh F, et al. Treatment of opioid-induced constipation with oral naloxone: a pilot study. Clin Pharmacol Ther. 1992;52:90–5.
38. Ahmedzai S, Brooks D. Transdermal fentanyl versus sustained release oral morphine in cancer pain: preference, efficacy, and quality of life – The TTS-Fentanyl Comparative Trial Group. J Pain Symptom Manage. 1997;13:254–61.
39. Payne R, Mathias SD, Pasta DJ, Wanke LA, Williams R, Mahmoud R. Quality of life and cancer pain: satisfaction and side effects with transdermal fentanyl versus oral morphine. J Clin Oncol. 1998;16:1588–93.
40. Bruera E, Chadwick S, Brenneis C, Hanson J, MacDonald RN. Methylphenidate associated with narcotics for the treatment of cancer pain. Cancer Treat Rep. 1987;71:67–70.
41. Bruera E, Brenneis C, Paterson AH, MacDonald RN. Narcotics plus methylphenidate (Ritalin) for advanced cancer pain. Am J Nurs. 1988;88:1555–6.
42. Bruera E, Brenneis C, Paterson AH, MacDonald RN. Use of methylphenidate as an adjuvant to narcotic analgesics in patients with advanced cancer. J Pain Symptom Manage. 1989;4:3–6.
43. Bruera E, Miller MJ, Macmillan K, Kuehn N. Neuropsychological effects of methylphenidate in patients receiving a continuous infusion of narcotics for cancer pain. Pain. 1992;48:163–6.
44. Bruera E, Fainsinger R, MacEachern T, Hanson J. The use of methylphenidate in patients with incident cancer pain receiving regular opiates: a preliminary report. Pain. 1992;50:75–7.
45. Wilwerding MB, Loprinzi CL, Mailliard JA, O'Fallon JR, Miser AW, van Haelst C, et al. A randomized, crossover evaluation of methylphenidate in cancer patients receiving strong narcotics. Support Care Cancer. 1995;3:135–8.
46. Bruera E, Franco JJ, Maltoni M, Watanabe S, Suarez-Almazor M, et al. Changing pattern of agitated impaired mental status in patients with advanced cancer: association with cognitive monitoring, hydration, and opioid rotation. J Pain Symptom Manage. 1995;10:287–91.
47. Galer BS, Coyle N, Pasternak GW, Portenoy RK. Individual variability in the response to different opioids: report of five cases. Pain. 1992;49:87–91.

48. Zylicz Z, Smits C, Krajnik M. Paroxetine for pruritus in advanced cancer. J Pain Symptom Manage. 1998;16:121–4.
49. Organisation Mondiale de la Santé. Traitement de la douleur cancéreuse : complétée par une analyse des problèmes liés à la mise à disposition des opioïdes. Genève: OMS; 1997.
50. Simonnet G, Rivat C. Opioid-induced hyperalgesia: abnormal or normal pain? Neuroreport. 2003;14(1):1–7.
51. Mercadente S, Lodi F, Sapio M, Calligara M, Serretta R. Long-term ketamine subcutaneous continuous infusion in neuropathic cancer pain. J Pain Symptom Manage. 1995;10:564–8.
52. Fitzgibbon EJ, Schroder C, Viola R. Low dose ketamine as an analgesic adjuvant in difficult pain syndromes: a strategy for conversion from parenteral to oral ketamine. J Pain Symptom Manage. 2002; 23:165–70.
53. Benitez-Rosario MA, Feria M, Salinas-Martin A. A retrospective comparison of the dose ratio between subcutaneous and oral ketamine. J Pain Symptom Manage. 2003;25:400–1.
54. Mercadante S. Ketamine in cancer pain: an update. Palliat Med. 1996;10:225–30.
55. Fitzgibbon EJ, Viola R. Parenteral ketamine as an analgesic adjuvant for severe pain: development and retrospective audit of a protocol for Palliative Care Unit. J Palliat Med. 2005;8(1):49–57.
56. Huot A-M. La kétamine dans le soulagement des douleurs. Pharmactuel. 2006;39(4):229–30.
57. Bauer C, Lahjibi-Paulet H, Somme D, Onody P, Saint Jean O, Gisselbrecht M. Tolerability of an equimolar mix of nitrous oxide and oxygen during painful procedures in very elderly patients. Drugs Aging. 2007;24(6):501–7.
58. Onody P, Gil P, Hennequin M. Safety of inhalation of a 50 % nitrous oxide/oxygen premix: a prospective survey of 35, 828 administrations. Drug Saf. 2006;29(7):633–40.
59. Sanders RD, Weimann J, Maze M. Biologic effects of nitrous oxide: a mechanistic and toxicologic review. Anesthesiology. 2008;109: 707–22.
60. PRIALT. HAS, Commission de la transparence. 14 mai 2008. www.has-sante.fr.
61. Schmidtko A, Lötsch J, Freynhagen R, Geisslinger G. Ziconotide for treatment of severe chronic pain. New drug class. Lancet. 2010;375 :1569.
62. Staats P. Intrathecal ziconotide in the treatment of refractory pain in patients with cancer or AIDS. JAMA. 2003;291:63–70.
63. Wallace MS, Charapata SG, Fisher R, Byas-Smith M, Staats PS, Mayo M, et al. Intrathecal ziconotide in the treatment of chronic nonmalignant pain: a randomised double blind placebo controlled clinical trial. Neuromodulation. 2006;9(2):75–86.

64. Rauck RL. A randomized, double-blind, placebo-controlled study of intrathecal ziconotide in adults with severe chronic pain. J Pain Symptom Manage. 2006;31:393–406.
65. Krakowski I, Theobald S, Balp L, Bonnefoi MP, Chvetzoff G, Collard O, et al. Summary version of the standards, options, and recommendations for the use of analgesia for the treatment of nociceptive pain in adults with cancer (update 2002). Br J Cancer. 2003;89 Suppl 1:S67–72.

# Chapter 19
# Totally Implanted Access Ports: Indications and Prevention of Complications

**Didier S. Kamioner**

**Abstract** Repeated venipunctures are often aggressive, painful, and sometimes dangerous, especially with the risk of severe extravasation during the administration of anticancer chemotherapy. An implanted central catheter (ICC) can be used for chemotherapy, infusions, transfusions, and blood samples and for the administration of various medications or parenteral nutrition requiring repeated access to the venous system. The installation must be done by a trained operator in surgical aseptic conditions. To prevent complications, training, information, protocols, and evaluation are recommended. Nevertheless, some important complications may occur during installation or use of the device (hematoma, pneumothorax, thrombosis, extravasation, infection, no reflux, etc.).

**Keywords** Totally implanted access ports • Venipuncture • Thrombosis • Catheter infection • Extravasation • Recall reaction • Huber needle • Venous reflux • Pinch-off syndrome • Costoclavicular clamp

D.S. Kamioner, M.D.
Department of Medical Oncology and Haematology,
Hôpital Privé Ouest Parisien, Trappes, France
e-mail: didier.kamioner@gmail.com

M.A. Dicato (ed.), *Side Effects of Medical Cancer Therapy,*
DOI 10.1007/978-0-85729-787-7_19,
© Springer-Verlag London 2013

# Introduction

Repeated venipunctures are often aggressive, painful, and sometimes dangerous, especially with the risk of severe extravasation during the administration of anticancer chemotherapy.

Externalized central catheters are used less frequently and are currently reserved for special situations such as short chemotherapy treatment (less than three cycles), terminal palliative care, and intensive care. Peripherally inserted central catheters (PICCs) are frequently used in some countries. This technique, developed in the 1990s in North America, has reduced the indication of conventional central venous insertion; however, it is not currently in use everywhere, due to the lack of familiarity with the equipment. In addition, the incidence rate of infection with PICCs is 1–2 infections in 1,000 catheter-days. In comparison, the incidence rate of infection with the ports is 0.1–0.2 infections per 1,000 catheter-days. Similarly, the incidence of thrombosis with the port is lower (OR = 0.43, 95: 0.23–0.80). Thus, the implantable central catheter (ICC) is currently the preferred central venous access [1].

The ICC can be used for chemotherapy, infusions, transfusions, and blood samples and for the administration of various medications or parenteral nutrition requiring repeated access to the venous system.

Instructions for the device must be observed rigorously according to the rules defined by tracing items (Code of Public Health). The information delivered to the patient is now largely enshrined in law.

# Installation

The installation [2] must be performed quickly, as soon as the decision of chemotherapy is made, to respect the peripheral venous capital.

It is not appropriate to insert an ICC after the start of chemotherapy because of organizational problems in health-care facilities. This can be done only in cases of true therapeutical emergency, such as enlarged mediastinum in lymphomas or small cell carcinoma. After one cycle of chemotherapy, the tumor mass will be reduced and the catheter easily inserted.

The management of antiplatelet agents and anticoagulants is subject to the same rules as any other surgery. Upon installation, the platelet count should be greater than 50,000/mm$^3$ and the INR (international normalized ratio) lower than 1.5.

The type of anesthesia – usually a local anesthesia – must take into consideration the preferences of the patient and his or her physical and mental state.

The choice of the site must be done in consultation with stakeholders: the patient, the surgeon, the anesthesiologist, and the users (including oncologists, nurses, and therapists). Insertion of an ICC in a pre-irradiated area (apart from controlateral breast cancer after evaluation) or near infected skin metastases is not recommended, and the equipment must be inserted on the opposite side of the tumor (ballistical reasons in case of radiotherapy). The choice of the vein has to be done according to the experience of the operator (preferred: superior vena cava, subclavian vein, or internal jugular vein). If implantation in the lower cave system increases the risk of thrombosis and infection, it must still be chosen in certain situations: compression or thrombosis of the superior vena cava, bilateral-jugulo-subclavian thrombosis, extensive skin metastasis, lymphangitis and bilateral cancers.

There are two implementation techniques: the percutaneous and the surgical denudation. The installation must be done in the operating room or in a room reserved specifically for this purpose, by a trained operator in surgical aseptic conditions, preferably under ultrasound guidance, and without antibiotic prophylaxis.

Before the patient is discharged from the operating room, the physician must verify the existence of a blood reflux and flush the ICC with saline serum to ensure the permeability of the system. A chest x-ray should be performed at the end of intervention to check the correct position of the catheter at the junction of the right atrium and superior vena cava and eliminate the risk of pneumothorax. The nurse may use the ICC just after the installation or within days.

The identification card of the equipment must specify the lot number and will then be given to the patient (a copy is kept in the patient's file and another is sent to the pharmacy). A book of his supervision is also provided. An educational approach tailored to the patient or his or her family is undertaken.

# Training, Information, Protocols, and Evaluation

The following procedures are recommended [3–5]:

- The existence of written protocols, shared in a network of care, regularly reviewed, brought to the attention of care-givers who apply them and whose compliance is assessed
- Staff training in the installation, manipulation, and maintenance of catheters
- Monitoring of infections associated with vascular catheters and their census

For the protection of personnel, it is imperative to:

- Prevent transmission of infectious agents carried by the blood or the body fluids of the patient.
- Respect general hygiene safety measures, in particular, to make rubbing alcohol first care.
- Provide a secure equipment in order to prevent accidental exposure to blood.

## *Asepsis*

It is recommended that the nursing staff wear sterile gloves during the assembly of infusion lines, during the installation of the Huber needle, and during the bandage change. It is also recommended that the caregivers and the patient wear a mask. If the patient is neutropenic, caregivers must wear a gown over clean business attire and cap.

It is necessary to ensure compliance with the closed system, to limit connections and valve manipulations, and never reconnect a disconnected infusion line.

Twenty-two-gauge type II Huber needles (fitted with an extender) with integrated security connector (with a pre-slit septum) should be used preferentially.

The length of the needle must be adapted to the chamber depth and build of the patient. It is recommended to use only syringes with a volume equal to or greater than to 10 mL in order to avoid excessive pressure that could damage the ICC. The site of needle insertion should be protected by a sterile bandage that is occlusive, transparent at best, and semipermeable.

The needle is changed every 8 days, maximum, as is the bandage, unless it is contaminated or has been removed. The main line is changed every 96 h. There is no evidence to recommend rinsing with heparin.

Given the risk of infection associated with the handling of a central venous line, maintenance of an implantable venous device table during the intercure or after the treatment is not recommended. A simple clinical surveillance (signs of infection and thrombosis) is necessary. However, a system check is desirable every 3–4 months to find a possible thrombosis of the catheter, a disinsertion of the catheter, a pinch-off syndrome with migration of a piece of the catheter into the heart chambers or a fibrin muff.

**Asepsis**
- Rinse three times.
- Rotate the needle 360° during flushing.
- Remove the needle while injecting to maintain a positive pressure.
- Immediately remove the needle into a collector, leaving the catheter in a column of saline.
- Place a sterile and occlusive dressing for 1 h.

**Indicators of Proper Functioning**
The absence of one of these four criteria requires immediate verification of the system:
• Presence of venous reflux
• No injection pain
• Good flux of infusion
• Easy injection with a syringe

# Major Complications

Despite compliance with the recommendations regarding the installation and use of ICC, complications may occur.

## *Mechanical Complications [1, 2, 6]*

### Absence of Reflux

The absence of reflux should always be explored and explained. It can be related to malposition of the needle, a rupture or displacement of the catheter, thrombosis, partial or total occlusion of the catheter, or a sleeve of fibrin. Required additional tests are a chest x-ray, a clouding of the catheter, particularly in the case of an associated painful injection, and a Doppler ultrasound.

### Pinch-Off Syndrome

The pinch-off must, no matter its rank, lead to a withdrawal and a change of catheter:

• Grade 1: narrowing of the catheter between the clavicle and the first rib with no narrowing of the lumen of the catheter.
• Grade 2: narrowing of the lumen of the catheter.
• Grade 3: fracture with embolization of the catheter. The broken fragment should always be removed using interventional radio-roping techniques.

In case of occlusion of the catheter by a cruoric fibrin deposit, the proper use of fibrinolytic agents according to procedures can "save" the catheter. The best prevention of catheter occlusions is "obsessive" rinsing between two injections and after use.

**Complications During Installation or Utilization of ICC [1, 2, 5]**
- Hematoma of the operation site
- Pneumothorax
- Hemothorax
- Arterial punctures
- Gaz emboly (exceptional cases 15/7,000)
- Pinch-off syndrome or costoclavicular clamp
- Thrombosis
- Infections
- Extravasation

## Ulceration of the Skin Above the Device [1, 6]

Ulceration of the skin occurs due to the situation of the subcutaneous injection site and may be secondary to a technical error during installation, to a lack of healing after the establishment of the device, to late ulceration of the skin in an emaciated patient, or to an un-noticed micro-extravasation, or even to a rejection of the material. In all cases, a surgical approach is necessary to change or replace the device and/or catheter.

## Extravasation [6]

Extravasation secondary to extravascular injection of cytotoxic molecules is often a serious complication that can cause tissue necrosis and ulceration with severe dammages to nerves, joints and tendons, which sometimes cause major repercussions (chronic pain, muscular dystrophy, loss of function, esthetic repercussions) (Table 19.1).

TABLE 19.1 Extravasation: potential necrosis risk

| Drugs Year of publication | I. Krämer 2002 | Cytotoxic handbook 2002 | Mader et al. 2002 | Quapos 3 2003 | CHNIM 2004 | CCO 2007 | AFSOS St. Paul 2009 |
|---|---|---|---|---|---|---|---|
| Bevacizumab? | – | – | – | – | – | Nonirritant | Nonirritant |
| Carboplatine | Irritant | Irritant | Nonirritant | Nonirritant | Vesicant | Nonirritant | Irritant |
| Cisplatine ≤ 0.4 mg/mL | Irritant | Exfoliant | Irritant | Irritant | Vesicant | Irritant | Irritant |
| Cisplatine > 0.4 mg/mL | – | – | Vesicant | Vesicant | – | – | Vesicant |
| Cyclophosphamide | Nonirritant | Nonirritant | Nonirritant | Nonirritant | Irritant | Nonirritant | Nonirritant |
| Docetaxel | Vesicant | Exfoliant | Irritant | Irritant | Irritant | Irritant | Irritant |
| Doxorubicine | Vesicant | Vesicant | Vesicant | Vesicant | Vesicant | Vesicant | Vesicant |
| Doxorubicine liposo. | – | Irritant | Irritant | Irritant | – | Irritant | Irritant |

|  |  |  |  |  |  |  |  |
|---|---|---|---|---|---|---|---|
| Epirubicine | Vesicant | Vesicant | Vesicant | Vesicant | Vesicant | Vesicant | Vesicant |
| Fluorouracil | Irritant | Inflammatory drug | Nonirritant | Nonirritant | Nonirritant | Nonirritant | Irritant |
| Méthotrexate | Nonirritant | Inflammatory drug | Nonirritant | Nonirritant | Nonirritant | Irritant-min. | Nonirritant |
| Paclitaxel | Vesicant | Vesicant | Vesicant | Vesicant | Irritant | Irritant | Vesicant |
| Trastuzumab | – | – | – | – | – | Nonirritant | Nonirritant |
| Vinorelbine | Vesicart | Vesicant | Vesicant | Vesicant | Vesicant | Vesicant | Vesicant |

It is a therapeutic emergency that is undervalued and undertreated. It may delay proper management of the disease by the interruption of chemotherapy and lead to medicolegal procedures. It is essential that the medical and nursing staffs be trained to prevent and manage extravasation.

The rapid establishment of early surgical techniques – drainage-washing and suction – is the key factor in preventing the development of irreversible soft tissue damage and/or disabling scarring. Ideally, this procedure should be initiated within 4–6 h following the incident. Without intervention, the lipophilic products (e.g., doxorubicin) may persist in the subcutaneous tissue for up to 5 months after the incident.

An emergency kit is essential in each service. The kit should contain a felt pen to mark the area of extravasation, a camera to visualize the area going forward, and the phone number of the surgical team to contact as soon as possible.

**Levels of Risk Associated with Extravasation [6]**
Vesicant drugs – responsible for severe necrosis (anthracyclines, vinorelbine, trabectedin, dactinomycin, mitomycin C, vinca alkaloids, etc.):
- Nonvesicant drugs (cyclophosphamide, liposomal doxorubicin, gemcitabine, methotrexate).
- Irritant drugs: responsible for irritations.
- Drugs known as nonirritating do not cause severe reactions.

In any case, the chemotherapy perfusion should be stopped immediately, but the needle should be left in place.

There is no specific antidote out of dexrazoxane for anthracycline, yet. However, the product has been approved to go to market (AMM), but is not refunded and cannot be replaced or substituted by another dexrazoxane (cardioxane), which is used to prevent cardiac toxicity of anthracyclines.

Reactivation of a preexisting skin lesion (recall reaction) [1, 6] on a previous extravasation site may occur during a subsequent injection through another site. The supposed phenomenon is a synergy between cytotoxic drugs and radiotherapy or between other cytotoxic drugs: anthracycline, cisplatin, mitomycin C, and paclitaxel.

## Infectious Complications [7, 8]

In oncology, the average incidence rate of infection was 0.2/1,000 catheter-days (0–2.7/1,000 days). Infection of the central venous line is a major cause of nosocomial infections and a source of excess morbidity and mortality. The catheter infection requires immediate management and prompt treatment, with or without preservation of the ICC.

Central and peripheral blood cultures with differential time of growth must be performed, but ICC can be retained, unless there are signs of severity (sepsis, local infection, deep thrombophlebitis, or useless equipment). After 48 h, the secondary attitude will depend on the clinical condition, the existence or absence of another focus of infection, the differential time of growth, and the nature of the germ.

About 13 % of infections are caused by nosocomial bacteriae. These infections prolong hospital stay, delay the administration of specific treatments, increase the problems of antibiotic resistance, and generate incremental hospitalization costs.

## Thromboembolic Complications [9–11]

The incidence of symptomatic thrombosis of ICC is around 4 %. Indications include pain, absence of reflux, arm edema, and so on. It is necessary to perform chest x-rays as well as a systematic echo Doppler to visualize the catheter and the casing when facing any type of dysfunction.

If the primary prevention of catheter thrombosis is not recommended, the curative treatment, however, is compulsory and is based on the prolonged use of low molecular weight heparins.

## Equipment Removal [1, 2]

If the ICC must be performed by a team that specializes in surgical aseptic conditions, it is also the case for its removal. The patient should therefore be informed of the reasons for (end of treatment, occurrence of complications, or poor tolerance) and the consequences of this removal. It seems legitimate to quickly remove a catheter that is no longer used.

## Summary

If the use of totally implanted catheters with subcutaneous chambers has grown considerably, it is important not to trivialize the techniques of both installation and use so as to avoid complications that can sometimes be very severe.

## References

1. Kamioner D, Kriegel I. Abord veineux de longue durée. Référentiels interrégionaux des réseaux de cancérologie. AFSOS Paris 2 et 3 décembre 2010.
2. Ackermann M, Cosset-Delaigue MF, Kamioner D, Kriegel I. L'abord veineux de longue durée dans le cancer du sein. Dispositifs veineux implantables (DVI): indications, pose et complications. Oncologie. 2009;11(12):621–34.
3. Marcy PY. Central venous access: techniques and indications in oncology. Eur Radiol. 2008;18(10):2333–44.
4. Vescia S, Baumgärtner AK, Jacobs VR, Kiechle-Bahat M, Rody A, Loibl S, et al. Management of venous port systems in oncology: a review of current evidence. Ann Oncol. 2008;19(1):9–15.
5. Biffi R, Orsi F, Pozzi S, Pace U, Bonomo G, Monfardini L, et al. Best choice of central venous insertion site for the prevention of catheter-related complications in adult patients who need cancer therapy: a randomized trial. Ann Oncol. 2009;20(5):935–40.
6. Ackermann M, Cosset-Delaigue MF, Kamioner D, Kriegel I. Extravasation. Oncologie. 2009;11(12):634–41.
7. Maki DG, Kluger DM, Crnich CJ. The risk of bloodstream infection in adults with different intravascular devices: a systematic review of 200 published prospective studies. Mayo Clin Proc. 2006;81(9):1159–71.

8. Crisinel M, Mahy S, Ortega-Debalon P, Buisson M, Favre JP, Chavanet P, et al. Incidence, prevalence and risk factors for a first infectious complication on a totally implantable venous-access port. Med Mal Infect. 2009;39(4):252–8.

9. Saber W, Moua T, Williams EC, Verso M, Agnelli G, Couban S, et al. Risk factors of catheter-related thrombosis (CRT) in cancer patients: a patient-level data (IPD) meta-analysis of clinical trials and prospective studies. J Thromb Haemost. 2011;9(2):312–9.

10. Beckers MM, Ruven HJ, Seldenrijk CA, Prins MH, Biesma DH. Risk of thrombosis and infections of central venous catheters and totally implanted access ports in patients treated for cancer. Thromb Res. 2010;125(4):318–21.

11. Debourdeau P, Kassab Chahmi D, Le Gal G, Kriegel I, Desruennes E, Douard MC, et al. 2008 SOR guidelines for the prevention and treatment of thrombosis associated with central venous catheters in patients with cancer: report from the working group. Ann Oncol. 2009;20(9):1459–71.

# Index

**A**

Aapro, M.S., 352, 353, 377
Acute myeloid leukemia
    amsacrine, 431–432
    clofarabine, 433–434
    cytarabine, 427–429
    daunorubicin, 431
    idarubicin, 429–431
    mylotarg, 434–436
Adenocarcinoma, first-line
    systemic therapy, 121
Adjuvant chemotherapy, 128–129
Ahles, T.A., 75
Alemtuzumab, lymphomas,
    450–451
Alkylating agents, 178–179
Aminobisphosphonates, 534
Amsacrine, acute myeloid
    leukemia, 431–432
Anagrelide, chronic
    myeloproliferative
    diseases, 437–439
Analgesics, 14–15
Androgen-deprivation therapy
    (ADT)
    and CTIBL
        bone mineral density, 258
        fragility fractures, 259, 260
        monitoring and prevention,
        259, 261–262
        pharmacologic prevention and
        treatment, 262

        external beam radiation
            therapy, 250
    long-term adverse events
        anemia, 253
        bisphosphonates, 262–263
        cardiovascular events, 253–257
        low-dose denosumab, 263–264
    short-term adverse events
        adrenal insufficiency, 253
        fatigue, 252
        hot flushes, 250–251
        psychological side effects, 252
        sexual dysfunction, 251
    before and during treatment,
        264–265
Anemia
    bevacizumab, 337
    causes of, 335, 336
    interleukin-1, 336
    interleukin-6, 336
    prevalence, 335
    therapy
        erythropoiesis-stimulating
            agents, 338–342
        iron, 342–344
        RBC transfusions, 337–338
    trastuzumab, 337
    treatment, side effects of
        erythropoiesis-stimulating
            agents, 347
        increased mortality, 350–354
        iron, 354–355

M.A. Dicato (ed.), *Side Effects of Medical Cancer Therapy,*     635
DOI 10.1007/978-0-85729-787-7,
© Springer-Verlag London 2013

Printed by Publishers' Graphics LLC
SO20121218.10.02.19